Adult Orthopaedic Nursing

Delores C. Schoen, PhD, RN, C, FAAN

Nurse Educator and Consultant
Harmon Enterprises, Inc.
State College, PA

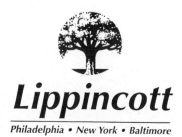

Lippincott

Philadelphia • New York • Baltimore

Acquisitions Editor: Susan M. Glover, RN, MSN
Editorial Assistant: Hilarie Surrena
Senior Production Manager: Helen Ewan

Design Coordinator: Doug Smock
Production Service: Shepherd Incorporated

9 8 7 6 5 4 3 2 1

Library of Congress Cataloging-in-Publication Data

Schoen, Delores C. (Delores Christina), 1938-
    Adult orthopaedic nursing / Delores C. Schoen.
        p. ; cm.
    Includes bibliographical references and index.
    ISBN 0-7817-1880-5
    1. Orthopedic nursing. 2. Musculoskeletal system--Diseases--Nursing. I. Title.
    [DNLM: 1. Musculoskeletal Diseases--nursing. 2. Orthopedic Nursing--methods. WY
157.6 S356a 2000]
    RD753.S355 2000
    610.73'69--dc21   99-050235

Care has been taken to confirm the accuracy of the information presented and to describe generally accepted practices. However, the authors, editors, and publisher are not responsible for errors or omissions or for any consequences from application of the information in this book and make no warranty, express or implied, with respect to the contents of the publication.

The authors, editors, and publisher have exerted every effort to ensure that drug selection and dosage set forth in this text are in accordance with current recommendations and practice at the time of publication. However, in view of ongoing research, changes in government regulations, and the constant flow of information relating to drug therapy and drug reactions, the reader is urged to check the package insert for each drug for any change in indications and dosage and for added warnings and precautions. This is particularly important when the recommended agent is a new or infrequently employed drug.

Some drugs and medical devices presented in this publication have Food and Drug Administration (FDA) clearance for limited use in restricted research settings. It is the responsibility of the health care provider to ascertain the FDA status of each drug or device planned for use in their clinical practice.

Contents

CHAPTER 7

Care of the Patient with an External Fixation Device — 195

CHAPTER 8

Care of Patients with Spinal and Pelvic Injuries — 217

CHAPTER 9

**Care of a Patient with Hip
and Femoral Surgery**   271

CHAPTER 10

The Knee and the Lower Leg 317

CHAPTER 11

Care of a Patient with Foot and Ankle Conditions 357

Preface

Adult Orthopaedic Nursing presents the nursing care of musculoskeletal conditions that affect the total adult body, from the neck to the toes, to provide the knowledge and skills necessary for a nurse to care for adult patients with common musculoskeletal conditions. Major conditions, and their potential complications, are presented through the use of the nursing process and clinical pathways, with numerous pictures and illustrations. The narrative portion of the book presents the content in a straightforward, easy to read style, and provides important information regarding the theory and principles underlying orthopaedic nursing. Nursing interventions are presented in step-by-step fashion with detailed instructions on how to do specific procedures. The numerous illustrations reinforce the written text and assist the nurse in mastering the procedures. The focus of the book is on preoperative care, postoperative care, and preparation for home care and rehabilitation. Where appropriate, the discussion also includes the care of outpatients in the clinic or physician's office, with follow-up home care and rehabilitation instructions.

Chapter 1 presents a brief historical review of orthopaedics and the major factors influencing orthopaedic nursing care. That chapter also presents a discussion of nursing care management focusing on the use of the nursing process and clinical pathways, the conceptual approaches that are utilized throughout the book.

Chapter 2, Assessment of an Orthopaedic Patient, presents taking a health history, doing a comprehensive physical assessment of the trunk and extremities, and implementing diagnostic procedures. The physical examination portion presents techniques for (1) testing range of motion, (2) measuring muscle mass and extremity length, (3) testing reflexes, and (4) assessing neurovascular status. In addition, diagnostic procedures (e.g., joint aspiration, biopsies, arthroscopies, x-ray examinations, and blood and urine tests) are discussed.

Chapter 3, Musculoskeletal Pathology, presents a brief overview of the major pathological conditions affecting the musculoskeletal system and the basic knowledge needed for clinical practice, including a discussion of such conditions as arthritis (rheumatoid arthritis, osteoarthritis, and gouty arthritis), infectious conditions (tuberculosis and osteomyelitis), neoplasms (both benign and malignant), and other pathological processes (osteoporosis, osteomalacia, and Paget's disease). In contrast to the later anatomical chapters, Chapter 3 gives a broader view of each condition and how it affects the entire body. General symptomatology, diagnostic tests, treatment methods, and complications are discussed. After the overview, arthritis (rheumatoid and osteoarthritis) and infectious conditions (tuberculosis and osteomyelitis) are discussed in relation to how the pathology affects specific areas of the body. That more specific discussion helps the nurse to understand exactly how each pathology affects specific joints, how to assess for each condition, and the specific treatment methods utilized.

Chapter 4 presents a discussion on the effects of trauma on the musculoskeletal system. It examines soft tissue trauma (including contusions, strains, sprains, and dislocations) and fractures, including first-aid measures, methods of repair, and complications related to fractures. The chapter discusses complications from imposed immobility and ways to restore ambulation through the use of assistive devices. There is a lengthy discussion, with numerous pictures, of the different types of crutches and walkers, how to measure and prepare the patient for using crutches, canes, or walkers, a demonstration of the different gaits, and how to ambulate up and down stairs. This comprehensive coverage will be a help to nurses on inpatient units, in the trauma area, and in outpatient and physician offices, as well as to home care and geriatric nurses.

Chapters 5 and 6 present discussions of the different types of casts and traction, with detailed nursing care. Chapter 5 presents information on the different types of casts and splints, providing step-by-step instructions on cast application, cast removal, and how to prevent potential complications. Nursing management of these patients is presented in a nursing process for each specific type of cast, demonstrating the hospital and home care of the patient. Numerous pictures are presented to assist the nurse in the application and care of patients with a cast or splint. Chapter 6 presents an in-depth discussion of the major types of traction, including the step-by-step process of traction application, how to move and care for a patient in traction, and patient exercises specific for the type of fracture and traction apparatus. Nursing management of these patients is presented as a nursing process for each specific traction, including both hospital and home care. Numerous pictures are presented to assist the nurse in traction application and nursing care.

Chapters 7 and 14 present information regarding external fixation devices and amputations respectively. Generic nursing processes are presented to illustrate the nursing care for those patients. Chapter 7 presents a discussion of the different types of external fixation devices, the nursing care involved, and potential complications. Chapter 14 focuses on the nursing and rehabilitaion process for different levels of amputations.

Chapters 8 through 13 focus on the care of specific areas of the body: the back and pelvis; hip and upper thigh; knee; ankle and foot; hand and wrist; and elbow and shoulder. In each chapter there is a discussion of the different pathologic and traumatic conditions, treatment methods, and nursing management. Nursing management is organized within a nursing process and is followed by a generic clinical pathway.

The book is appropriate for use by nurses new to orthopaedics, non-orthopaedic nurses caring for orthopaedic patients in an acute care setting (e.g. medical/surgical units), subacute care nurses, home care nurses, rehabilitation nurses, geriatric care nurses, outpatient care nurses, orthopaedic clinic or physician office practice nurses, as well as undergraduate student nurses learning the basic care of orthopaedic patients. It can also serve as a resource book for hospital units, nursing homes and extended care facilities (specifically those caring for patients following total joints and fractured hips) and home health care providers. The book is an excellent resource for faculty teaching students in orthopaedics, medical/surgical nursing, and geriatrics. The book would also be appropriate for students at the graduate level who want to specialize in orthopaedics.

ACKNOWLEDGMENTS

I would like to express my appreciation to all of my past students, faculty and clinical colleagues, and patients whose questions and suggestions have influenced the content and motivated me to write it. I would also like to thank the reviewers and editors whose comments helped to improve the book.

My greatest debt is to my husband, Robert Schoen, for his encouragement, support, and critical review of the manuscript. His help was invaluable.

Chapter
1
Orthopaedic Nursing Today

The health care industry in the United States has experienced numerous changes in recent decades as the result of scientific, demographic, economic, and political developments. The industry's restructuring, downsizing, and rightsizing reflect (1) the increasing age of the population, (2) the changing pattern of diseases, (3) the changing diversity of the population, and (4) the rising cost of health care. The health care system has been pressed to increase its efficiency and effectiveness. As a result, there has been an increase in outpatient care services, a decrease in length of hospital stays, an increase in the amount of care provided in the home, and an expansion of the role of the nurse. Nursing has been changing to meet these new demands.

Nursing care is now provided to orthopaedic patients in a larger number of settings. These include acute care, extended care, inpatient and outpatient care, subacute care, nursing home, home care, ambulatory care, operating room, and office facilities. In different practice areas, nursing care is carried out through different organizational structures. Some areas use team nursing, which had it origins in the 1950s and 1960s; others employ more recent forms of care delivery such as primary nursing and case management.

Primary nursing (not to be confused with primary health care) refers to comprehensive, individualized care that is provided by the same nurse throughout the course of care. It allows the nurse to implement the practitioner and leadership roles while providing direct patient care, rather than managing and supervising the functions of others who provide the care. The nursing process, the problem-solving model utilized by nurses, gained prominence at the same time as primary nursing, though it is applicable in all settings. The nursing process comprises the assessment of the patient, the formulation of a nursing diagnosis, the formulation of patient-centered goals, the planning of nursing care, the implementation of nursing interventions, the evaluation of outcomes of care, and the reassessment of nursing care based on that evaluation (American Nurses Association, 1975). Today the steps utilized by nurses are less formal but still include assessment, nursing diagnosis, planning and implementing nursing interventions based on the nursing diagnosis, and the evaluation of outcomes of care.

In the early 1990s, the case management model, utilized in the public health sector, was brought into the acute care setting. Case management is a method for coordinating health care services to provide cost-effectiveness, accountability, and quality care. It has gained prominence in part because of shorter hospital stays coupled with rapid and frequent transfers from specialty to standard care units. The role of the nurse manager, instead of emphasizing direct patient care, focuses on managing the care of a number of patients and collaborating with all members of the health team who care for those patients.

With the expansion of managed care nationwide, a new approach to health care has developed: critical pathways. The critical pathways tool represents the interdisciplinary treatment plan and includes vital elements designed to both positively affect patient outcomes and promote timely care delivery (Leininger, 1996). The tool is used for tracking a patient's progress with respect to the achievement of positive outcomes within a specified time frame. It identifies certain key events that must occur for the desired outcome to be attained in a timely manner. With case management and the use of critical pathways, patients and the care they receive are continually assessed from preadmission to discharge and, in many cases, postdischarge as well. Thus, nurses utilize both the nursing process and critical pathways to provide effective, cost-contained, continuity of care.

This chapter presents a brief historical perspective on orthopaedics, the major factors influencing orthopaedic nursing, and the nursing management of the orthopaedic patient.

HISTORICAL PERSPECTIVE ON ORTHOPAEDICS

Orthopaedics is derived from two Greek words, *orthos* meaning "straight" and *paidos* meaning "child." It was introduced in 1741 by Nicholas Andre in a two-volume work entitled *Orthopaedia, or The Art of Correcting and Preventing Deformities in Children*. The first Orthopaedic Institute was founded in Switzerland in 1780.

For many years, orthopaedic practitioners were known as "strap-and-buckle" doctors because of the appliances they used to straighten body and limbs. In Liverpool, Hugh Owen Thomas (1834–1891, see Fig. 1–1) became known for his ability to set broken bones and reduce dislocated joints. A number of appliances in use today, including the Thomas splint, bear his name. His nephew, Sir Robert Jones (1857–1933), was an orthopaedic surgeon who helped to establish orthopaedic surgery as a specialty. In the United States, orthopaedic surgery was pioneered by Dr. Virgil P. Gibney, Surgeon-in-Chief of the New York Hospital for the Ruptured and Crippled; and, in 1887, the American Orthopaedic Association was founded as a professional society for orthopaedic surgeons.

Relatively little is known about the pioneers of orthopaedic nursing, but one name, Agnes Hunt (1862–1948), stands out. Known as the "Florence Nightingale of orthopaedic nursing," she suffered an orthopaedic deformity in childhood but went on to open the "Baschurch Home" in Oswestry, England, in 1900. From modest beginnings, the home grew into a large orthopaedic hospital with a school for training orthopaedic nurses.

The first professional association of orthopaedic nurses in the United States, the Orthopedic Nurses Association (ONA), was not established until 1972. The ONA dissolved and was succeeded in 1980 by the National Association of Orthopaedic Nurses (NAON).

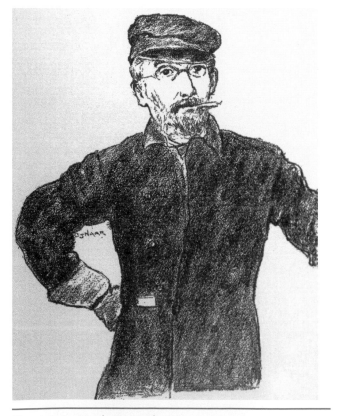

Figure 1–1   Hugh Owen Thomas.   *(Callaghan, et. al. (1998). The Adult Hip: Philadelphia: Lippincott. p. 358.)*

NAON seeks to meet the professional needs of orthopaedic nurses by promoting high standards of practice, encouraging continuing education, and furthering research in orthopaedic nursing.

MAJOR FACTORS INFLUENCING ORTHOPAEDIC NURSING CARE

Six important factors influence orthopaedic nursing care. They are (1) Standards of Practice, (2) philosophy of rehabilitation, (3) aging, (4) nutrition, (5) health teaching, and (6) interrelations between the musculoskeletal system and the rest of the body.

STANDARDS OF PRACTICE

Standards of Practice are objective criteria established by the profession by which the quality of nursing practice can be measured. Since 1973, the American Nurses Association (ANA) Congress for Nursing Practice and several ANA Divisions of Practice (e.g., Medical-Surgical, Gerontological, and Community Health) have published materials setting forth the baselines of acceptable practice, the rationales for the establishment of those Standards, and the specific criteria by which practice in any setting can be evaluated to determine whether the Standards are being met.

The Standards emphasize the nursing process as the means by which nursing care should be delivered. Although the setting in which care is provided and the observable outcomes of care are considered, the focus of the Standards is on evaluating the implementation of the nursing process. The Standards state that to implement the nursing process effectively, nurses should (1) base nursing practice on principles and theories of biophysical and behavioral sciences; (2) continuously update knowledge and skills, applying new knowledge generated by research, changes in health care delivery systems, and changes in social profiles; (3) determine the range of practice by considering the patient's needs, the nurse's competence, the setting for care, and the resources available; and (4) ensure patient and family participation in health promotion, maintenance, and restoration. The Standards explicitly recognize that ongoing revisions of their contents will be necessary to reflect changes in the scope of practice and the extent of knowledge.

Standards of Orthopaedic Nursing Practice were established by the National Association of Orthopaedic Nurses (NAON) and the ANA Division of Medical-Surgical Practice in 1975 and revised in 1996. (From those Standards, NAON also has developed Guidelines for Orthopaedic Nursing for future publication.) Orthopaedic nursing practice was defined as the nursing care of individuals with known and/or predicted neuromusculoskeletal alterations. Orthopaedic nursing takes into account related physiological, social, and behavioral problems resulting from or affecting the individual's response and adjustment to the neuromusculoskeletal alterations. Modern orthopaedic nursing has moved well beyond dealing with broken or malformed bones. It has grown rapidly as technological innovations have expanded the field of orthopaedics, which today is one of the most demanding and challenging fields of nursing practice.

PHILOSOPHY OF REHABILITATION

Rehabilitation has been defined as the restoration of the individual to the fullest physical, mental, social, vocational, and economic capacity attainable. Broadly speaking, rehabilitation seeks to prevent further disability, to maintain the patient's remaining abilities, and to restore lost functions. It is a dynamic process that begins with the onset of a disabling injury or disease and continues throughout its presence.

A disabling injury or disease is one of three major types: temporary, permanent, or progressive. A temporary disability is typically one of short duration, with rapid improvement and ultimate removal of all etiological factors, for example, recovery from a simple fracture. In a permanent disability, the individual never fully regains premorbid levels of function, as in the case of an amputation following trauma. A progressive disability is a nontemporary affliction that produces a continuing and irreversible loss of function. As is the case in rheumatoid arthritis, there may be periods of both exacerbation and remission, but the patient never returns to premorbid status.

In all types of disabling injury or disease, the patient goes through a period of adjustment and even grieving. Those psychological stages of adaptation to a disability are closely related to those described in the literature on death and dying. Five stages are usually described: psychological shock, denial, depression, anxiety, and acceptance. The stages may overlap, there may be progression and regression, and the length in any stage may vary from days to months and even years. Not all individuals go through all of the stages, but most exhibit grief, which is believed to be necessary to adapt to a disability. Only by carefully observing the patient's behavior can the nurse determine the stage the patient is in and help the patient through to final acceptance. Some individuals may require the assistance of a mental health professional to assist in the adjustment. The nurse must show a willingness to listen and talk about the disability.

A number of factors can affect the impact of a disability and how a person will move through the five stages of adjustment. Significant personal characteristics include (1) age and sex, (2) marital/family status, (3) occupation, (4) educational level, and (5) personality before the disability. Significant characteristics of the disability include (1) suddenness of onset, (2) severity and prognosis, and (3) degree of physical dependency. Important environmental factors include (1) the degree of family and community support available and (2) the financial resources available. The role of the patient's family and significant others is often crucial. They, like the nurse, should adopt the philosophy that "It is never how high one rises that determines one's merit, but rather how far one has come, considering the difficulties" (Brenner & Suddarth, 1980, p. 179).

SOCIETAL AGING

Orthopaedic nurses provide care to patients of all ages, race/ethnic groups, and socioeconomic statuses. However, the bulk of the patients who receive care related to fractured hips, joint replacements, amputations, arthritis, and osteoporosis are 65 years and older. A discussion of adult orthopaedic nursing would not be complete without a discussion of the current demographic situation and how it impacts the health care system and orthopaedic nursing.

In 1990, the authors of *Healthy People 2000* presented a profile of the U.S. population for the year 2000. They predicted that (1) the overall population will grow to nearly 270 million people; (2) the median age will increase from 29 years in 1975 to age 36; (3) in contrast to 8% in 1950, there will be 13% of the population (35 million persons) over age 65; and (4) the population of those over age 85 will be about 30% of those over age 65, or some 4.6 million persons. The authors also predicted changes in the race and ethnic composition as (1) whites (excluding Hispanic Americans) will decline from 76% to 72%; (2) Hispanics, the fastest growing population group will rise from 8% to 11.3% (more than 31 million persons); (3) blacks will increase from 12.4% to 13.1%; and (4) other racial groups (including American Indians, Alaska Natives, and Asians and Pacific Islanders) will increase from 3.5% to 4.3% of the total. It is also estimated that the U.S. population will gain some 6 million net migrants over the decade.

The Census Bureau predicts that by the year 2020, the average life expectancy will be 82.0 years for women and 74.2 years for men. It has been customary to use age 65 to define the elderly. With the increase in the percentage of older people, those age 85 and older have been named the "oldest-old" (Fig. 1–2).

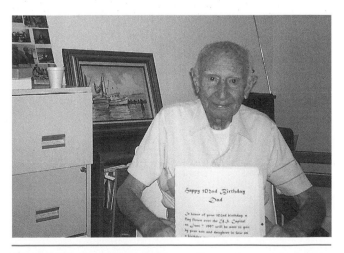

Figure 1–2   Age 102 and still counting.   *(Courtesy of Robert Schoen.)*

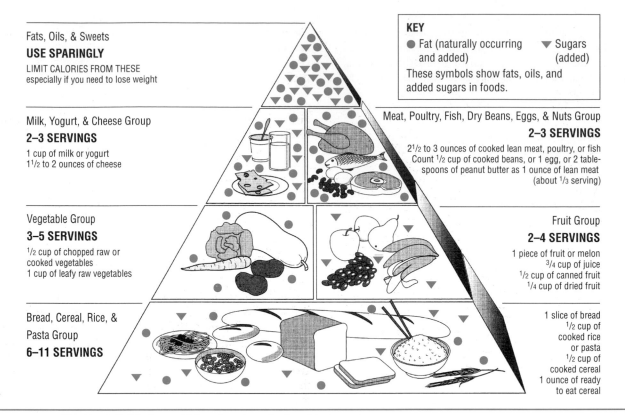

Figure 1–3   The Food Guide Pyramid (serving sizes depicted in boxes).   *(Dudek,* Nutrition Handbook for Nursing Practice, *3/e p. 203.)*

With more elderly persons, there will be an increase in hip fractures. It is estimated that 250,000 hip fractures occur in the United States each year. Some have predicted that the number of hip fractures in the elderly will double or even triple over the next 20 years. According to Daleiden (1990), there has been an increase in fractures in individuals living in nursing homes, and each year it is estimated that perhaps one fourth of the elderly living in the community suffer a fracture. The increase in fractures is due primarily to the elderly's predisposition to falling and to the progressive bone loss associated with osteoporosis. Physiological changes of the musculoskeletal system due to aging are that (1) muscle mass and elasticity diminish, resulting in decreased strength and endurance and thus a decrease in reaction time and coordination; (2) bone demineralizes, causing skeletal instability and shrinkage of intervertebral discs resulting in a less flexible spine and spinal curvatures; and (3) joints undergo degenerative changes, resulting in pain, stiffness, and loss of range of motion. As people age, they tend to develop a stooped posture (kyphosis) and a shuffling and broad-based gait. The change in gait, slowed reflexes, and loss of muscle strength make it difficult to prevent a fall. Medications (e.g., antihypertensives and diuretics), sensory impairments, confusion, and an unsafe environment (e.g., slippery and uneven walking surfaces, unstable railings, loose rugs, and inadequate lighting) increase the risk for falls. Other pathologies (e.g., osteoporosis, osteoarthritis) related to aging are discussed in Chapter 3.

NUTRITION

A good diet is important in preventing and managing musculoskeletal problems. A well-balanced diet, rich in proteins and minerals, will help maintain the structure of the bones and muscles. Daily food guidelines for nutritional support provided by the U.S. Departments of Agriculture and Health and Human Services (Edge & Miller, 1994) are (1) 6–11 servings from the bread, cereal, rice, and pasta groups; (2) 2–4 servings from the fruit group; (3) 3–5 servings from the vegetable group; (4) 2–3 servings from the meat, poultry, fish, dry beans, eggs, and nuts group; (5) 2–3 servings from the milk, yogurt, and cheese group; and (6) sparing use of fats, oils, and sweets (Fig. 1–3).

Factors influencing body weight include intake of food, activity, size and body type, metabolism, and genetics. Weight gain occurs when energy intake (food) exceeds energy output. It is necessary to know the individual's basal metabolic rate (BMR) in order to determine calories needed to maintain, reduce, or increase weight. First, obtain the person's height and weight and then determine the person's activity level (i.e., calories expended in muscular movement during a typical day). Activity levels are as follows: (1) sedentary (e.g., desk job, sitting during most of work or leisure time), 40% to 50%; (2) light activity (e.g., teacher, assembly line worker or walks 2 miles regularly), 55% to 65%; (3) moderate activity (e.g., waitress), 65% to 70%; and (4) heavy activity (e.g., construction worker), 75% to 100%. Calculations for

---

Box 1–1
Calculating the Basal Metabolic Rate

Using the example of a 154-lb, 5'2" woman with a sedentary lifestyle:

1. Convert body weight to kilograms:

   154 lbs ÷ 2.2 = 70 kg

2. Multiply weight by the gender constant:

   70 kg × 0.9 cal/kg/h = 63 cal/h

3. Multiply calories per hour by 24 hr (day):

   63 cal/h × 24 h = 1,512 cal/24 h

4. The BMR is 1,512 calories per day.
5. Multiply the BMR by the level of activity:

   1,512 × 0.40 = 604.8
   1,512 × 0.50 = 756.0

6. Add BMR calories to the level of activity calories to get total:

   1,512 + 604.8 (756.0) = 2,116.8 (2,268) calories

---

estimating an individual's BMR use different constants for men and women. The constant for men is one calorie per kilogram (2.2 lbs) per hour and for women 0.9 calorie per kilogram per hour. Consider a woman 5 feet 2 inches tall weighing 154 pounds with a sedentary activity level. To determine the total calories required to maintain that body weight, follow the steps shown in Box 1–1 (Edge & Miller, 1994, p. 276). To decrease her weight, she would need to reduce that number of calories and/or increase her activity level.

It has been recommended that an older women should reduce her caloric intake to 1,800 calories until age 75 and to 1,600 calories thereafter; for the older man, the recommendations are for 2,400 calories, reduced to 2,050 after age 75. However, it must be emphasized that these figures are general guidelines only, and each person will have a unique caloric need based on individual body size, metabolism, health status, and activity level.

The diet for elderly persons should reflect a lower quantity and higher quality of food, and should include fewer carbohydrates and fats. The decreased ability of the older person to maintain a regular blood glucose level emphasizes the need for reduced carbohydrate intake. A high carbohydrate diet can stimulate an abnormally high release of insulin, leading to hypoglycemia. At least one gram of protein per kilogram of body weight is necessary for the renewal of body protein and protoplasm and for the maintenance of enzyme systems. Protein supplements may be added to the older person's diet to meet that daily requirement.

With the reduced amount of intracellular fluid available in the older person, attention must be given to ensuring a good fluid intake. The usual recommended fluid consumption for an older adult is from 1,500 to 2,000 ml daily. (Note if there is any fluid restriction due to other health problems.)

Although the ability to absorb calcium decreases with age, calcium is still required in the diet to maintain a healthy musculoskeletal system and to promote the proper functioning of the body's blood-clotting mechanisms. The use of calcium supplements may benefit the older person but needs to be discussed with a physician to ensure that other medical problems do not contraindicate them.

HEALTH TEACHING

Health teaching should take into account the perceptions, feelings, and specific needs of the learner, and should be responsive to feedback. Learning is the development of new behavior patterns as a result of acquiring new knowledge, skills, or attitudes. Learning is active, not passive, and requires the full participation of the learner. It is through the teaching-learning process that the nurse assists patients in acquiring necessary behaviors to meet their own health needs. Although adults are certainly not a homogeneous group, there are four basic principles of adult learning that are broadly applicable (Kidd, 1973). These are that (1) adult learners see themselves as responsible, self-directing, capable individuals who will resent being treated like children; (2) adults have accumulated a great many experiences on which to base new learning, but some of those experiences may interfere with new learning; (3) adults are interested in learning what is relevant to them "here and now"; and (4) teachers of adult learners should relate to them as individuals with individual needs.

Health teaching is an integral part of health care. It is the responsibility of all nurses, individually and collectively, to provide relevant, effective, and consistent health education to the patient and to the patient's family or significant others. With today's short hospital stays, it is imperative for nurses and other members of the health care team to take every opportunity, no matter what the setting, to teach patients about their health care. For patients having elective surgery, both the initial nursing assessment and organized patient teaching need to be done in the physician's office or outpatient clinic.

Health teaching requires a well-developed plan that includes (1) an assessment of the patient's needs and readiness for health teaching, (2) a diagnosis of why and in what areas the patient is deficient in knowledge, (3) a formulation of short- and long-term educational goals, (4) planning to properly present the material to the patient, (5) intervention in carrying out the presentation, (6) an evaluation of the effectiveness of the presentation by such means as written or verbal responses or a return demonstration, and (7) a reassessment to renew the effort if the goals are not met. In other words, the nursing process is central to health teaching as it is to all other aspects of nursing care.

INTERRELATIONS BETWEEN THE MUSCULOSKELETAL SYSTEM AND THE REST OF THE BODY

The musculoskeletal system is composed of bones, muscle, cartilage, joints, ligaments, tendons, fascia, and bursa, organized into a complex system that protects the body, gives it shape and structure, and provides its ability to move. Muscle mass accounts for approximately half of normal body weight, and associated body structures and connective tissue add an additional 25%. Thus, the musculoskeletal system collectively constitutes the largest organ system in the body.

There are 206 bones in the human body (Fig. 1–4). They can be divided into four categories: long bones (i.e., the humerus), short bones (i.e., the tarsals), flat bones (i.e., the sternum), and irregular bones (i.e., the vertebrae). More than 99% of total body calcium and a substantial portion of body phosphorus are present in bones. Bone also works as a chemical buffer to prevent rapid changes in hydrogen ion concentrations in body fluids. After birth, the red bone marrow is the only tissue capable of red blood cell formation, and the yellow bone marrow produces some white blood cells. Muscles serve as a repository for glycogen, the body's stored energy.

Bones as living tissue have the characteristics of all living material, including respiration, nutrition, excretion, reproduction, and response to stimulation. Respiration for bone cells is the taking in of oxygen and the giving off of carbon dioxide. Nutrition in the form of protein, fat, carbohydrates, water, mineral salts, and vitamins must reach bone cells in a steady supply for growth, replacement of worn cells, and other activities to occur. Excretion of the by-products of metabolism, (i.e., excess water, carbon dioxide, lactic acid, and urea) occurs continuously. Reproduction in the adult skeleton is the steady process of cell division and production of new bone cells to replace worn out cells. The skeletal system responds to stimulation or stress by improving its strength and by repairing itself when broken or damaged.

Because the musculoskeletal system serves to support the other systems of the body, a disabling injury or illness to the musculoskeletal system can greatly affect other systems of the body. In particular, immobility has serious and far-reaching consequences. With regard to the cardiovascular system, immobility can lead to orthostatic hypotension, increased workload on the heart, and thrombus formation. The respiratory system may be affected by decreased respiratory movement, decreased movement of secretions, and disturbed oxygen–carbon dioxide balance. The gastrointestinal system may encounter dysfunctions in ingestion, digestion, and elimination, which can result in a stress ulcer, a paralytic ileus, or constipation. In the urinary system, there may be difficulty in urine formation, urinary tract stones, and difficulty in micturition. The psychosocial effects can also be severe, as boredom, loss of morale, loss of independence, and negative self-image take their toll (Olson, 1967; Asher, 1983).

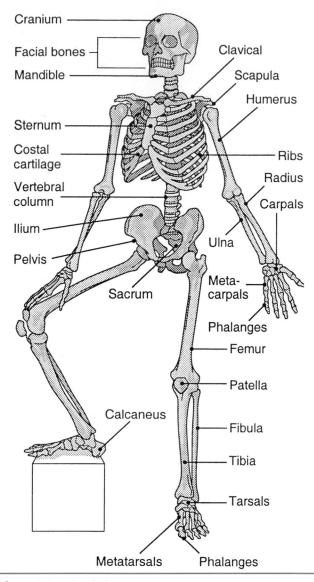

Figure 1–4   The skeleton.   *(Memmler,* Structure & Function of the Human Body, *6/e, p. 59.)*

NURSING MANAGEMENT

The four major areas of concern confronting orthopaedic nurses are (1) alleviating the patient's pain, (2) increasing patient mobility, (3) preventing complications, and (4) providing patient teaching. The orthopaedic patient may have soft tissue, muscle, nerve, or bone pain due to trauma, surgery, or a disease process. The type and degree of pain vary greatly, and a wide variety of nursing measures must be utilized.

Orthopaedic patients frequently have greatly decreased mobility, whether it be in their ability to walk and bear weight, to move their arms to care for themselves, or to have the spinal flexibility to work and earn a living. Preventing complications includes averting problems due to surgery, trauma, disease, or immobility. Those potential problems involve not only the musculoskeletal system but all other systems of the body.

Patient teaching strives to increase the patient's knowledge of the disease or injury, the methods of care, and the rehabilitation process; to help reduce the patient's anxiety; and to enable the patient to become an active participant in the recovery effort. The teaching plan includes the patient, family, and significant others and focuses on (1) care in the hospital setting, (2) at-home care, and (3) ways to prevent the occurrence of future injuries. To provide the highest quality of care in the most efficient and cost-effective manner, nurses generally utilize the problem-solving approach of the nursing process and the interdisciplinary treatment plan of the critical pathway.

NURSING PROCESS

The nursing process is a problem-solving approach, a systematic method for organizing nursing care. Several variations of the nursing process are being used. Although the American Nurses Association identified seven steps in the *Standards of Nursing Practice* 1975, this book will follow an abbreviated version with five steps, i.e., assessment, nursing diagnosis, goal formulation and planning, intervention, and evaluation/outcomes. Even in crisis situations, when nurses will rarely consciously articulate each step in the nursing process, professional standards require that the nursing process underlie the actions taken.

ASSESSMENT

The assessment step of the nursing process involves the collection of information relevant to the patient's health status. The necessary data are obtained in several ways. The most direct is by interviewing, observing, and examining the patient. Other methods include reviewing available records, including the results of diagnostic tests, and obtaining information from family, significant others, and other health care providers. The data are usually classified into two categories: subjective and objective. Subjective data can be observed or obtained directly or indirectly from the patient, but not measured. Objective data are observable and measurable by others. When an individual who has had a total hip replacement complains of severe pain in the hip following a turn to the unaffected side, subjective information is being given. The nurse cannot measure the pain, but the nurse can objectively observe and measure whether the affected leg is shorter, internally rotated, or abducted.

The nursing history is the part of the assessment that assembles information about the patient's past and present health status. The nursing history frequently includes information on the patient's (1) previous experience with illness and hospitalization, (2) understanding of their health problems and treatments, (3) educational level and ability to learn, (4) ability to communicate, (5) occupation, (6) usual behavioral patterns (e.g., diet, exercise routines, religious observances, hours of sleep, personal hygiene practices, and recreational activities), (7) ability to deal with stress, and (8) significant others who might provide support.

At first, one might think that conducting a lengthy assessment, which includes a nursing history, is too time consuming to be practical. On the contrary, the nurse-patient relationship is begun during the assessment, which should convey the nurse's interest and concern, and the effort helps to establish a sense of mutual trust. During the first contact with the patient, family, or significant other, the initial or "first-level" assessment may focus on determining the perceived health threat, the patient's adjustment to the threat, and the information needed for immediate nursing actions. In some instances, depending on the health status of the patient, this assessment is very brief. The ongoing or "second-level" assessment is the assessment that continues throughout the time the nurse is in contact with the patient. The patient needs time to build a relationship of trust with the nurse before a complete nursing history can be taken, and changes in the patient's condition must be continually observed. Assessment, no matter how thorough, is never complete, because the patient and the patient's environment are constantly changing.

NURSING DIAGNOSIS

Once the data have been collected in the assessment step, they need to be analyzed and interpreted so that explicit statements about the patient's health can be made. A diagnosis has been defined as "a careful examination and analysis of the facts in an attempt to understand or explain something" (*Webster's Ninth New Collegiate Dictionary*, 1986). Accordingly, nursing diagnosis involves the identification of existing or potential threats to the patient's health.

Although nurses have been making judgments about existing or potential health problems for many years, it is important to distinguish between nursing diagnoses and medical diagnoses. A key distinction is that different courses of action are open to each professional after the judgment is made. In March 1990, at the Ninth Conference of the North American Nursing Diagnosis Association (NANDA), the General Assembly approved the following official definition of nursing diagnosis:

> Nursing diagnosis is a clinical judgment about individual, family, or community responses to actual or potential health problems/life processes. Nursing diagnosis provides the basis for selection of nursing interventions to achieve outcomes for which the nurse is accountable (Carpenito, 1993, p. 5).

The nurse needs to state the nursing diagnosis in a sufficiently precise way so that goals can be established, nursing interventions planned, and the underlying problem identified. For example, a nursing diagnosis of "skin breakdown" is not specific enough. A more complete nursing diagnosis, which specifically states what, where, and why, would be "sacral decubitus related to immobility."

GOAL FORMULATION AND PLANNING

After assessment and diagnosis, various nursing actions need to be considered to develop a plan of care for promoting, maintaining, and restoring the patient's health. Based on the collected and analyzed data, the goal formulation phase establishes patient-centered goals, which describe the observable outcomes that, in consultation with the patient and the patient's significant others, are considered desirable and attainable.

Once they have been formulated, priorities are set to meet the patient's needs. Specific plans to meet those needs are set forth, identifying (1) what is to be done, (2) how it is to be done, (3) when it is to be done, (4) where it is to be done, and (5) who is to do it. Thus, the planning step prescribes the nursing actions necessary to achieve the desired outcomes.

INTERVENTION

Intervention is the action step and includes all therapeutic actions taken by the nurse on behalf of the patient. These include nursing procedures; measures for patient comfort; teaching, counseling, and purposeful socializing; and coordinating or collaborating with other health team members. Whenever possible, the patient and the patient's significant others should be encouraged to take an active part in the intervention and the rationale for the measure should be explained. Every nursing intervention must be properly authorized. In areas where independent nursing action is permitted, nurses can act on the basis of their own professional abilities. In other areas, the nurse must work in conjunction with the physician or on the basis of the standing medical orders.

EVALUATION/OUTCOMES

The evaluation compares the postintervention health status of the patient with observations relative to the desired outcomes. The patient, the patient's family, and significant members of the health team should contribute to the evaluation, and they should be kept informed of the progress toward the achievement of the desired outcomes. If the patient is not making satisfactory progress, a reorientation and renewal of the nursing process needs to be initiated. The nursing process is thus continuing and dynamic and, typically, is repeated in its entirety many times in the course of caring for a patient.

COLLABORATIVE PROBLEMS

Since working collaboratively with other members of the health team is now an essential nursing responsibility, a discussion of "collaborative problems" is incorporated into the nursing process framework of this book. Collaborative problems can be defined as patient abnormalities or dysfunctions for which nurses must assess and monitor/manage, but for which nurses have no independent nursing interventions. Thus, nursing assessment includes assessment for collaborative problems, and goal formulation and planning and evaluation/outcomes include those steps for collaborative problems (Fig. 1–5).

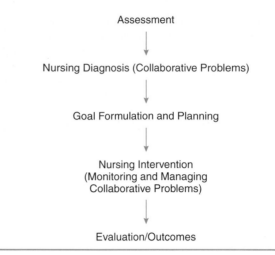

Figure 1–5   Steps of the nursing process.

Box 1–2
Clinical Pathway Categories

1. Assessment
2. Consultations
3. Treatments
4. Medications
5. Tests (including laboratory and x-rays)
6. Diet/nutritional needs
7. Patient activities
8. Patient teaching
9. Discharge planning
10. Outcomes

CLINICAL PATHWAYS

Clinical pathways have been defined by Zander (1997, p. 20) as "clinical management tools that organize, sequence, and time the major interventions of nursing staff, physicians, and other departments for a particular case type, subject, or condition." Alfaro-LeFevre (1998, p. 249) has a similar definition: "a standard plan that predicts the course of recovery and day-by-day care required to achieve outcomes for a specific health problem within a specific time frame." The term *clinical pathway* has also been used by some individuals and organizations synonymously with critical pathway, care map, care path, or care management plan.

Although there are key events such as patient education, diagnostic tests, treatments, activities, medications, and consultations that must be included, the clinical pathways format has not been standardized. Because health care providers and health care institutions have different practice patterns, it is best for an institution to develop its own clinical pathways format. Some of the more common categories to include in a clinical pathway tool are present in Box 1–2. This book will use those 10 categories.

The pathway process can begin in the hospital, but it is possible to begin the process in the physician's office, preoperative teaching clinic, or preadmission clinic. The sequence of patient care can be written in different ways, such as in a daily format or in a phases of care format. The body of the clinical pathway identifies the treatment plan/care plan for the patient. Although the nurse does much more, it is usually recommended that only required nursing activities be included in the clinical path. Examples of clinical pathways are presented in later chapters as they relate to the care of specific conditions.

References

Adler, S. L., Bryk, E., Cesta, T. G., & McEachen, E. (1995). Collaboration: The solution to multidisciplinary care planning. *Orthopaedic Nursing, 14*(2), 21–29.

Adsit, K. I. (1996). Multimedia in nursing and patient education. *Orthopaedic Nursing, 15*(4), 59–63.

Alfaro-LeFevre, R. (1998). *Applying nursing process: A step-by-step guide* (4th ed.). Philadelphia: J. B. Lippincott.

Applegate, V. E. (1995). Moving from the operating room to home care. *Orthopaedic Nursing, 14*(2), 30–31.

American Nurses Association. (1975). *Standards of Nursing Practice*. Kansas City: Author.

Asher, R. (1983, May). The dangers of going to bed. *Critical Care Update*, 40–41, 51.

Bates, B. (1995). *A guide to physical examination and history taking* (6th ed.). Philadelphia: J. B. Lippincott.

Brunner, L. S. & Suddarth, D. S. (1980). Medical-Surgical Nursing 4th ed. Philadelphia: J. B. Lippincott. p. 179.

Bulechek, G. M., & McCloskey, J. C. (1992). *Nursing interventions: Essential nursing treatments*. Philadelphia: W. B. Saunders.

Carpenito, L. J. (1993). *Nursing diagnosis: Application to clinical practice*. Philadelphia: J. B. Lippincott.

Cohen, E. (1996). *Nurse case management in the 21st century*. St. Louis: Mosby Year Book.

Daleiden, S. (1990). Prevention of falling: Rehabilitative or compensatory interventions. *Topics in Geriatric Rehabilitation, 5*(2), 44–53.

Devereaux, S. D. (1997). Managed care 101: A practical instruction guide to managed care for the orthopaedic office. *Orthopaedic Nursing, 16*(1), 11–15.

Edge, V., & Miller, M. (1994). *Women's health care*. St. Louis: Mosby Year Book.

Eliopoulos, C. (1995). *Manual of gerontological nursing*. St. Louis: Mosby Year Book.

Humphrey, C. J., & Milone-Nuzzo, P. (1996). *Orientation to home care nursing*. Gaithersburg, MD: Aspen Publishers, Inc.

Hymovich, D. P., & Hagopian, G. A. (1992). *Chronic illness in children and adults*. Philadelphia: W. B. Saunders.

Johnson, M., & Maas, M. (Eds.). (1997). *Nursing outcomes classification (NOC)*. St. Louis: Mosby Year Book.

Jones-Walton, P. (1994). Orthopaedic health promotion 2000. *Orthopaedic Nursing, 13*(3), 29–35.

Kidd, J. R. (1973). *How adults learn*. New York: Association Press.

Koval, K. J., & Zuckerman, J. D.(Eds.). (1998). *Fractures in the elderly*. Philadelphia: Lippincott-Raven.

Leininger, S. M. (1996). Tools for building a successful orthopaedic pathway. *Orthopaedic Nursing, 15*(2), 11–19.

Leininger, S. M. (1997). *Building clinical pathways*. Pitman, NJ: National Association of Orthopaedic Nurses.

Masear, V. R. (1996). *Primary care orthopaedics*. Philadelphia: W. B. Saunders.

McCloskey, J. C. (1992). *Nursing interventions classification (NIC)*. St. Louis: Mosby Year Book.

Miller, J. F. (1992). *Coping with chronic illness: Overcoming powerlessness* (2nd ed.). Philadelphia: F. A. Davis Company.

Murrow, E. J., & Oglesby, F. M. (1996). Acute and chronic illness: Similarities, differences, and challenges. *Orthopaedic Nursing, 15*(5), 47–51.

National Center of Health Statistics. (1997). *Health people 2000 review*. Hyattsville, MD: U.S. Public Health Service.

Neal, L. J. (1997). Publication excerpt: Orthopaedic home care independent study. *Orthopaedic Nursing, 16*(5), 76–79.

Needham, J. F. (1993). *Gerontological nursing: A restorative approach*. Albany, NY: Delmar Publishers, Inc.

Olson, E. V. (Ed.). (1967). The hazards of immobility. *American Journal of Nursing, 67*(4), 779–797.

Rockwood, C. A., Green, D. P., Bucholz, R. W., & Heckman, J. D. (Eds.). (1996). *Rockwood and Green's fractures in adults*. Philadelphia: Lippincott-Raven.

Ross, D.(Ed.). (1996). *NAON scope and standards of orthopaedic nursing practice*. Pitman, NJ: National Association of Orthopaedic Nurses.

U.S. Department of Health and Human Services Public Health Service. (1990). *Healthy people 2000: National health promotion and disease prevention objectives*. Washington, DC: Author.

Webster's Ninth New Collegiate Dictionary (1986) Merriam-Webster Inc, Publishers, Springfield, MA

Zander, K. (1997). Use of variance from clinical paths: Coming of age. *Clinical Performance and Quality Health Care, 5*(1), 20–30.

Assessment is the first step in the nursing process and the clinical pathway and thus influences all phases of nursing practice. Even before the nursing process was articulated, nurses were expected to assess patients, but the recognition of assessment as a nursing skill and a nursing responsibility was not appreciated.

The musculoskeletal system is very complex and is usually evaluated in conjunction with other systems. This chapter concentrates on the musculoskeletal system alone. Its assessment includes both objective and subjective elements and is directed toward both function and structure. The assessment is conducted primarily by inspection and palpation of the tissue surrounding joints, the determination of active range of motion, and the determination of muscle strength against resistance. The musculoskeletal assessment of the patient can be done in its entirety or be focused on specific areas of concern. When interpreting the data, special consideration should be given to different age, gender, and cultural groups. Here, the focus is on the healthy, "normal" patient and the identification of abnormalities. Assessments for specific pathological and traumatic conditions afflicting different areas of the body are discussed in depth in later chapters. Here, history taking is simply defined, diagnostic procedures are discussed briefly, and the emphasis is placed on the physical examination of the patient.

HEALTH HISTORY

The health history serves as the foundation for the physical and laboratory assessment by directing the examiner toward the areas that should be examined. In the health history, patients are asked to give information on their past and present health status and their present concerns. During the interview, the examiner evaluates the patient's ability to carry out normal activities of daily living, their bodily proportions, and ease in movement. It is also important to determine the patient's perception of how symptoms affect their ability to carry out normal activities of daily living. In a musculoskeletal assessment, there are four specific areas that must be examined in detail: (1) onset of symptoms, (2) deformity, (3) paralysis, and (4) pain.

ONSET OF SYMPTOMS

Important points to know about the onset of symptoms are (a) when the symptoms started, (b) how they started, (c) what they were, (d) whether the onset was gradual or sudden and whether anything specific was associated with the onset of the symptoms, (e) how the symptoms have progressed, (f) what has increased or decreased symptoms, and (g) what specific treatments have been used and whether they have been effective in the immediate or long term.

DEFORMITY

In obtaining information about a deformity, it is essential to know when the changes were first noted and whether there was any pain, swelling, or stiffness associated with the onset. Determine if there is family history of those or similar symptoms. Deformities may occur as the result of dislocations, fractures, spurs, or the enlargement of bones caused by hypertrophic bone formation. Typical sites for bony enlargement due to arthritic conditions are the distal and proximal interphalangeal joints, the knees, and the feet. The fingers may deviate laterally at the distal joints, and nodules develop on the dorsum of the distal interphalangeal joints of individuals with osteoarthritis. Both lateral or ulnar deviations of all fingers at the metacarpophalangeal joint and swan-neck and boutonnière deformities are common for individuals with rheumatoid arthritis. Ganglia (fluid-filled cysts that develop along joint capsules and are attached to a tendon sheath) are typically found at the wrist. Rheumatoid arthritis nodules are often found on the extensor surfaces or bony prominences. Tophi nodules can occasionally be found near joints that contain urate deposits. Bursitis (an inflammation of a bursa) occurs over areas subject to friction, such as an elbow or shoulder.

PARALYSIS

In collecting data about paralysis, it is important to note the time of onset, the extent of involvement, progression or regression, and the presence or absence of sensory disturbances.

PAIN

Pain, the most common symptom in orthopaedics, must be evaluated closely. The critical features of pain are (1) type, (2) location, (3) severity, (4) duration, and (5) precipitating factors (Meinhart & McCaffery, 1983, p. 174ff.).

TYPE

Have the patient describe in his or her own words just what the pain is like. Use the patient's own words (e.g., sharp, dull, stabbing, or aching) to describe the character of the pain. Pain may be described as "being stabbed with an ice pick" or with such words as "heavy," "sharp," "burning," and "throbbing." Deep as opposed to superficial pain is a diffuse aching sensation such as that produced by squeezing the Achilles tendon and is often described by expressions like "being in a vise," or "having an iron band around my chest." You may have to ask the patient for more details if you receive an answer such as "like a headache," because there are many types of headaches.

LOCATION

Try to ascertain where the patient's pain is perceived. The patient may need help in locating the exact point of the pain, in part because of different degrees of sensitivity in different areas of the body. On the fingertip, two pinpoints can be distinguished from one another when they are only 3 mm apart, but, on the back, the minimum distance for distinguishing two pinpricks may be 50 mm. Often the patient will add nonverbal descriptions such as pointing with a fingertip or spreading an outstretched hand over an area. The location of the pain should include whether it is superficial or deep and whether or not it radiates to another anatomical side (e.g., pain radiating from the lower back down the posterior thigh is associated with the sciatic nerve).

SEVERITY

In some diseases, pain is characteristically severe, whereas in others it is mild or may vary in severity. Individuals vary so much in their tolerance to pain that a mere statement of severity is insufficient. Thus, severity is generally best described by having the patient tell how the pain affects the patient's lifestyle and ability to perform activities of daily living. Another way to help determine the severity of the patient's pain is to use a pain scale. Patients identify their level of pain on a scale of 1 to 10 with 10 being the most severe (or by visual tools such as a face scale, which demonstrates the same concept). In evaluating severity, it must be remembered that the intensity of pain depends greatly upon the patient's state of mind. Mental depression, anxiety, and introspection tend to aggravate pain.

DURATION

The assessment of pain should include its duration and frequency. Estimates made without actual measurements are often very inaccurate, but even such estimates may be helpful. In some instances, pain occurs at regular intervals. It is sound practice to ask if the pain recurs at any special times (e.g., at night or upon wakening). Soft-tissue pain, for example, is generally more severe after activity, whereas bone pain occurs more often at night.

PRECIPITATING FACTORS

Many factors are associated with the onset and relief of pain. Find out what precipitates or relieves the pain, the frequency of occurrence, how long the pain lasts, and if there are any associated symptoms. The patient's accounts should be carefully assessed for reliability. For example, if bending is alleged to bring on pain, questions should determine whether bending is always painful, whether it is always the same type of pain, and so on. Ask questions that can be answered by "yes" or "no." Remember that patients may believe their condition has improved from treatment or activities that have had no real effect.

Besides these four areas of concern, the present and past medication history is important. Be clear about what has been prescribed, what the patient is actually taking, and why past medications were discontinued. For an in-depth discussion of history taking, see the references on assessment at the end of this chapter.

PHYSICAL EXAMINATION

TECHNIQUES

Inspection and palpation are the principal techniques used to examine the musculoskeletal system. Inspect and palpate each body part, then test its range of motion and muscle strength. Examine each muscle and joint bilaterally, comparing the two sides of the patient's body. Remember that both sides of the body must be in the same position before a comparison can be made.

Inspection of the musculoskeletal system includes visual scanning of the two sides of the body for symmetry, contour, and size. Look for gross deformities, areas of swelling or inflammation, skin changes such as ecchymosis or other discolorations, and muscle atrophy. The patient's posture and body alignment should be viewed from both front and back. Note the structural relationship of the feet to the legs, the hips to the pelvis, the hands to the arms, the arms to the shoulders, and the shoulders to the upper trunk. Inspect the shape of the spine and its structural opposition to the shoulder girdle, thorax, and pelvis. When a deformity is present, another body part may shift to compensate for the imbalance (e.g., the pelvis may tilt when one leg is shorter than the other). The nurse should look for such compensatory changes.

Palpation is utilized to detect pain, tenderness, swelling, localized temperature changes, and marked changes in shape and muscle tone. Palpate all bones, joints, and surrounding muscles. Note any heat, tenderness, swelling, crepitus, and resistance to pressure. No discomfort should occur when pressure is applied to bones and joints. Muscle tone should be firm, not hard or doughy. Pain and tenderness in a bone may indicate a tumor, inflammation, or the aftermath of trauma. An angulated bone, one that is out of its original alignment, may be the result of abnormal bone development, injury, or an old fracture that healed in an improper alignment. While palpating a muscle, the examiner should be alert to fasciculations, which are involuntary contractions or twitchings of groups of muscle fibers. The examiner should ask patients about any sensation that they feel while their muscles and tendons are being palpated and note any facial grimacing. Their physical reaction and descriptions of pain or tenderness on palpation should be recorded.

MEASURE RANGE OF MOTION
After inspecting and palpating each body part with the patient at rest, test the active and passive range of motion of the joints. During passive range-of-motion testing, evaluate the patient's muscle tone by feeling the movements of the muscles with your hands. Although not all joints have all possible motions, there are six basic types of joint motion (Fig. 2–1): (1) flexion, bending and decreasing the joint angle; extension, straightening and increasing the joint angle; and circumduction, moving the joint in a swinging fashion; (2) adduction, moving toward the midline, and abduction, moving away from the midline; (3) inversion, turning inward, and eversion, turning outward; (4) pronation, turning downward, and supination, turning upward; (5) internal rotation, turning toward the midline, and external rotation, turning away from the midline; and (6) dorsiflexion, movement toward the dorsum or posterior aspect, and plantar flexion, extension of the foot so the forepart of the foot is depressed with respect to the ankle. The range-of-motion measures add to the information obtained during the earlier palpation of the muscles at rest.

To measure the patient's range of motion, use a goniometer (Fig. 2–2). Place the center, or zero point, on the joint to be measured, and the axis (the fixed part of the goniometer) along the zero-degree line. Use the movable arm to measure degrees of movement. For example, in measuring degrees of flexion at the elbow, place the zero point on the lateral epicondyle of the humerus, align the axis with the shaft of the humerus, and use the movable arm to measure the number of degrees the forearm departs from the fully extended position.

ASSESS MUSCLE STRENGTH
Knowledge of muscle strength and tone is helpful in diagnosing musculoskeletal conditions and gives information about the amount of assistance a patient may need when ambulating or doing activities of daily living. Muscle strength is assessed throughout the full range of motion for each muscle or group of muscles. Muscle strength is tested by asking the patient to resist movement or to move against restrictions applied by the examiner. Strength is graded according to the examiner's subjective judgment in observing muscular contraction and feeling the patient's muscle strength exerted. Grading is usually based on a scale of 0 to 5, as shown in Table 2–1. Disability is considered to exist if muscle strength is less than grade 3 and external support may be required to make the involved part functional. It is expected that muscle strength will be greater in the dominant arm and leg (e.g., the right arm and leg for right-handed persons).

MEASURE MUSCLE MASS
The difference between the firm, hypertrophic muscle of the athlete and the limp, atrophic muscle of the paralytic is obvious both on inspection and by palpation. Only in the very obese patient is muscle mass difficult to assess. Although muscle size is largely a function of the use or disuse of muscle fibers, a change in the size of a muscle may be indicative of disease. Malnutrition tends to reduce muscle size and weaken the strength of muscle contraction. Lack of neural input due to lesions of the spinal cord may also lead to a reduction in muscle size.

Measurements taken of extremities at their maximum circumference provide a basis for comparison when swelling or atrophy are suspected. In making such a comparison, the measurements are taken with the extremities placed in the same position and with the muscles in the same state of tension. Measurements should be made at several corresponding points above and below, for example, the patella or the olecranon process. For example, authorities routinely measure 5 cm below and 5 cm and 10 cm above or 10 cm below and 10 cm and 20 cm above the midpatella (Fig. 2–3). Differences in symmetry or extremity size of less than one cm are not significant.

MEASURE EXTREMITY LENGTH
Measurements of patient extremity lengths are best made with the patient lying relaxed on an examining table with pelvis level, hips and knees fully extended, and both hips equally adducted. The length of the lower extremity is the distance from the lower edge of the anterosuperior iliac spine to the tibial malleolus

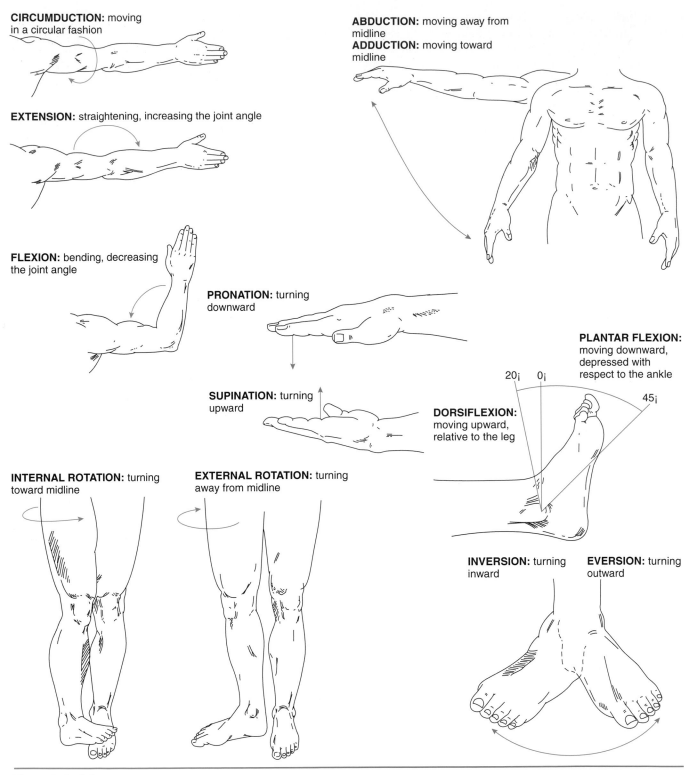

CIRCUMDUCTION: moving in a circular fashion

EXTENSION: straightening, increasing the joint angle

FLEXION: bending, decreasing the joint angle

PRONATION: turning downward

SUPINATION: turning upward

INTERNAL ROTATION: turning toward midline

EXTERNAL ROTATION: turning away from midline

ABDUCTION: moving away from midline
ADDUCTION: moving toward midline

PLANTAR FLEXION: moving downward, depressed with respect to the ankle

DORSIFLEXION: moving upward, relative to the leg

20ᵢ   0ᵢ   45ᵢ

INVERSION: turning inward   **EVERSION:** turning outward

Figure 2–1   Joint movements.

(Fig. 2–4). The length of the upper extremity is the distance from the tip of the acromion process to the tip of the middle finger with the shoulder adducted and the other joints in neutral position. See Table 2–2 for specific points of measurement for the upper and lower extremities.

TEST REFLEXES

In the musculoskeletal system, there are five major reflexes to evaluate. They are the biceps, brachioradialis, triceps, patellar, and Achilles tendon reflexes. The biceps reflex tests the C5–C6 spinal nerve response. The patient's arm is flexed at the elbow and held by the

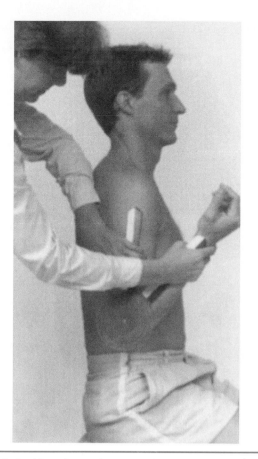

Figure 2–2 Use of a goniometer to measure range of motion. *(B. Bates (1996). Physical Examination and History Taking. Philadelphia: Lippincott.)*

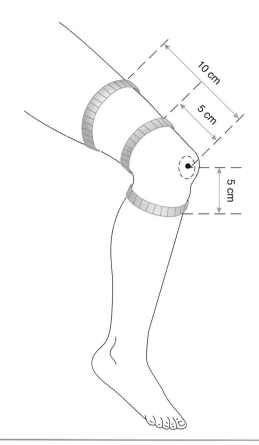

Figure 2–3 The sites at which a limb is measured are carefully noted so that they may be accurately located for future comparative measurements.

Table 2–1	Criteria for Grading Muscle Strength				
Grade	**Lovett Scale**	**Percent**	**Muscular Reaction of Normal**		**Notation in Charting**
0	0 (zero)	0	No evidence of contractility seen		0/5
1	T (trace)	10	Only slight contractility, no joint motion		1/5
2	P (poor)	25	Complete range of motion with gravity eliminated		2/5
3	F (fair)	50	Complete range of motion against gravity		3/5
4	G (good)	75	Complete range of motion against gravity and some resistance		4/5
5	N (normal)	100	Complete range of motion against gravity and full resistance		5/5

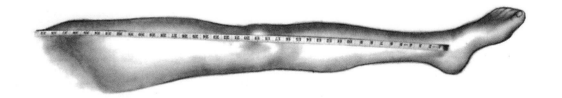

Figure 2–4 Measuring lower extremity length. *(B. Bates (1996). Physical Examination and History Taking. Philadelphia: Lippincott.)*

examiner. The examiner then places his or her thumb horizontally over the biceps tendon. A blow on the examiner's thumb is delivered with a percussion hammer (Fig. 2–5). There will be slight flexion of the elbow, and the examiner will be able to feel the bicep's con-

traction through the thumb. Spinal nerve responses can be graded using the scale in Table 2–3.

The brachioradialis reflex also tests the C5–C6 spinal nerve response. The patient's forearm can rest on either the examiner's forearm or the patient's leg. A percussion

Table 2–2   Measuring Extremity Length

Extremity	Points of Measurement
Arm	
Arm length	Tip of acromion process to tip of middle finger
Upper arm length	Tip of acromion process to tip of olecranon process
Forearm length	Tip of acromion process to styloid process of ulna
Leg	
Leg length	Lower edge of anterosuperior iliac spine to tibial malleolus
Thigh length	Lower edge of anterosuperior iliac spine to medial aspect of the knee
Lower leg length	Medial aspect of knee to tibial malleolus

(Adapted from Malasanos et al. (1990). Health assessment (4th ed.). St. Louis: C. V. Mosby.)

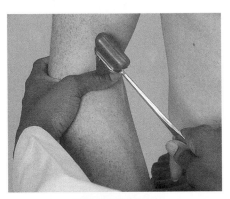

PATIENT SITTING

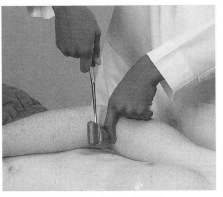

PATIENT LYING DOWN

Figure 2–5   Biceps reflex sitting and lying down. *(B. Bates (1996). Physical Examination and History Taking. Philadelphia: Lippincott.)*

hammer strikes the radius 2 to 5 cm (1 to 2 inches) above the wrist (Fig. 2–6). The patient is observed for flexion and supination of the forearm, and the fingers of the patient's hand may also extend slightly.

The triceps reflex tests the C7–C8 spinal nerve response. The patient's arm is flexed at the elbow. The

Table 2–3   A Scale for Reflex Responses

Rating	Description of Reflex
U	No reflex response or absence of reflex
+1	Below normal or present but diminished
+2	Average or normal
+3	Stronger than average or hyperactive
+4	Very intense response or markedly hyperactive (may resemble clonus, a rhythmic contraction of muscles initiated by stretching)

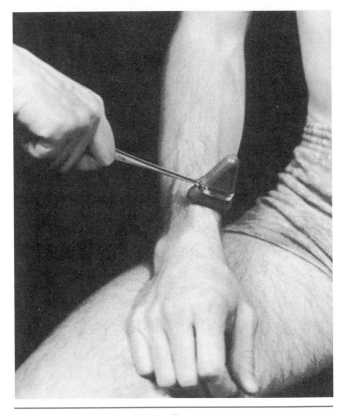

Figure 2–6   Brachioradialis reflex. *(B. Bates (1996) Physical Examination and History Taking. Philadelphia: Lippincott.)*

examiner palpates the triceps tendon about 2 to 5 cm (1 to 2 inches) above the elbow and then delivers a blow with a percussion hammer directly to the tendon (Fig. 2–7). The patient is observed for a contraction of the triceps tendon and a slight extension of the elbow.

The patellar (knee jerk) reflex tests the L2–L4 spinal nerve response. The patient should be sitting up with legs dangling over the side of a bed or table. If the patient is unable to sit up, the examiner should slide his or her arm under the patient's knee and lift the patient's leg to flex the knee. The patellar tendon is then tapped with a percussion hammer (Fig. 2–8). The tendon is usually found directly below the patella itself. If no response is obtained, the patient's legs may not be relaxed enough. In that case, ask the patient to interlock the fingers and pull. That allows the patient to relax the legs so that the reflex can be elicited.

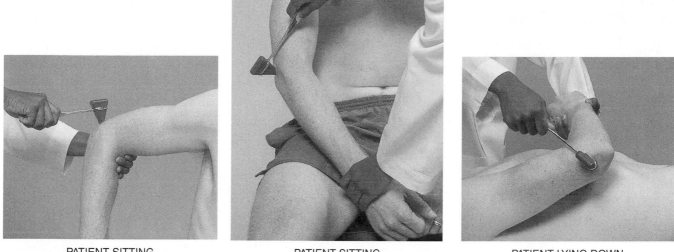

| PATIENT SITTING | PATIENT SITTING | PATIENT LYING DOWN |

Figure 2–7   Triceps reflex.   *(B. Bates (1996). Physical Examination and History Taking. Philadelphia: Lippincott.)*

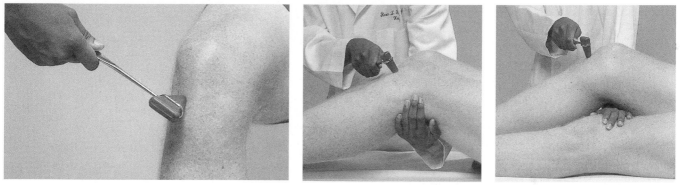

| PATIENT SITTING | PATIENT LYING DOWN | PATIENT LYING DOWN |

Figure 2–8   Patellar reflex.   *(B. Bates (1996). Physical Examination and History Taking. Philadelphia: Lippincott.)*

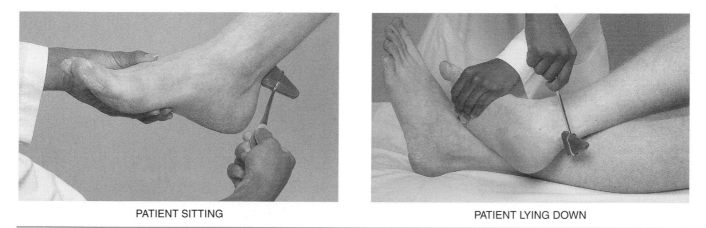

| PATIENT SITTING | PATIENT LYING DOWN |

Figure 2–9   Achilles tendon reflex.   *(B. Bates (1996). Physical Examination and History Taking. Philadelphia: Lippincott.)*

The Achilles tendon reflex tests the S1–S2 spinal nerve response. That reflex should be checked after the patellar reflex so that the patient can remain in the same position. With the patient's foot dorsiflexed, the examiner strikes the Achilles tendon with a percussion hammer just above the heel (Fig. 2–9). The examiner should see and feel the foot plantar flex. If the patient is unable to sit up, the examiner can take the foot and place it on the patient's other shin, which will dorsiflex the foot.

ASSESS NEUROVASCULAR FUNCTION

Neurological Assessment. In doing a neurological assessment of the upper extremities (Fig. 2–10), it is important to check the five major nerves, that is, the circumflex, the musculocutaneous, the median, the ulnar, and the radial. The *circumflex nerve* supplies sensation to the skin over the deltoid and is the motor nerve to the deltoid muscle. Check the sensory portion of the nerve by determining the patient's sensation over the deltoid area. Have the patient do an abduction of the arm at the shoulder to test the motor function of the circumflex nerve. The *musculocutaneous* nerve supplies motor function to the biceps and the brachioradialis muscles. To check the sensory portion, determine the patient's sensation at the radial side of the forearm. The patient's ability to flex the arm at the elbow is the test for motor function. The *median nerve* innervates most of the flexor muscles of the forearm, particularly the muscles of the thenar eminence. To determine the sensory portion of the *median nerve,* check the sensation of the entire palmar surface of the thumb, index, and long finger. To check motor function, have the patient oppose the thumb to the little finger. The *ulnar nerve* supplies motor function to the flexor muscles of the ulnar side of the arm and to the intrinsic muscles of the hand, particularly the interossei and the lumbricals of the third and fourth fingers. For sensory function, check the patient's sensation along the palmar surface of the little finger. To determine motor function, have the patient abduct and adduct all of the fingers. The *radial nerve* has a small sensory distribution and an extensive motor function. Virtually all of the extensor muscles of the arm from the triceps down are supplied by the radial nerve. To assess the sensory portion, determine sensation in the area over the web space between the patient's thumb and index finger. For an assessment of the motor function of the radial nerve, have the patient extend the wrist and fingers.

In doing a neurological assessment of the lower extremities (Fig. 2–10), it is important to check the three major nerves: the sciatic, the femoral, and the obturator. Each *sciatic nerve*—with its two major divisions, the posterior tibial and the common peroneal—supplies motor and sensory function to much of the entire leg. The sciatic nerve supplies the hamstring muscles in the thigh and the division of those muscles below the knee. The *tibial nerve* supplies the gastrocnemius muscle, the soleus muscle, and the flexor of the toes; and it provides sensation along the dorsum of the foot. Check the motor function of the tibial nerve by having the patient plantarflex the ankle and flex the toes. To assess the sensory portion, prick the medial and lateral surfaces of the sole of the foot. The *common peroneal nerve* innervates the peroneal and anterior tibial muscles of the leg and provides sensation along the lateral aspect of the leg below the knee and to the sole of the foot. To determine the motor function of the peroneal nerve, have the patient dorsiflex the ankle and extend the toes. Assess the sensory portion

by pricking the lateral surface of the great toe and the medial surface of the second toe.

If the major trunk of the sciatic nerve is injured, the site of the injury is usually in the buttock or thigh. The patient will have an anesthetic foot and be unable to move that foot and its toes. If the nerve is injured high in the thigh, loss of hamstring function and weakness of knee flexion may also occur. Injury to the tibial branch usually occurs at the posterior calf or the popliteal space and produces anesthesia over the lateral aspect of the calf and the foot. The patient has a loss of sensation over the heel and sole of the foot and cannot plantarflex the ankle. Eversion and dorsiflexion of the foot at the ankle are also lost.

The *femoral nerve* supplies motor function to the quadriceps femoris and sensation along the medial side of the foot and leg, extending as low as the medial malleolus. The femoral nerve is usually injured at the inguinal ligament in the anterior aspect of the thigh. Loss of femoral nerve function produces anesthesia along the medial aspect of the foot and an inability to extend the knee.

The *obturator nerve* supplies the adductor muscles of the thigh, with a small sensory distribution along the medial side of the thigh. The obturator nerve is rarely injured, as it lies deep in the pelvis. However, injury to the obturator nerve should be kept in mind when penetrating wounds of the perineum occur. Injury to that nerve can result in an inability to adduct the thigh.

Vascular Assessment. To assess the vascular function of the extremities, check the patient's pulse, color, and temperature. The first steps in assessing circulatory status are to note if there is any swelling of the hands and fingers or of the feet and toes, any abnormal color (i.e., pallor or cyanosis), or any abnormal temperature (i.e., coldness or increased warmth). Determine circulation to the fingers and toes by checking capillary refill (by blanching). Pinch the end of a finger or toe and then let go. The patient's nail bed should first turn white and then return to pink in less than 3 seconds. Take the patient's pulse, and note if there is any weakness or disappearance of the pulse. Compare the vascular status of one side of the body with the other.

There are three major pulses in the upper extremity: the radial, the ulnar, and the brachial (Fig. 2–11). The radial artery extends down the radial side of the forearm to the wrist. The *radial pulse* is the most commonly palpated and is located on the flexor surface of the wrist laterally. (To describe the strength of a pulse, see Table 2–4.) The ulnar artery extends down the ulnar side of the forearm to the wrist. It then divides into two branches, which anastomose with branches of the radial artery to form the arterial arches of the hand. The *ulnar pulse* is located on the flexor surface of the wrist medially. It is usually palpated only when arterial insufficiency is suspected. The *brachial pulse* is palpated in the groove between the biceps and triceps muscles. It too is usually palpated only when arterial

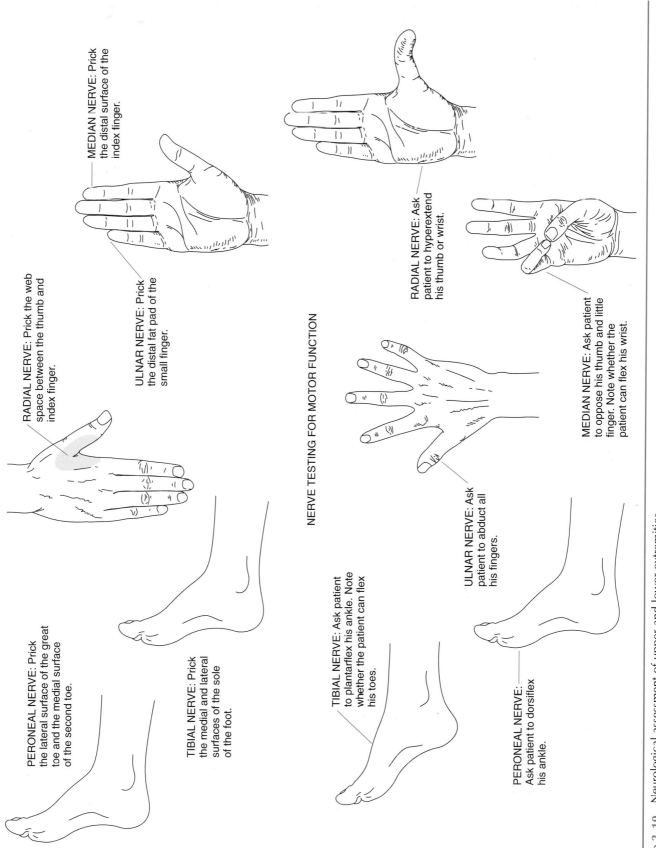

MEDIAN NERVE: Prick the distal surface of the index finger.

RADIAL NERVE: Prick the web space between the thumb and index finger.

ULNAR NERVE: Prick the distal fat pad of the small finger.

RADIAL NERVE: Ask patient to hyperextend his thumb or wrist.

MEDIAN NERVE: Ask patient to oppose his thumb and little finger. Note whether the patient can flex his wrist.

PERONEAL NERVE: Prick the lateral surface of the great toe and the medial surface of the second toe.

TIBIAL NERVE: Prick the medial and lateral surfaces of the sole of the foot.

NERVE TESTING FOR MOTOR FUNCTION

TIBIAL NERVE: Ask patient to plantarflex his ankle. Note whether the patient can flex his toes.

ULNAR NERVE: Ask patient to abduct all his fingers.

PERONEAL NERVE: Ask patient to dorsiflex his ankle.

Figure 2–10 Neurological assessment of upper and lower extremities.

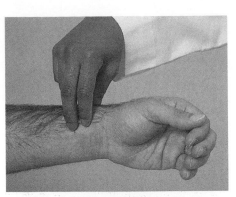

RADIAL PULSE

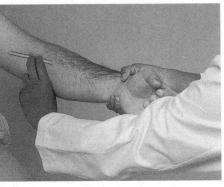

BRACHIAL PULSE

Figure 2–11   The radial pulse and the brachial pulse are located in the upper extremity as shown.   *(B. Bates (1996). Physical Examination and History Taking. Philadelphia: Lippincott.)*

Table 2–4 **Pulse Strength**	
Rating	**Description of Pulse**
0	No pulse.
1+	Pulse is thready, weak, and difficult to palpate; it may fade in and out and is easily obliterated with pressure.
2+	Pulse is difficult to palpate and may be obliterated with pressure, so light palpation is necessary; once located, it is moderately strong.
3+	Pulse is easily palpable, does not fade in and out, and is not readily obliterated by pressure; it is considered to be a normal pulse.
4+	Pulse is strong and bounding, easily palpated, and not obliterated with pressure; it may reflect a pathological condition such as aortic regurgitation.

(Adapted from Bates, B. (1995). Physical examination and history taking (6th ed.). Philadelphia: J. B. Lippincott.)

Table 2–5 **Severity of the Edema**	
Grade	**Descriptions**
1+	Slight pitting on depression, no visible distortion.
2+	A somewhat deeper pit than in 1+, but again no readily detectable distortion.
3+	The pit is noticeably deep; the dependent extremity looks fuller and swollen.
4+	The pit is very deep, lasts awhile, and the dependent extremity is grossly distorted.

insufficiency is suspected. Just below the elbow, the brachial artery branches into the radial and ulnar arteries.

There are four major pulses in the lower extremity: the femoral, the popliteal, the posterior tibial, and the dorsalis pedis (Fig. 2–12). The femoral artery arises at the level of the inguinal ligament and extends downward through the thigh. The *femoral pulse* is palpable at the inguinal ligament midway between the anterior-superior iliac spine and the pubic tubercle. The popliteal artery is a continuation of the femoral artery and is located behind the knee. To palpate the *popliteal pulse*, the patient should be asked to slightly flex the knee. The examiner then presses the fingers of both hands deeply into the popliteal fossa. This pulse is often difficult to locate. The posterior tibial artery extends down the posterior aspect of the leg around the medial malleolus to the side of the foot. The *posterior tibial pulse* is palpable behind and below the medial malleolus. The *dorsalis pedis pulse* is felt in the groove between the first two tendons on the medial side of the dorsum of the foot. It is congenitally absent in approximately 10% of the population.

EXAMINE SWELLING AND INFLAMMATION

Inflammation results from injury to tissues, and swelling occurs as exudate forms to defend the tissues from further injury. Swelling within the musculoskeletal system may be local or diffuse. Localized swelling is most often present as a lump or a small, specific mass under the skin, for example, as in a swollen olecranon bursa, where swelling is confined to the area of the bursa. Diffuse swelling is more widespread. As a general rule, localized swelling is contained within a joint capsule or bursa and does not extravasate into nearby tissues, whereas diffuse swelling may involve the entire region (Table 2–5). A joint appears swollen when there is a thickened synovial membrane; an increase in synovial fluid, blood, or purulent material within the joint capsule; or swelling in the surrounding soft tissue. Inflammation of a joint typically produces pain and an increase in temperature and erythema (redness).

It is important to know whether a joint is enlarged from soft-tissue swelling or from an increase in fluid within the joint. This is especially true for the knee, because many knee injuries involve swelling that may be due to either cause. To check for increased fluid, the examiner can "milk" the medial aspect of the knee by two or three upward strokes with the ball of the hand.

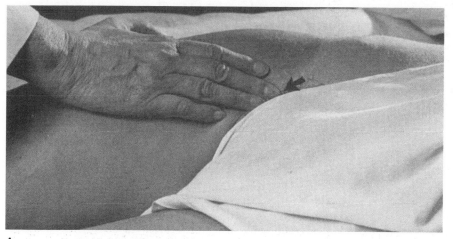

A

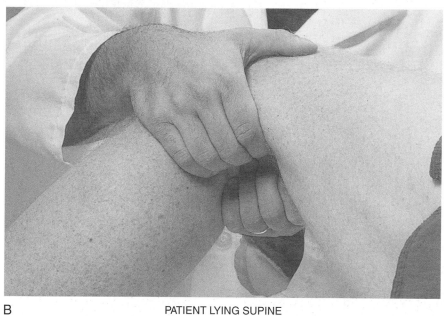

B

PATIENT LYING SUPINE

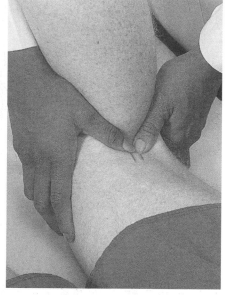

PATIENT LYING PRONE

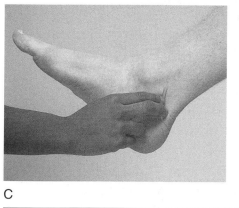

C

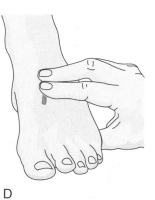

D

Figure 2–12   The four major pulses in the lower extremity are (A) the femoral pulse, (B) the popliteal pulse, (C) the posterior tibial pulse, and (D) the dorsalis pedis pulse.   *(B. Bates (1996). Physical Examination and History Taking. Philadelphia: Lippincott.)*

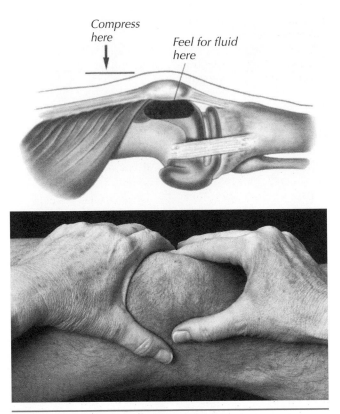

Compress here

Feel for fluid here

The knee is then tapped just behind the lateral margin of the patella. A bulge on the median side indicates fluid returning to the hollow area medial to the patella. Another method of checking for fluid in the knee joint is ballottement for a "floating patella" (Bates, 1995, p. 483). Firmly grasp the thigh just above the knee with one hand, forcing any fluid out of the superior portion of the joint space into the space between the patella and femur. With the fingers of the other hand, push the patella sharply back against the femur. A palpable tap indicates fluid within the knee joint (Fig. 2–13).

Figure 2–13   Ballottement for a "floating patella."   *(B. Bates (1996) Physical Examination and History Taking. Philadelphia: Lippincott.)*

DETECT CREPITUS (CREPITATION)

Crepitus is a palpable or even audible crunching or grating produced by movement of a joint or tendon. Crepitus is more significant when it is associated with other signs and symptoms than when it exists by itself. Cracking or snapping sounds that result from movement of tendons or ligaments over bone may occur in normal joints such as the knees. Fine, soft crepitus may be felt over inflamed joints, while coarser crepitus usually suggests roughened articular cartilages, as in an inflamed or osteoarthritic joint. A creaking, leathery crepitus may arise in inflamed tendon sheaths. To detect possible crepitus, place your hand over the joint while taking the joint through normal range of motion. The crepitus can be heard and usually felt through your hand.

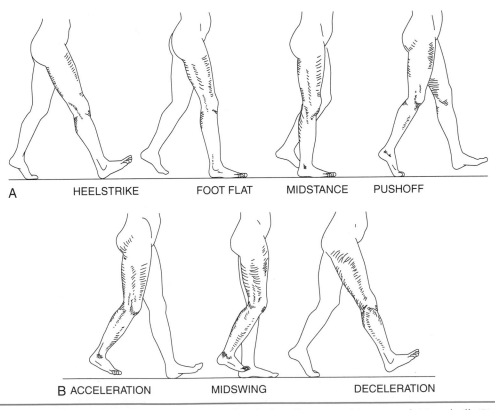

A   HEELSTRIKE   FOOT FLAT   MIDSTANCE   PUSHOFF

B ACCELERATION   MIDSWING   DECELERATION

Figure 2–14   The phases of gait. (A) Stance phase: *(1)* heelstrike, *(2)* foot flat, *(3)* midstance, and *(4)* pushoff. (B) Swing phase: *(1)* acceleration, *(2)* midswing, and *(3)* deceleration.

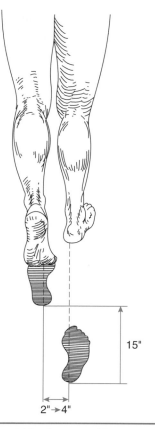

Figure 2–15   The width of a normal base measures from 2 to 4 inches. Normal step length is approximately 15 inches.

ASSESSMENT

When doing a complete musculoskeletal assessment, organize the examination so that it progresses smoothly with minimal position changes for the patient. A good way is to begin with the patient sitting so that you can examine the neck, shoulders, and upper extremities. Then examine the back, ilium, and gait with the patient both standing and walking. Finally, have the patient lie supine while you examine the hips, knees, ankles, and feet. *Note: For clarity of presentation, a slightly modified order is followed in subsequent sections.*

GAIT AND POSTURE

Observe how the patient sits, stands, and walks. The assessment of the patient should begin when the patient walks into the room, because the patient is less apt to be conscious that his or her gait is being assessed. Gait varies from person to person, but normally there is a certain rhythm to a person's walk. Observe the patient's posture, swing of the arms, the stride length and rhythm, and any associated movements (Fig. 2–14). A distance of 2 to 4 inches should separate the patient's heels as they pass during walking, and the stride length should be about 15 inches, depending on the patient's height and body structure (Fig. 2–15). The patient's arms should swing freely at the side, the body should be well balanced, and posture should be erect. When the patient turns, the face and head should turn before the rest of the body. For examples of abnormal gait patterns, see Table 2–6.

THORACIC AND LUMBAR SPINE

With the patient's back and buttocks exposed, inspect the curvature of the spinal column from both posterior and lateral views. Note any prominence of the scapulae and whether the shoulders are level. Palpate the spinous processes and paravertebral muscles, noting any tenderness or swelling. Use the flat of your hand to detect muscle hardening from spasms. Have the patient perform active range of motion of the trunk (Fig. 2–16). Examples of assessment procedures are

Name	Gait Pattern	Associated Disorder
Table 2–6 Gait Disturbance		
Ataxia	Unsteady, uncoordinated, feet staggering, feet raised high while stepping and then stepped flat onfloor, wide-based walk with difficulty turning	Disease of cerebellum or associated tracts; intoxication
Steppage	Feet either dragged or lifted high and then brought down with a slap; appears as if climbing stairs; one or both sides involved	Lower motor neuron disease; footdrop
Spastic hemiplegic	Unilateral footdrop and foot dragging or leg circumducted; arm flexed and held close to side	Unilateral upper motor neuron disease
Parkinsonian	Trunk leans forward, slight flexion of hip and knees, no arm swing while stepping, short and shuffling steps, starts slowly and then increases in speed	Basal ganglia deficit
Scissors	Slow, stiff, short steps; thighs tend to cross while stepping forward; appears to be walking through water	Bilateral spastic paraplegia, dementia
Spastic	Uncoordinated, jerking, short steps with legs stiff, toes dragging	Neurogenic, cerebral palsy
Old age	Decreased speed and balance, steps short or shuffling, flexed hip and knee, stooped posture	Aging process

(Adapted from Bates, B. (1995). Physical examination and history taking, (6th ed.). Philadelphia: J. B. Lippincott.)

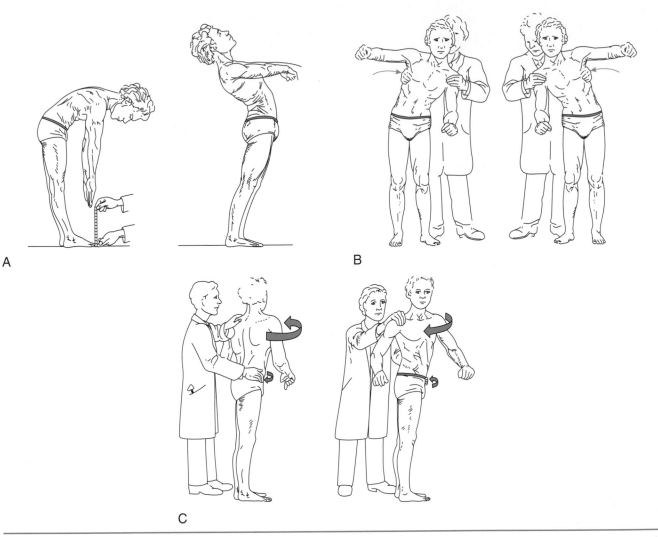

A   **B**

C

Figure 2–16   (A) *Left.* Range of flexion in the lumbar spine. *Right.* Range of extension in the lumbar spine. (B) Range of lateral bending in the lumbar spine should be equal on both sides. (C) Range of rotation in the lumbar spine.

Table 2–7 Assessing Range of Motion in the Thoracic and Lumbar Spine		
Spinal Movements and Normal Range of Motion	**Instructions to the Patient**	**Procedure for Testing Muscle Strength**
Flexion: 70–90 degrees	"Bend over and touch your toes without flexing your knees."	With one hand stabilizing the patient's pelvis, apply resistance with the other hand to the center of the patient's chest.
Extension: 30 degrees when standing; 20 degrees when prone	"Bend your head and shoulders back as far as you can."	With the pelvis stabilized, apply resistance between the patient's scapulae.
Lateral: 35 degrees	"Bend your trunk as far to the side as possible."	With the pelvis stabilized, apply resistance to the deltoid area.
Rotation: 30–45 degrees	"Twist your shoulders as far to the left as possible."	With the pelvis stabilized, apply resistance to the shoulders.

shown in Table 2–7. Deviations in the spine include (1) kyphosis, an increased convex curve ("hunchback") in the thoracic spine; (2) lordosis, an increased concave curve ("swayback") in the lumbar spine; and (3) scoliosis, a lateral curve of the spinal column.

CERVICAL SPINE

Inspect the front, back, and sides of the neck for size and for symmetry of the patient's neck muscles. Compare the neck muscles, particularly the sternocleidomastoid and trapezius. Note any abnormalities, such as deviations in

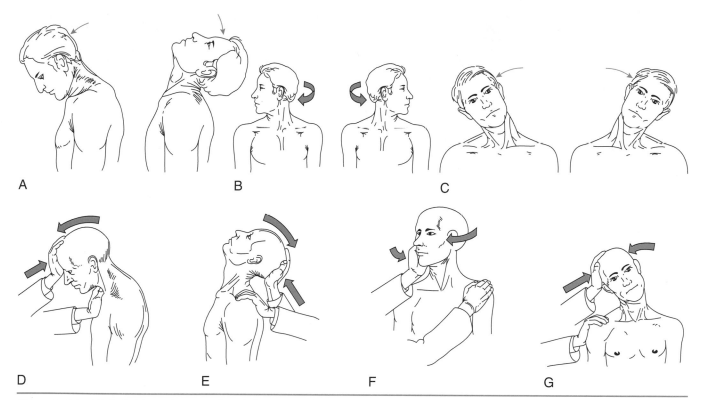

Figure 2–17 (A) *Left.* Normal range of neck flexion. *Right.* Normal range of neck extension. (B) Normal range of neck rotation. (C) Normal range of lateral bending. (D) Hand positions for neck flexion muscle test. (E) Hand positions for neck extension muscle test. (F) Hand positions for testing the sternocleidomastoid muscles for lateral rotation. (G) Muscle test for lateral bending of the neck.

Table 2–8	Assessing Range of Motion in the Cervical Spine	
Spinal Movements and Normal Range of Motion	**Instructions to the Patient**	**Procedure for Testing Muscle Strength**
Flexion: 45 degrees	"Bend your head down to touch your chest."	Apply resistance to the forehead.
Extension: 55 degrees	"Lift your head and bend it back as far you can."	Apply resistance to the occipital prominence.
Lateral bend: 40–45 degress	"Bend your head so that your ear touches your shoulder. Do not bring your shoulder up to meet your ear."	Apply resistance to the temporal bone.
Rotation: 70 degrees	"Turn your head as far as you can to the right and then turn it as far as you can to the left."	Apply resistance to the temple.

the cervical spine and along the supraclavicular fossa for any nodules or points of tenderness and swelling. Have the patient perform active range of motion of the cervical spine (Fig. 2–17). See Table 2–8 for examples of assessment procedures.

SHOULDER

Inspect and compare the patient's shoulders and shoulder girdle anteriorly, noting bony or muscular asymmetry, swelling, masses, deformities, muscular atrophy, discolorations, and scars. Inspect and compare the clavicles for alignment. Inspect the scapulae and related muscles posteriorly. Inspect the deltoid muscles for atrophy, for prominence of the greater tuberosity of the humerus, and for the presence of hollows in the muscle (which could indicate displacement of the humerus). Observe the rhythm of the patient's shoulder movements. Normal motion has a smooth, even flow with no jerky or irregular movements. Palpate the shoulder to determine bony landmarks, and note any tenderness, bogginess, or crepitation around the joint. Have the patient perform active range of motion of the shoulder (Fig. 2–18). See Table 2–9 for examples of assessment procedures.

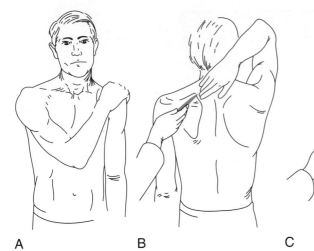
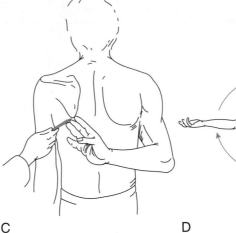
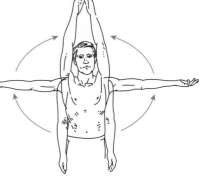

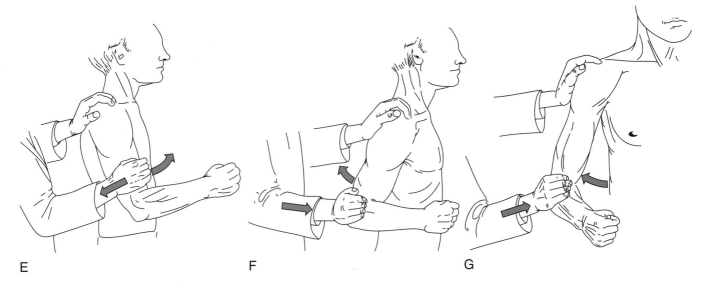

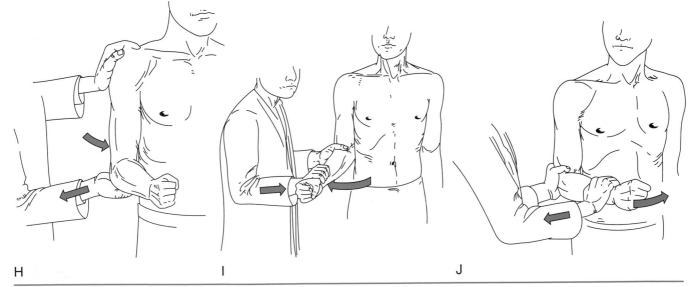

Figure 2–18   (A) Test for internal rotation and adduction. (B) The Apley scratch test; external rotation and abduction. (C) Internal rotation and adduction. (D) Test for shoulder flexion. (E) Test for shoulder extension. (F) Range of motion (G) Test for shoulder adduction. (H) Test for shoulder adduction. (I) Test for external rotation of the shoulder. (J) Test for internal rotation of the shoulder.

Table 2–9	Assessing Range of Motion in the Shoulder	

Shoulder Movements and Normal Range of Motion	Instructions to the Patient	Procedure for Testing Muscle Strength
Forward flexion: 180 degrees	"Move your arms forward and up."	Apply resistance to the anterior aspect of the arm proximal to the elbow.
Backward extension: 50–60 degrees	"Move your arms downward and back; clasp your arms behind your back."	Apply resistance to the posterior aspect of the arm proximal to the elbow.
Abduction: 120 degrees	"Lift your arm straight out from your side, away from your body."	Apply resistance to the lateral aspect of the arm proximal to the elbow.
Horizonal adduction: 45 degrees	"Bring your straight arm over your chest."	Apply resistance to the medial side of the arm proximal to the elbow.
Horizontal abduction: 180 degrees	"Keeping your straight arm at shoulder height, move it backward as far as you can."	Apply resistance to the posterior surface of the arm proximal to the elbow.
Internal rotation	"Rotate your shoulder inward and swing your arm backward with your palm upward, pointing your fingers toward the ceiling."	Apply resistance to volar surface of the wrist.
External rotation	"Rotate your shoulder outward with your palm down and bring your arm up."	Apply resistance to dorsum of the wrist.

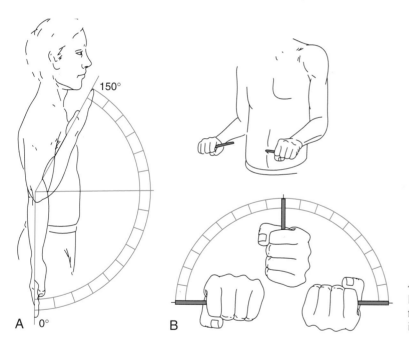

Figure 2–19   (A) The elbow range of motion in flexion and extension. (B) the elbow range of motion in supination and pronation. *(continued)*

ELBOW AND FOREARM

Flex the patient's elbow to 90 degrees, noting any redness, swelling, nodules, or deformities. Compare the two elbows, noting any differences between the elbow joint angles and the muscular structures of the forearm and upper arm. Palpate the elbow in positions of flexion and extension, checking for subcutaneous nodules, bogginess, crepitation, and tenderness or enlargement of the supracondylar lymph nodes. (Lymph nodes are located above the epicondyle and are not palpable unless there is an infection below the elbow.) Palpate the muscle bodies for tenderness

or muscle spasm. Have the patient perform active range of motion of the elbow (Figure 2–19 and Table 2–10).

The terms valgus and varus describe deviations of the joints of the extremities. Valgus is a deformity in which the distal portion of a joint is angulated away from the midline of the body; for example, cubitus valgus is when the forearm deviates laterally (at a "carrying angle"). Varus is a deformity in which the distal portion of a joint is angled toward the midline of the body; for example, cubitus varus is when the forearm deviates medially (the "gunstock deformity").

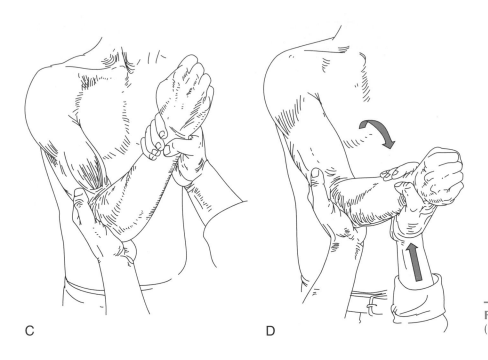

C   D

Figure 2–19   (C) Muscle test for flexion.
(D) Muscle test for extension.

Table 2–10   Assessing Range of Motion in the Elbow and Forearm

Elbow and Forearm Movement Range of Motion	Instructions to the Patient	Procedure for Testing Muscle Strength
Elbow		
Flexion: 150 degrees	"Move your right (left) hand to your right (left) shoulder."	Apply resistance to the lower arm.
Extension: 0 degrees	"Straighten out your right (left) arm."	Apply resistance to the dorsal surface of the arm.
Forearm		
Pronation: 90 degrees	"Rotate your right (left) hand inward so that your palm is downward."	Apply resistance at the base of the thumb on the volar surface.
Supination: 90 degrees	"Rotate your right (left) hand outward so that the palm is upward."	Apply resistance to the dorsal surface of the hand.
Hyperextension: 0–15 degress	Motion not present in all individuals	

Table 2–11   Assessing Range of Motion in the Wrist

Wrist Movements and Normal Range of Motion	Instructions to the Patient	Procedure for Testing Muscle Strength
Flexion: 80 degrees	"Bend your right (left) hand down toward you."	Apply resistance to the surface of the hand.
Extension: 70 degrees	"Bend your right (left) hand back on itself."	Apply resistance to the dorsum of the hand.
Lateral (ulnar) deviation 30–50 degrees (Ulnar deviation is usually measured with the wrist in pronation. When measured in supination, ulnar deviation is increased.)	"Rotate your hand laterally outward from your body (toward the ulna)."	Apply resistance to the ulnar surface of the hand.
Lateral (radial) deviation 20 degrees	"Rotate your hand laterally and inward toward your body (toward the radius)."	Apply resistance to the radial surface of the hand.

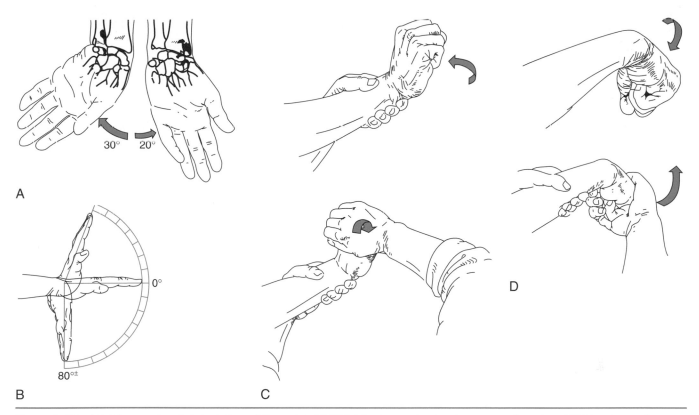

Figure 2–20   (A) Ulnar and radial deviation of the wrist. (B) Wrist flexion and extension range of motion. (C) Muscle test for wrist extension. (D) Muscle test for wrist flexion. *(continued)*

WRIST
Inspect each wrist for shape, deformity, swelling, lumps, or redness; then compare their contour and bony prominences. Palpate both wrists, checking for bogginess, crepitation, tenderness, and enlargement. Have the patient perform active range of motion of the wrist (Table 2–11 and Fig. 2–20).

HAND AND FINGERS
Inspect and compare the hands in terms of their bony and muscular structures, noting any swelling, redness, nodules, and deformities, such as extra fingers (polydactyly), missing fingers, partially amputated fingers, or webbing between fingers (syndactyly). Inspect the thenar and hypothenar eminences for atrophy, which deepens the palmar depression. Palpate the hand and fingers for bony landmarks, noting any tenderness, bogginess, or nodules. Have the patient perform active range of motion of the hand and fingers (Fig. 2–21 and Table 2–12).

HIP AND PELVIS
Observe the patient's ability to move, sit, get out of a chair, get onto the examination table, and lie supine.

Note if the movements are smooth or if the patient has any difficulty performing them. Look for any bruising, abrasions, or swelling. With the patient's legs aligned symmetrically, check for equal leg length (if they appear unequal, measure). With the patient lying supine, palpate the iliac crests, the anterior spines of the pelvis, and the symphysis. With the patient lying prone, palpate the ischial tuberosities and feel along the spine for tenderness, swelling, or nodules. Have the patient perform active range of motion of the hip and pelvis (Fig. 2–22 and Table 2–13).

KNEE
Inspect the patient's knee while the patient is supine, observing the contour and alignment. Note any deformities (such as knock-knees or bowlegs), redness, swelling, or nodules; observe the quadriceps muscles for contour, symmetry, and atrophy; and look for the normal hollows around the patella. If muscle atrophy is present, measure the circumference of the leg (Fig. 2–3); it is normal for the dominant leg to be up to one cm (0.4 inches) larger. Palpate each knee by placing your thumb and forefinger over the suprapatellar pouch on both sides of the quadriceps. Check for any bogginess

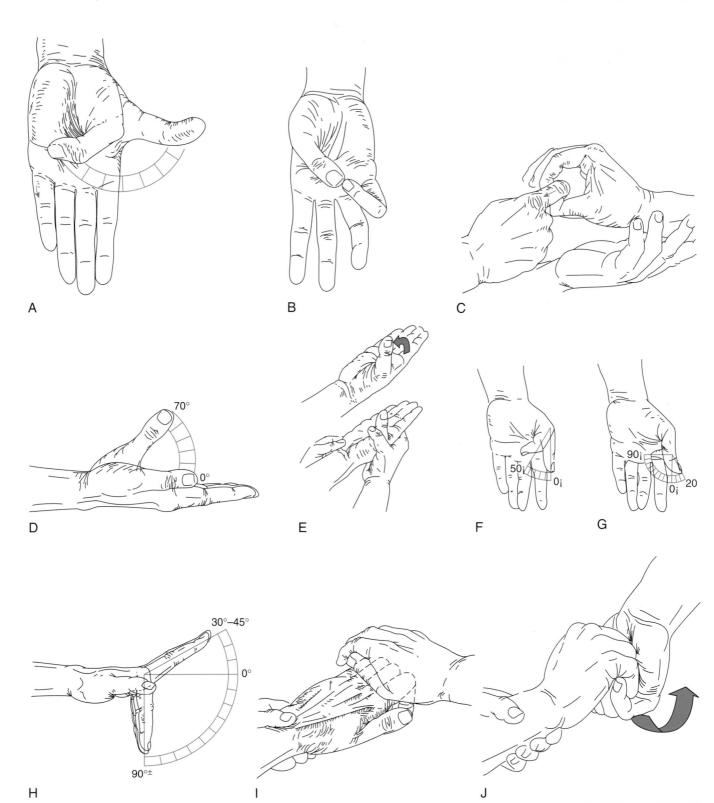

Figure 2–21   (A) Thumb flexion and extension. (B) Opposition to the thumb and fingertips. (C) Muscle test for the pinch mechanism. (D) Palmar abduction-adduction of the thumb. (E) A muscle test for thumb abduction. (F) Thumb flexion and extension, metacarpophalangeal joint. (G) Thumb flexion and extension, interphalangeal joint. (H) Metacarpophalangeal joint range of motion, flexion-extension. (I) Muscle test for finger extension. (J) Muscle test for finger flexion. *(continued)*

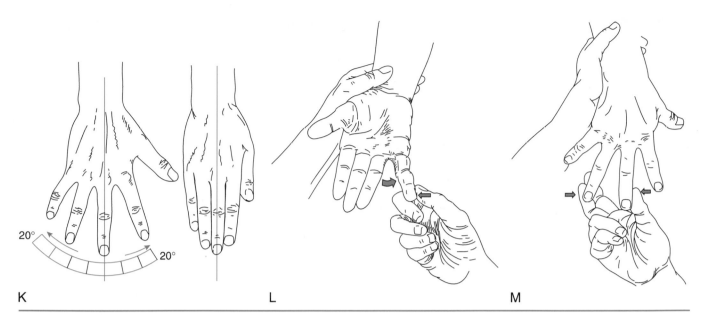

K   L   M

Figure 2–21   (K) Finger abduction and adduction. (L) Muscle test for finger abduction. (M) Muscle test for finger abduction.

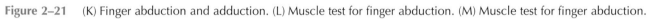

Table 2–12	Assessing Range of Motion in the Hand and Fingers	

Movements and Normal Range of Motion	Instructions to the Patient	Procedure for Testing Muscle Strength
Thumb		
Metacarpophalangeal joint		
Flexion: 50 degrees	"Bend your thumb to touch your palm."	Apply resistance to the volar surface of the thumb.
Extension: 0 degrees	"Straighten out your thumb as if thumbing a ride."	Apply resistance to the dorsal surface of the thumb.
Abduction: 70 degrees	"With your palm up, raise your thumb to the ceiling."	Apply resistance to the lateral surface of the thumb.
Adduction: 0 degrees	"Bring your thumb against the index finger."	Apply resistance to the medial surface of the thumb.
Opposition—touching each fingertip with the tip of the thumb	"Touch the top of the right (left) thumb to the tip and then to the base of the little, ring, middle, and index fingers."	Apply resistance to the volar surfaces of the thumb and fingers.
Interphalangeal joint		
Flexion: 90 degrees		
Extension: 20 degrees		
Hand		
Metacarpophalangeal joint		
Flexion: 90 degrees	"Bend your fingers at the first joint."	Apply resistance to the volar surface of the the proximal and distal phalanges.
Extension: 30–35 degrees	"Straighten out your fingers."	Apply resistance to the dorsal surface of the proximal and distal surface of the fingers being tested.
Adduction: fingers should touch	"Put your fingers together."	Apply resistance by attempting to pull the fingers apart.
Proximal interphalangeal joint		
Flexion: 100–120 degrees	"Bend your fingers at the middle joint."	Apply resistance to the volar surface of the middle phalanx.
Extension: 0 degrees		
Distal interphalangeal joint		
Flexion: 80–90 degrees	"Bend your distal finger joint."	Apply resistance to the volar surface of the fingertip.
Extension: 20 degrees	"Straighten your finger as much as possible."	Apply resistance to the fingernails.

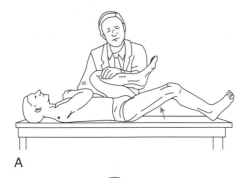

A

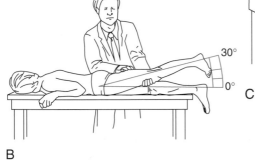

B

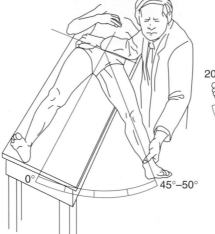

C

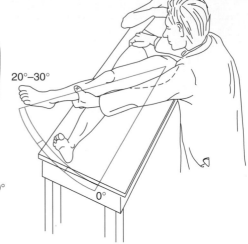

D

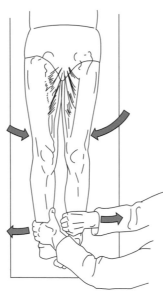

E

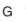

F

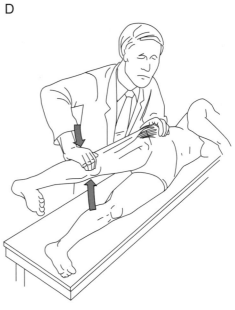

G

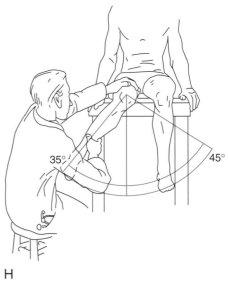

H

Figure 2–22   (A) The normal limit for hip flexion is approximately 135 degrees. (B) Test for hip extension. (C) Normal limits for hip abduction are 45 to 50 degrees. (D) Normal limits for hip adduction are 20 to 30 degrees. (E) Alternate muscle test for abduction (gluteus medius). (F) Test for adductor muscle strength. (G) Muscle test for abduction. (H) Test for internal and external femoral rotation on the flexed position.

Table 2–13   Assessing Range of Motion in the Hip and Pelvis

Movements and Normal Range of Motion	Instructions to the Patient	Procedure for Testing Muscle Strength
Flexion: 110–120 degrees	"Draw your knees up to your chest." (while sitting or supine)	Apply resistance to the anterior surface of the leg proximal to the knee.
Extension: 30 degrees or less	"Lift your leg toward the ceiling." (while lying prone)	Apply resistance to the posterior surface of the leg proximal to the knee.
Abduction: 45–50 degrees	"Move your upper leg toward the ceiling." (while lying on a side)	Apply resistance to lateral surface of the upper leg.
Adduction: 20–30 degrees	"Try to bring your legs together."	Apply resistance to the medial surface of the upper legs.
Internal rotation: 45 degrees (with knee extended)	"Pivot your hip inward by turning your foot away from your body." (while sitting)	Apply resistance against the lateral surface of the ankle and foot.
External rotation: 35 degrees (with knee extended)	"Rotate your hip outward by turning your foot toward your body." (while sitting)	Apply resistance to the medial ankle and foot.

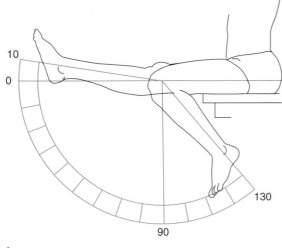

A

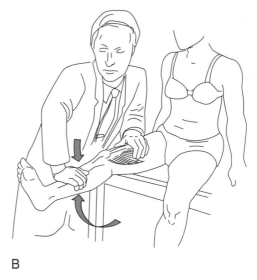

B

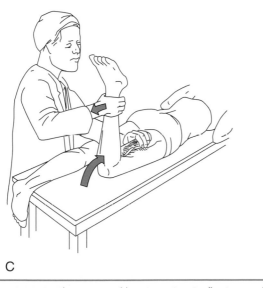

C

Figure 2–23   (A) The range of knee motion in flexion and extension. (B) Quadriceps muscle test. (C) Hamstring muscle test.

or tenderness in the synovial membrane. Observe the muscle structures around the knee, and note any bony enlargements or points of tenderness in the joint, muscles, and tendons. Compare the two knees. Palpate the quadriceps muscles, starting at the uppermost aspect of each thigh and moving lengthwise in a circular motion to cover the anterior, posterior, medial, and lateral aspects. The thigh muscles should be firm and continuous from origin to insertion. Palpate the popliteal space to check for swelling or cysts. Have the patient perform active range of motion of the knee (Fig. 2–23 and Table 2–14).

The terms valgus and varus describe deviations of the knee joints. Valgus is a deformity in which the distal portion of a joint is angulated away from the midline of the body (e.g., genus valgus describes "knock-knees"). Varus is a deformity in which the distal portion of a joint is angled toward the midline of the body (e.g., genus varus describes "bowlegs").

Table 2–14 Assessing Range of Motion in the Knee		
Knee Movements and Normal Range of Motion	**Instructions to the Patient**	**Procedure for Testing Muscle Strength**
Flexion: 130 degrees	"Bend your right (left) leg. Try to touch your heel to the back of your leg." (while prone or sitting)	Apply resistance to the posterior ankle.
Extension: 10 degrees	"Straighten out your right (left) leg as far as you can."	Apply resistance to the anterior ankle.
Internal rotation: 10 degrees	"Turn your foot inward toward the midline."	Apply resistance against the medial side of the foot.
External rotation: 10 degrees	"Turn your foot outward from the midline."	Apply resistance against the lateral side of the foot.

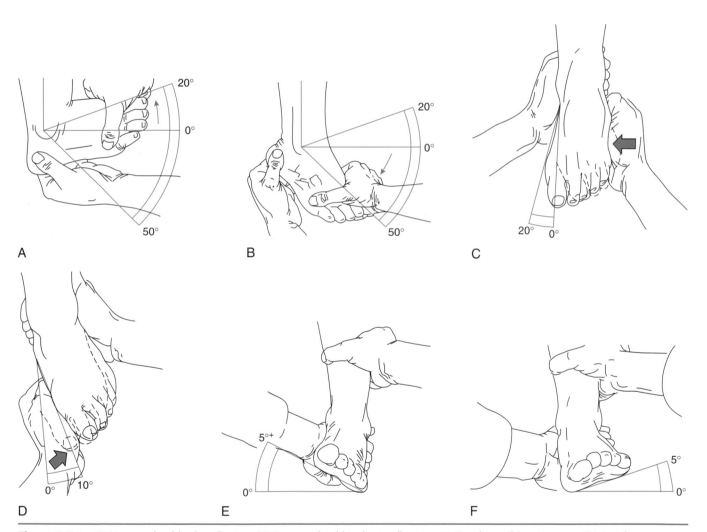

Figure 2–24   (A) Range of ankle dorsiflexion. (B) Range of ankle plantar flexion. (C) Forefoot adduction test. (D) Forefoot abduction test. (E) Foot inversion test. (F) Foot eversion test. *(continued)*

ANKLE AND FOOT

Inspect the patient's ankles and feet for swelling, tenderness, redness, nodules, and other deformities. Check the arch of each foot, look for any toe deformities, and note any skin changes. Check the position of the ankles, noting whether the medial malleolus angles in or out abnormally. Note any edema, calluses, bunions, corns, ingrown toenails, plantar warts, trophic ulcers, hair loss, or unusual pigmentation. Palpate the bony and muscular structures of the patient's ankles and feet and check for any areas of tenderness. Ask the patient to perform active range of motion of the ankle, foot, and toes. Several of the motions may need to be done passively, or at least with assistance (Fig. 2–24 and Table 2–15).

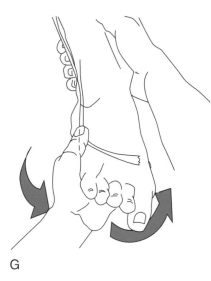

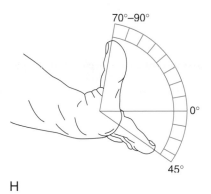

70°–90°

0°

45°

H

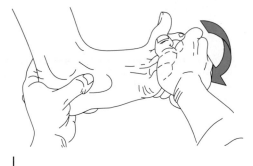

I

G

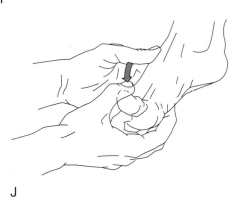

J

Figure 2–24 (G) The peronel muscle test. (H) The normal flexion-extension range of the first metatarsophalangeal joint. (I) Testing the strength of the digitorum longus muscle. (J) The extensor hallucis longus muscle test.

Table 2–15	Assessing Range of Motion in the Ankle and Foot	

Movements and Normal Range of Motion	Instructions to the Patient	Procedure for Testing Muscle Strength
Ankle		
Flexion (dorsiflexion): 20 degrees	"Bend your toes toward your knees."	Apply resistance to the dorsal aspect of the foot.
Extension (plantarflexion): 45–50 degrees	"Point your toes away from you (downward) as far as you can."	Apply resistance to the ball of the foot.
Inversion: 5 degrees (passive)	"Point your toes and rotate them inward along the long axis of your foot."	Apply resistance against the medial aspect of the first metatarsal.
Eversion: 5 degrees (passive)	"Point your toes and rotate them outward along the long axis of your foot."	Apply resistance against the lateral aspect of the fifth metatarsal.
Abduction: 10 degrees (passive)	"Point your toes; then move them outward."	Apply resistance against the fifth metatarsal.
Adduction: 20 degrees (passive)	"Point your toes; move them inward."	Apply resistance against the first metatarsal.
Great Toe		
Metatarsophalangeal joint		
Flexion: 45 degrees	"Bend your big toe downward."	Apply resistance to the plantar side of the great toe.
Extension: 70–90 degrees	"Bend your big toe upward."	Apply resistance to the dorsum of the great toe.
Toes		
Metatarsophalangeal joints		
Flexion: 40 degrees	"Bend all your toes downward."	Apply resistance to the plantar surface of the proximal phalanges.
Extension: 40 degrees	"Straighten out your toes and point them upward."	Apply resistance to the dorsum of the proximal phalanges.
Interphalangeal proximal joints		
Flexion: 35 degrees	"Bend your toes downward."	Apply resistance to the plantar surface of the medial phalanges.
Extension: 0 degrees		
Interphalangeal distal joints		
Flexion: 60 degrees	"Bend your toes downward."	Apply resistance to the plantar surface of the distal phalanges.
Extension: 30 degrees	"Point your toes upward."	Resistance is applied to the dorsum of the distal phalanges.
Adduction: degrees vary	"Try to spread your toes apart."	

The terms eversion and inversion are used to describe abnormal positionings of the foot. Eversion is a "turning out" position where the foot is rotated along its longitudinal axis so that increased weight is borne on the medial side. Inversion is a "turning in" position where the foot is rotated along its longitudinal axis so that increased weight is borne on the lateral side. The terms valgus and varus also describe deviations of the joints of the foot. Valgus is a deformity in which the distal portion of a joint is "angulated away from the midline" of the body (e.g., talipes valgus describes the feet as turned outward). Varus is a deformity in which the distal portion of a joint is "angled toward the midline of the body" (e.g., talipes varus describes the feet as turned inward as in "pigeon toes").

DIAGNOSTIC PROCEDURES

A third source of information on the patient is gained from diagnostic procedures. The major orthopaedic diagnostic techniques are (1) joint aspirations, (2) biopsies, (3) arthroscopies, (4) roentgenographic examinations, (5) electromyographies, and (6) laboratory tests.

JOINT ASPIRATION

Joint aspiration (arthrocentesis) is performed as an inpatient or outpatient procedure to obtain samples of synovial fluid from within the joint cavity. The procedure is performed by introducing a needle into the joint cavity and withdrawing fluid. It aids in determining the presence of aseptic inflammatory processes, such as rheumatoid arthritis, and septic processes, such as bacterial arthritis.

The synovial fluid samples are cultured and examined microscopically and chemically. Synovial fluid is normally straw-colored and clear. Its viscosity resembles that of motor oil. In the presence of inflammation, it becomes turbid and more watery; the number of white blood cells, the protein content, and the number of polymorphonuclear cells are increased; and the glucose content is decreased.

A local anesthetic is usually administered before the procedure. After the procedure, the joint is often dressed and an elastic bandage applied for 8 to 24 hours. If infection is present in the joint and there is drainage from the joint following aspiration, precautions should be taken with the wound dressings to prevent the possible spread of infection. Teach the patient the signs and symptoms of infection. Continued or additional joint swelling, elevated temperature, purulent drainage, redness, and increased pain or tenderness at the aspiration site should be reported to the physician.

BIOPSY

A biopsy is the removal of tissue for purposes of microscopic examination to confirm a diagnosis, to follow the course of a disease, or to determine the effectiveness of treatment. Specimens may be obtained by means of a special needle or punch, a surgical incision, or the aspiration of fluid. Needle or punch biopsies may be done at the patient's bedside, in a physician's office, in an outpatient clinic, or in surgery. When a needle biopsy is done on an internal lesion, however, there is no certainty that the area sampled contains cells from the lesion. Therefore, an open incision, where the lesion is visualized, may be the method of choice. The incisional biopsy is an operative procedure under general or local anesthesia.

MUSCLE BIOPSY

A muscle biopsy is performed to aid in the diagnosis of myopathic disorders. In most instances, the muscle to be biopsied has previously been examined by gross muscle testing and electromyography (EMG). Histochemical staining of biopsied muscle tissue may reveal features of lower motor neuron disease (such as atrophy of groups of fibers innervated by single motor units), degeneration, inflammatory reactions, or involvement of specific fibers that indicate myopathic disease.

A muscle biopsy is an operative procedure usually performed under a local or general anesthetic. Following the procedure, the patient will experience minor to moderate discomfort, depending on the location of the muscle biopsied. The discomfort may be in the form of stiffness or pain at or around the operative site. If the muscle biopsied is in the lower extremity (i.e., one of the gluteal or quadriceps), the patient is usually encouraged to resume ambulation within hours to avoid stiffness.

SYNOVIAL BIOPSY

A synovial biopsy is helpful in differentiating various forms of arthritis. The specimen of synovium is examined histologically for evidence of inflammation, and a sample of the synovial fluid obtained at the same time is sent for culture and other studies. The biopsy may be performed as a closed biopsy with a special synovial biopsy needle (such as the Parker-Pearson) or as an open biopsy done in surgery. When a closed biopsy is performed, the patient is given a local anesthetic. Afterward, a small compression dressing with an elastic bandage is usually applied around the joint, and the patient is asked to rest the joint for 24 hours to prevent hemorrhage or effusion.

OTHER BIOPSIES

In the musculoskeletal system, biopsies also involve bone, skin, the buccal mucosa, and the temporal artery. A bone biopsy may be accomplished by an open or needle biopsy to diagnose connective tissue disorders. The buccal mucosa may be biopsied to help diagnose Sjögren's syndrome, and the temporal artery may be biopsied to diagnose temporal arteritis.

ARTHROSCOPY

Arthroscopy, a procedure performed in surgery, is the examination of a joint through a special fiberoptic endoscope called an arthroscope. The arthroscopy allows for extensive, accurate visualization of a joint cavity and can be done on an inpatient or outpatient basis. The most common joint for an arthroscopy is the knee, but other joints such as the ankle, hip, fingers, wrist, elbow, shoulder, and temporomandibular joint can be scoped.

The instrument (arthroscope) has lenses and a light source that permits visualization, photography, and surgical procedures within the joint. After the administration of a local anesthetic and the application of a tourniquet (to reduce the blood flow), the endoscope is inserted into the joint cavity through a small incision. Normal saline is instilled to provide a viewing medium, enabling the physician to see the structure and contents of the joint. The procedure permits biopsy or removal of a torn meniscus, removal of loose bodies, and in some instances biopsy of a synovium or cartilage.

Once the procedure is completed, a compression dressing with an Ace bandage is applied. The patient needs to keep the extremity elevated as much as possible for the first 48 hours to reduce edema. Ice packs should also be applied for at least 24 hours to help prevent swelling. Following a knee arthroscopy, the patient is usually allowed partial weight bearing using crutches, but must avoid excessive use of the joint for 24 to 48 hours. Because an arthroscopy is frequently done on an outpatient basis, make sure the patient knows the signs of infection and who to contact if a problem should arise. Range of motion is usually started on the second or third day with physical therapy for muscle strengthening. The patient can usually take a shower in 48 hours but no tub bath for 4 days. A mild analgesic is usually ordered for pain control, with a return appointment to the physician in 7 days. A return to work and limited sports activities (e.g., swimming and biking) are usually possible within a week. However, pain is the patient's best guide. If the joint becomes more painful, the patient is usually doing too much and needs to reduce activities and advance more slowly.

ROENTGENOGRAPHIC EXAMINATIONS

ROENTGENOGRAM OF BONE AND JOINTS

Roentgenographic (x-ray) examination provides data important to the identification and treatment of fractures and the identification and observation of a number of pathological conditions, including rheumatoid arthritis, spondylitis, avascular necrosis, and tumors. Joint changes such as erosion of joint margins, joint space narrowing, bone spurs, loose bodies, and dislocations can also be detected. Injuries to soft tissues such as tendons and ligaments do not show on roentgenograms, but soft-tissue swelling can be observed.

No special preparation is required for roentgenograms of bones and joints. Some orthopaedic patients have significant mobility restrictions, however, and may be unable to lie on a hard x-ray table for any length of time. In particular, persons with arthritis, who frequently experience joint stiffness and pain, may require extensive roentgenographic examinations. Careful planning should be given in scheduling their roentgenograms, and several sessions with 1 or 2 days of rest in between may be required in cases with severe joint involvement. Analgesics before, and analgesics or local heat applications afterward, may be necessary for relief of joint pain. When a fracture is suspected, the patient should be carefully moved to and from the x-ray table to prevent further injury. Having the suspected extremity splinted is very helpful.

ARTHROGRAM

An arthrogram is a roentgenographic and fluoroscopic examination of a joint (usually the knee, but shoulder, ankle, and other joints can be also be examined). Following the injection of air (pneumoarthrography), a radiopaque contrast medium is injected into the joint space, which permits the imaging of components within the joint that are not normally seen on bone and joint roentgenograms. This imaging helps to detect injuries of the meniscus, cartilage, and ligaments of the knee, and structures of the joint capsule, rotator cuff, and subacromial bursa of the shoulder.

An arthrogram of the knee is accomplished by first cleansing the skin around the puncture site and then anesthetizing the area. A needle is inserted into the joint space between the patella and the femoral condyle, and synovial fluid is aspirated. The needle is not withdrawn, and a fluoroscopic examination is done to verify correct needle placement. Dye is then injected into the joint space. After the needle is removed, the puncture site is cleansed and sealed with collodion. The patient is asked to walk a few steps or to move the knee through its normal range of motion to distribute the dye throughout the joint space. A series of films is then taken with the knee in various positions before the contrast medium is absorbed by the joint tissue. Once the film series is completed, a dressing with an elastic bandage is applied to the knee. Postcare involves keeping the knee joint at rest for at least 6 to 12 hours (which may include immobilization) and keeping the dressing in place for several days. The patient may experience some swelling, discomfort, crepitus, or squishing sounds in the joint, but the symptoms usually disappear after a day or two. Ice applied to the knee helps reduce swelling, and analgesics help reduce pain. Instruct the patient on the signs and symptoms of infection.

MYELOGRAM

A myelogram is the roentgenographic and fluoroscopic examination of the spinal cord and subarachnoid space following the injection of a contrast medium. A myelogram is helpful in the identification of lesions in the intradural and extradural compartments of the spinal canal and in the diagnosis of abnormalities such as a herniated disc, tumor, degenerative arthritis, or spinal stenosis.

The myelogram involves a cisternal or lumbar spinal puncture, the removal of cerebrospinal fluid for analysis, and the injection of a radiopaque contrast medium into the subarachnoid space. The flow of the

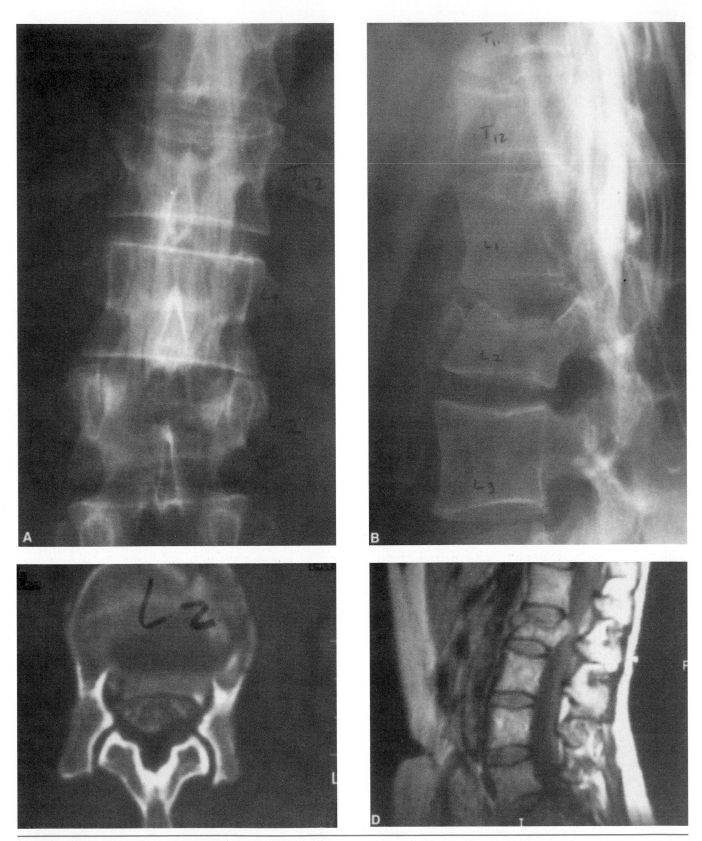

Figure 2–25 A 30-year-old female involved in a motor vehicle accident presented to the emergency room complaining of back pain and had no obvious neurological deficit (A, B) Pre-operative myelography shows an obvious burst fracture of 1.2 with retropulsed bone into the neural canal and complete block on myelography. There is also a mild compression fracture of T12 (C) Post myelographic CT reveals retropulsed bone causing compromise of the neural canal. (D) Sagittal and axial MRI show compromise of the neural canal due to retropulsed bony fragments and a small epidural hematoma.   *(Rockwood, et al. (1996).* Rockwood & Green's Fractures in Adults. *Philadelphia: Lippincott. p. 1557.)*

radiopaque dye through the subarachnoid space is observed using fluoroscopy. Lesions in the spinal cord or the subarachnoid space usually produce a complete or incomplete blockage in the spinal canal. The exact configuration of the defect causing the blockage is helpful in determining whether the lesion is intramedullary or extramedullary. Turning the patient in various positions helps to secure a more complete visualization. See Figure 2–25 to note the differences between the myleogram, a computerized tomography (CT) scan, and a magnetic resonance imaging (MRI) of the spine.

Preprocedure, discontinue phenothiazines and neuroleptics for at least 48 hours, and only restart them after at least 24 hours postprocedure. The patient NPO for approximately 4 hours before the procedure. In some instances, a cleansing enema may be ordered to help reduce the appearance of gas shadows on the x-rays. Pre-existing allergies to iodines need to be documented. For lumbar myelograms, instruct the patient that they will be positioned on their side and draped as for a lumbar puncture.

After the fluoroscopic examination and roentgenogram are completed and oil-based dye removed (to help reduce irritation to the meninges), maintain the patient in a supine position for 12 to 16 hours. If the patient had a nonionic, water-soluble dye used, maintain the patient for 6 to 8 hours with the head elevated 45 degrees. Observe the patient for signs of meningeal irritation. Complaints of headache, fever, nausea and vomiting, or convulsions should be reported to the physician and treated. Adverse reactions usually occur 3 to 8 hours after injection and generally disappear within 24 hours. However, in some instances, patients with persistent headaches are referred to the anesthesia department for epidural blood patching. Postprocedure care varies with physician and institutional policies; most have the patient push fluids to filtrate the dye.

RADIOISOTOPE SCAN

A radioisotope scan (bone scan) permits an imaging of the skeleton by a scanning camera following the intravenous injection of a radioactive tracer compound. The tracer of choice is usually a photon-emitting radionuclide, technetuim –99m (^{99m}Tc), which concentrates at sites of abnormal bone metabolism, such as sites of abnormal osteoblastic activity. In malignancies, osteoblastic activity is accelerated, and those sites appear as "hot spots" 3 to 6 months before roentgenography can reveal any lesion. A bone scan is primarily indicated in patients with symptoms of metastatic bone disease, but it is helpful for bone trauma patients, patients with bone grafts, and patients with known degenerative disorders that require monitoring for signs of progression. Bone scans can also help detect an infection after a total hip arthroplasty. See Figure 2–26 to note the differences between an x-ray and a bone scan to detect a fibrosarcoma.

To reduce patient anxiety and make the procedure more comfortable, describe it to the patient, family, and significant others. The patient is required to drink several glasses of water or tea in the 1- to 3-hour period after the injection of the tracer and before the scan to facilitate excretion of tracer that is not absorbed by bone tissue. Advise the patient not to drink large amounts of fluid before the injection. The scan itself takes about an hour and is painless. The patient will need to lie still on a hard, flat surface for the entire examination. Postcare involves checking the injection site for redness or swelling. If a hematoma develops, discomfort may be eased by warm compresses. Once more, have the patient drink large quantities of fluid and void frequently over the next 24 to 48 hours to eliminate the Tc99m via the kidneys. The patient's urine is radioactive. It should be handled wearing latex gloves and discarded according to institutional policy for radioactive materials.

COMPUTERIZED AXIAL TOMOGRAPHY

Computerized axial tomography (CAT or CT scan) provides cross-sectional views of the body by passing a narrow roentgenographic beam from a computerized scanner through the body at different angles. CT scanning may be done with or without an injected radioiodine contrast agent, which highlights blood vessels and allows greater visual discrimination. The CT scan is a series of x-ray photographs, translated by a computer and displayed on an oscilloscope, representing the cross-sectional images of various layers (or slices) of the body. The technique can reconstruct cross-sectional, horizontal, and sagittal plane images. See Figure 2–27 to compare an x-ray with a CT scan of the hip.

CT scans are at least a hundred times more sensitive than ordinary roentgenograms and can discriminate even slight variations in tissue densities to help diagnose a disease at an early stage in the disease process. For example, a lumbar CT scan presents sharper images than a myelogram and provides cross-sectional displays that are not possible with myelograms (Fig. 2–25).

The CT scan can be done on an outpatient or inpatient basis. For a scan without a contrast medium, there is no physical preparation of the patient, but educating the patient about the procedure is essential. The patient lies on a hydraulically adjustable couch, which is moved into a doughnut-like scanner opening. When the patient is positioned, the scanner revolves around the body. The patient usually lies supine. During the scan, the patient will hear clicking noises that are normal scanner sounds. The procedure is painless, but the patient may become uncomfortable as the scan takes 10 to 45 minutes. If the patient is very restless or claustrophobic, the physician may order a sedative; movements during the scan cause a streaking of the image.

TOMOGRAM

Tomography is any x-ray method that produces images of single tissue planes. In conventional radiology, tomographic images (body section radiographs) are produced by motion of the x-ray tube and film

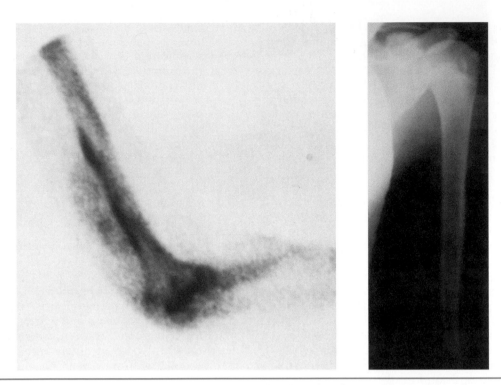

Figure 2–26   Fibrosarcoma of the left arm. The soft tissue tumor is faintly outlined on a technetium-99m bone scan. The intense activity in the adjacent humerus, however, denotes bone involvement by the tumor. Radiograph of the arm is unremarkable for bone involvement.   *(Weinstein & Buckwalter (1994).* Turek's Othropaedics: Principles and Their Application *5th ed. Philadelphia: Lippincott. p. 110.)*

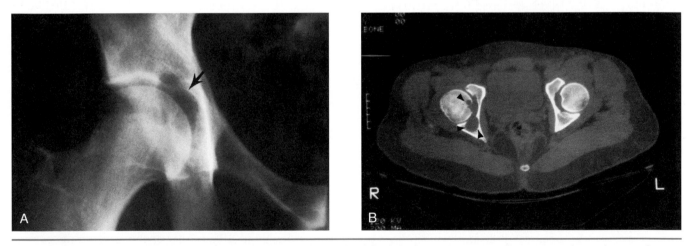

Figure 2–27   Pigmented villonodular synovitis. (A) AP radiograph of the hip showing a geographic region of osteolysis in the acetabulum suspected to represent neoplasm. (B) Noncontrast CT examination of the hip showing osteolysis of the posterior acetabulum and perifoveal femoral head (*arrowheads*), suggesting a synovial rather than osseous origin of the process. Pigmented villonodular synovitis was found at biopsy.   *(Callaghan, et. al. (1998).* The Adult Hip: *Philadelphia: Lippincott. p. 358.)*

(which are moved in opposite directions) or by motion of the patient, which blurs the image except for a single plane of tissue that remains in focus during the exposure.

Although conventional tomograms have been obviated by the advent of computerized axial tomography, they retain an important, though limited, role in spinal trauma. Odontoid fractures, in which the plane of the fracture may be in the imaging plane of the CT scan, are sometimes best seen by anteroposterior or lateral tomogram. For the same reason, flexion-distraction fractures of the thoracolumbar spine may be best demonstrated by conventional tomography. Multiplaner CT with sagittal and coronal reconstructions are rapidly supplanting tomography in this regard.

MAGNETIC RESONANCE IMAGING (MRI)

Magnetic resonance imaging (MRI) is a noninvasive examination that uses a magnetic field and radio waves to depict the hydrogen density of tissues in the body. Different tissues in the body have different hydrogen densities; thus, the MRI can differentiate among tissues based on their differing hydrogen content. MRI is considered more sensitive than the CT (Fig. 2–25), especially in conditions involving a change in tissue with water content, such as disc disease, strokes, and tumors.

For patient safety, individuals with cardiac pacemakers, electric neurostimulators, and intracranial aneurysm clips should be excluded from MRI examination. There is a risk of displacement or dislocation of the metals, and the metals can also produce distorted images. Any patient requiring life support equipment should also be excluded. An individual weighing 300 pounds or having a 52-inch abdominal girth may also be excluded because the scanner may not accommodate individuals of that size, unless it is an "open" MRI.

The procedure takes at least 20 minutes (usually 30 to 90 minutes), and the patient must lie supine without any movement. Verbal communication is maintained, but the patient is out of visual sight during the procedure. All metal devices and objects (e.g., watches, hearing aids, rings, hair and safety pins, and brassieres and boxer shorts with metal fasteners must be removed. If the patient has an IV line, it must be switched to a heparin lock. The patient's bladder should be at least half full if it is to be a pelvic examination. If it is not a pelvic examination, the patient needs to void preprocedure. Postprocedure, normal diet and activities are resumed. However, patients may experience some discomfort from lying quietly on a hard surface for such a long time.

BONE MINERAL DENSITY (BMD)

The bone mineral density (BMD) test is a noninvasive and accurate measurement of BMD based on the fact that mineralized bone absorbs x-rays at different rates than soft tissue. Two standardized scores are provided. The T-score is the patient's score in standard units based on values from young adult populations. The Z-score is the patient's score in standard units based on a population of the same age and sex. This is the patient's standard deviation from other people of the same age.

The World Health Organization (WHO) defines osteoporosis in terms of BMD. Normal bone density is a T-score between +1 and –1. Osteopenia is defined as a T-score between –1 and –2.5. Osteoporosis is considered present when the T-score is below (i.e., more negative than) –2.5; it is considered severe if the patient already has had a fracture. The WHO definitions are based on a population of Caucasian women and are not necessarily applicable to all groups.

The "gold standard" for BMD testing is dual energy x-ray absorptiometry (DXA), which is used for testing the hip and spine. DXA predicts fractures, better than blood pressure predicts stroke, or cholesterol level predicts a myocardial infarction (MI). However, the DXA scanner can give elevated readings (i.e., T-scores that are too large) if the patient is taking calcium. A number of smaller machines are presently in use that utilize sites such as the forearm, heel, and fingers. Bone density by any method at any site predicts the risk of osteoporotic fracture.

ELECTROMYOGRAPHY

Electromyography measures electrical activity across muscle membranes by means of needle electrodes. The procedure yields information on the condition of nerve impulses to muscles, as well as the response of those muscles to the nerve impulses. No electrical activity is present in normal muscles at rest, but electrical activity can be detected during volitional movements. During the procedure, electrical activity is recorded with the muscle at rest, during voluntary movement, and during electrical stimulation. The electrical activity can be heard over a loudspeaker, viewed on an oscilloscope, or printed on a graph called an electromyogram (EMG). In primary myopathic and neuropathic disorders, there are specific patterns of electrical activity, and in neurogenic atrophy there may be fibrillations in resting muscles. An EMG is thus particularly helpful in the diagnosis of lower motor neuron disease, primary muscle disease, and diseases involving defects in the transmission of electrical impulses across neuromuscular junctions, such as myasthenia gravis. However, electromyography cannot be used to differentiate specific disease entities in either the myopathic or neuropathic categories.

There is no special preparation for the procedure. The patient should be informed, however, that small needles will be inserted into the skin and muscles, which may cause some discomfort, though there is no danger of an electrical shock. The procedure can last from 30 minutes to 2 hours. With modern-day computers, the results can be interpreted immediately.

BLOOD AND URINE TESTS

Tests on the patient's blood provide information useful in diagnosing and following the course of many disease processes. Even though routine blood tests, such as white blood counts and hematocrits, are used in orthopaedic practice, only tests that are commonly used (although not inclusive) for musculoskeletal conditions are presented in Table 2–16.

Table 2–16 Diagnostic Tests Used for Musculoskeletal Conditions

Laboratory Test	Normal Values	Indications for Abnormal Values
Blood		
Acid phosphatase	0.5–2.0 Bodansky units/dl 1–5 King-Armstrong units/dl	Increased in Paget's disease and carcinoma of the bone
Aldolase	1.0–7.5 units/100ml	Increased in skeletal muscle necrosis
Alkaline phosphatase	1.5–4.0 Bodansky units/dl 4–13.5 King-Armstrong units/dl	Increased in osteoblastic bone tumors (osteogenic sarcoma and metastatic carcinoma), inflammatory conditions, rickets, osteomalacia, hyperparathyroidism, and during fracture healing
Calcium (Ca)	7–12 mg/dl 4.5–5.5 mEq/l	Increased in metastatic bone cancer, acute osteoporosis, multiple myeloma, prolonged immobilization, and during fracture healing Decreased in hypoparathyroidism, osteomalacia, and rickets
Creatine phosphokinase (CPK),	15–57 units/L in women 23–99 units/L in men 0–12 Sigma units/cc	Increased in necrosis or atrophy of skeletal muscles, traumatic muscle injury, strenuous exercise, and progressive muscular dystrophy
Lactic dehydrogenase (LDH)	80–120 Wacker units 48–115 IU/l 150–450 Wroblerskin units	Increased in muscle dystrophy, damage to skeletal muscles (0–14 days postinjury), after a pulmonary embolism, and during skeletal muscle malignancy
Phosphorus (P)	3.0–4.5 mg/dl 1.8–2.6 mEq/l	Increased in fracture healing, osteoporosis, and hypoparathyroidism
Serum glutamic oxaloacetic transaminase (SGOT)	8–20 units/l 5–40 Karmen units	Increased in skeletal muscle damage and muscular dystrophy
Serum glutamic pyruvic transaminase (SGPT)	5–40 Karmen units	Increased in skeletal muscle damage
Uric acid	2.3–6.0 mg/dl in women 4.3 mg–8.0 mg/dl in men	Increased in gout, multiple myeloma, arthritis, and hyperparathyroidism Decreased in acromegaly
Creatine	0–40 mg/24 hours in men 0–100 mg/24 hours in women	Increased in active rheumatoid arthritis and skeletal muscle damage
C-Reactive protein	Negative	Positive in any acute inflammatory change or necrosis, widespread metastasis, and rheumatoid arthritis
Antinuclear antibodies (ANA)	Negative	Positive in rheumatoid arthritis
Human lymphocyte and antigen B27 (HLA-27)	Negative	Positive in ankylosinspondylitis and rheumatoid arthritis
Lupus erythematosis cell preparation (LE prep)	Negative	Positive in rheumatoid arthritis
Serum rheumatoid (RF)	Negative	Positive (titers in the factor 1:100 to 1:150 range) in rheumatoid arthritis and some chronic inflammatory diseases
Urine		
Calcium	1+ to 2+ 275 mg/24 hours in men 250 mg/24 hours in women	Increased in hyperparathyroidism, osteolytic bone disease, and osteoporosis Decreased in hypoparathyroidism and osteomalacia

References

Bates B. (1995). *A guide to physical examination and history taking* (6th ed.). Philadelphia: J. B. Lippincott.

Greenberger, N. J., Hinthorn, D. R. (1993). *History taking and physical examination.* St. Louis: Mosby Year Book.

Hoppenfeld, S. (1976). *Physical examination of the spine and extremities.* New York: Appleton-Century-Crofts.

Maher, A. B. (1998). Assessment of the musculoskeletal system. In A. B. Maher, S. W. Salmond, & T. A. Pellino (Eds.), *Orthopaedic nursing* (2nd ed., pp. 168–189). Philadelphia: W. B. Saunders.

Malasanos, L., Barkauskas, V., Moss, M., & Allen, K. S. (1990). *Health assessment.* St. Louis: Mosby.

Moye, C. E. (1998). Diagnostic modalities for orthopaedic disorders. In A. B. Maher, S. W. Salmond, & T. A. Pellino

(Eds.), *Orthopaedic nursing* (pp. 190–211). Philadelphia: W. B. Saunders.

Meinhart, N. T. & McCaffery, M. (1983). Pain: A nursing approach to assessment and analysis. Norwalk, Conn: Appleton-Century-Crafts.

Salmond, S. W., Mooney, N. E., & Verdisco, L. A. (1996). *NAON core curriculum for orthopaedic nursing.* Pitman, NJ: National Association of Orthopaedic Nurses.

Seidel, H. M., Ball, J. W., Dains, J. E., & Benedict, G. W. (1998). *Mosby's guide to physical examination* (3rd ed.). St. Louis: Mosby Year Book.

Sims, L. K., S'Amico, D., Stiesmeyer, J. K., & Webster, J. A. (1995). *Health assessment in nursing.* Redwood, CA: Addison-Wesley.

Chapter

3

Musculoskeletal Pathology

A brief overview of the major pathological conditions affecting the musculoskeletal system is presented in this chapter. These conditions include arthritis; osteoporosis; infections due to tuberculosis, osteomyelitis, and other causes; neoplasms; and other orthopaedic abnormalities such as osteomalacia and Paget's disease. In contrast to the later anatomical chapters, this chapter gives a broader view of each condition and how it affects the entire body. General symptomatology, diagnostic tests, treatment methods, and complications are discussed, but neither a nursing process nor a clinical pathway is presented. After an overview, arthritis (rheumatoid arthritis and osteoarthritis) and infections (tuberculosis and osteomyelitis) are discussed in relation to how the pathology affects specific areas of the body. Neoplasms are first discussed in general and then as malignant and benign lesions.

ARTHRITIS

Arthritis, a singular and nonspecific term, refers to a variety of diseases and conditions. These include, but are not limited to, osteoarthritis, rheumatoid arthritis, lupus, juvenile arthritis, gout, bursitis, rheumatic fever, Lyme arthritis, and carpal tunnel syndrome. Osteoarthritis and rheumatoid arthritis, the two most common forms of arthritis, have the greatest public health implications.

Arthritis and musculoskeletal disorders are the most common chronic conditions in the United States. Arthritis affects more than 42.7 million Americans, or almost one out of every six people, making it one of the most prevalent diseases in the United States (Lawrence, Helmick & Arnett, 1998). Women and certain racial and ethnic groups (e.g., American Indians and Alaska Natives) are particularly at risk. It is not just an "old person's disease"; nearly three out of five people with arthritis are younger than 65 years of age. Arthritis is the leading cause of disability, limiting everyday activities for more than 7 million Americans. It is second only to heart disease as a cause of work disability. In many cases, arthritis deprives individuals of their freedom and independence and disrupts the lives of family members and other caregivers. Severe arthritis can shorten life expectancy.

Disabilities from arthritis result in enormous health care costs for individuals. Edward Yelin, a professor of Medicine and Health Policy at the University of California at San Francisco (Arthritis Foundation, 1999) stated that "arthritis and other rheumatic conditions have an annual economic impact on the nation roughly equivalent to a moderate recession, with an aggregate cost of about 1.1% of the gross national product". Each year, arthritis results in 39 million physician visits and more than half a million hospitalizations. Estimated medical care costs for people with arthritis total $15 billion annually, and total costs (medical care and lost productivity) are estimated at almost $65 billion annually. The impact of arthritis is expected to increase dramatically as the "baby boomers" age. An estimated 60 million Americans, or almost 20% of the population, will be affected by 2020. More than 11 million of these individuals will be disabled as a result of arthritis.

Who gets arthritis and why are two questions that still remain to be answered, although research has made substantial progress. If an individual has a sibling with rheumatoid arthritis, they are 2 to 10 times more likely to develop the disease than someone in the general population. If that sibling is an identical twin, the risk rises to one in three. Researchers have also linked race/ethnicity to the chance of developing musculoskeletal and rheumatic diseases. Links between racial groups and several arthritis-related conditions that have been firmly established are (1) Asian American women have an increased risk of developing osteoporosis, a disease marked by fragile bones; (2) African Americans are affected more often and more severely with sarcoidosis, an inflammatory disease of the joints, skin, lungs, and eyes; and (3) people of Mediterranean descent, such as Sephardic Jews, Armenians, and Arabs, are more likely to develop Familial Mediterranean Fever (FMF), a rheumatic disease marked by recurrent fever and abdominal pain.

A recent breakthrough answered an important question about one rheumatic disease. In 1998, the FMF gene was identified for the first time. The gene holds the code for making pyrin, a protein that influences the control of inflammation (Dunkin & Reese, 1999). FMF is believed to be the only rheumatic disease with a simple genetic structure. Researchers hope that studying how pyrin works will lead to improved treatments for FMF and perhaps for other inflammatory diseases as well. Although other genetic links are not likely to be as direct, researchers believe that genetics plays some role in most forms of arthritis and related conditions. Even osteoarthritis, the most common form of arthritis, caused largely by wear and tear of joints, has a genetic link in as many as one quarter of the people who have it. The culprit in at least some of those cases is a genetic mutation in type II collagen, a key component of joint cartilage.

The complexity of genetic and environmental factors underlying arthritis makes the identification of specific genes quite difficult. Scientists first discovered in the mid-1970s that rheumatoid arthritis (RA) is associated with a genetic marker called HLA-DR4. *Human leukocyte antigens,* or HLAs, play a role in the body's immune response. The HLA-DR4 can facilitate the development of disease in people with rheumatoid arthritis by causing the immune system to attack one's own body. HLA-DR4's prevalence varies from race to race. It appears in approximately 25% of Caucasians but in less than 10% of African Americans, which might explain why fewer blacks than whites report having rheumatoid arthritis (Dunkin & Reese, 1999). Only a small fraction of individuals with HLA-DR4, no matter their race, will develop rheumatoid arthritis.

Other research includes (1) linking the probability of developing lupus-related kidney disease to genetic makeup, helping to explain why lupus affects three to four times as many Africans as Caucasians; (2) showing that among full-blooded Choctaws, the incidence rate for scleroderma, a condition marked by a tightening of skin and organ tissue and a high mortality rate, is more than 20 times higher than in the general population; and (3) demonstrating the genetic links between ankylosing spondylitis, an inflammatory form of arthritis in which the vertebrae may become fused, and the genetic marker HLA-B27. It appears in about 96% of people diagnosed with the disorder. Eskimos and Native Alaskans carry the HLA-B27 genetic marker almost twice as often as Caucasians, and their rates of the disease are also much higher (Dunkin & Reese, 1999). However, the fact that not all people with that genetic marker actually develop the disease and the fact that a small percentage of the people with the disease do not have the genetic marker suggest that other factors must be present for the disease to develop. In fact, for almost all forms of arthritis and related diseases, scientists believe that factors other than genetics are involved. Environmental or lifestyle factors, such as diet, viral or bacterial infection, injury, smoking, or exposure to chemicals, also play an important role.

RHEUMATOID ARTHRITIS

Rheumatoid arthritis (RA) is a chronic systemic inflammatory disease characterized by recurrent inflammations involving the synovia or linings of joints and leading to destructive changes in the joints. Although any synovial joint can be affected, the small bones of the hands and feet usually are affected first.

RA is the most virulent form of arthritis and affects more than 2 million people in the United States. It afflicts all racial and ethnic groups, and the prevalence is particularly high among several Native American tribes. Women are affected 2 to 3 times more often than men. Although RA can occur at any age and has been diagnosed in children only a few months old, the primary ages of onset are 20 to 40.

In spite of intensive research, the exact etiology of RA is still unknown. Besides the HLA-DR4 discussed earlier, other causes hypothesized are a virus or other microorganism (e.g., mycoplasma) and a metabolic aberration. The condition is seen in families and has a higher concordance rate in identical twins (32%) than in fraternal twins (9%) (Smith & Arnett, 1991).

PATHOLOGY

RA commonly involves the peripheral joints, but it is a systemic disease, attacking connective tissues throughout the body. Degenerative lesions may occur in collagen in the lungs, heart, muscles, blood vessels, pleura, and tendons. Vasculitis may occur in the eyes, nervous system, and skin, producing ischemia and thrombosis. In most patients, the disease follows an intermittent course with periods of remission and exacerbation. Some patients experience a relatively brief period of illness, lasting only a few days or months, and then have their symptoms subside for several months or even years. Periods of remission, which allow normal activity, tend to appear more frequently in the early course of the disease. Occasionally, permanent spontaneous remissions occur. In general, however, the disease becomes more severe over time, with the development of nodules, vasculitis, and high titers of rheumatoid factors. RA usually requires lifelong treatment and, in some instances, surgery.

RA usually develops insidiously, but onset often coincides with disturbances that deplete the patient's physical and emotional reserves (e.g., worry, exposure, overwork, divorce, and acute illness). Initially, RA produces nonspecific symptoms, such as malaise, early afternoon fatigue, vasomotor disturbances, anorexia, weight loss, persistent low-grade fever, enlarged lymph nodes, enlarged spleen, mental depression, vague articular symptoms, and subcutaneous nodules. Then more specific localized articular symptoms develop, such as joint deformities and ocular manifestations. Atrophy of the muscles and the skin around the involved joint ensues. The patient develops flexion contractures from spasms of the flexor muscles around the inflamed joints and atrophy of the antagonistic extensor muscles. Typically, RA initially involves the proximal interphalangeal (PIP), metacarpophalangeal (MCP), and metatarsophalangeal (MTP) joints of the hands and feet. Those symptoms occur bilaterally and symmetrically and may extend to the wrists, knees, elbows, and ankles. The pain produced by RA is variable in intensity and tends to be most persistent upon use of the involved joints. Stiffness

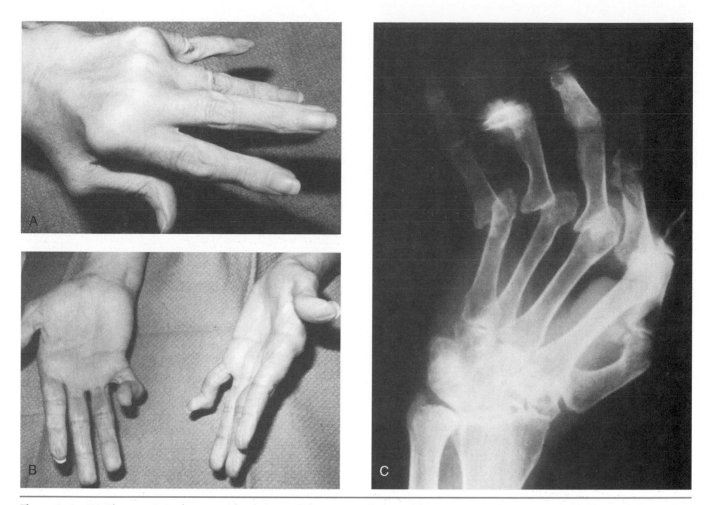

Figure 3–1 (A) Characteristic rheumatoid soft-tissue deformities include prolific synovitis at the wrist and metacarpophalangeal joints, Z-collapse of the thumb, and extensor tendon ruptures to the ring and small fingers. (B) Collapse deformities in rheumatoid arthritis often form a Z-collapse pattern. Note the ulnar shift of the carpal bones, radial deviation of the wrist, intercarpal fusions, and metacarpophalangeal joint subluxations with ulnar drift of the digits. (C) Although rheumatoid changes in the hand are often symmetric, a boutonnière deformity is noted in the right little finger, and a swan-neck deformity in the left little finger. *(Weinstein & Buckwalter (1994).* Turek's Othopaedic: Principles and Their Applications: *Philadelphia: J.B. Lippincott Company.)*

is often the most constant symptom, especially upon rising in the morning. The fingers may assume a spindle shape from marked edema and congestion in the joints. The joints become tender and painful, at first only when the patient moves them, but eventually even at rest. The involved joints often feel hot to the patient, a sign of active disease. Ultimately, joint function is diminished.

If unarrested, the disease process within the joint passes through four main stages: (1) synovitis, (2) pannus formation, (3) fibrous ankylosis, and (4) bony ankylosis. In the stage of synovitis, the involved joint develops a proliferative type of inflammation that is initially localized in the joint capsule, primarily in the synovial membrane. Edema and congestion then thicken the synovial tissue. In the second stage, pannus formation, a layer of granulation develops in the inflamed synovial tissue. The pannus extends over the surface of the articular cartilage into the interior of the joint and adheres tightly to the underlying cartilage of the joint. The rough, granular pannus erodes and destroys the cartilage

of the joint by invasion, lysis, and decreased nutrition. Additional destruction occurs as granulation develops in the subchondral bone. In the third stage, fibrous ankylosis, there is subluxation and distortion of the affected joint as the granulation spreads throughout the joint. The fibrous tissue of the joint is toughened and scarred by the continuing inflammation. The result is a joint with decreased motion due to subluxation and the inhibiting effects of the fibrous tissue. In the fourth stage, bony ankylosis (union) develops as the fibrous tissue becomes calcified and changes into osseous tissue.

Deformities are inevitable if the disease process is allowed to progress. In the hand, the PIP joints can develop flexion or hyperextension deformities. The MCP joints can swell dorsally, and volar subluxation and stretching of tendons can pull the fingers to the ulnar side ("ulnar drift"). The fingers may develop "swan-neck" or "boutonnière" deformity (Fig. 3–1). The hands may appear shortened and the wrists boggy. Carpal tunnel syndrome may develop from synovial pressure on the median nerve, causing tingling paresthesia in the fingers.

A less common complication is degeneration of the odontoid process, a part of the second cervical vertebra. In rare instances, cord compression occurs, particularly in patients with long-standing, deforming RA. Upper motor neuron weakness and a positive Babinski sign occur infrequently. RA can also cause temporomandibular disease, which impairs chewing and causes earaches.

The most common extra-articular symptom is the gradual appearance of rheumatoid subcutaneous nodules. The nodules, which may be present for weeks or months, most commonly develop over bony prominences, especially near the elbow. Vasculitis can lead to skin lesions, leg ulcers, and multiple complications. Peripheral neuropathy may produce numbness, tingling, weakness, and loss of sensation in the feet and hands. Stiff, weak, or painful muscles are common. Other extra-articular effects include pericarditis, pulmonary nodules or fibrosis, pleuritis, scleritis, and behavioral changes (e.g., depression and anxiety). General body reactions to treatment can include renal calculi, cushingoid features from steroids, and gastrointestinal bleeding from salicylates.

DIAGNOSIS

Besides the typical features of RA observed on physical examination, laboratory findings and diagnostic tests (see Chapter 2) are necessary to confirm the diagnosis. Serum protein electrophoresis frequently shows elevated serum globulin. Rheumatoid factors (RF), large antibody-like protein molecules, are found in 75% to 80% of the patients, as indicated by a titer of 1:160 or higher. The erythrocyte sedimentation rate (ESR) is elevated in 85% to 90% of the patients with RA. C-reactive protein indicates the presence of abnormal plasma protein (i.e., glycoprotein) from a trace to 6 mg/ml. C-reactive protein and ESR are both elevated during acute and chronic phases. A complete blood count (CBC) usually shows a moderate anemia and a slight leukocytosis. A hypochromic, normocytic anemia is common. Usually the white blood cell (WBC) count is slightly elevated or normal, though leukopenia may be present (e.g., with splenomegaly). When synovial (joint) fluid is aspirated, abnormalities are found. Roentgenograms show soft-tissue swelling early in the course of the disease. As the disease progresses, roentgenograms can reveal osteoporosis around the involved joint, erosion of the cartilage at the periphery of the joint surface, joint space narrowing due to erosion of cartilage, and bony cysts from the invasion of granulated tissue. After several years, degenerative changes from secondary osteoporosis become apparent.

TREATMENT

As RA is a chronic and potentially crippling disease, it is difficult for a patient to accept. When the diagnosis is presented to the patient, attempts should be made to realistically discuss how the illness will affect the patient's life. Given the variable nature of the disease process, precise forecasts cannot be made, but it should be emphasized that many persons with RA continue to lead active, productive lives and that with early, intensive treatment only slight modifications in life style may be necessary. Arthritis does not need to be a hopeless disease. If treatment is delayed or avoided, however, the condition typically worsens, and patients who cannot or will not accept their limitations and modify their lives accordingly tend to do more poorly than those who are able to adapt.

Treatment goals are the preservation of function, the reduction of pain and inflammation, and the prevention or correction of deformities. Initially, the treatment of RA is usually conservative, employing salicylates, rest, and physical therapy. An important aspect of that treatment is a successful patient education program that teaches the patient about the illness and the best methods for dealing with it. Patients with RA should be alerted to the pitfalls of "quack" cures and should be informed of local assistance efforts, such as those of the Arthritis Foundation, which may be of help.

Medications. In the initial treatment phase of patients with RA, salicylates (e.g., aspirin) have been effective drugs. They have analgesic and anti-inflammatory properties, in addition to being relatively safe and inexpensive. Aspirin is available in plain, enteric-coated, or buffered tablets and as a suppository. Aspirin should be taken with food because of its irritating effects on the stomach.

With the advancement of the disease, additional medications are used and the patient's list of medications may become quite extensive. Besides aspirin, the list may include (1) nonacetylated salicylates such as magnesium salicylate (Magan, 1,500 to 4,000 mg daily in 2 to 4 divided doses), diflunisal (Dolobid, 500 to 1,500 mg daily in 2 divided doses), and meclofenamate sodium (Meclomen, 200 to 400 mg daily in 4 divided doses); (2) nonsteroidal anti-inflammatory drugs (NSAIDs); (3) indoles such as indomethacin (Indocin, 50 to 200 mg daily in 2 to 4 doses), sulindac (Clinoril, 300 to 400 mg daily in 2 divided doses), and tolmetin (Tolectin, 800 to 1,600 mg daily in 4 to 6 divided doses); (4) propionic acid derivatives such as ibuprofen (Motrin, 1,200 to 3,200 mg daily in 3 to 6 doses), naproxen (Naprosyn, 250 to 1,500 mg daily in 2 doses), fenoprofen (Nalfon, 1,200 to 3,200 mg daily in 3 to 4 doses), and ketoprofen (Orudis, 100 to 4,000 mg daily in 3 to 4 doses); (5) oricams such as piroxicam (Feldene, 20 mg daily); (6) pyrazoles such as phenylbutazone (Butazolidin, 200 to 800 mg daily in 1 to 4 doses) and oxyphenbutazone (Tandearil, 400 to 600 mg daily in 2 to 3 divided doses); (7) antimalarials such as hydroxychloroquine (Plaquenil, 200 to 400 mg daily) and chloroquine (Aralen, 20 mg once daily); (8) gold compounds such as gold sodium thiomalate (Myochrysine, dose individualized for the patient and weeks on the drug), aurothioglucose (Solganal, dosage same as Myochrysine), and auranofin (Ridaura, 6 to 9 mg daily in 2 to 3 divided doses); (9) disease-modifying drugs such as penicillamine (Cuprimine and Depen, 250 to 750 mg daily), methotrexate (Rheumatrex 7.5 to 40 mg weekly), and azathioprine (Imuran, 1 to 2.5 mg/kg daily); and (10) corticosteroids such as hydrocortisone (Cortef), prednisolone (Delta-Cortef), and prednisone (Deltasone), all with highly individualized dosages (Holmes, 1998). Since all of these drugs have a high incidence of adverse side effects, it is best to check the insert with the medication, the formulary or pharmacy in the facility, or the *Physician's Desk Reference* for side effects. For example, side effects of NSAIDs and propionic acid derivatives are gastrointestinal irritation, fluid retention and edema, diarrhea, interstitial nephritis, central nervous system changes (dizziness, blurred vision, and headaches), hematologic changes, bone marrow depression, prolonged bleeding time, skin reactions, and rashes.

Over the last couple of years, there have been several new medications and devices approved by the Food and Drug Administration (FDA) for the treatment of rheumatoid arthritis. Two biologic agent drugs are infliximab (Remicade) and etanercept (Enbrel). They inhibit the action of tumor necrosis factor (TNF), a chemical believed to play an important role in driving the process of inflammation and tissue damage in RA. Remicade is administered intravenously by a health care professional in a 2-hour outpatient procedure with the dosage based on the patient's weight. Remicade will be given along with methotrexate. Enbrel, 25 mg, is administered twice weekly by subcutaneous injections and is sold in prefilled syringes that patients can administer themselves; the cost is approximately $1,300 per month. A third drug, leflunomide (Arava, 10-, 20-, or 100-mg tablets), is a disease-modifying antirheumatic drug that affects the function of immune cells called T lymphocytes. Leflunomide is administered orally once a day and costs $8 per pill. Two other drugs that are COX-2 inhibitors, a subcategory of NSAIDs, are celecoxib (Celebrex) and Vioxx (5-, 12.5-, 25-, or 50-mg doses).

Rest. Rest for a patient with RA should include complete physical and emotional rest, not just rest of the involved joints. The amount of systemic rest needed depends on the stage of the disease and the number of joints involved. With mild RA, 2 to 4 hours of rest daily (in addition to the normal 8 to 10 hours of rest at night) is usually adequate. That amount of rest may be reduced as the patient's condition improves. For rest to be effective, the bed needs to be firm and the patient should lie in correct body alignment to prevent flexion or extension deformities. Sandbags, splints, footboards, pillows, and other supportive devices may be used to maintain correct body alignment.

Physical Therapy. Physical therapy helps to (1) prevent and correct deformities, (2) control pain, and (3) strengthen weakened muscles and improve joint function. Physical therapy helps to prevent or correct deformities by

teaching positioning and an active exercise program and, sometimes, by splinting and casting. Pain control is accomplished by teaching the patient methods of regulating activities so as to minimize pain. Strengthening of weakened muscles is accomplished by isometric exercises. Improved joint function can be obtained by identifying patient needs and teaching patients more effective methods of daily living. A variety of self-help appliances are also available to help the patient maintain a high level of independence.

Other treatment modalities are hot and cold applications. Heat has an analgesic effect and helps to relax muscles. Heat may also relieve joint stiffness and swelling. After heat, exercises can usually be performed more effectively. Various forms of heat therapy that can be used are moist heat (whirlpools, Jacuzzis, hot tubs, showers, hot packs, and hot towels), dry heat (electric heating pads, hot water bottles, and infrared heat lamps), diathermy, ultrasound, and paraffin baths. Cold applications (e.g., crushed ice packs) induce a local anesthesia. They are effective during acute episodes.

Advanced stages of the disease may require surgical repair, often including arthroplasties of major joints. Other useful surgical procedures include metatarsal head and distal ulnar resection arthroplasties; insertion of a silastic prosthesis between MCP and PIP joints to free and stabilize them; arthrodesis (joint fusion), usually in the wrists, feet, or spine; synovectomy (removal of a destructive, proliferating synovium), usually in the wrists, knees, and fingers to delay the course of the disease; osteotomy (cutting or excising bone) to realign joint surfaces and redistribute stresses; and tendon transfers to prevent deformities or relieve contractures.

SPECIFIC JOINTS

The following section presents a discussion of different areas of the body, how different joints are affected by RA, and what care and treatment is involved.

Cervical Spine. Patients with RA of the cervical spine typically have a more generalized pattern of RA. Approximately 30% of patients having chronic RA with severe peripheral joint involvement show evidence of cervical spine subluxation (Fig. 3–2) on roentgenography. Often the patient with a cervical spine abnormality does not have associated neurologic symptoms. Only about 5% of patients with significant cervical subluxation have signs of neurologic involvement or spinal cord compression. These abnormal neurologic findings vary from quadriplegia to minimal proprioceptive loss in either the upper or lower extremities.

When RA affects the upper levels of the cervical spine, it usually produces cervical spine fusion in children and cervical spinal subluxation in adults. The most common subluxation is an anterior subluxation of C1 or C2. Patients with a significant C1–C2 subluxation are usually at risk from falls, whiplash injuries, and excessive head movements, especially during anesthesia. When a cervical spine subluxation leads to neurologic involvement or spinal cord compression, treatment

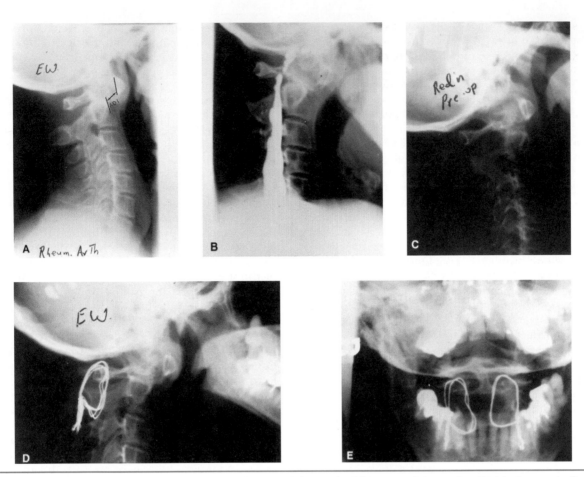

Figure 3–2   (A) C1–C2 instability, adult rheumatoid arthritis with forward subluxation of C1 on C2. (B) Myelogram in flexion, adult rheumatoid arthritis, demonstrating C1–C2 instability. (C) Preoperative reduction in extension, adult rheumatoid arthritis, exhibiting C1–C2 instability. (D) Postoperative Brook-type fusion, C1–C2 with reduction. (E) AP view, C1–C2, Brooks fusion.
(Weinstein & Buckwalter (1994). Turek's Othopaedic: Principles and Their Applications: *Philadelphia: J.B. Lippincott Company.)*

includes the use of a firm cervical support, a halo apparatus (see Chapter 6), or surgical fusion of the subluxed vertebrae (see Chapter 8). Long-term studies of patients with cervical spine subluxation due to RA indicate that 25% will worsen, 25% will improve, and 50% will remain stable.

Hip. Surgery plays an important role in the treatment and rehabilitation of patients with RA of the hip who do not respond adequately to nonoperative measures. Operations on the joints can be effective in preventing some deformities, in relieving pain, and in improving overall function. Many types of operations have proved successful in the past, and new procedures are being developed that promise success in the future. It is no longer necessary to wait until the disease has run its course in the hip if it is believed surgery can help the patient.

For patients with RA, persistent pain unrelieved by conservative methods is the most demanding reason for surgery. Pain during activities can be controlled by the patient through restricting those activities, but pain at rest and at night may convince the patient and the physician of the need for surgical intervention. A second

important indicator is the restriction of movement in the hip.

Over the years, many surgical procedures have been used for RA of the hip, but few have been very successful. A brief description follows (for more information, see Chapter 9):

* *Synovectomy* (removal of the synovial membrane), effective on a number of other joints, was found to be unsuitable for the hip joint.
* *Arthrodesis* (surgical fusion) of the hip was found to be an excellent procedure if the other hip, lumbar spine, and knees work well. Because this is rarely the case, arthrodesis is usually contraindicated.
* The *Girdlestone procedure* (removal of the lip of the acetabulum, the greater trochanter, the neck and head of the femur, and creating a gliding surface between the two bones), originally introduced for tuberculosis of the hip, requires a long convalescence, and active control of the joint is slow to develop. After recovery, passive range of motion is good and pain at rest is relieved, but discomfort persists on activity. More importantly, the hip joint is unstable, and the patient must use

crutches or canes to ambulate, a serious problem for patients with upper extremity RA.

- A *subtrochanteric* or *femoral osteotomy* (cutting a wedge into the femur to allow a change in the position of weight bearing in the joint) does not materially improve the stability of the hip, and the femoral head has been known to collapse after such procedures.

- A *hemiarthroplasty with an Austin-Moore, Bateman, Thompson, or other endoprosthesis* (removal of the head and neck of the femur and replacement with a metallic component with the metallic head the same size as the one removed) is of value only if the acetabulum is healthy; so, for patients with RA, this procedure is not useful because the acetabulum is always involved.

- Some patients who cannot withstand extensive surgery can benefit from an operation that severs the muscles that move the hip joint. This *hanging hip procedure* permits some limited ambulation while providing symptomatic relief.

- The *cup arthroplasty* or *mold arthroplasty* (where the acetabulum is reamed down to untraumatized surface and a metal cup is fitted over the head of the femur), which has been used since 1943, has a long rehabilitative period, with 12 or more months of non- or partial-weight bearing. It is still considered in adolescents or young adults where the disease has not progressed to the stage of severe bone involvement and where symptoms with disability persist despite a full and fair trial of conservative treatment.

- A *total hip arthroplasty* (removing the head and neck of the femur, reaming out the femoral canal and acetabulum, and implanting a polyethylene acetabular cup and a metallic femoral component) has become the surgery of choice for most adult RA patients. For patients considered too young for a total hip replacement, a total joint surface replacement, which involves only the joint surfaces and not the joint itself, is indicated. The joint surface of the femoral head is capped by a metallic shell held in place by methyl methacrylate, and a plastic cup is cemented into the acetabular cavity. The main advantage of this technique is that the femoral head and neck are preserved rather than resected. It allows the retention of adequate bone stock for further reconstructive hip surgery should these implants fail.

Knee. Usually, RA has been clinically evident and diagnosed before the knee joints are involved. Synovial fluid drawn from a knee effusion is turbid with elevated specific gravity, slightly decreased sugar, and increased cellular inclusion. The disease process usually follows a sequence of events in which all of the tissue in and about the joint are involved sequentially. In the first phase, there is usually only soft-tissue involvement. This is primarily synovial hyperemia with joint effusion. The surrounding ligaments and capsule are stretched, swollen, and tender; and roentgenographic evidence reveals only soft-tissue swelling with no articular changes. In the second phase, there is pannus formation and evidence of nonarticular bone destruction, along with the continuation of synovitis. It is during this phase that the synovitis begins to invade the cartilage and the adjacent bone. Roentgenograms become diagnostic in this phase as there is now noticeable bone destruction (erosion) at the margins of the articular cartilage under the collateral ligaments and the appearance of decalcification. The knee-joint space appears to remain intact on the roentgenogram, but, by arthroscopic examination, the presence of pannus and some erosion of cartilage is usually revealed. The third phase involves the beginning of the destruction of the cartilage and the erosion of subchondral bone. The joint space is now narrower, especially on the lateral aspect of the joint, and the knee joint is unstable. Soft-tissue swelling usually lessens by the third phase, because by then the synovial tissue is more fibrotic and less inflamed. The periarticular swelling is firmer and feels thicker on examination. By the fourth phase, there is joint destruction of varying degree with marked destruction of cartilage, which is apparent on the roentgenogram. There is marked joint laxity because of ligamentous involvement that causes subluxation and decreased joint function.

Treatment of a knee afflicted with RA consists of physical methods with prevention of deformity as the goal. Unlike other joints for which complete rest of prolonged duration is valuable, complete rest and immobilization are not appropriate in the knee because flexion contractures, quadriceps atrophy, fibrous adhesions with possible ankylosis, and subluxation are frequent and severe complications of immobility.

The position of flexion must be avoided during periods of exacerbation. Unfortunately, flexion is the position most comfortable to the patient, because it is promoted by both muscle spasms and joint capsule inflammation. Pillows under the knee during bed rest are not permitted. Posterior mold splints are sometimes used both to protect the extended knee and to help with comfort measures. The leg must be exercised periodically while in the splints. To do range-of-motion exercises to the knee, assist the patient in removing the leg from the splint and in doing gentle active and passive flexion and extension of the knee several times daily. This simple routine helps to prevent intra-articular fibrosis and capsular contractures. Heat or ice applications as tolerated by the patient can also be included in the exercise routine.

The quadriceps are to be exercised frequently. The exercises best tolerated during periods of exacerbation are the quadriceps-setting and straight leg raises, either while in the splint or during periods when the splint is removed. A gradual increase in quadriceps activity to active resistive exercises should be done as tolerated. Weight bearing is to be avoided except with the aid of crutches or a walker and usually is not advisable if any flexion contracture exists. In general, the use of a brace to immobilize the extended knee is discouraged because it adds to further atrophy and dependence.

With the decrease of inflammation and associated spasm and painful joint motion, active exercises should be instituted. Once resistive exercises are initiated, they should be carefully supervised and done frequently during the day with both the time and amount of exercise gradually increased. A patient's fear and low threshold of pain are strong factors that delay progress in rehabilitation efforts. Fear that pain means aggravation of the disease should be allayed and realistic encouragement given. Some patients may require surgical treatment to relieve pain, correct deformity, or restore joint motion. The choice of surgical treatment depends upon the individual patient, the patient's physician, and the aims for the surgery. The surgical alternatives are a synovectomy, a total knee arthroplasty, or an arthrodesis (see Chapter 10).

Ankle and Foot. The ankle is a joint with a sizable synovium that can become inflamed. With RA, the synovitis may also injure the adjacent ligaments so that the ankle joint slips or subluxes, the ligaments are strained, and pain and instability result. Walking on an unstable ankle increases trauma to the joint, but if the ankle is stabilized, walking is to be encouraged to prevent stiffness. Unless the ankle is carefully supported by splints during the acute stage of RA of the ankle, an equinus deformity can develop and rapidly become fixed. An equinus deformity of long duration is corrected by lengthening the tendo calcaneus and dividing the posterior capsule. If the joint is ankylosed, an osteotomy is made to realign the foot, the tendo calcaneus is lengthened if necessary, and the ankle is then fused.

The development of a stiff, flat foot and a valgus heel deformity produce symptoms in patients with RA. Painful RA of the ankle can be relieved by a period of nonweight bearing and local steroid injections. A painful ankle may also be helped by wearing supportive ankle boots or ankle braces rather than regular shoes. Crutches or a cane are often a help during a period of exacerbation, as they take weight off a painful ankle.

Ankle fusion for severe RA has been a satisfactory procedure. However, careful evaluation of the ipsilateral subtalar and knee joints should be done before the ankle is fused. When the subtalar joint is involved, using the ankle joint can concentrate the stresses on that joint and cause considerable pain. In such a situation, a total ankle arthroplasty may be indicated. For RA of the talar joint for which surgical treatment is necessary, a triple arthrodesis (see Chapter 11) is usually the procedure of choice, but the functional status of the ankle joint influences the decision.

Rheumatoid tenosynovitis about the ankle and the subtalar joint may be symptomatic and disabling. Excision of diseased sheaths or of an exostosis associated with the tibialis posterior or peroneal tendons can often relieve symptoms sufficiently to avoid an ankle fusion.

Forefoot and Toes. RA frequently affects the forefoot and leads to the development of stiff, painful feet. With RA, there is inflammation and subluxation of the metatarsophalangeal (MTP) joints. Typically, the forefoot broadens and the metatarsal heads are depressed into the sole of the foot. The subluxation is upward, producing a clawing of the toes. The skin under the subluxed joints becomes thickened to form calluses, producing a sensation that has been compared to walking on marbles. The arthritis may also affect the ankle joint, producing pain and decreased movement, especially when walking. The subtalar and tarsal joints may become involved, causing a stiff, flat foot with a valgus heel deformity.

The problem of MTP subluxation and callus formation can be dealt with in a number of ways. Simple paring of the callus can reduce discomfort, but that has to be repeated. Wearing pads that lie just behind the MTP heads takes some of the weight off the MTP joints. Attaching a transverse metatarsal bar to the patient's shoe can serve the same purpose. Another nonsurgical approach is to provide surgical shoes, which are designed to fit the sole of the patient's foot so that body weight is well distributed and every part of the foot is well supported.

In many patients, Fowler's operation, where the painful MTP joints (or the metatarsal heads) are excised, may be necessary to allow toes to drop down into a more functional position.

Shoulder. Rheumatoid synovial disease often involves the shoulder joint (Fig. 3–3A and Fig. 3–3B), and, when it does, it almost invariably extends beyond the confines of the joint to the subacromial bursa and the synovial sheath about the bicipital tendon. The main destructive force in RA is an inflamed, proliferating synovium. The four stages in joint destruction are (1) the initial acute synovitis, (2) the stage of synovial proliferation, (3) the fibrous stage, and (4) the final stage of destruction.

In the first stage, there are episodes of acute synovial inflammation associated with effusions of a thin, cellular fluid. Eventually, the subacromial bursa and bicipital synovial sheath become involved in the inflammatory process and are distended with a thin, turbid fluid. The subacromial bursal distention is almost always an extension of an intra-articular synovitis. In the second stage, the inflammation becomes less acute and the synovial tissue proliferates and extends, destroying the joint capsule. In the third stage, the swollen mass of tissue extends into the subacromial bursa and along the bicipital sheath. Slowly, the capsule and surrounding muscles contract and produce an adduction and internal rotation deformity (Fig. 3–4). In the final stage, joint destruction occurs when the proliferated synovium forms a pannus that destroys the articular cartilage and the subchondral bone. The same process invades and destroys the bicipital tendon, which may rupture or become fixed in its groove by peritendinous adhesions. The rotator cuff and capsule are weakened by synovial distention and invasion, which cause them to rub against the coracoacromial arch. The resulting capsular defect provides a direct communication between the subacromial bursa and the glenohumeral

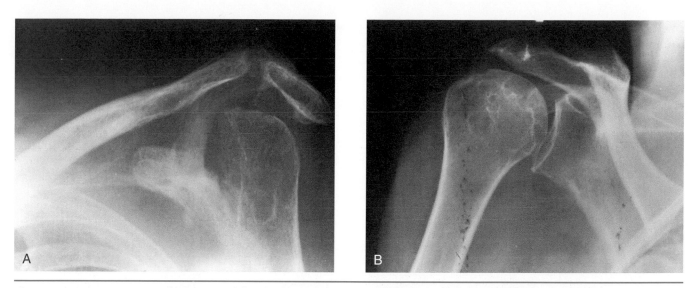

Figure 3–3   (A) More severe destruction of the glenohumeral joint in rheumatoid arthritis. There is marked collapse of the humeral head, medial and central glenoid wear, and a fracture of the acromion. (B) Rheumatoid arthritis of the shoulder with marginal erosion, cystic changes in the humeral head, pathology in the acromioclavicular joint, and reasonable preservation of the glenohumeral joint space.   *(Weinstein & Buckwalter (1994).* Turek's Othopaedic: Principles and Their Applications: *Philadelphia: J.B. Lippincott Company.)*

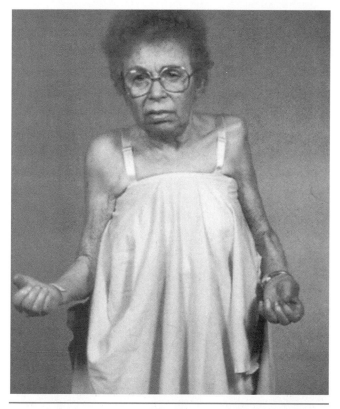

Figure 3–4   A patient with rheumatoid arthritis, bilateral shoulder disease, and bilateral elbow and hand disease. The condition of the muscles (rotator cuff and deltoid) is highly variable in rheumatoid arthritis. With marked weakness of the rotator cuff and deltoid, even though shoulder replacement can eliminate pain, active motion may be limited by the muscle disease.   *(Weinstein & Buckwalter (1994).* Turek's Othopaedic: Principles and Their Applications: *Philadelphia: J.B. Lippincott Company.)*

joint. Disintegration of the glenohumeral articulation and the development of capsular adhesions and contractures permanently restrict shoulder motion.

RA of the shoulder assumes a wide variety of forms. The acute inflammation may be limited to the glenohumeral joint where it almost always starts, or it may appear as an acute subacromial bursitis and/or bicipital tenosynovitis, both of which are almost invariably associated with intra-articular diseases. Recurrent acute inflammatory episodes may be interspersed with symptom-free intervals when the joint may appear normal. The condition may develop insidiously, producing synovial proliferation that appears as persistent, painful, boggy swellings about the shoulder joint, extending along the course of the bicipital tendon. Capsule disease and disintegration are reflected in rotator cuff insufficiency. In about 10% of the cases of advanced disease, a disabling adduction and internal rotation contracture develop.

The aim of treatment is to halt the synovial inflammatory process before it proceeds to destroy the articular surfaces and para-articular structures. If the spread of the synovial disease process is unrelenting and cannot be controlled by conservative means, a synovectomy of the joint and removal of the subacromial bursa and bicipital tenosynovium sometimes stop or greatly retard the disease. However, such surgery needs to be done early in stage two for best results.

Because early diagnosis is not available in most cases, surgery is usually not done until the disease has advanced and involves tendinous structures, causing persistent pain and restricting glenohumeral motion by pain and contractures. In addition to a synovectomy, other surgical procedures are (1) excision of the subacromial bursa, (2) repair of the rotator cuff, (3) capsular release, and (4) resection of the intra-articular position of the biceps tendon. To overcome adduction and internal rotation contractures, the subscapularis tendon is lengthened, the adductors sectioned, and the cora-coacromial ligament and the anterior portion of the acromion are removed. When RA of the shoulder has caused a deterioration of the joint, some function can be restored by a hemiarthroplasty (i.e., the insertion of a prosthesis for the humeral head) or a total shoulder joint replacement. Arthrodesis is rarely indicated because it completely restricts motion and may even encourage further deterioration of other joints of the extremity.

Elbow. RA of the elbow develops insidiously, is tenacious and progressive, and often proceeds toward joint destruction (Fig. 3–5) in spite of local and systemic treatment. RA of the elbow is often associated with RA of the shoulder, the wrist, and the hand. As a general rule, other joints are already involved and the diagnosis established before elbow involvement.

Early in the disease process, the elbow is painful and somewhat limited in movement, particularly in the morning and at the extremes of motion. There is minimal diffuse soft-tissue swelling; tenderness about the joint margins; and slight restriction of flexion, extension, and forearm rotation. Later in the disease process, the pain becomes more intense and persistent, movement is voluntarily restricted to guard against provoking pain,

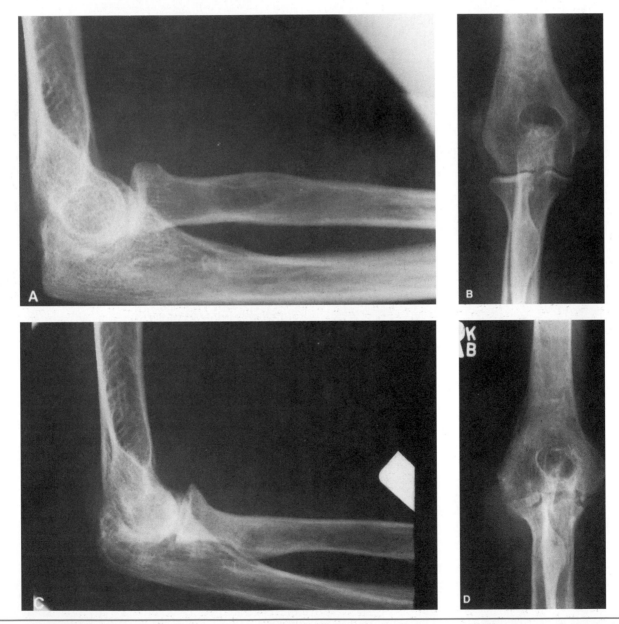

Figure 3–5   Significant rheumatoid destruction in this elbow occurred over a 3-year period. In the initial films (A and B), the joint appears normal except for slight anterior subluxation of the radius on the capitellum. In the later films (C and D), cartilage loss is noted both in the radial capitellar joint and in the ulnar trochlear portions of the joint, along with further deformity of the radial head.   *(Weinstein & Buckwalter (1994). Turek's Othopaedic: Principles and Their Applications: Philadelphia: J.B. Lippincott Company.)*

the soft-tissue swelling about the joint becomes more pronounced, and the joint becomes extremely tender. The joint is warm and usually held in a semiflexed position. Soft-tissue swelling usually develops adjacent to the medial and lateral humeral condyles.

Remissions and exacerbations are the rule. Repeated effusions into the joint occur but gradually lessen as the inflammatory process becomes less intense and the course of the disease more chronic. As destruction and deformity develop, marked grating and crepitus reflect articular disintegration. Motion in flexion, extension, and forearm rotation becomes increasingly limited, and mediolateral instability occurs with destruction of the capsuloligamentous structures. In the latter stages of joint destruction, the muscles of the arm and forearm atrophy. The disease process may involve the capsule at various sites. When it proceeds posteromedially, it may encroach on the ulnar nerve, and, unless that is recognized and the nerve decompressed, permanent nerve damage may ensue.

Subcutaneous rheumatoid nodules that develop over the proximal aspect of the ulna and recurring olecranon bursitis are both characteristic of RA of the elbow. RA causes bursal swelling and distention and a thickening of the bursal wall.

In the elbow joint, the intra-articular destruction may predominantly affect the humeroradial joint or the humeroulnar joint, either of which will interfere with flexion and extension. The synovial extension may invade the radioulnar articulation, and rotation movement of the forearm may become impeded and painful. Pressure may cause the radial head to collapse and the articular fossa of the ulna to become ragged and deeply excavated. Destruction of the capsuloligamentous structures results in subluxations and dislocations. When the annular ligament has been destroyed, the radius is displaced anteriorly by the pull of the biceps, creating a mechanical block to flexion and preventing extension. The tendons, particularly the biceps and the brachialis, become elongated and may even rupture. Despite severe destructive changes (that can be observed on a roentgenogram) and fibrous ankylosis, some degree of motion is usually preserved.

RA of the elbow is but one part of a generalized disease; therefore, the patient will be on a generalized medical regime. Local treatment for the elbow may consist of rest, a splint to prevent deformity, and intra-articular injection of corticosteroids. With advanced disease, reconstructive surgical procedures may be indicated. Possible procedures are a synovectomy, a resection of the radial head, or even the removal of the proximal end of the ulna. For an extensively destroyed and markedly unstable joint, a total joint replacement of the elbow may be done.

Wrist. RA of the wrist is often associated with arthritis of the hands and the fingers. Synovial inflammation and proliferation distend the joint capsule by effusion and destroy the capsuloligamentous structures. All degrees of the disease are seen in the wrist. The inflammation may be acute and recurring and may present effusion and swelling in the joint, in the tendon sheaths, or in both at the same time. At the other extreme, it may be

chronic, progressive, and ultimately destructive to all wrist joint structures and neighboring tendons, with resultant deformity and tendon disintegration.

Clinically, the disease involves the wrist joint and adjacent tendons. At first, there are recurring episodes of swelling, heat, tenderness, limitation of motion, and pain in the wrist. Between these episodes, the wrist may appear normal. Involvement of the adjacent tendons (tenosynovitis) may occur at the same time but may appear unrelated. With advancing rheumatoid disease, swelling, stiffness, and deformity become pronounced and persistent. The wrist usually becomes fixed in flexion. The distal ulna is loose and prominent dorsally. The flexor tendons, digitorum superficialis and digitorum profundis, may rupture, causing loss of extension at the metacarpophalangeal joint of the little, ring, and middle fingers. Less often, there are ruptures of the extensor pollicis longus or the flexor pollicis longus.

The principles of medical treatment are (1) immobilizing the wrist with a removable plaster splint and applying heat to aid in the resorption of inflammatory swelling, (2) exercising the wrist at least twice daily to prevent adhesions, (3) injecting hydrocortisone if swelling persists, and (4) intervening surgically. This surgical intervention may be a synovectomy, an arthrodesis, or an arthroplasty. An early synovectomy helps prevent local destruction of the wrist joint and tendon rupture. However, the proliferative synovium needs to be removed before it can seriously damage cartilage, ligaments, and tendons. After destruction of the wrist joint has occurred, only an arthrodesis or an arthroplasty may be able to restore function.

Hand. Severe RA may cause grotesque and disabling deformities of the hand. RA of the hand principally affects the synovial lining of the joints and the tendon sheaths, and the disease process also invades and destroys ligaments and tendons (Fig. 3–6). The synovial

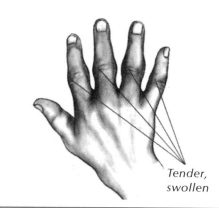

Tender,
swollen

Figure 3–6   Tender, painful, stiff joints characterize rheumatoid arthritis. Symmetrical involvement on both sides of the body is typical. The proximal interphalangeal, metacarpophalangeal, and wrist joints are frequently affected; the distal interphalangeal joints are rarely so. Patients with acute disease often have fusiform or spindle-shaped swelling of the proximal interphalangeal joints.   *(Bates, B. (1995).* A Guide to Physical Examination and History Taking. *6th ed. Philadelphia: J.B. Lippincott Company.)*

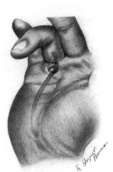

Figure 3–7   A trigger finger is caused by a painless nodule in a flexor tendon in the palm, near the head of the metacarpal. The nodule is too big to enter easily into the tendon sheath when the person tries to extend the fingers from a flexed position. With extra effort or assistance, the finger extends with a palpable and audible snap as the nodule pops through the narrow area. This snap may also be evident during flexion. Watch and listen as the patient flexes and extends the fingers, and feel for both the nodule and the snap.   *(Bates, B. (1995).* A Guide to Physical Examination and History Taking. *6th ed. Philadelphia: J.B. Lippincott Company.)*

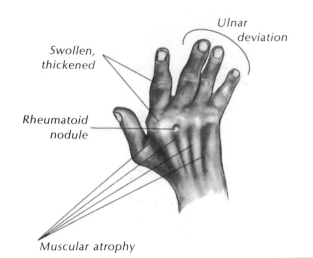

Figure 3–8   As the arthritic process continues and worsens, chronic swelling and thickening of the metacarpophalangeal and proximal interphalangeal joints appear. Range of motion becomes limited, and the fingers may deviate toward the ulnar side. The interosseous muscles atrophy.   *(Bates, B. (1995).* A Guide to Physical Examination and History Taking. *6th ed. Philadelphia: J.B. Lippincott Company.)*

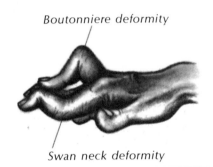

Figure 3–9   The fingers may show *"swan-neck" deformities* (i.e., hyperextension of the proximal interphalangeal joints with fixed flexion of the distal interphalangeal joints). Less common is *boutonnière deformity* (i.e., persistent flexion of the proximal interphalangeal joint with hyperextension of the distal interphalangeal joint).   *(Bates, B. (1995). A Guide to Physical Examination and History Taking. 6th ed. Philadelphia: J.B. Lippincott Company.)*

covering of the flexor tendons in the hands may become inflamed and thickened and obstruct the easy sliding of tendons within the fibrous canal on the volar surface of the fingers, preventing full-finger flexion. The thickening of the synovial lining may be palpable in the hands, and nodular protrusions may develop.

The development of "trigger fingers" may be the earliest evidence of rheumatoid disease (Fig. 3–7). This condition is due to diffuse synovitis of the flexor sheath and thickening of the flexor superficialis tendon where it passes through the canal over the metacarpal heads. Distally within the finger, nodular thickening of the profundis may prevent its gliding through the bifurcation of the superficialis (sublimis).

The disease process may directly invade the tendons, which become frayed, fragile, attenuated, and ruptured. Any tendon may rupture, but rupture is more likely where bony compression and friction occur. Therefore, one of the most commonly ruptured tendons is the extensor pollicis longus. Other finger extensor ruptures are also seen, especially in patients with involvement of the distal radioulnar joint and dorsal dislocation of the ulna. The protruding flexor pollicis longus tendon is the most commonly ruptured tendon among the flexors, and the disruption usually takes place within the carpal tunnel.

RA usually exists in the wrist as well as in the hands. A volar flexion deformity at the wrist increases the tension on the extensors, which pulls the MCP joints into hyperextension. The distal joints in the fingers are flexed secondarily, resulting in a "clawhand" deformity. The ulnar drift (i.e., a deviation of the fingers toward the ulnar side of the hand) tends to develop, which involves a subluxation of the MCP joints and a slipping of the extensor tendons off the top of the joints of the ulnar side (Fig. 3–8). Ulnar deviation does not cause a great loss of function but may be unsightly.

As the disease process in the MCP joints invades and destroys the fascia and collateral ligaments, subluxation occurs because of the unopposed pull of the flexors. Increased tension in the extensors may lead to a buttonhole or boutonnière deformity of the fingers (Fig. 3–9). Flexion and subluxation of a proximal finger joint, followed by hyperextension of the middle joint, produces a swan-neck deformity. The distal joints of the fingers may also develop a flexion deformity due to hyperextension of the middle joint, though it is not particularly disabling. The joints of the thumb may develop subluxation, hyperextension, and flexion deformities. Most commonly, the MCP joint is flexed and subluxed, the interphalangeal joint is hyperextended, and the carpometacarpal joint is subluxed. Joint replacement may be needed to restore function.

OSTEOARTHRITIS

Osteoarthritis (also known as osteoarthrosis, degenerative arthritis, and hypertrophic arthritis) is an idiopathic, slowly progressive, noninflammatory disease of diarthrodial (synovial-lined) joints, characterized by deterioration and erosion of articular cartilage and the formation of new bone, or spurs, at the articular margins. It is a localized disorder with no systemic effects. Osteoarthritis generally occurs later in life and is the most frequent of all forms of arthritis, estimated to afflict well over 40 million people in the United States. Only a small fraction of that number, however, are significantly incapacitated.

Aging is the single most important factor in the development of osteoarthritis, and virtually all persons over the age of 50 have at least a trace of it. However, some older persons have little evidence of the disease, whereas other, relatively young persons may become incapacitated. The precise nature of the aging influences is uncertain, but the condition has generally been attributed to cumulative stress and mechanical trauma. It is twice as prevalent in the obese and mainly affects the weight-bearing joints. In men, a single weight-bearing joint is usually involved, but in obese men the disease often assumes the generalized pattern more typical of women. Osteoarthritis tends to appear earlier and to be more severe in patients with diabetes, ochronosis, and acromegaly, and there are some indications of a familial tendency.

PATHOLOGY

Osteoarthritis may involve one joint or many joints. The hips and knees are particularly susceptible. The spine is a common site, especially in the midcervical, midthoracic, and midlumbar areas, which are the regions of greatest movement in the spine. Osteoarthritis of the first metatarsophalangeal (MTP) joint of the foot and the distal interphalangeal joints of the hand is common. In the hand, osteoarthritis leads to Heberden's nodes in the distal joints and Bouchard's nodes in the proximal joints.

Osteoarthritis principally involves degeneration of cartilage rather than inflammation of the synovia. The first changes are fissuring and irregularity of the articular cartilaginous surfaces, followed by microfractures and the separation of small fragments of cartilage. After the destruction of the articular cartilage, the underlying bone is exposed. That subarticular bone is thickened by compression and new bone formation. The narrow spaces become filled with fibrous tissue and small pieces of cartilage. Some cartilage fragments become ossified and project above the surface of the articular cartilage, usually at the margins, producing the characteristic bony spurs of osteoarthritis. Those spurs are responsible for the "lipping" found in the vertebral body when the spine is affected. The calcific spurs may break off to form free intra-articular foreign bodies known as "joint mice." The capsule and ligaments of the joints often undergo calcification that further limits mobility.

TREATMENT

Osteoarthritis progresses slowly. Even though there is no "cure" for the disorder, effective joint function can usually be maintained. Treatments include the reduction of stress on the joints, medications, physical therapy, orthopaedic appliances, and orthopaedic surgical procedures that may completely relieve the discomforts of osteoarthritis for some patients.

Reduction of Stress. Reducing the stress on affected joints can be accomplished in a number of ways. First, weight reduction in obese patients greatly relieves the strain on affected weight-bearing joints. The involved joint should be rested to reduce compression and shear stress and to allow any synovial inflammation to subside. During an acute inflammatory episode, the patient may be placed on bed rest with the involved joint positioned to relax the capsule and ligamentous structures, thereby minimizing compression of the articular surfaces. In rare instances, traction may be used to separate the joint surfaces and stretch the contracted capsule until the inflammation subsides.

Vertical loads on weight-bearing joints in the legs may be reduced by using assistive devices. A cane can be used in the hand on the uninvolved side to reduce stress. With advanced disease or bilateral joint involvement, the patient may require two canes, crutches, or a walker. The patient will need instruction on the proper gait (Chapter 4).

Medications. There are a number of medications that help to relieve the pain of osteoarthritis. Those drugs are classified as (1) salicylates (e.g., aspirin); (2) nonsalicylates (e.g., Magan and Meclomen); (3) indoles (e.g., Indocin, Clinoril, and Tolectin); (4) propionic acid derivatives (e.g., Motrin, Naprosyn, Nalfon, and Orudis); and (5) pyrazoles (e.g, Butazolidin and Tandearil). Nonsteroidal anti-inflammatory drugs (NSAIDs) are most commonly used. These drugs all have a high incidence of adverse reactions. They are rapidly absorbed in the gastrointestinal tract but frequently cause gastric irritation, so patients need to be instructed to take them with food or antacids. Muscle spasms may be relieved with diazepam (Valium), methocarbamol (Robaxin), or other such antispasmodics. Check the medication inserts, the formulary or pharmacy in the facility, or the *Physician's Desk Reference* for side effects.

Systemic corticosteroid therapy is not usually given for osteoarthritis, but intra-articular injections (e.g., of hydrocortisone acetate) may be helpful in treating inflamed areas in and around large joints. Local injections can be made into the inflamed periarticular sites of tendon insertions, bursae, or joint capsules. The patient needs to be aware that in the beginning there will be increased pain in the joint. Because of the potential for steroid-induced arthropathy to develop in joints due to the injections, some physicians resist injecting a joint, and most limit the number of injections to one or two a year.

Two viscosupplement/hyaluronic acid substitute drugs, sodium hyaluronate (Hyalgan) and hylan G-F 20 (Synvisc) have become available for the treatment of osteoarthritis. They serve as a substitute for natural hyaluronic acid in the joint fluid, as that natural acid loses its effectiveness in people with osteoarthritis. Hyaluronic acid is believed to lubricate the joint and act as a shock absorber. Hyalgan treatment is given in a series of five injections directly into the knee joint(s), one shot per week. Because Hyalgan is a thick substance requiring a large-gauge needle, a local anesthetic is injected beforehand to ease the discomfort. Presently the cost of the five-injection series is over $600, not including the office and physician charges. Synvisc is administered into the knee by three injections, one week apart. Synvisc presently costs over $500, not including physician and office charges. They have not been approved for use in any other joints besides the knee, nor have they been approved for a repeat injection series in the same knee.

Recently, two dietary supplements, glucosamine (500 mg) and chondroitin (250 mg) have become widely available. The drugs may be combined in a single capsule, with the patient taking one to two tablets three times a day. The supplements are extracted from animal tissue. Glucosamine comes from crab, lobster, or shrimp shells; chondroitin sulfate most often comes from cattle tracheae or shark. These dietary supplements are being touted as wonders that will bring relief to individuals with osteoarthritis. As dietary supplements, they are not regulated by the Food and Drug Administration, but in Europe they have been used in humans since the 1980s with no known side effects. Some well-known and respected physicians advocate them for their patients, others say no, while still others remain "on the fence." The jury is still out.

Physical Therapy. Physical therapy is of major importance in the management of osteoarthritis to help relax muscles and relieve aching and stiffness. Physical therapy usually consists of moist heat followed by massage and range-of-motion exercises, both passive and active. Forcible attempts to regain lost range of motion should be avoided, as excessive motion will put too much pressure on the joint surfaces. Isometric rather than isotonic exercises are usually preferred to build muscle power while minimizing joint stress.

Orthopaedic Appliances. A number of orthopaedic appliances may be used to eliminate faulty posture and maintain joint function. Supportive shoes can improve posture. A removable plaster or plastic splint can rest a joint while permitting daily physical therapy. An ordinary elastic bandage applied about an affected joint restricts motion while permitting some use. A simple plastic or fabric corset may provide sufficient support to the lower back, though a brace is a more effective form of immobilization. A long, ischial-weight-bearing caliper brace may be used to reduce stress on the joints of the leg, and a leather cuff about the knee can provide additional support.

Surgical Procedures. Surgical procedures are aimed at the relief of pain, improving and maintaining joint movement, correcting deformity and malalignment, reducing vertical loads and shear stresses, removing intra-articular causes of erosion of articular surfaces, or creating a new joint with artificial implants. Arthrodesis is the only certain way of relieving pain and providing joint stability and should be considered when other forms of surgery are not feasible or have failed. Special surgical considerations are applicable to each joint and are described in later chapters.

SPECIFIC JOINTS

The following section presents a discussion of different areas of the body, how different joints are affected by osteoarthritis, and what care and treatment is involved.

Cervical Spine. Osteoarthritis of the cervical spine involves the simultaneous deterioration of intervertebral disc, vertebral bodies, ligamentous structures, and apophyseal joints. With multiple disc degeneration and a narrowing of multiple disc spaces, hypertrophic bone changes appear in the form of osteophytes or spurs. Those osteophytes form along the margins of the vertebral bodies and are usually more prominent anteriorly than posteriorly. As the narrowing process continues, the apophyseal joints sublux, resulting in additional degeneration of those joints.

The typical patient with osteoarthritis of the cervical spine is past middle age and complains of stiffness and neck pain. The stiffness is worse following periods of immobility of the head and is partially relieved by slow movement of the head and certain sleeping positions (e.g., sleeping with the arms above the head). The pain may be localized in the neck but may also radiate to the head, the anterior chest, the thoracic spine region, and the shoulders. Motions of the cervical spine are restricted by pain and stiffness, and there is usually tenderness over the posterior neck and the trapezius muscles. If the patient complains of pain radiating to the arm or hand, it may be an indication of cervical nerve root compression by bony impingement on adjacent spinal nerve roots. The C4–C5, C5–C6, and C6–C7 interspaces are the most frequently involved.

In most instances, the symptoms caused by osteoarthritis of the cervical spine can be alleviated by nonoperative measures, such as supporting the head in a cervical collar, particularly during periods of sleep, applying moist heat to the neck muscles, and using anti-inflammatory drugs to relieve pain and stiffness. Surgery is rarely required unless the patient develops an intractable cervical radiculitis. Spinal fusion may then be necessary to control chronic neck pain.

Lumbar Spine. The lumbar spine is a common site for osteoarthritis (lumbago) in patients over age 50. In younger patients, osteoarthritis may involve the thoracic or lumbar spine, particularly as a complication of a malalignment of the vertebrae, such as from Scheuermann's disease or scoliosis. Osteoarthritis may affect a number of vertebrae as part of a generalized disease process or be localized to one spinal segment as a result of trauma or repeated stress. Patients may remain pain free for long periods only to have symptoms reappear after a trauma to the back. Osteoarthritis, discogenic degenerative disease, and spondylosis are morbidly and mechanically similar as sequelae to intervertebral disc degeneration.

Characteristically, patients with osteoarthritis of the lumbar spine have stiffness and an ache in the low back area. Stiffness following periods of inactivity is common, particularly first thing in the morning or after long periods of sitting. The sensation of stiffness may be somewhat relieved by activity, but prolonged activity will bring back the pain. Discomfort is usually aggravated by cold, damp weather and is frequently relieved by rest and local heat. Many patients have associated muscular and ligamentous radiation of pain into the buttocks, anterior thigh area, pelvis, and along the tensor fasciae latae to the lateral aspect of the knee. If spurs impinge on the lower spinal nerve roots in the root canals, the patient will have sciatic symptoms of lumbosacral nerve root compression syndrome. A trochanteric bursitis often may be associated with osteoarthritis of the lumbar spine.

Effective relief of pain and stiffness requires treatment of the underlying osteoarthritis. Salicylates and anti-inflammatory drugs are beneficial, though oral steroids have had little positive effect. In addition to medication, conservative treatment includes weight reduction (if indicated), adequate rest, use of local heat, and exercises to maintain muscle tone and joint mobility. Brace and corset use is usually contraindicated, as these patients benefit more if kept flexible. Various physical therapeutic measures such as diathermy and massage may also be helpful. Surgery has a limited role in the treatment of osteoarthritis. However, surgical decompression of a spinal nerve root is occasionally necessary if osteoarthritis spurs impinge on it and cause sciatica (see Chapter 8).

Hip. Osteoarthritis of the hip (Fig. 3–10) produces pain, a limp, limited joint motion, and deformity in the affected leg. Pain is usually felt in the region of the groin and may be referred along the anterior surface of the thigh to the knee, along the lateral aspect of the thigh, or posteriorly to the buttock or low back area. Pain is invariably associated with a sensation of stiffness. In severe hip joint involvement, the affected leg tends to shorten and turn into external rotation. The leg is usually flexed and adducted at the hip joint. A limp may be due to pain, stiffness, shortening of the leg, or disturbance in gluteus medius function. Often, several of these factors operate to produce an abnormal gait in a patient with an externally rotated leg.

The presence of flexion contractures of the hip and limited joint motion are detected by comparing the passive range of motion obtained in both hips, as patients with osteoarthritis of the hip joint usually lose hip joint motion sequentially. The ability to rotate the hip joint

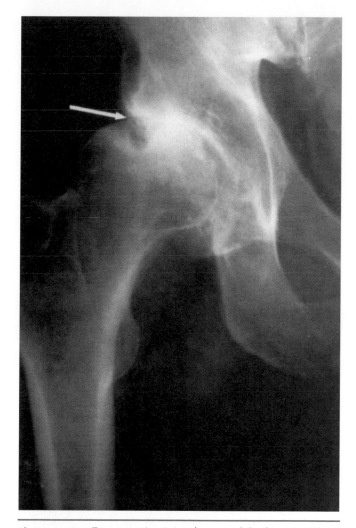

Figure 3–10 Degenerative joint disease of the hip. An AP view of the hip joint illustrates superolateral migration of the femoral head (*arrow*) with asymmetric joint space narrowing. *(Weinstein & Buckwalter (1994). Turek's Othopaedic: Principles and Their Applications: Philadelphia: J.B. Lippincott Company.)*

internally or externally is always lost first. The motions of abduction and adduction are lost next, with hip flexion maintained longest.

Surgical procedures are becoming more important as part of the treatment program for patients with osteoarthritis of the hip. A variety of procedures may be performed to relieve general symptoms, decrease pain, improve function, and correct deformities. For example, an osteotomy of the femoral neck may relieve symptoms by changing the position of the head of the femur when it is being subjected to impact stress against the acetabulum. Persons with advanced joint destruction and intractable pain may benefit from surgical procedures such as arthrodesis or arthroplasty. Arthrodesis sacrifices function of the joint but relieves pain in severely damaged joints. The hanging hip procedure, which permits some limited ambulation while providing symptomatic relief, has been effective in some elderly persons. Arthroplasty (total joint replacement) is used when the destructive process has involved both the acetabulum and the femoral head (see Chapter 9).

Knee. Osteoarthritis involving the knee joint (Fig. 3–11) is a common and frequently progressive disorder seen mainly in middle-aged and older patients. It is characterized by deterioration of the articular cartilage, narrowing of the joint space, and overgrowth of the juxta-articular bone.

The knee, a major weight-bearing joint, is frequently affected. Even though only one knee may be involved, it is not uncommon for osteoarthritis to affect both knees. Quite frequently, osteoarthritis affects one side of a knee joint more severely that the other, resulting in the development of an angular deformity of the knee. Narrowing of the medial side may lead to a varus deformity; narrowing of the lateral side may lead to a valgus deformity of the joint. A long-standing or severe angular deformity may cause knee-joint instability. Osteoarthritis of the knee may also occur as a later complication of an intra-articular fracture of the joint or the removal of a torn meniscus.

Clinical assessment reveals an osteoarthritic knee that causes the patient to complain of pain, grating, and stiff-

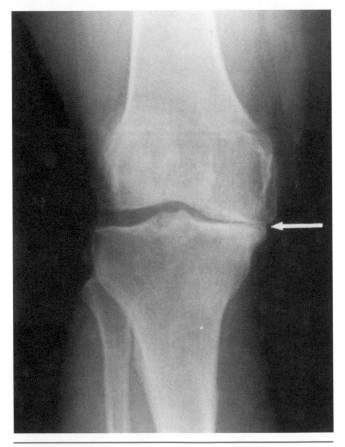

Figure 3–11 Degenerative joint disease of the knee is manifested by asymmetric joint space narrowing. The medial compartment (*arrow*) is affected primarily over the lateral compartment. *(Weinstein & Buckwalter (1994).* Turek's Othopaedic: Principles and Their Applications: *Philadelphia: J.B. Lippincott Company.)*

ness in the joint and, on occasion, a joint deformity with instability. Pain may be referred to the thigh and calf muscles. Synovial effusion in the knee is frequently present, and the patient may complain of a tightness in the back of the joint. The joint outlines may be distorted by the synovial effusion or by thickening of the synovial membrane. Some limitation of joint motion usually occurs, and a flexion contracture may develop. Roentgenographic examination of the knee joint may disclose narrowing of the joint space associated with sclerotic changes in the subchondral bone. Bone spurs may be seen along the joint margins and at the distal end of the patella. Changes may be more marked on one side of the joint than the other, as already discussed. In advanced cases of osteoarthritis, the tibia may appear subluxed on the femur.

Symptoms produced by osteoarthritis in the knee joint frequently may be relieved by the use of intra-articular hydrocortisone, following aspiration of any effusion present. Systemic use of anti-inflammatory drugs is helpful in relieving symptoms of pain and stiffness. Locally applied moist heat, mild support of the joint, and the occasional use of a cane to relieve stress to the joint may also be helpful in relieving symptoms.

Some patients require surgical treatment to relieve pain, correct deformity, or restore joint motion. The choice of surgical treatment depends on the specific findings, the history, the physical and roentgenographic examination, and the intended outcome. The surgical procedure may be a tibial osteotomy, a total knee arthroplasty, or an arthrodesis. See Chapter 10 for a discussion of the procedures.

Ankle and Foot. Osteoarthritis rarely becomes as advanced in the ankle as it does in the hip or the knee unless intensified by an underlying disease process or trauma. Consequently, when advanced osteoarthritic changes develop in the ankle joint, contributory factors are sought in determining an appropriate corrective regime. The main underlying factors could be idiopathic, trauma, infection, other forms of arthritis, neoplasia, deformity, or blood dyscrasia.

Most patients with osteoarthritis of the ankle give a history of sustaining a fracture, fracture-dislocation, or infection of the ankle joint some years previously. Gradually, symptoms typical of osteoarthritis appear, namely pain and stiffness, pronounced at rest and relieved by activity, heat, and salicylates. Swelling in the joints may be due to increased joint fluid (which can be confirmed by aspiration) or may be caused by thickening of the capsular tissues. There is usually moderate generalized tenderness, and joint motion is often restricted. The gait is typically antalgic (see Chapter 2), short and halting, with a painful dorsiflexion just before the toes are lifted off.

Roentgenography demonstrates that the joint space becomes gradually narrowed as the subchondral cortex becomes dense and irregular. Beneath the subchondral cortices, cysts may develop. Marginal bony outgrowths appear, particularly at the anterior tibial border. There may be evidence of an older, malunited fracture; a deformed, dense astragalus suggesting an older avascular necrosis; a punched out gouty lesion; or severe demineralization and erosive defects that suggest an infectious or rheumatoid process. Locally, arthrography may demonstrate intra-articular soft-tissue pathology.

Osteoarthritis of the ankle joint is not necessarily painful and disabling. Intermittent episodes can often be controlled by conservative means, such as rest, no weight bearing, application of heat, and salicylates, but these means are only temporarily effective in most cases. The ankle can be immobilized in a bivalved cast or plaster support or placed in a brace that limits the motion of the ankle. Injections of corticosteroids into the joint space can provide temporary symptomatic relief. Persistence of symptoms, particularly pain severe enough to constitute a continuous disability, is an indication for surgical intervention. The surgery may be (1) debridement and synovectomy to maintain joint motion by removing loose bodies and part of the synovium; (2) denervation of the ankle joint, particularly the distal branches of the posterior tibial nerve and the lateral terminal division of the deep peroneal nerve to relieve pain; (3) arthrodesis or fusion of the ankle joint to eliminate motion and relieve pain; and (4) total ankle replacement (see Chapter 11).

Toes. The joint in the foot that most frequently develops osteoarthritis is the big toe joint (i.e., the first metatarsophalangeal [MTP] joint). The condition, which is more common in men, is characterized by spurring (osteophytosis) around the MTP joint, producing a stiff and painful toe known as hallux rigidus. Treatment is by adapting shoes to prevent the bending of the first MTP joint during walking. If that is ineffective, fusion of the joint or Keller's operation may be indicated.

Hallux valgus is associated with the development of osteoarthritis of the first MTP joint together with bunion formation. This deformity is more common in women and is aggravated by wearing shoes with high heels or shoes that do not provide proper support to the forefoot. Pain is common and is usually due to an inflammation of the associated bunion. (For further discussion about hallus valgus, see Chapter 11.)

Shoulder. Osteoarthritis of the shoulder (Fig. 3–12A and Fig. 3–12B) may affect the sternoclavicular joint and give rise to a painful thickening and swelling of the joint. A patient may seek medical attention because of a "lump" in the neck area. In the acute stage, the joint may be warm, thickened, and tender. Later, all signs and symptoms may subside, but the thickness and enlargement usually remain. Pain may be relieved by warm applications and by use of oral anti-inflammatory agents. Sometimes, if pain persists, hydrocortisone is injected into the sternoclavicular joint. Surgical treatment is usually not required.

Osteoarthritis in the acromioclavicular (AC) joint is a major cause of shoulder area pain, especially in older patients. The condition is more frequent in men, particularly those who have subjected the joint to repeated trauma from either athletic or occupational demands.

Adduction of the arm across the chest and abduction above the horizontal are motions that cause shoulder pain when the AC joint is involved. Thus, patients frequently experience pain in the affected shoulder when they sleep on that side.

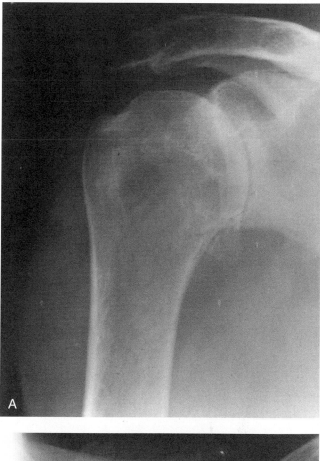

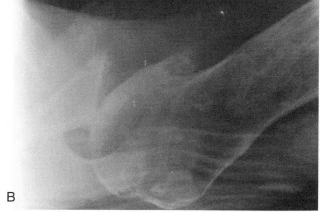

Figure 3–12 (A) Primary osteoarthritis of the shoulder. There is joint space narrowing, sclerosis of the humeral head, and a large inferior osteophyte, which is a classic radiographic finding. The osteophyte is, in fact, circumferential. (B) Axillary radiographic view. There is asymmetric posterior wear of the glenoid fossa with resultant posterior subluxation of the humeral head. This finding is common in primary osteoarthritis of the shoulder.   *(Weinstein & Buckwalter (1994). Turek's Othopaedic: Principles and Their Applications: Philadelphia: J.B. Lippincott Company.)*

In most patients, the joint margins become palpably enlarged and roughened, and visible enlargement of the joint is frequently observed. When direct pressure is applied to the joint, pain is felt by the patient. Often, there is little damage to the joint that can be demonstrated on roentgenographic examination, because the majority of the changes involve the soft tissue and the cartilage components of the joint. The pain due to osteoarthritis of the AC joint usually can be relieved by local heat applications, oral anti-inflammatory drugs, and, in some instances, injection of hydrocortisone into the joint. If the symptoms cannot be controlled by these measures, the distal end of the clavicle may be removed by surgery. This widens the joint and relieves the pain.

Osteoarthritis of the glenohumeral joint can result from wear and tear on the joint or from infection, trauma, fractures, or abnormalities of the joint. As the disease progresses, the articulating cartilage gradually becomes inelastic and develops a pitted, irregular surface. Eventually, those irregularities deepen, ulceration into the bone occurs, and there is spurring around the edge of the joint and destruction of surrounding soft tissues.

Pain is the main symptom, usually in the form of an ache associated with joint motions. Rest may relieve the pain for a short while, but stiffness usually follows. Range of motion is not affected, but the patient may consciously restrict movement to avoid pain. This can lead to muscle, tendon, and soft-tissue shortening. Treatment consists of heat applications, physical therapy, oral anti-inflammatory drugs, and, in some instances, local injection of hydrocortisone. If the symptoms cannot be controlled by these measures, a shoulder arthroplasty may be done. (See Chapter 13 for discussion of shoulder arthroplasty.)

Wrist. Osteoarthritis of the articular surfaces of the distal radioulnar joint usually occurs when the articular cartilage of the joint has been damaged, but the joint surfaces are held tightly opposed by intact ligaments. The damaged articular cartilage may have been produced by trauma, or, rarely, by a generalized degenerative process.

Clinically, there is pain and stiffness at rest, especially after extensive use of the wrist, which is relieved to some extent by heat. Pain is intensified by rotary motions and by extreme supination and pronation. There is usually swelling of soft tissues about the joint, tenderness, limitation of supination and pronation, palpable crepitus with motion, and, occasionally, bony prominences due to spur formation.

Surgical intervention may consist of resecting the distal end of the ulna. If the carpals are affected by degenerative arthritis, radiocarpal arthrodesis may also be required. (For more information on the surgical procedures, see Chapter 12.)

Fingers. The joints most frequently affected by osteoarthritis of the hands (Fig. 3–13) are the distal

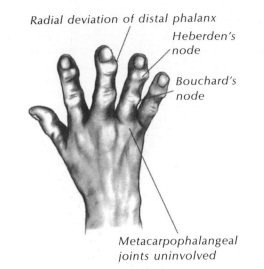

Radial deviation of distal phalanx

Heberden's node

Bouchard's node

Metacarpophalangeal joints uninvolved

Figure 3–13   Nodules on the dorsolateral aspects of the distal interphalangeal joints (*Heberden's nodes*) are due to the bony overgrowth of osteoarthritis. Usually hard and painless, they affect the middle-aged or elderly and often, although not always, are associated with arthritic changes in other joints. Flexion and deviation deformities may develop. Similar nodules on the proximal interphalangeal joints (*Bouchard's nodes*) are less common. The metacarpophalangeal joints are spared.   *(Bates, B. (1995). A Guide to Physical Examination and History Taking. 6th ed. Philadelphia: J.B. Lippincott Company.)*

interphalangeal joints, the proximal interphalangeal joints, and the first carpometacarpal joint (i.e., the base of the thumb). The osteophytes that develop around the finger joints produce characteristic deformities known as Heberden's nodes at the distal interphalangeal joints and Bouchard's nodes at the proximal interphalangeal joints (Fig. 3–14). Those conditions are more common in women, and the onset often coincides with menopause. Osteoarthritis of the hand may or may not be painful. Commonly, there is pain when the nodes appear, and, occasionally, pain may be severe and associated with redness and tenderness. Eventually, the pain subsides leaving a stiffer digit and a somewhat less dexterous but still functioning hand. Osteoarthritis of the first carpometacarpal joint is frequently asymptomatic, though occasionally there is temporary but severe pain.

Treatment consists primarily of anti-inflammatory drugs. In cases of severe pain in the thumb, the first carpometacarpal joint may be splinted to allow the fingers to function. Occasionally, local injections of a steroid into the first carpometacarpal joint produce relief. Paraffin baths are also useful in producing temporary relief from pain in some patients. It is important to reassure patients with osteoarthritis of the hand that they do not have rheumatoid arthritis and will not develop major deformities of the hand. Surgical fusion or removal of one of the carpal bones is occasionally used in difficult cases of osteoarthritis of the first carpometacarpal joint.

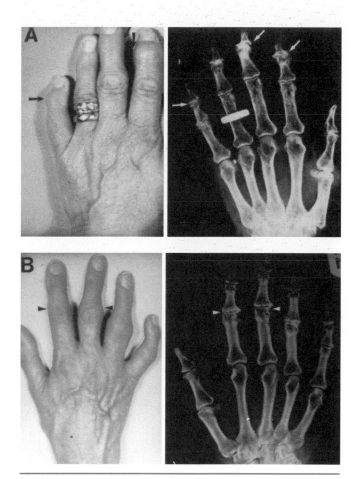

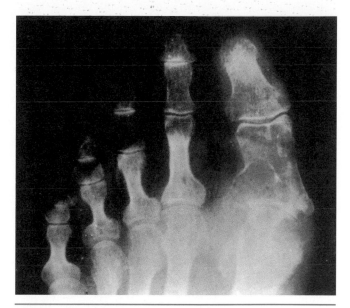

Figure 3–15 Gout. A radiograph of the first metatarsophalangeal joint shows a lytic lesion that destroys the joint space. There is an adjacent soft-tissue tophus, as well as surrounding edema. *(Rubin & Farber (1994). Pathology. 4th ed. Philadelphia: J.B. Lippincott.)*

Figure 3–14 Heberden's and Bouchard's nodes. (A) Enlargement of the distal interphalangeal joint (*arrow*) is termed a *Heberden's node* when caused by osteophytes. (B) A similar deformity at the proximal interphalangeal joint is called a *Bouchard's node* (*arrowhead*). *(Weinstein & Buckwalter (1994). Turek's Othopaedic: Principles and Their Applications: Philadelphia: J.B. Lippincott Company.)*

GOUT (GOUTY ARTHRITIS)

Gout is a hereditary condition of abnormal purine metabolism, which produces urate deposits in articular, periarticular, and subcutaneous tissues that cause painfully arthritic joints. It is characterized by recurring acute attacks, intervals of freedom from pain, and, in the later stages, by crippling, deforming arthritis, nephritis, urinary calculi, and cardiovascular lesions. Gout can affect any joint but tends to involve those in the feet and legs. Primary gout occurs predominately in men over 40 years of age. It rarely occurs in women (about 5%), and when it does the women are usually postmenopausal. Secondary gout occurs in the elderly. Even though gout can lead to chronic disability or incapacitation, prognosis is good with treatment.

Gout can result from (1) overproduction of purine, (2) augmented catabolism of nucleic acids as a result of increased cell turnover, (3) decreased salvage of free purine bases, or (4) decreased excretion of uric acid. Uric acid is the end product of the catabolism of purines and is eliminated from the body in the urine. The level of uric acid in the blood (normally less than 7.0 mg/dl in men and 6.0 mg/dl in women) reflects the difference between the amount of purines ingested and synthesized and the extent of renal excretion. Increased dietary intake of purine-rich foods, particularly meat, in an otherwise normal person does not lead to hyperuricemia and gout.

Gout develops in four stages: (1) asymptomatic hyperuricemia, (2) acute gouty arthritis, (3) intercritical gout, and (4) chronic tophaceous gout (Schiller, 1994, p. 1337). In asymptomatic gout, serum urate levels rise but produce no symptoms. The first acute "attack" of gout usually occurs suddenly and peaks quickly. Although it generally involves only one or two joints, it is extremely painful. Affected joints appear hot, tender, inflamed, and dusky red or cyanotic. The MTP joint of the great toe usually becomes inflamed first (Fig. 3–15), but the disease frequently affects the joints of the instep, ankle, heel, knee, and wrist. The patient may develop a low-grade fever. Mild acute episodes often subside quickly but tend to recur at irregular intervals. Severe episodes may persist for days or weeks. As the disease progresses, it may cause hypertension, nephrolithiasis, and severe back pain.

Intercritical periods are the symptom-free intervals between gout attacks. Most patients have a second attack within 6 months to 2 years, but in some the attack is delayed for 5 to 10 years. Subsequent attacks are more common in those who are untreated, and they tend to be longer and more severe than initial attacks. Such attacks are sometimes accompanied by fever. Some attacks are migratory, sequentially affecting various joints and the Achilles tendon and are associated with either subdeltoid or olecranon bursitis.

Swollen

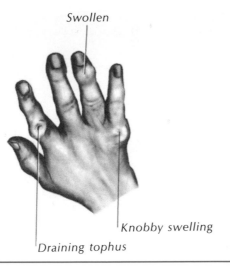

Knobby swelling

Draining tophus

Figure 3–16   The deformities that develop in long-standing chronic tophaceous gout can sometimes mimic those of rheumatoid and osteoarthritis. Joint involvement is usually not so symmetrical as in rheumatoid arthritis. Acute inflammation may be present. Knobby swellings around the joints sometimes ulcerate and discharge white chalk-like urates. *(Bates, B. (1995). A Guide to Physical Examination and History Taking. 6th ed. Philadelphia: J.B. Lippincott Company.)*

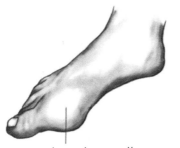

Hot, red, tender, swollen

Figure 3–17   The metatarsophalangeal joint of the great toe may be the first joint involved in acute gouty arthritis. It is characterized by a very painful and tender, hot, dusky red swelling that extends beyond the margin of the joint. It is easily mistaken for a cellulitis. Acute gout may also involve the dorsum of the foot.   *(Bates, B. (1995). A Guide to Physical Examination and History Taking. 6th ed. Philadelphia: J.B. Lippincott Company.)*

Eventually, chronic polyarticular gout develops. That final, unremitting stage of the disease is marked by persistent painful polyarthritis, with large, subcutaneous, tophaceous deposits in cartilage, synovial membranes, tendons, and soft tissue. A tophus is a chalky, cheesy, yellow-white, pasty deposit of monosodium urate crystals. The classic site is the helix of the ear (above the ear lobe), but urate deposits also form in fingers, hands (Fig. 3–16), knees, feet (Fig. 3–17), ulnar sides of the forearms, Achilles tendons, and, rarely, in internal organs such as the kidneys. The skin over the tophus may ulcerate and release a chalky, white exudate or pus. Chronic inflammation and tophaceous deposits cause joint degeneration with eventual deformity and disability. Kidney

involvement, with associated tubular damage, leads to chronic renal dysfunction. Hypertension and albuminuria occur in some patients; urolithiasis is common.

DIAGNOSIS

The main factors in making a diagnosis of gout are family history, repeated attacks with intervals of freedom from pain, renal disturbances such as urate calculus, and hyperuricemia. Urate deposits in or near affected joints, bursae, the helixes of the ears, distal finger joints, Achilles tendons, or elsewhere strongly suggest chronic gout. Aspiration of synovial fluid (arthrocentesis) or of tophaceous material reveals needle-like intracellular crystals of sodium urate. Serum uric acid is above normal; urinary uric acid values are usually higher in secondary gout than in primary gout.

Roentgenograms show clearly defined "punched out" areas of bone lysis. Similar erosions occur in other diseases (including rheumatoid arthritis, degenerative joint disease, and tuberculosis), but only gout manifests outward displacement of the overhanging margin from the bone contour. A positive test for the rheumatoid factor also distinguishes RA from gout.

TREATMENT

The objectives of gout management are (1) relieve acute discomfort by decreasing the severity of acute attacks, (2) prevent the development of chronic gouty arthritis by lowering serum urate levels, (3) prevent future attacks, (4) promote the dissolution of urate deposits, and (5) decrease urinary acidity to prevent stone formation and renal damage. The treatment of gout falls into two categories: acute and long-term management.

During the acute attack, treatment is directed toward relieving pain and inflammation by means of anti-inflammatory drugs. The patient is placed on bed rest and the affected extremity immobilized in a soft pillow splint. An ice pack effectively reduces pain. A bed cradle over the foot of the bed helps to relieve pressure from the bed linen on the affected leg. Occasionally, hot packs may be used. Medications such as colchicine (an analgesic and diuretic), ACTH, phenylbutazone, indomethacin, oxyphenbutazone, most steroidal anti-inflammatory agents, ibuprofen, naproxen, and fenoprofen are used to reduce inflammation. Narcotics or analgesics may be used for severe pain until anti-inflammatory therapy becomes effective. The patient should eat a diet high in carbohydrates and fluids and avoid alcohol. The patient may be allowed to rest in a chair with the affected extremity protected and elevated. Weight bearing is to be avoided until the attack subsides.

Long-term management is to lower serum uric acid levels to the normal range. The therapy involves either inhibiting production of uric acid or increasing the excretion of uric acid. Drugs that result in increased excretion of uric acid are probenecid (Benemid) and sulfinpyrazone (Anturane). The effectiveness of both drugs can be reduced if the patient receives aspirin or other salicylates. Allopurinol (Zyloprim) is a xanthine oxidase inhibitor that reduces the production of uric acid.

INFECTIONS

The following section presents a discussion of extrapulmonary tuberculosis, as it affects the musculoskeletal system, and osteomyelitis.

EXTRAPULMONARY TUBERCULOSIS

Tuberculosis in areas other than the lungs is called extrapulmonary tuberculosis. In the past, tuberculosis was the most common chronic joint disease, and this is still the case in many underdeveloped countries. Tuberculosis of bones and joints is always secondary to a focus of tuberculosis elsewhere in the patient's body. The mycobacteria are spread to the bone hematogenously; only rarely is there direct spread into bone from a lung or lymph node. When the bone infection is caused by the rare bovine type of tubercle bacillus, the initial focus is often the gut or tonsils (Schiller, 1994, p. 1296). For further discussions on primary tuberculosis, see the references at the end of the chapter.

The onset of tuberculosis is usually insidious. The patient has loss of weight and general malaise followed by the gradual development of pain, muscle spasms, restricted movement, and deformity in the affected joint. The classic joint symptom is night pain. There is marked wasting of the muscles adjacent to the joint, substantial limitation of joint movement, and, ultimately, the development of a fixed deformity. To prevent the deformity, it is essential that the diagnosis be made and treatment started at an early stage in the disease process. When tuberculosis of a joint is found on clinical and roentgenographic examination, diagnostic studies must be done to determine the primary focus of the disease. A direct biopsy of the synovial membrane may be done to confirm a diagnosis of joint tuberculosis.

TREATMENT

The treatment of bone and joint tuberculosis involves (1) rest, (2) drug therapy, (3) other forms of disease control, and (4) nutrition. In the early stages, apart from diagnostic measures, surgical procedures are rare, but, if there is a chronic thickening of the synovial membrane, it is usually excised. If there is extensive destruction of the bone and joint cartilage, an arthrodesis of the joint may be done, or, if the joint has assumed a position of fixed deformity, a corrective osteotomy may be necessary. For more details on the treatment and nursing care of tuberculosis of different parts of the skeletal system, see later portions of this chapter.

Rest. In general, the patient is placed on bed rest, particularly in the acute stage of the infection. When it is demonstrated that antituberculin drugs are effective and the patient's condition is improving, limited activity is allowed. The involved joint is placed at rest, usually in a splint, until roentgenographic and clinical examination show that the infection is subsiding and movement can be permitted. If the progress of the infection is

arrested in time and proper immobilization is maintained, the prognosis for restoration of joint function is good.

Drug Therapy. Isoniazid, ethambutol, rifampin, and streptomycin are often referred to as the first-line drugs against tuberculosis. However, other effective drugs are viomycin, capreomycin, kanamycin, ethionamide, pyrazinamide, para-aminosalicylic acid, and cycloserine. Currently there is no medication that can be given in amounts large enough to completely destroy all of the tubercle bacilli in the body. However, persons receiving antituberculosis drug therapy rapidly become noninfectious. Drug therapy for patients with active tuberculosis requires uninterrupted, intensive, and prolonged administration. It may require 2 to 3 years or even longer if the lesions respond slowly.

Other Forms of Disease Control. Tuberculosis can spread through pus produced by bone and joint lesions. Dressings, exudate from sinuses or abscesses, and the debris obtained from the site at the time of surgery must be treated with the same care as any infected dressing. For the protection of the staff, other patients, and the patient's relatives and friends, all patients with tubercular joints are investigated for a possible pulmonary lesion.

Irradiation of the upper room air with ultraviolet light is the most effective method of decontaminating the immediate environment. This procedure can rapidly make room air noninfectious. Good ventilation is important but is usually much slower than ultraviolet light in reducing the concentration of airborne organisms.

Nutrition. Patients with tuberculosis may have had a loss of appetite for some months before the pathology was diagnosed; alternatively, they may have come from an environment where there was insufficient food. Good nutrition is part of the treatment regime and involves a diet high in protein, especially meat, fish, and dairy products. Patients with poor appetites should be encouraged to eat frequent small meals. The patient's fluid intake should be higher than normal because of the drug therapy and the nature of the disease. Fluids facilitate discarding toxins from the infection and prevent stasis and crystal deposits in the tubules of the kidney, which can lead to stone formation.

COMPLICATIONS OF TUBERCULOSIS
OF THE SKELETAL SYSTEM

A common complication of tubercolosis of the skeletal system is the formation of a cold abscess, a painless collection of pus and debris. An abscess may occur at the site of the lesion or may appear some distance away (e.g., in spinal tuberculosis, an abscess may form in the psoas sheath and appear in the groin). Another complication is the formation of a sinus. If an abscess is not surgically aspirated, the phagocytes of the blood create their own channel to the surface of the body. A third complication is Pott's paraplegia, in which tuberculosis of the vertebral column results in the formation of an abscess that impinges upon the cord. A fourth complication is an amyloid disease, the presence of a chronic tubercular body. This disease is associated with vitamin and protein deficiency and is rarely seen today in developed countries. Amyloid disease primarily affects the kidneys, liver, intestines, and (rarely) the peripheral nerves.

SPECIFIC JOINTS

The following section presents a discussion of different areas of the body, how different joints are affected by tuberculosis, and what care and treatment is involved.

Spine (Pott's Disease). Tuberculosis should be considered when there is a spinal infection. A tubercular infection of the spine, by far the most common form of skeletal tuberculosis, is known as Pott's disease. It commonly affects the segment from the tenth thoracic to the first lumbar vertebra, the segment of the spine that possesses the greatest mobility. Although spinal tuberculosis may strike any age group, about half of the patients are between 3 and 5 years of age at the time of onset. In general, spinal infections tend to be more serious than those in the peripheral joints, because the spinal cord may become involved. Pott's disease is more serious in instances where there are tubercular lesions elsewhere in the body; where the primary focus of infection is virulent; where the patient is very old, very young, has AIDS, or is homeless; or where associated debilitating conditions, such as diabetes, nephritis, and anemia are present.

A spinal infection usually begins in the vertebral body along the anterior aspect of the bone. The tuberculous granulomas first produce necrosis of the bone marrow, an effect that leads to slow resorption of bony trabeculae and, occasionally, to cystic spaces in the bone. Thus, because there is little or no reactive bone formation, this bone destruction leads to the collapse of the vertebral body. The collapse of one or more vertebral bodies can lead to compression of the spinal cord at any level from the foramen magnum to the upper lumbar region. It occurs most often in the thoracic spine where the spinal canal is narrow and the cord occupies most of the space, so that even a small abscess or bone sequestrum may produce cord pressure and paraplegia. Spinal cord compression is less likely in the cervical region, as the infected material can follow the fascial plane, or in the lumbar region where it can go along the psoas muscle sheath toward the groin. The intervertebral disc becomes crushed and destroyed by the compression fracture instead of by the invasion of organisms.

If the infection ruptures, the necrotic material is then forced out into the soft tissue anteriorly, forming paravertebral abscesses, and the infection may spread beneath the anterior longitudinal spinal ligament to involve several vertebrae. Pus and necrotic debris drain along the spinal ligaments and form a cold abscess. A psoas abscess forms near the lower lumbar vertebrae and dissects along the pelvis to emerge through the skin of the inguinal region as a draining sinus. Such a process

may occur without any prior symptoms and may be the first manifestation of tuberculous spondylitis. In this case, paraplegia is secondary to vascular insufficiency of the spinal nerves rather than to direct pressure.

The patient with Pott's disease complains of back pain that restricts spinal movement. He or she tends to squat rather than bend to retrieve an object from the floor. Because of the pain, spinal movements are guarded and the patient tends to walk with a protective gait. If there is a marked anterior collapse of several vertebral bodies in the thoracic region, the patient develops a pointed protuberance of the spine called a gibbus. In the days when spinal tuberculosis was common, it was the chief cause of the "hunchback" deformity.

Tuberculous meningitis is the result of a rupture of a tubercular abscess through the dura mater. Before the development of antituberculin drugs, tuberculous meningitis was frequently fatal. Immobilization of the spine by bed rest or spinal brace, coupled with prolonged drug therapy, is usually considered the treatment for spinal tuberculosis. At times, posterior spinal fusion of the involved vertebrae may be required to obtain complete immobilization of the spinal column.

Hip. Tuberculosis of the hip is the second most common form of skeletal tuberculosis, and the majority of patients with tuberculosis of the hip are young children. In most cases, a previous infection in the lung acts as the source, although genitourinary or intrapelvic tuberculosis abscesses can extend directly into the hip or reach it through the lymphatic system. Because there does not have to be a pulmonary focus for tuberculosis to exist in the hip, its diagnosis is sometimes difficult.

When tuberculosis is diagnosed early, before joint destruction, immobilization and chemotherapy may induce healing and preserve joint mobility. Bed rest with traction can then be done to counteract muscle spasm and pain. For irreparable joint destruction, operative fusion for control of infection and relief of pain is necessary. The joint is surgically cleansed of all tubercular tissues and articular cartilage, and the denuded cancellous bone of the femoral head and acetabulum are placed in contact. An iliac bone graft is usually placed between the ilium and the femur to promote osteogenesis. If an abscess or draining skin sinuses are present, some physicians will do an extra-articular fusion, that is, bypass the hip joint and run the iliac graft from the trochanteric area of the femur to the ischium.

Foot and Ankle. As tuberculosis spreads through the blood from a primary source, usually in the lungs, it often lodges simultaneously in various sites throughout the foot. Both the ankle and the foot are almost always simultaneously involved as the disease moves through intercommunicating synovial channels or along soft tissue planes. The first and most common manifestation of infection is a synovitis of the ankle or tarsal joints.

Certain bones appear more predisposed to tuberculosis. In infants, they are the metatarsals; in children, the tarsal bones; and in adults, the ankle bone. In older adults, the talus is the bone most often involved with simultaneous infection of the subtalar and sometimes the talonavicular joint.

The onset of the disease is insidious and may appear as a synovitis of the ankle joint, causing effusion, periarticular soft-tissue swelling, limitation of ankle motion, pain, limpness, local warmth, and tenderness. Characteristically, the soft-tissue swelling is doughy, only slightly tender, and barely warm. It tends to subside at rest and reappears with walking. Eventually, the swelling becomes persistent, pain increases in intensity, and ankle motion becomes progressively restricted. As the subastragalar joint becomes increasingly involved, pain occurs with each step at heelstrike. The pain is situated in the hindfoot and the peroneal areas and can be reproduced by passive side-to-side movement of the heel. The swelling extends about the dorsolateral aspect of the tarsal area, and the infection extends toward the tarsometatarsal joint. One can reproduce the pain and demonstrate involvement of the distal joint by torsion (i.e., twisting the forefoot while the heel is held immobilized). More often the presence of tuberculosis is discovered on roentgenograms.

Antituberculosis drug regime is instituted even if surgery is indicated and may be started several months before surgery. To immobilize the ankle, a cast is applied from the upper thigh to the toes with the ankle at 10 degrees of equinus so that a functional position is attained in the event that fusion takes place as healing occurs. When drug therapy and immobilization are instituted early, these nonoperative treatments produce an apparent "cure" in 90% of the patients, and many will regain normal function.

The objectives of surgery for tuberculosis of the ankle area are to remove grossly diseased tissue, to improve the effectiveness of antituberculosis drugs, and, if possible, to prevent involvement of adjacent joints, thereby preserving motion. A highly variable degree of involvement and distribution of infective foci requires a wide variety of applicable procedures, including (1) arthrotomy for synovial biopsy, partial synovectomy, and debridement and curettage of the surface lesions; (2) excision of an isolated large-bone lesion, with or without bone grafts; (3) total ostectomy of one or several bones (e.g., astragalectomy, metatarsectomy); (4) arthrodesis; and (5) amputation.

Tuberculosis of the bones of the foot, particularly the calcaneus and the talus, may occur at any age. When several bones of the foot are involved, amputation has been the procedure of choice for adults, because the extensive excisions required usually leave a deformed and worthless extremity. Alternative surgical procedures, which may be used for less extensive infections, are curettage and bone excision.

Shoulder. Tuberculosis of the shoulder is rare. When present, tubercular lesions are usually found in the anatomical neck of the humerus and the glenoid of the scapula. A synovitis develops, and the joint capsule becomes filled with masses of granular tissue. Early in the disease, only osteoporosis is evident, cortical margins are indistinct, and the capsular shadow is expanded and denser than normal. The localized osteolytic lesions and a narrowing of the articular space become apparent when the disease is well advanced.

Muscle weakness, a sensation of heaviness, and pain on motion are the earliest symptoms. Later, the pain becomes severe, and muscle spasms fix the shoulder in adduction. The soft tissue becomes swollen, thickened, and generally tender. Motion in all directions, particularly external rotation and abduction, is restricted. Marked muscle atrophy becomes evident, and the axillary lymph nodes become enlarged.

In the beginning, treatment focuses on conservative measures (i.e., rest and a nutritious diet), drugs, and immobilization by a shoulder spica cast or brace, as a shoulder bony ankylosis will arrest the disease process. The shoulder is placed in a functional position, usually 90 degrees of abduction, 60 degrees of external rotation, and 30 degrees of forward flexion, in the event that ankylosis occurs while the shoulder is immobilized. In some adults, abduction may be limited to 60 to 70 degrees to allow the arm to be brought down to the side.

A surgical procedure that is used to treat tuberculosis of the shoulder is the resection of abnormal tissues and joint arthrodesis. Once the shoulder is fused, a shoulder spica cast is applied, and immobilization is continued until the bony bridging of the joint is demonstrated by roentgenograms. Under rare conditions, shoulder motion may be preserved by the resection of the upper end of the humerus, leaving a movable but weakened shoulder.

Elbow. Osseous tuberculosis of the elbow is relatively uncommon. Like tuberculosis of other bony structures, it may be mild or severe, depending upon the intensity of the disease and the body's response to it. At first there is an acute exudative inflammation that produces a clinical picture of pain, muscle spasm, generalized joint tenderness, swelling that consists of boggy edema of the periarticular tissues, increased synovial effusion, and marked limitation of motion. The infection slowly spreads, destroying the intra-articular tissues, but the body may be able to seal it off by means of a fibrous ankylosis (or rarely, a bony ankylosis). If not, destructive changes continue with the formation of persistent draining sinuses in the bones and loss of all joint motion.

When roentgenograms reveal diffuse osteoporosis and the exudative reaction, conservative treatment by immobilization and antituberculin drugs may be sufficient. Surgical procedures to excise the focus of the disease may be necessary to halt the destructive process. If the infection has spread to the coronoid process or joint destruction has been extensive, an arthrodesis may be required.

After an arthrodesis, the position of immobilization depends upon the functional needs of the patient. Ankylosis in a position of approximately 120 degrees presents the best cosmetic result. One can type, reach into a back pocket, and have the arm and hand naturally at the side. For eating, however, fusion at not more than a right angle is best.

Wrist. Tuberculosis of the wrist is uncommon. The synovial membrane may be the first to show signs of the disease, or it may first be demonstrated by an osseous lesion in one of the bones of the wrist joint, usually the lower end of the radius. There may be pain, swelling, local heat and tenderness, limitation of movement, and deformity. The wrist is usually held in palmar flexion. Abscesses are usually superficial and quickly break down and form sinuses. Roentgenographic examination demonstrates generalized osteoporosis or the presence of an osseous focus of infection.

Treatment begins with the generalized treatment for tuberculosis. Local treatment for tuberculosis of the wrist includes immobilization in a cast from the metacarpals and the transverse crease of the palm to just below the elbow, or above the elbow when complete immobilization of the wrist is necessary. The wrist is usually held in approximately 30 degrees of dorsiflexion, and, if the thumb is included in the cast, it is held in opposition. Cast immobilization and chemotherapy are continued until the disease is quiescent (inactive).

Most patients require surgery because of the spread of the disease or the bony destruction present. Surgically treated lesions may heal even when other lesions in the body resist generalized treatment. Surgery for tuberculosis of the wrist is usually undertaken when the lesion is at least momentarily quiescent, and the most common procedure is an arthrodesis. After an arthrodesis, the wrist is immobilized in a cast until union is complete. Amputation is indicated in tuberculosis of the wrist when the disease is so extensive that a permanent cure appears impossible.

Hand. Tuberculosis of the hand is more common in children, is usually hematogenous, primarily involves the bony structures, and secondarily involves the joints. The tubercular infection is mainly in the subperiosteum of the bone. It interferes with the blood supply to the distal portion of the bone, causing necrosis. The infection also causes the bone to enlarge at the infection site, shortening it before a bony involucrum (new bony sheath) can develop. The course of the disease is chronic. Cold abscesses form within the bone and may rupture; persistent draining and secondarily infected bone sinuses result. The infected finger joints become ankylosed, and a spindle-shaped distended bone is characteristic.

Treatment consists of curettage of the bone, closure of the wound without drainage, prolonged immobilization of the finger, and the administration of antibiotics and chemotherapeutic agents specific for tuberculosis. The prognosis is good only in children. Obstinate drainage and crippling of the finger justify amputation.

OSTEOMYELITIS

Osteomyelitis is an inflammation of the bone, bone marrow, and surrounding soft tissue caused by pyogenic (pus-producing) bacteria. Despite the common use of antibiotics, osteomyelitis is still a major diagnostic and therapeutic problem. Osteomyelitis is most often

caused by *Staphylococcus aureus*, with hemolytic *Streptococcus* the second most common cause. Other organisms that can cause osteomyelitis are *Escherichia coli*, *Salmonella*, *Neisseria gonorrhea*, *Hemophilus influenzae*, *Proteus*, and *Pseudomonas*. The infection may reach the bone directly (e.g., through an open fracture), through the bloodstream, or from infections in adjacent soft tissues. It can cause bone destruction, mobility limitations, and severe pain and can be an acute or chronic condition.

When the bacteria enter the bone, they multiply and destroy bone cells. In response, the body's macrophages enter to kill the bacteria. The collection of debris and the resulting edema cause a rise in pressure within the rigid bone, and, if the pressure reaches arterial pressure, blood and antibiotics cannot enter. Eventually, the infection extends from the marrow cavity through the cortex of the bone. Pressure elevates the periosteum, destroying the blood vessels and causing bone necrosis. The dead bone tissue (sequestrum) collapses. The body's response is to attempt to protect the infected bone by laying down new bone cells over the sequestrum, forming a new covering called the involucrum. Even though healing appears to take place, the involucrum interferes with normal phagocytosis, acts as a barrier to antibiotics, and thus preserves a chronically infected sequestrum that can produce recurring abscesses through the life of the individual. The course of chronic osteomyelitis is characterized by asymptomatic remissions and exacerbations when pain and inflammation reoccur as the body tries to rid itself of sequestra. Sinus tracts may form between the sequestra and the skin or may lead into an adjacent joint, draining the purulent abscesses into that joint.

Infection by direct penetration is now the most common cause of osteomyelitis in the United States (Rubin & Farber, 1994). Bacteria are introduced directly into the bone by penetrating wounds, fractures, or surgery, with *Staphylococcus aureus* being the most common bacteria associated with surgery without preoperative antibiotics. When preoperative antibiotics are given, *Staphylococcus epidermidis* is usually the cause. However, approximately 25% of the postoperative infections are anaerobic organisms.

Infectious organisms may reach the bone from a focus elsewhere in the body through the bloodstream. The most common sites affected by hematogenous osteomyelitis are the joints of long bones, such as the hip, knee, and ankle. The infections principally affect boys 5 to 15 years of age, but are occasionally seen in older age groups. Drug addicts may develop hematogenous osteomyelitis from infected needles.

CLINICAL MANIFESTATIONS

Local symptoms of acute osteomyelitis are a sudden onset of severe pain in the affected bone, tenderness over the bone, heat, redness, swelling, painful movement, and involuntary restriction of movement. Muscle spasms may occur and cause the patient to hold the extremity in flexion and resist attempts to touch the painful area. General symptoms that often occur with acute severe bone infection are chills, high fever, headache, nausea, diaphoresis, rapid pulse, marked leukocytosis, an elevated erythrocyte sedimentation rate (ESR), and a positive blood culture. Evidence of bone infection may not appear on roentgenograms for at least 2 weeks after onset.

In the chronic phase, an exacerbation is characterized by low-grade fever, pain, and persistent drainage from a sinus. A sinogram (a roentgenogram with dye) may be used to reveal the location of the sinus and the site of the primary infection.

TREATMENT

Early diagnosis is extremely important to prevent chronic osteomyelitis. With early treatment, the chances of effectively controlling acute osteomyelitis are quite good. Once osteomyelitis is suspected, antibiotics (usually a penicillinase-resistant penicillin) are given immediately. After blood cultures are obtained and the causative organism is identified, antibiotics specific to that organism are begun and continued for several weeks. It is important that the specific antibiotic reach the bone before bone necrosis occurs. If treatment is delayed, bone necrosis may develop and prevent the antibiotic from effectively combating the infection. With the patient on bed rest, the infected bone should be immobilized using a cast or traction until evidence of acute infection disappears.

In acute infectious osteomyelitis, if the response to antibiotics is slow and an abscess develops, an incision and drainage (I and D) may be done. If the patient has internal fixation devices for fracture repair or total joint replacement, they may be removed at the time of the I and D. After an I and D, antibiotics may be instilled into the bone cavity daily. Catheters may also be placed in the wound for continuous drip instillation of an antibiotic solution or for irrigation of the wound. A closed irrigation and drainage system with low-pressure suction is frequently used.

If chronic osteomyelitis develops, the wound usually needs to be exposed and all infected dead bone and cartilage carefully removed so permanent healing can take place. This operation, called a sequestrectomy, consists of the removal of the sequestrum and the overlying involucrum. The procedure is followed by continuous wound irrigation with an antibiotic solution. The joints above and below the affected part may be immobilized with a splint to decrease pain and muscle spasm until the wound heals. Hot packs may also be utilized to reduce swelling.

COMPLICATIONS

According to Schiller (1994, pp. 1295–1296), complications of osteomyelitis include the following:

- *Septicemia* is a dissemination of organisms through the bloodstream that may occur secondary to bone infection. However, it is unusual for osteomyelitis to occur secondary to septicemia.

- *Acute bacterial arthritis* is a joint infection that arises as a result of osteomyelitis in children and in adults and represents a medical emergency. As a result of the bacteria, there is a direct digestion of cartilage by inflammatory cells that destroys the articular cartilage of the joint and leads to osteoarthritis. Rapid intervention to prevent this complication is necessary.

- *Pathologic fractures* can result from osteomyelitis. They frequently heal poorly and may require surgical drainage.

- *Squamous cell carcinoma* develops in the bone or in the sinus tract of long-standing chronic osteomyelitis, often years after the initial infection. In such cases, squamous tissue arises from the epithelialization of the sinus tract and eventually undergoes malignant transformation.

- *Amyloidosis* is a systemic disease that is now rare in industrialized countries. In the preantibiotic era, it was a common complication of chronic osteomyelitis, leading to death from cardiac and renal disease.

- *Chronic osteomyelitis* is a chronic infection of bone that may follow acute osteomyelitis. Chronic osteomyelitis, especially that involving an entire bone, is incurable, because necrotic bone or sequestra function as foreign bodies in avascular areas and antibiotics do not reach the bacteria. Chronic osteomyelitis is therefore treated symptomatically with surgery or antibiotics for the duration of the patient's life.

SPECIFIC JOINTS

The following section presents a discussion of different areas of the body, how different joints are affected by osteomyelitis, and what care and treatment is involved.

Vertebral Body. Pyogenic infection of the spine is called vertebral osteomyelitis or pyogenic spondylitis. The infecting organism is *Staphylococcus aureus* 50% or more of the time; in some 20% of cases, it is *Escherichia coli* and other enteric organisms. The organism is usually blood borne to the spine from some primary focus of infection elsewhere in the body, such as a pelvic inflammatory disease or a genitourinary tract infection. The condition rarely develops following spinal surgery or a spinal puncture. The most common predisposing factors are intravenous drug abuse, upper urinary tract infections, urologic procedures, and hematogenous spread of organisms from other sites. Diabetics are especially susceptible.

The intervertebral disc is not a barrier for bacterial osteomyelitis, particularly staphylococcal infection. Infections travel from one vertebra to the next by directly invading and traversing the intervertebral disc. (Some physicians consider the intervertebral disc as the primary source of infection, so called discitis.) In most cases, two adjacent vertebrae and their intervening disc are involved. An abscess may be formed as the result of the infection, and there may be neurologic involvement.

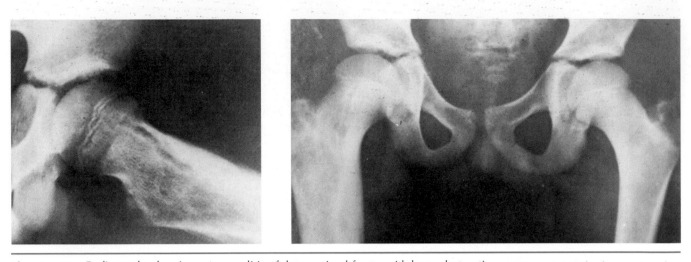

Figure 3–18   Radiographs showing osteomyelitis of the proximal femur with bone destruction.   *(Weinstein & Buckwalter (1994).* Turek's Othopaedic: Principles and Their Applications: *Philadelphia: J.B. Lippincott Company.)*

The onset is insidious, and a chronic infection usually develops. The patient may initially complain of a "non-specific" backache. The pain may or may not be associated with systemic signs of infection. The back pain is usually moderate to severe, with more severe pain at night, and is frequently associated with functional disability. All movement may be painful with marked guarding of the paravertebral and hamstring muscles. The involved vertebrae are usually exquisitely sensitive to percussion. Roentgenography usually shows evidence of bone destruction involving one or more vertebral bodies, accompanied by a narrowing or loss of intervertebral disc space. Diagnostic tests that may be indicated if performed early in the disease process are white blood counts (elevated), sedimentation rates, and blood cultures. Occasionally a paravertebral abscess draining the bone may emerge in the groin or elsewhere.

Before treatment begins, the organism is usually isolated by a biopsy or needle aspiration. Antibiotic treatment is then dependent on sensitivity studies. Bed rest with or without a body cast or brace may be necessary for as long as 3 to 6 months. Fusion occurs in about 50% of the patients. If an abscess forms, surgery may be needed to drain it. Vertebral osteomyelitis may lead to (1) vertebral collapse with paravertebral abcesses; (2) spinal epidural abcesses, with cord compression from the abcess or from displaced fragments of the infected bone; and (3) compression fractures of the vertebral body, leading to neurologic deficit.

Hip. Osteomyelitis is an infection in or around bone (Fig. 3–18). In the hip, it is caused by *Staphylococcus aureus* in 70% to 80% of the cases, but can also be caused by *Streptococcus* and *Pneumococcus*. The condition can be either acute or chronic, though the acute form is rare in adults. The infection is most often blood borne from another infected area, but it can develop directly as a result of an open fracture, a surgical procedure, a puncture, or a gunshot wound. Osteomyelitis can cause the nonunion of fractures, and both the

infection and the nonunion of the fracture may follow an unsuccessful open reduction. In most instances, the infection tends to remain medullary, progressing to cancellous and cortical bone. When the suppurative process reaches the periosteum, erosion occurs and a soft-tissue abscess forms. If the infection invades the bone itself, the bone undergoes necrosis and has a tendency to retain the infection, resulting in retardation of the healing process. The necrotic area can become a potential focal point for reinfection. The sequestrum or necrotic bone can be surgically separated from normal bone, and, following that procedure, new bone begins to form as the body attempts to repair itself. However, some remaining sequestrum may be covered by new bone. Although healing seems to occur, the remaining sequestrum becomes chronically infected and is prone to repeated abscess formation. In the hip joint, this may lead to resecting the joint and the surrounding tissue. Prevention is the most critical factor in eliminating osteomyelitis.

Most adults with osteomyelitis of the hip who are candidates for surgery have had the infection for some time, and medical management with antibiotics, even by the closed-irrigation method, has been ineffective. Those patients have been having pain for some time and may even appear physically debilitated because the pain has caused loss of appetite. They tend to hold the affected leg in a position of hip flexion because it reduces the strain on the hip, and, thus, they may have a hip flexion contracture. They are usually extremely apprehensive, especially of having the affected leg moved. If moving the leg is necessary, handle it gently, securely, and slowly. Another realistic fear the patient has is the uncertainty of the outcome. Their self-image is impaired by the prospect of scars, deformity, and limitation of motion. The most common surgery, the Girdlestone procedure, generally does leave the patient with some degree of limited mobility. At best, recovery and rehabilitation from surgery will be prolonged, difficult for the patient to adjust to, and probably expensive.

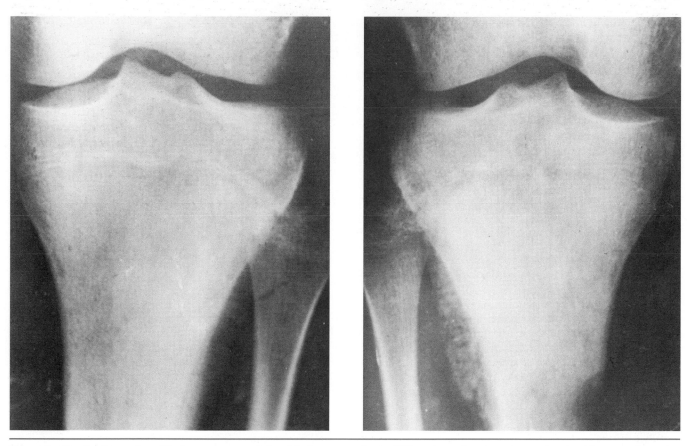

Figure 3–19 Radiographs of Ewing, sarcoma of the tibia in two patients. Diffuse bone involvement and a prominent periosteal reaction can be seen.   *(Weinstein & Buckwalter (1994). Turek's Othopaedic: Principles and Their Applications: Philadelphia: J.B. Lippincott Company.)*

NEOPLASMS

Tumors involving the skeleton are by no means rare and are frequently malignant. Bone neoplasms may occur as primary benign or malignant lesions or as secondary (i.e., metastatic) lesions. The most common benign tumors include osteomas, chondromas, giant-cell tumors (the most common), cysts, and osteoid osteomas. Benign tumors are usually well circumscribed, grow slowly, and seldom spread. Primary malignant bone tumors include osteogenic sarcoma (the most common), Ewing's sarcoma (Fig. 3–19), and multiple myeloma (Fig. 3–20). However, multiple myeloma is considered by some authorities to be a disorder of the blood-forming organs (i.e., bone marrow) rather than a primary bone tumor. In adults, the most common bone tumors are metastatic, with the primary lesion frequently in the breast, lung, prostate, kidney, ovary, or thyroid. Among tumors, carcinomas tend to metastasize to bone more frequently than sarcomas.

Certain bone tumors tend to occur at specific ages. For example, osteogenic sarcomas generally appear below age 25; giant-cell tumors usually occur between the ages of 21 and 35; and multiple myelomas occur more frequently between the ages of 50 and 70. In general, bone tumors interfere with mobility and comfort. The major symptoms are a local swelling or mass, pain,

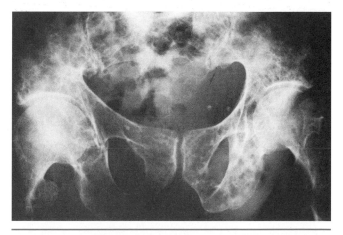

Figure 3–20 Radiograph showing the multiple round bone defects in the pelvis of a patient with multiple myeloma. *(Weinstein & Buckwalter (1994). Turek's Othopaedic: Principles and Their Applications: Philadelphia: J.B. Lippincott Company.)*

restricted motion, aching, and fractures due to the weakening of the bone. In tumors of the lower extremity, the patient may walk with a limp due to pain. The bone pain may range from mild to severe and is frequently described as persistent. Pain usually occurs before the tumor is detectable on roentgenography.

The diagnostic measures for detecting bone tumors are based on personal history, signs and symptoms, roentgenography, and bone biopsies with frozen sections. Once a malignant tumor is suspected, roentgenography such as a radioisotope scanning or computerized axial tomographic scan is done to look for additional lesions. The precise identification of the tumor type is extremely important in determining treatment. Bone tumors are usually treated by either chemotherapy, irradiation, or surgery. Sometimes a combination of treatments is required. Surgical procedures may range from small resections to radical amputations.

BENIGN TUMORS

Benign neoplasms of bone and soft tissue occur more commonly than malignant neoplasms. All of the benign lesions result at least in part from cell proliferation and matrix synthesis that produce new tissue, but their behavior varies considerably. Because of those behavioral differences, they require different treatments. Most osteochondromas and enchondromas should be left untreated (Buckwalter, 1994); but others, like giant cell tumors and osteoblastomas, usually require surgical removal. Some lesions may be capable of metastasizing despite their benign histologic appearance; in particular, rare patients with giant-cell tumors and chondroblastomas have developed lung lesions with the benign histologic appearance of the primary bone neoplasm (Buckwalter, 1994).

HEMANGIOMAS

A hemangioma is an uncommon benign bone tumor composed of vascular channels of varied patterns occurring most often in the skull, the vertebral bodies, and the long bones of patients over age 40. It weakens the structure of the bone, leading to a pathologic fracture. When seen in the spine, the hemangioma usually occurs in two or more contiguous vertebral bodies. The lesion tends to cause symptoms by applying direct pressure on the spinal cord or on spinal nerve roots. Hemangiomas are not believed to undergo malignant transformations, and radiation therapy is usually the treatment of choice.

ANEURSYMAL BONE CYST

An aneurysmal bone cyst is a benign, solitary lesion of bone occurring most often in the metaphysis of long bones, flat bones, and vertebrae (Fig. 3–21). The growth of the lesion causes a ballooning of the overlying cortex, which tends to expand the host bone and destroy the overlying periosteum.

The bone cyst occurs most commonly during the second and third decades of life. The patient's chief complaints are usually pain and a mass. Extensive bleeding may result if the overlying cortical bone shell is broken and a pathologic fracture occurs. Cysts of a vertebral body are usually treated by radiation to sclerose the blood vessels of the tumor.

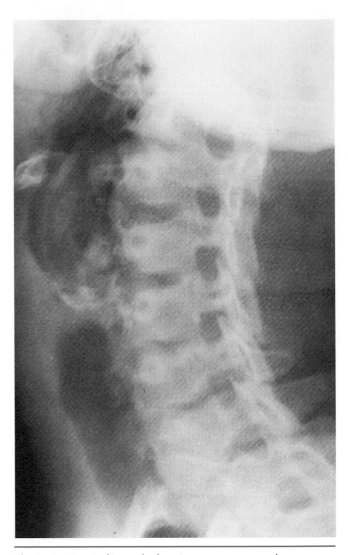

Figure 3–21   Radiograph showing an aneurysma bone cyst of the cervical spine. The aneurysma bone cyst in the body of the C4 vertebra produced an unusually large soft-tissue mass that extends along the anterior aspects of the bodies of C3, C4, and C5.   *(Weinstein & Buckwalter (1994).* Turek's Othopaedic: Principles and Their Applications: *Philadelphia: J.B. Lippincott Company.)*

OSTEOID OSTEOMAS

An osteoid osteoma is a small, rare lesion of the cartilaginous tissue of bones, composed of vascular fibrous tissue, proliferating fibroblasts, and minute formed osteoids. It occurs most frequently in young men 10 to 25 years of age. Osteoid osteoma has a predilection for the diaphyses and metaphyses of the long bones, particularly the tibia and the femur, but the small bones of the hands and the feet are involved in many instances.

There is usually a solitary lesion that causes pain, mild at first but then increasingly severe and continuous, especially at night. There is a localized swelling that gradually becomes palpable as a spindle-shaped bony enlargement. When the lesions involve bone near synovial joints, they can cause joint effusions, muscle spasm, and joint contractures. Complete excision

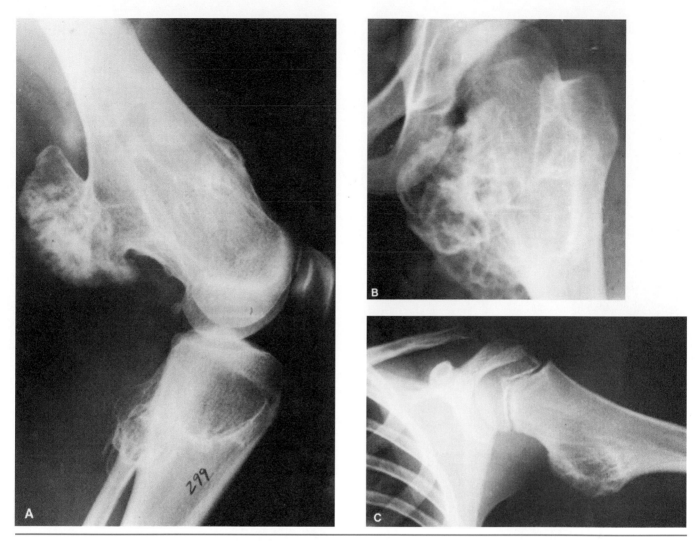

Figure 3–22 Plain radiographs showing typical osteochondromas of long bone metaphyses. The bony bases of the lesions extend directly from normal bone, and the medullary cavity of the normal bone extends into the lesion. Plain radiographs do not show the cartilage portion of an osteochondroma, so the lesions may be much larger than the plain radiographic images. (A) Osteochondromas of the distal femoral and proximal tibial metaphyses. (B) An osteochondroma of the proximal femoral metaphysis. (C) An osteochondroma of the proximal humeral metaphysis. *(Weinstein & Buckwalter (1994).* Turek's Othopaedic: Principles and Their Applications: *Philadelphia: J.B. Lippincott Company.)*

immediately relieves the pain. Amputations are rarely warranted because surrounding sclerotic bone recedes once the center of the tumor is removed.

OSTEOBLASTOMAS

A benign osteoblastoma (or osteogenic fibroma of bone, or giant osteoid osteoma) is an uncommon vascular osteoid and bone-forming tumor. The behavior of osteoblastomas varies from slow enlargement to rapid aggressive growth that resembles the behavior of an osteosarcoma, occasionally causing pathologic fractures.

Young men, usually younger than 20, are predisposed, and the majority of the tumors occur in the spine, in the metaphyseal or diaphyseal areas of the long bones of the lower extremities, and in the small bones of the hands and the feet. The patient usually complains

of a dull, aching pain, not nocturnal and not relieved by aspirin. Symptoms are caused by the encroachment of the tumor on neighboring structures and generally occur from a few months to 2 years before the tumor is diagnosed. Surgical resection or meticulous curettage eradicates most osteoblastomas.

OSTEOCHONDROMAS

The largest group of benign bone tumors are osteochondromas (or osteocartilaginous exostoses), which are composed of spongy bone covered by a cartilaginous cap. Osteochondromas (Fig. 3–22) appear and grow during the individual's growth period, but rarely thereafter. Tumors typically occur in long tubular bones, especially about the knee and ankle, the hip, the shoulder, and the elbow. They are usually located in the bone at the site of tendinous attachments of strong

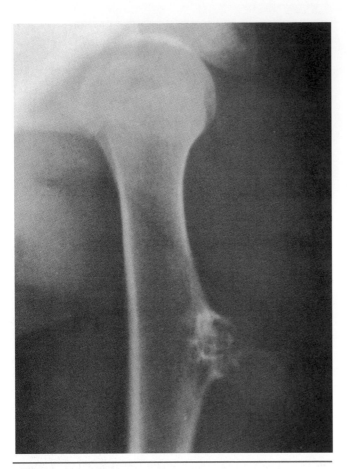

Figure 3–23   Osteochondroma. A radiograph of an osteochondroma of the humerus shows a lesion that is directly contiguous with the marrow space.   *(Rubin & Farber (1994). Pathology. 4th ed. Philadelphia: J.B. Lippincott.)*

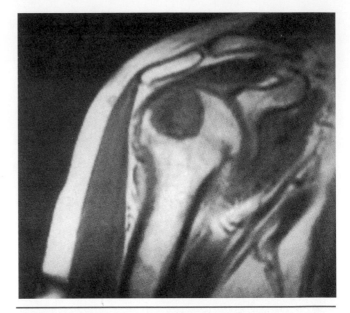

Figure 3–24   Chondroblastoma. A magnetic resonance image of the shoulder of a child shows a prominent lytic lesion of the head of the humerus, which involves the epiphysis and extends across the epiphyseal plate.   *(Rubin & Farber (1994). Pathology. 4th ed. Philadelphia: J.B. Lippincott.)*

muscles (Fig. 3–23). They are solitary or multiple, firm, fixed, asymptomatic bony masses.

Occasionally, osteochondromas fracture through their bony stalk or develop a soft-tissue bursa. Pain for a patient with osteochondroma is usually mild and is due to an overlying bursitis. Enlargement of the osteochondromas may cause nerve compression or skeletal deformity. Surgical removal is indicated if there is interference with joint function, repeated painful bursitis, a fracture of the bone through the tumor, or a suspicion of malignant change. The tumor is not sensitive to radiation.

ENCHONDROMAS

An enchondroma (or chondroma) is a benign hyaline cartilage mass formed in the medullary cavities of otherwise normal bone that causes destruction of the surrounding bone. It is most common in young adults and usually occurs in bones of the hands and feet, but may appear in almost any part of the skeleton, including the large long bones of the limbs, especially the femur, tibia, and humerus. There is usually a single lesion, with only slight soreness. However, some patients may develop multiple enchondromas that can cause severe deformities and stunting of growth. That increases the probability of a

lesion becoming a chondrosarcoma (Ollier's disease). Severe pain can occur suddenly as the result of a pathologic fracture, or slowly from malignant transformation.

Unless they cause pathologic fractures or show signs of malignant transformation, enchondromas generally do not require treatment. However, if treatment is required, it consists of the excision or curettage of the tumor and the cauterization of the tumor cavity. If a large defect develops, bone grafting is necessary. When there is a suspicion that the tumor is malignant, a radical resection is done.

CHONDROBLASTOMAS

A chondroblastoma (Fig. 3–24) is a cellular, vascular, and cartilaginous tumor of young adults, which occurs about the epiphyseal lines of long bones, destroys cancellous bone, and characteristically contains multiple calcium deposits. However, the lesions rarely involve more than half the epiphysis and only occasionally extend into the metaphysis. Chondroblastomas occur most commonly in the proximal humeral epiphysis, but they have occurred in multiple other sites. They typically occur in males between the ages of 10 and 20.

The patient usually gives a history of trauma, pain, tenderness, swelling, and joint effusion. Conservative surgical treatment is usual and consists of curettage and obliteration of the tumor cavity by the use of bone grafts.

GIANT-CELL TUMOR

A giant-cell tumor (Fig. 3–25) is an osteophytic tumor (osteoclastoma) that occurs in young adults after the epiphyseal plate has ossified and longitudinal bone growth is completed, usually between ages 15 and 35.

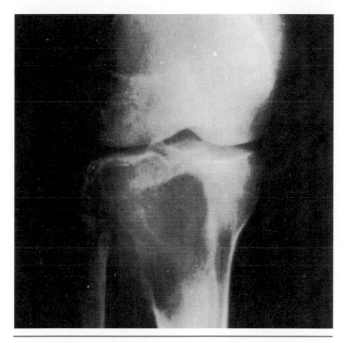

Figure 3–25   Giant-cell tumor of bone. A radiograph of the proximal tibia shows an eccentric lytic lesion with virtually no new bone formation. The tumor extends to the subchondral bone plate and breaks through cortex into the soft tissue. *(Rubin & Farber (1994).* Pathology. *4th ed. Philadelphia: J.B. Lippincott.)*

The most common location is an asymmetric position in the epiphyses of the ends of the long bones, especially the distal femur, proximal tibia, and distal radius (Fig. 3–26). The cause is unknown.

The manifestation of the tumor is chronic, constant pain in the region of the joint. Pain becomes progressively more severe at night and with increased activity. Usually, there is swelling and the overlying skin is stretched. In contrast to osteogenic sarcoma, the skin displays no dilated vessels. Pressure over the swelling produces audible and palpable crackling as the bone cortex is ruptured. Limitation of joint motion is not observed until late in the disease process, as the tumor expands and distorts the end of the bone. A pathologic fracture may also occur at a later stage after a large amount of cancellous and cortical bone is destroyed. The diagnosis is based on the patient's personal history, signs and symptoms, and roentgenograms. Positive roentgenograms show a circumscribed osteolytic growth.

The focus of treatment is to preserve the extremity when possible. The surgical procedure is usually to remove the tumor by curettage and then cauterize the cavity walls or fill the cavity with bone chips. When the tumor is extensive, a resection of the bone is done and the remaining shaft may be arthrodesed to other bones at the joint. An intramedullary pin is sometimes utilized in the arthrodesis. Other methods are cryotherapy after

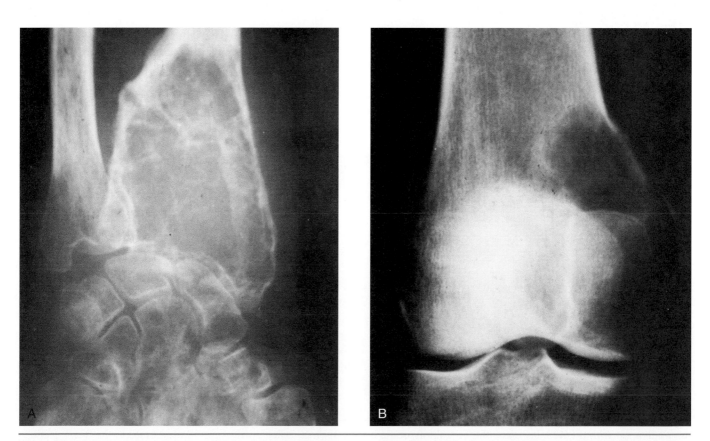

Figure 3–26   Radiographs of giant-cell tumors. (A) A giant-cell tumor of the distal radius that has destroyed bone and expanded the cortex. (B) A giant-cell tumor of the distal femur. Bone destruction and expansion of cortex by the eccentric lesion can be seen. *(Weinstein & Buckwalter (1994).* Turek's Othopaedic: Principles and Their Applications: *Philadelphia: J.B. Lippincott Company.)*

tumor excision, or cryotherapy and filling the cavity with methyl methacrylate bone cement. Depending upon the extent of the tumor and its recurrence, amputation may be indicated.

MALIGNANT TUMORS

Except for plasma cell myeloma, primary malignant bone tumors of the vertebral column are quite rare. More frequently, the spine is the site of metastatic cancer from primary tumors in the breast, prostate, thyroid, kidney, and lungs. Secondary involvement of the vertebral column may also accompany leukemia, Hodgkin's disease, and malignant lymphoma.

CHORDOMA

A chordoma is an uncommon tumor that occurs in bone primarily at either end of the vertebral column. It develops from remnants of embryonic notochord, such as the nucleus pulposus or abnormal "rests" of notochordal tissue, and affects most patients in the middle years of life. More than half of the tumors occur in the sacrococcygeal region. The tumor is slow growing, and is considered malignant because it is locally invasive. Treatment is usually surgical excision.

PRIMARY CHONDROSARCOMA

Primary chondrosarcoma is a virulent, malignant tumor composed of cartilage and myxomatous tissue and occurring subperiosteally, at first without involvement of the cortex of the bone. It is usually found at points where muscles attach to the bone near a joint and where

cartilage formation continues throughout life. The most common areas are the knees, the shoulders, and the pelvis.

Patients are usually 14 to 21 years of age, with pain in the affected area that becomes progressively more severe. The pain is worse at night than during the day. Upon examination, there is swelling at the site. The course of the disease is one of rapid growth of the tumor and severe and persistent pain. A fatal outcome within a year is usual. The tumor is not radiosensitive, so that most radical form of amputation is usually attempted.

SECONDARY CHONDROSARCOMA

Secondary chondrosarcoma is a very slow-growing malignant tumor, occurring as a result of malignant degeneration of an enchondroma or a cartilaginous exostosis. Long bones (Fig. 3–27), especially the proximal end of the humerus (Fig. 3–28), the ribs, and the innominate bone are the usual sites.

The onset is usually in third decade or later in life. The patient usually gives a history of mild, intermittent ache and swelling that suddenly increases in severity. There may be persistent pain, pain at night, and edema due to venous and lymphatic obstruction. Treatment usually consists of amputation, as local removal and irradiation are ineffective.

OSTEOSARCOMA

Osteosarcoma (osteogenic sarcoma) is the most common primary malignant bone tumor. It is a highly malignant, rapidly growing bone tumor characterized by the production of neoplastic osteoid directly from anaplastic,

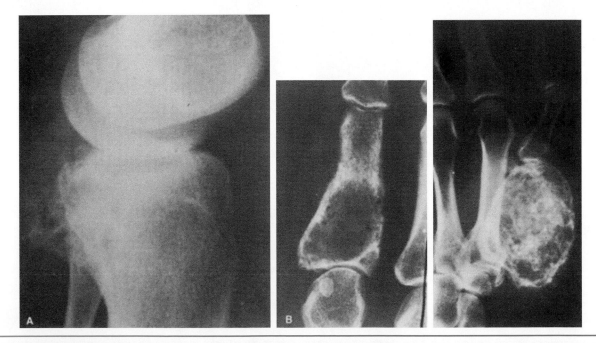

Figure 3–27   Plain radiographs of chondrosarcomas. (A) Plain radiograph of a chondrosarcoma of the proximal tibia. Notice the mineralization with the neoplasm and the irregularity of the bone. (B) Plain radiographs of chondrosarcomas in the hand. (*Left*) Chondrosarcoma of the proximal phalanx. The lesion has destroyed the medullary bone and invaded the cortical bone. (*Right*) A chondrosarcoma of a metacarpal has invaded the soft tissues. *(Weinstein & Buckwalter (1994). Turek's Othopaedic: Principles and Their* Applications: *Philadelphia: J.B. Lippincott Company.)*

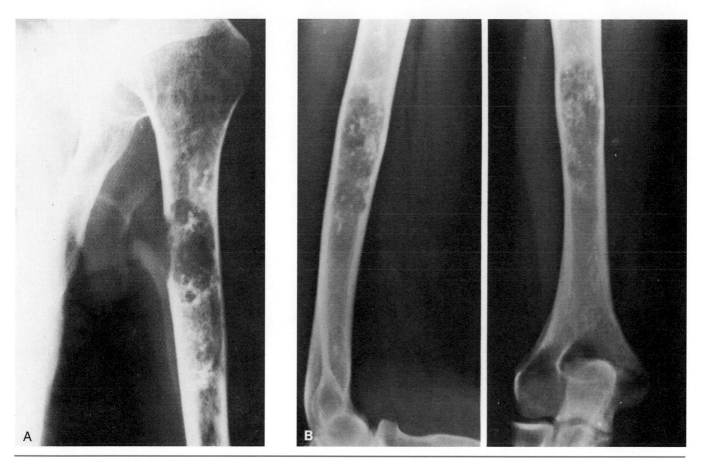

Figure 3–28   Plain radiographs showing central chondrosarcomas. These lesions cause bone destruction and often produce regions of mineralization. (A) A central chondrosarcoma of the humerus showing an irregular area of central bone destruction with mineralization and erosion of the inner bone cortex. (B) Radiographic features include osteolysis, scalloping erosion of inner cortex, central areas of calcification, and no reactive bone formation about the periphery.   *(Weinstein & Buckwalter (1994).* Turek's Othopaedic: Principles and Their Applications: *Philadelphia: J.B. Lippincott Company.)*

osteoblast-like cells. Osteosarcoma is found predominantly in the metaphyseal region of a large long bone, occasionally in the midshaft. It is most common in the distal femur (Fig. 3–29), proximal tibia (Fig. 3–30), and proximal end of the humerus. It is slightly more common for men than for women, and its incidence peaks in the second decade of life (usually between ages 10 and 25). However, it has been known to occur later in life secondary to Paget's disease, and in some instances following osteomyelitis or bone irradiation.

Osteosarcoma is manifested by pain, swelling, limitation of motion, and weight loss. There is intermittent pain at first (usually noted at night), but pain eventually becomes continuous and incapacitating. The bone mass may be palpable and tender, with venous dilation leading to increased skin temperature over the mass. The patient may complain of fatigue. The onset is gradual and spontaneous, but occasionally trauma precipitates symptoms or, infrequently, a pathologic fracture. Osteosarcomas that originate within bone almost always behave aggressively (Buckwalter, 1994). They rapidly destroy normal bone and invade and destroy

soft tissue, and, in approximately 90% of the patients, the osteosarcomas metastasize to the lungs within 2 years (Buckwalter, 1994). Sometimes the metastases extend to other skeletal sites. If untreated, the median time for survival after the onset of pulmonary metastases is 2 to 3 months.

The tumor is visible on roentgenograms, and bone scans and MRIs can be used to demonstrate increased tumor growth. In 50% of patients, there is an elevation in the serum alkaline phosphatase. The primary lesion may involve any bone. The most common sites, however, are the distal femur, the proximal tibia, and the proximal humerus.

The goal of the treatment is to destroy or remove the malignant tissue. The most effective method usually requires a combination of treatments. The surgical removal of the tumor may involve local bone resection, resection and implantation of metallic prostheses or allografts as bone replacement, or amputation. Chemotherapy and high-voltage radiation may also be utilized. Large pulmonary tumors may be surgically resected.

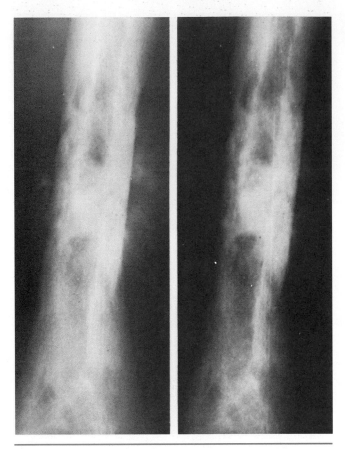

Figure 3–29   Radiograph showing a femoral osteogenic sarcoma in an area of pagetoid bone. The neoplasm has formed new bone and extended outside the bone cortex. *(Weinstein & Buckwalter (1994). Turek's Othopaedic: Principles and Their Applications: Philadelphia: J.B. Lippincott Company.)*

OTHER PATHOLOGIC PROCESSES

This section presents a discussion on other pathologic processes that include osteoporosis, osteomalacia, and Paget's disease.

OSTEOPOROSIS

Osteoporosis has been defined as "a disease characterized by low bone mass and microarchitectural deterioration of bone tissue, leading to enhanced bone fragility and a consequent increase in fracture risk" (National Osteoporosis Foundation, 1998a). Osteoporosis occurs when the rate of bone resorption exceeds the rate of bone formation. With rare exceptions, it is a systemic disorder that effects the patient's entire skeleton. It can occur locally when part of the body is immobilized by a fracture or paralysis.

Osteoporosis represents a major health problem for 28 million people in the United States, 80% of whom are women. It is also responsible for over 1.5 million osteoporosis-related fractures occurring annually in the United States, including more than 300,000 hip and 700,000 vertebral fractures. Approximately 70% of

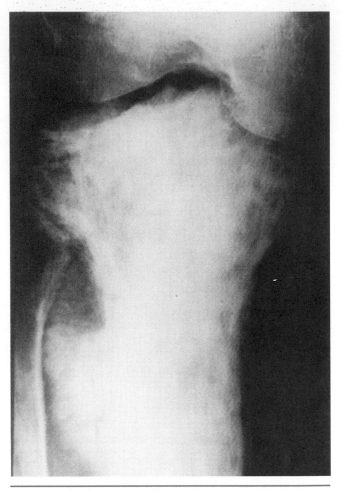

Figure 3–30   Radiograph showing a tibial osteogenic sarcoma in an area of pagetoid bone. The neoplasm has disrupted the cortex and formed a mass outside the bone. *(Weinstein & Buckwalter (1994). Turek's Othopaedic: Principles and Their Applications: Philadelphia: J.B. Lippincott Company.)*

fractures in persons older than 45 are related to osteoporosis, and more than half of all postmenopausal women will develop a spontaneous fracture as a result of osteoporosis. In 1994, it was estimated that the annual direct costs of osteoporosis-related fractures in the United States was $13.3 billion. It is also estimated that one quarter of all women over age 60 will develop vertebral deformities related to osteoporosis.

Systemic osteoporosis appears to be most marked in the spine and pelvis. Bone changes are characterized by a thinning of the cortical bone, resorption of cancellous bone, enlargement of the medullary cavity, and an overall loss of bone mass. Bones become porous, brittle, and subject to fractures from minimal trauma. Compression fractures of the vertebrae are most common, but the ribs, wrist, and hip are also frequently fractured.

PRIMARY OSTEOPOROSIS

Osteoporosis has been classified as either primary or secondary. In primary osteoporosis, there is no clearly identifiable cause, though the two major determinants of bone loss are believed to be postmenopausal estrogen deficiency and the aging process. The following presents the major potential factors that influence bone mass development and the rate of bone loss. They are

- *Gender.* While osteoporosis affects both sexes, women are more likely to develop the disease, primarily as the result of the accelerated bone loss that occurs in women after menopause. In addition, women tend to have less bone mass than men to begin with and, therefore, less bone to lose before the fracture threshold is reached.
- *Hormones.* Estrogen helps to regulate the bone-remodeling process in women, and an estrogen deficiency at any age can result in increased bone loss. However, the precise mechanism by which estrogen withdrawal results in bone loss remains rather obscure. One theory suggests that bones may become more sensitive to parathyroid hormone and therefore more susceptible to calcium resorption. Another theory is that estrogens antagonize the release of interleukin 1 (IL-1), which stimulates bone resorption. Thus, a reduction in estrogen levels might allow the production of IL-1 to go unchecked.
- *Aging.* The precise reason for the increased rate of bone loss after age 40 is unknown. Either factors intrinsic to bone or extrinsic to metabolism may be responsible. It is known that the absorption of calcium in the intestine decreases with age and is largely under the control of vitamin D (Schiller, 1994).
- *Calcium.* During the developmental years, calcium is important for the development of good peak bone mass by age 30. The average calcium intake of adults and especially postmenopausal women in the United States is well below the recommended value of 1,000 to 1,500 mg/day. However, whether this dietary deficiency contributes to the development of osteoporosis is controversial, because a number of studies have not found such a relationship.
- *Exercise.* Physical activity is necessary for the development and maintenance of bone mass. Research has shown that weight bearing and exercise increase lumbar spine bone density. Decreased activity with age may lead to a decrease in bone mass.
- *Body type/genetics.* Slender individuals have a higher risk of osteoporosis because they have less bone mass to lose. Less body weight and muscle mass mean less stress on the skeleton, hence lower bone mass. Women who have less body fat also tend to produce less estrogen. Genetic influences (from multiple genes) determine 75% to 80% of the variability, and the vitamin-D receptor gene has a significant effect in the development of bone mass. In general, peak bone mass is greater in men than women and greater in blacks than in whites.
- *Race/ethnicity.* Non-Hispanic white and Asian individuals tend to have less bone mass and a higher risk of osteoporosis than African Americans or Hispanics.
- *Environmental factors.* Both tobacco and alcohol are believed to have a toxic effect on bone or on the cells that make bone, and both have been linked with low bone mass and a higher risk of fractures. Studies have shown that smoking increases low bone mass in both sexes and is known to reduce estrogen levels in women. Alcohol is a direct inhibitor of osteoblasts and may also inhibit calcium absorption. The caffeine in tea, coffee, and sodas has also been linked to low bone density and higher risk of fracture in several studies.

Senile osteoporosis is the most common type of primary osteoporosis. Many are postmenopausal women, as women with osteoporosis outnumber men by a ratio of 4:1. They usually seek medical attention because of back pain related to minor trauma. The most common treatment is to improve the patient's protein, calcium, and vitamin D intake. Exercise, estrogen replacement, and high fluoride intake have also been used effectively. New medications have recently been introduced. For more information, see the section on medications later in this chapter.

SECONDARY OSTEOPOROSIS

Secondary osteoporosis has an identifiable cause. The list of known causes is long, but the three major ones are nutritional deficiencies, abnormal endocrine function, and disuse. Various abnormal nutritional states are known to cause osteoporosis, including vitamin C deficiency (scurvy), mild malabsorption syndrome (lactose intolerance), gastrointestinal and hepatic diseases (which cause impaired absorption of calcium, phosphate, and vitamin D), acid diets, and calcium-deficient diets. High-protein diets used for weight reduction may also increase bone resorption, because the increased acidity resulting from a nitrogen imbalance is buffered by calcium from the bones. Chronic alcohol abuse may contribute, since alcohol is a direct inhibitor of osteoblasts and may directly inhibit calcium absorption (Schiller, 1994).

Endocrine osteoporosis is caused by abnormal functioning of an endocrine gland. Persons with hyperthyroidism, hyperparathyroidism, Cushing's syndrome, acromegaly, and hypogonadism are likely to have endocrine osteoporosis. Some medications, such as corticosteroids, cause an osteoporotic reaction similar to endocrine osteoporosis. Disuse osteoporosis, caused by bed rest or inactivity, is well known, and elderly people who become less active are subject to it. Lack of sufficient stresses and strains appears to be the main factor, as stressing bones by exercise is known to strengthen them and increase bone mass.

SYMPTOMS

Osteoporosis may be present for a long time before it is detected. Postmenopausal osteoporosis usually becomes recognizable within 10 years after the onset of menopause, whereas senile osteoporosis generally becomes symptomatic after the age of 70. The symptoms of osteoporosis may occur suddenly or insidiously. However, most patients are unaware of their disease until they suffer a fracture. The patient usually has initial symptoms that include weakness, pain, unsteady gait, stiffness, and poor appetite. Back pain, usually in the lower thoracic or lumbar region, is the most common complaint. Other painful areas are the hips, pelvis, and legs. Physical changes in the spine cause a loss of height and a round back (kyphosis).

DIAGNOSTICS

Laboratory studies are usually within normal limits, and only after there has been a 30% bone loss is the loss visible on roentgenograms. The development of the bone mineral density (BMD) test became very important in the diagnosis of osteoporosis. The BMD test is a noninvasive and accurate measurement of BMD based on the fact that mineralized bone absorbs x-rays at different rates than soft tissue. Two standardized scores are provided. The T-score is the patient's score in standard units based on values from young adult populations. The Z-score is the patient's score in standard units based on a population of the same age and sex. This is the patient's standard deviation from other people of the same age.

The World Health Organization (WHO) defines osteoporosis in terms of BMD. Normal bone density is a T-score between +1 and −1. Osteopenia is defined as a T-score between −1 and −2.5. Osteoporosis is considered present when the T-score is below (i.e., more negative than) −2.5; it is considered severe if the patient already has had a fracture. The WHO definitions are based on a population of Caucasian women and are not necessarily applicable to all groups.

The quantitative computed tomography (QCT) scanning to assess bone mineral density of the vertebrae has an accuracy of 3% to 5% in measuring bone loss. The QCT is costly and delivers a considerable amount of radiation. The "gold standard" for BMD testing is dual energy x-ray absorptiometry (DXA), which is used for testing the hip and spine. It is precise, economical, and increasingly available. Quantitative ultrasound (QUS) is another technique that offers a lower-cost, ultra fast, portable, and radiation-free method for assessment of bone density, especially of the os calcis, wrist, and hand.

TREATMENT

Medical treatment is prescribed according to the cause and type of osteoporosis. Unfortunately, once osteoporosis has developed and fractures have occurred, few treatment options exist. Although some promising pharmacologic therapies have recently been approved by the Federal Drug Administration (FDA), these medications cannot erase the effects of fractures, eliminate kyphosis, compensate for losses in functional capability to carry out activities of daily living, or eliminate pain. However, treatment usually includes a well-balanced diet, exercise, frequent rest periods, avoidance of severe fatigue, hormone replacement, calcium (daily intake of 1,000 to 1,500 mg), fluoride (which in combination

with calcium and vitamins stimulates osteoblastic activity and increases bone strength, which helps to decrease fracture risks), and vitamin C and D supplements. Two drugs that have recently become available for osteoporosis treatment or prevention are calcitonin and alendronate sodium. Drug research and development is a major focus of at least three major pharmaceutical companies, and it is expected that more drugs will soon be approved.

Estrogen. Estrogen replacement therapy (0.3–0.625 mg/d PO is commonly prescribed for postmenopausal osteoporotic women, although the exact mechanism by which it suppresses bone mineral loss is unclear. Estrogen remains controversial because it increases the risk of breast cancer and endometrial carcinoma and has also been shown to aggravate certain preexisting conditions, such as gallbladder, hepatic disease, and hypertension. The use of the transdermal patch (0.05–0.1-mg patch applied twice a week) for the delivery of estrogen reduces some of the latter problems because this route bypasses the digestive system and delivers the estrogen directly from the skin to the vascular system. Patient teaching needs to include how to do monthly breast self-examinations, the need for yearly mammography, and the need to report any vaginal bleeding. Patients who smoke should be advised to stop.

Alendronate Sodium (Fosamax). Alendronate is a fairly new drug that was approved in 1995 by the FDA for the treatment of osteoporosis. Fosamax (10 mg for treatment and 5 mg for prevention) is an aminobisphosphonate suppressive agent that is used to decrease the rate of bone resorption and reduce the serum alkaline phosphatase levels by decreasing osteoclastic activities. Fosamax is poorly absorbed from the gastrointestinal tract. Patients need to follow instructions closely and take it in the morning with 6 to 8 ounces of plain water at least 30 minutes before they eat or drink anything else. The patient also needs to be instructed to remain in an upright position (standing or sitting) for 30 minutes after taking the morning dose. Side effects of abdominal pain and gastric distress are rare if the drug is taken properly. The patient must also continue to have a daily intake of adequate calcium. Alendronate is not recommended for patients taking estrogen.

Calcitonin. Calcitonin (human, 0.5 mg subcutaneously or intramuscularly) is administered daily or 2 to 3 times a week, and salmon calcitonin (50–100 IU/d subcutaneously or intramuscularly) is administered daily or 3 times a week. It is recommended that the patient administer it at bedtime to reduce the side effects of nausea and vomiting, anorexia, and mild transient flushing of the palms of the hands and soles of the feet (Hunt, 1998). The two major disadvantages of calcitonin are its cost and that it has to be taken by injection because it is a peptide hormone and is destroyed in the gastrointestinal tract. The patient must learn how to administer the injections.

To dispense with the injection requirement for calcitonin, Miacalcin, a synthetic salmon calcitonin nasal spray (200 to 400 IU/d daily in alternating nostrils) was developed and approved for the treatment of women at least 5 years postmenopause who have low bone density and who are not candidates for estrogen replacement therapy. The side effects are mild nasal discomfort and rhinitis.

PREVENTION

Prevention strategies are effective to deter osteoporosis if they are started before bone loss occurs. Ninety percent of individual bone mass is achieved by 25 to 35 years of age. The accelerated bone loss that occurs in the first 5 years after menopause is detrimental to the body skeleton, but less detrimental and less likely to cause osteoporosis if the person has good bone mass before menopause. Strategies to develop peak bone mass and reduce risk factors must be implemented in youth and maintained through adulthood to be effective at menopause. These include a well-balanced diet with adequate calcium, exercise, and vitamin D from birth, and abstaining from caffeine, alcohol, and smoking during adolesence through adulthood. Preventive strategies include an adequate calcium intake throughout life, a moderate physical activity level, avoiding smoking, and avoiding excessive alcohol or large amounts of caffeinated beverages. If these strategies fail, active treatment of osteoporosis is required.

OSTEOMALACIA

Osteomalacia, now a rare condition, literally means "softness of bone." It is the adult counterpart of childhood rickets and is characterized by inadequate mineralization of newly formed bone matrix. The difference between rickets and osteomalacia is that in adults the mechanisms of bone growth are not involved, and only bone turnover mechanisms are affected, so that the bones become softer and more fragile than normal. Fractures are common, but bending and stress deformities also develop because the bones have decreased rigidity.

It is overly simplistic to say that osteomalacia is merely the result of a dietary deficiency of vitamin D. There are other possible mechanisms leading to inadequate mineralization of bone. They can be divided into three categories. First, there may be insufficient intake of vitamin D, which is the most common cause. In industrialized countries, it is more often caused by diseases that are associated with intestinal malabsorption than by poor nutrition (Rubin & Farber, 1994). Diseases of the small intestine, cholestatic disorders of the liver, biliary obstruction, and chronic pancreatic insufficiency are most frequent in the United States. Second, there are patients with hypophosphatemia, principally familial hypophosphatemia (vitamin-D–resistant rickets), but also including Fanconi's syndrome and renal tubular acidosis. Third, there are patients with defective nucleation of preformed bone matrix, such as hypophosphatasia and fluoride and strontium intoxication. All three categories produce skeletal changes that cannot readily be distinguished from one another.

In all cases, osteomalacia is characterized by a prolongation of the time interval between osteoid synthesis and mineralization. Instead of the normal 6 to 10 days, the time lag for mineralization may be as long as 2 to 3 months. Moreover, some areas completely fail to mineralize, leaving osteoid residuals. Osteomalacia develops insidiously. It may be identified by reduced serum calcium and phosphorus levels, reduced urine calcium, bone deformities, bone pain and tenderness, and roentgenographic changes. A biopsy of the bone may help establish the diagnosis. The bones most commonly involved are the spine, pelvis, and lower extremities. Usually, there is a history of bone or spinal pain from crush fractures.

Treatment of osteomalacia may involve large amounts of vitamin D and dietary measures to ensure adequate intake of calcium and phosphorus, for example, diets high in eggs, milk, fish, and vegetables. Calcium salts and phosphate supplements may also be given.

PAGET'S DISEASE

Paget's disease of the bone (osteitis deformans) is an acquired disorder of unknown etiology. According to Rubin and Farber (1994), when James Paget coined the term *osteitis deformans* for this disease over a century ago, he thought it was an infection of the bone. More recent research indicates the structure of a virus in the osteoclasts. There is also evidence of a familial tendency, as 25% to 40% of the patients with Paget's disease have at least one relative with the disorder (Kaplan & Singer, 1995). It occurs in England, Canada, Europe, Australia, New Zealand, and the United States but is almost nonexistent in the indigenous populations of Asia, Africa, and South America.

PATHOLOGY

Paget's disease is characterized by hyperactive bone destruction (osteoclastic activity) and formation (osteoblastic activity), with replacement of normal bone by expanded, soft, poorly mineralized, "honeycombed" osteoid tissue (Fig. 3–31). Although the affected bones are increased in size, they are usually light, soft, and porous and almost have the consistency of dry bread. The bones are highly vascular, structurally weak, and susceptible to deformity and fractures (Kaplan & Singer, 1995). The bone disease occurs in two patterns, monostotic and polyostotic. The tibia (Fig. 3–32) is the most common site in the monostotic pattern, and the pelvis and sacrum are typically the first bones involved in the polyostotic form. Long bones, pelvis, lumbar vertebrae Fig. 3–33), and skull are the predominant bones that are affected. The entire skeleton is rarely involved. Paget's disease rarely occurs in patients under the age of 40, and is more common in men than in women by a ratio of about 2:1.

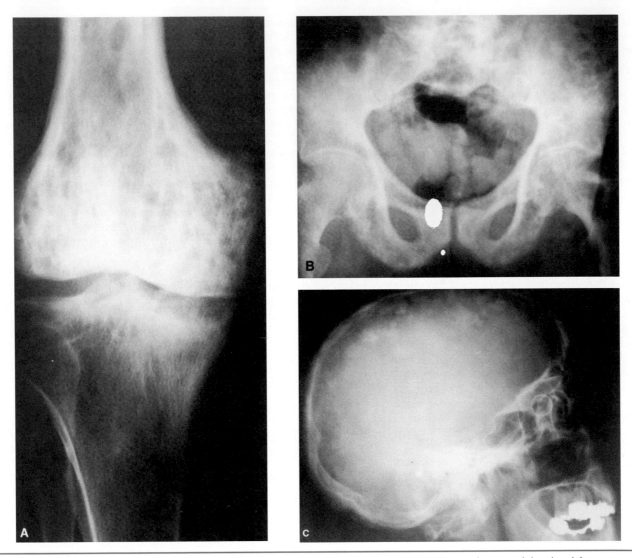

Figure 3–31   Radiographs showing the lytic and blastic changes of Paget's disease. (A) Paget's disease of the distal femur. (B) Paget's disease of the pelvis. (C) Paget's disease of the skull.   *(Weinstein & Buckwalter (1994).* Turek's Othopaedic: Principles and Their Applications: *Philadelphia: J.B. Lippincott Company.)*

When multiple bones are involved, Paget's disease usually produces readily identifiable characteristic deformities. The bone becomes shorter, broader, and weaker than normal bone and is more easily fractured. When the vertebral column is involved, grotesque dwarf-like distortions result. In the generalized form of the disease, the patient becomes shorter and, because the skull expands, may require a larger hat.

If only one or two bones are involved, the disease is commonly asymptomatic and is only discovered accidentally on roentgenographic examination. The onset of the disease is insidious. The initial complaint may be pain in the involved bone. It is unclear as to the cause of the pain, but Rubin and Farber (1994) state that the pain may be related to microfractures, to stimulation of free nerve endings by dilated blood vessels adjacent to the bones, or to weight bearing in weaker bone. The pain may be a dull ache, neurologic

discomfort, or a sharp stabbing sensation and may be intermittent or constant. When pain is felt over the tibia, the bone may be found to be enlarged and bowed. The overlying skin is often warm to the touch, but the bone is not tender. Skull lesions may cause headaches, facial pain, and enlargement of the skull. Backache is a common accompaniment of spinal involvement.

Over time, the enlarged head contrasts with the relatively small face. One or both legs or thighs become bowed anterolaterally as the enlarged tibiae increase the circumference of the legs. The femurs bend, and the femoral necks may yield under pressure. The width of the chest narrows, and a kyphosis develops from compression of the vertebral bodies. The bones affected, in decreasing order of frequency, are the pelvis, skull, femur, spine, tibia, humerus, scapula, and, only occasionally, other bones including the mandible.

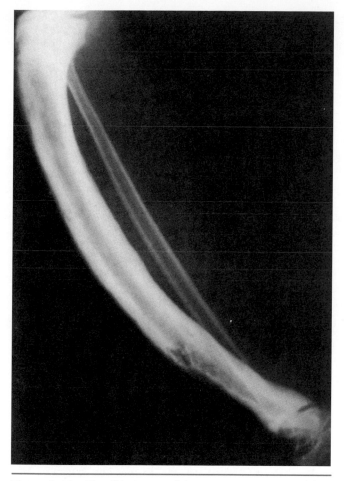

Figure 3–32 The tibia is one of the most common sites of the monostotic pattern in Paget's disease. *(Rubin & Farber (1994). Pathology. 4th ed. Philadelphia: J.B. Lippincott.)*

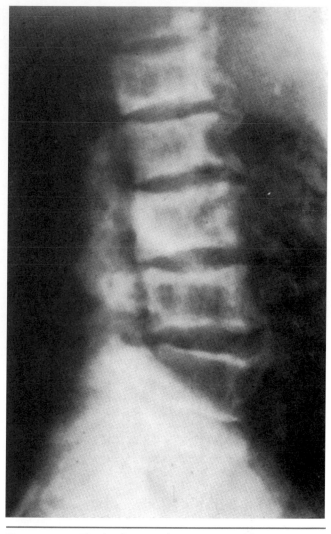

Figure 3–33 The lumbar vertebrae are one of the sites commonly affected in the polyostotic form of Paget's disease. *(Rubin & Farber (1994). Pathology. 4th ed. Philadelphia: J.B. Lippincott.)*

TREATMENT

The treatment consists of drug therapy. Calcitonin (human, 0.25–0.5 mg subcutaneously or intramuscularly) and salmon calcitonin (50–100 IU/d subcutaneously); etidronate disodium (Didronel), pamidronate disodium (Aredia, 15–90 mg intravenous), and tiludronate sodium (Skelid, 400 mg); and alendronate (Fosamax, 40 mg/d) are used to retard bone resorption and reduce serum alkaline phosphatase and urinary hydroxyproline secretions. Although calcitonin, a suppressive agent that inhibits the osteoclastic resorption of bone, involves long-term therapy, there is usually noticeable improvement after the first few weeks of treatment. However, there is the disadvantage that calcitonin is not available in oral form. Etidronate, a bisphosphonate suppressive agent that blocks bone resorption and bone formation by coating the bone surfaces with a slippery, soap-like substance, produces a decrease in serum calcium, urinary hydroxyproline, and serum alkaline phosphatase. Etidronate is available in oral form but should not be taken within 2 hours of any food and must be cycled on and off every 6 months. Pamidronate, also a bisphosphonate suppressive agent for bone resorption, inhibits the effect of osteoclasts, especially their ability to bind with calcium phosphate crystals in the bone and block calcium resorption. However, it is available only in IV form and must be given in 1,000 cc of IV solution over 4 to 24 hours and repeated every 7 days. Tiludronate is a bisphosphonate suppressive and is effective as a strong inhibitor of bone resorption. It is available in oral form and may be administered over a 3-month period either in the morning or evening with 6–8 ounces of water at least 2 hours before meals. Fosamax is an aminobisphosphonate suppressive agent that decreases the rate of bone resorption by decreasing bone formation. It is available in oral form, and must be taken with 6–8 ounces of water on an empty stomach at least 30 minutes before the first food or drink of the day. The patient must remain in an upright position for at least 30 minutes after taking Fosamax (Hunt, 1998). Mithramycin produces remission of symptoms within

2 weeks and biochemical improvement in 1 to 2 months. However, mithramycin may destroy platelets or compromise renal function and is not widely used today. Drugs that usually help to control pain are aspirin, indomethacin, and ibuprofen.

Patients may need surgery to reduce or prevent pathologic fractures, correct secondary deformities, and relieve neurologic impairment. Drug therapy may precede surgery to reduce the risk of excessive bleeding from hypervascular bones. Other treatments are symptomatic and supportive and vary according to the symptoms.

COMPLICATIONS

The most common complication of Paget's disease is a fracture, especially of weight-bearing long bones, which usually occurs in the vascular soft (osteoblastic) stage of the disease process. Those fractures are usually found over the apex of the convexity of the bowed shaft. The fractures heal rapidly, although with a minimum of callus. When fractures occur in dense bone during the osteoclastic stage, union is delayed.

In at least 5% of patients with Paget's disease, the involved bone will undergo malignant degeneration. The tumors are either osteogenic sarcoma, fibrosarcoma, or round-cell sarcoma. The development of a tumor is usually preceded by an increase in pain and a rapid increase in the size of the bone.

References

Agency for Health Care Policy and Research. (1994). *Management of cancer pain: Adults. Quick reference guide for clinicians.* No. 9 (AHCPR Publication Number 94-0593). Rockville, MD: Agency for Health Care Policy and Research. U.S. Department of Health and Human Services, Public Health Service.

Altizer, L. L. (1998). Degenerative disorders. In A. B. Maher, S. W. Salmond, & T. A. Pellino (Eds.), *Orthopaedic nursing* (2nd ed., pp. 480–544). Philadelphia: W. B. Saunders.

Arthritis Foundation, Association of State and Territorial Health Officials, and Centers for Disease Control and Prevention (1999). *National Arthritis Action Plan: A Public Health Strategy,* Atlanta, GA: Arthritis Foundation.

Bailey, J. M., & Nielson, B. I. (1993). Uncertainty and appraisal of uncertainty in women with rheumatoid arthritis. *Orthopaedic Nursing, 12*(2), 63–67.

Bates, B., Bickley, L. S., & Hoekelman, R. A. (1995). *A guide to physical examination and history taking* (6th ed.) Philadelphia: J. B. Lippincott.

Boutaugh, M. L., & Brady, T. J. (1996). Meeting the needs of people with arthritis: Quality of life programs of the Arthritis Foundation. *Orthopaedic Nursing, 15*(5), 59–70.

Buckwalter, J. A. (1994). Musculoskeletal neoplasms and disorders that resemble neoplasms. In S. L. Weinstein & J. A. Buckwalter (Eds.), *Turek's orthopaedics: Principles and their application* (5th ed., pp. 289–338). Philadelphia: J. B. Lippincott.

Campbell, B., & Morwessel, R. (1998). *Osteoporosis: Time to bone up.* Rosemont, IL: Ruth Jackson Orthopaedic Society.

Childs, S. (1996). Osteoarticular mycobacterium tuberculosis. *Orthopaedic Nursing, 15*(3), 28–33.

Craig, E. V. (1994). The shoulder and arm. In S. L. Weinstein & J. A. Buckwalter (Eds.), *Turek's orthopaedics: Principles and their application* (5th ed., pp. 359–400). Philadelphia: J. B. Lippincott.

Dowd, S. B. (1993). The radiographic appearance of gout. *Orthopaedic Nursing, 12*(1), 53–55.

Dunkin, M. A., & Reese, K. (1999, January–February). Your heritage, your health. *Arthritis Today,* 40–45.

Enzinger, F. M., & Weiss, S. W. (1995). *Soft tissue tumors.* St. Louis: Mosby.

Gray, M. A. (1993). Medications for a growing concern: Tuberculosis. *Orthopaedic Nursing, 12*(2), 75–79.

Gray, M. A. (1994). Osteoporosis medications: What's your source of information? *Orthopaedic Nursing, 13*(5), 55–58.

Gray, M. A. (1995). NSAIDs revisited. *Orthopaedic Nursing, 14*(1), 52–54.

Halverson, P. B. (1995). Extraarticular manifestations of rheumatoid arthritis. *Orthopaedic Nursing, 14*(4), 47–50.

Haynes, K. (1998). Neoplasms of the musculoskeletal system. In A. B. Maher, S. W. Salmond, & T. A. Pellino (Eds.), *Orthopaedic nursing.* (pp. 769–803). Philadelphia: W. B. Saunders.

Herzberg, M. A. (1998). Publication excerpt: Osteoporosis independent study. *Orthopaedic Nursing, 17*(2), 63–70.

Holmes, S. B. (1998). Autoimmune and inflammatory disorders. In A. B. Maher, S. W. Salmond, & T. A. Pellino (Eds.), *Orthopaedic nursing* (pp. 351–430). Philadelphia: W. B. Saunders.

Hunt, A. H. (1996). The relationship between height change and bone mineral density. *Orthopaedic Nursing, 15*(3), 57–64.

Hunt, A. H. (1998). Metabolic conditions. In A. B. Maher, S. W. Salmond, & T. A. Pellino (Eds.), *Orthopaedic nursing* (2nd ed., pp. 431–179). Philadelphia: W. B. Saunders.

Jones, E. T., & Mayor, P. (1994). The neck. In S. L. Weinstein & J. A. Buckwalter (Eds.), *Turek's orthopaedics: Principles and their application* (5th ed., pp. 341–358). Philadelphia: J. B. Lippincott.

Kaplan, F. S., & Singer, F. S. (1995). Paget's disease of bone: Pathophysiology, diagnosis, and management. *Journal of the American Academy of Orthopaedic Surgeons, 3,* 336–344.

Kessenich, C. R., & Rosen, C. J. (1996). Vitamin D and bone status in elderly women. *Orthopaedic Nursing, 15*(3), 67–71.

Krug, B. (1997). Rheumatoid arthritis and osteoarthritis: A basic comparison. *Orthopaedic Nursing, 16*(5), 73–75.

Lawrence, R. C., Helmick, C. G., Arnett, F. C., (1998). Estimates of the prevalence of arthritis and selected musculoskeletal disorders in the United States. *Arthritis Rheum.* 41: 778–99.

Lewis, M. L. (Ed.). (1992). *Musculoskeletal oncology: A multidisciplinary approach.* Philadelphia: W. B. Saunders.

Liscum, B. (1992). Osteoporosis: The silent disease. *Orthopaedic Nursing, 11*(4), 21–25.

Meads, R. A. (1994). The elbow and forearm. In S. L. Weinstein & J. A. Buckwalter (Eds.), *Turek's orthopaedics: Principles and their application.* (5th ed., pp. 401–416). Philadelphia: J. B. Lippincott.

Naides, S. J., Olson, R. R., Ashman, R. F., Janes, M. M., Field, E. H., Rochow, J. W., Strattman, M. P., Sparks, L. H., Cowdery, J. S., Croock, A. D., and Karr, R. W. (1994). Rheumatic diseases: Diagnosis and management. In S. L. Weinstein & J. A. Buckwalter (Eds.), *Turek's orthopaedics: Principles and their application.* (5th ed., pp. 151–212). Philadelphia: J. B. Lippincott.

National Osteoporosis Foundation. (1996). *Osteoporosis: The silent disease.* Slide presentation. Washington, DC: National Osteoporosis Foundation.

National Osteoporosis Foundation. (1998a). *Physician's guide to prevention and treatment of osteoporosis.* Washington, DC: National Osteoporosis Foundation.

National Osteoporosis Foundation. (1998b). *Pocket guide to prevention and treatment of osteoporosis.* Washington, DC: National Osteoporosis Foundation.

Orr, P. M. (1993). Salmon calcitonin. *Orthopaedic Nursing, 12*(5), 45–47, 70.

Piasecki, P. A. (1992). Update in orthopaedic oncology. *Orthopaedic Nursing, 11*(6), 36–43.

Piasecki, P. A. (1996). Nursing care of the patient with metastatic bone disease. *Orthopaedic Nursing, 15*(4), 25–33.

Pigg, J. S. (1997). Case management of the patient with arthritis. *Orthopaedic Nursing* (Suppl.), 33–40.

Proctor, M. C., Greenfield, L. J., & Marsh, E. E. (1997). Prophylaxis for thromboembolism in elective orthopaedic surgery. *Orthopaedic Nursing, 16*(5), 51–56.

Rankin, J. A. (1995). Pathophysiology of the rheumatoid joint. *Orthopaedic Nursing, 14*(4), 39–46.

Rubin, E., & Farber, J. L. (1994). Neoplasia. In E. Rubin & J. L. Farber (Eds.), *Pathology* (2nd ed., pp. 142–199). Philadelphia: J. B. Lippincott.

Salmond, S. W., Mooney, N. E., & Verdisco, L. (Eds.). *Core curriculum for orthopaedic nursing.* Pitman, NJ: National Association of Orthopaedic Nursing.

Schiller, A. L. (1994). Bones and joints. In E. Rubin & J. L. Farber (Eds.), *Pathology* (2nd ed., pp. 1273–1346). Philadelphia: J. B. Lippincott.

Smith, C. A., & Arnett, F. C. (1991). Epidemiologic aspects of rheumatoid arthritis: Current immunogenetic approach. *Clinical Orthopaedics and Related Research, 265,* 23–34.

Tresolini, C. P., Gold, D. T., & Lee, L. S. (Eds). (1996). *Working with patients to prevent, treat, and manage osteoporosis: A curriculoum guide for the health professions.* San Francisco, CA: National Fund for Medical Education.

Windsor, R. E. (1994). The adult knee. In S. L. Weinstein & J. A. Buckwalter (Eds.), *Turek's orthopaedics: Principles and their application* (5th ed., pp. 585–614). Philadelphia: J. B. Lippincott.

Chapter

4

Musculoskeletal Trauma, Immobility, and Ambulation

Chapter 4 discusses the effects of trauma on the musculoskeletal system. It examines soft-tissue trauma (including contusions, strains, sprains, and dislocations) and fractures (including first-aid measures, methods of repair, and complications related to fractures). The chapter also discusses complications from imposed immobility and ways to restore ambulation through the use of assistive devices.

Musculoskeletal injuries are relatively common occurrences. Many injuries occur at home from lifting heavy objects, slipping in the bathtub or on a wet or waxed floor, tripping over rugs or pets, falling off chairs or ladders, and falling down stairs. Other injuries occur in motor vehicle accidents, during recreational activities, and on the job. Musculoskeletal injuries can even occur during "normal" activities, as when violent coughing fractures a rib. Factors that increase the possibility of musculoskeletal injuries are age (because older persons have more fragile bones) and pathological conditions that weaken the musculoskeletal system.

MUSCULOSKELETAL TRAUMA

Trauma to the musculoskeletal system can involve either soft tissue or bone. It is not always the location or type of injury that produces the greatest concern for repair and healing, because the type of tissue involved is also of crucial importance.

SOFT-TISSUE TRAUMA

Trauma to the soft tissue of the musculoskeletal system may occur alone or in conjunction with a fracture. The more common soft-tissue injuries—contusions, strains, and sprains—tend to occur around joints.

CONTUSIONS

A contusion is a soft-tissue injury or bruise produced by a blunt force such as a blow, kick, or fall. There is always some hemorrhage into the injured tissue due to the rupture of small blood vessels. Those hemorrhages produce skin discolorations (ecchymoses or "black-and-blue" marks), which gradually turn purplish, then yellow, and finally disappear as absorption becomes complete. When the hemorrhage is sufficient to cause an appreciable collection of blood, a hematoma forms with local symptoms of pain, swelling, and discoloration.

Treatment of a contusion consists of elevating the affected part and applying moist or dry cold for the first 8 to 10 hours to produce vasoconstriction and a consequent decrease in hemorrhage and edema. Cold applications should be kept in place for 20 to 30 minutes at a time. After the first 24 hours, heat is usually applied for 20 minutes at a time to promote absorption and repair. Because heat can cause swelling and increase tissue fluid, hot compresses may be followed by cold applications to minimize those effects. Pressure in the form of an elastic bandage can also help reduce hemorrhage and swelling.

STRAINS

A strain is an injury to the musculotendinous structures surrounding a joint, produced by an excessive force or stretching, which causes hemorrhage into the tissues. Strains may be classified as first-degree strains (mild strains or slightly pulled muscles), second-degree strains (moderate strains or moderately pulled muscles), and third-degree strains (severely pulled muscles).

A first-degree strain causes a low-grade inflammation and some disruption of muscle-tendon tissue, but little hemorrhage. The patient has local pain in the area, which is aggravated by movement or muscle tension. Other symptoms include swelling, ecchymosis, local tenderness, and a minor loss of function and strength in the affected joint. Complications that can occur following a mild strain are recurrence of the strain, tendinitis, and periostitis at the tendinous attachment site. A second-degree strain involves the tearing of musculotendinous fibers without a complete disruption of the muscle or the tendon. The patient has local pain, which is aggravated by movement or muscle tension, moderate muscle spasm, swelling, ecchymosis, local tenderness, and impaired muscle function. Complications are the same as those for a first-degree strain.

Patients with a third-degree strain have a ruptured muscle or tendon with the separation of muscle from muscle, muscle from tendon, or tendon from bone. There is severe pain and disability, severe spasm, swelling, ecchymosis, hematoma, tenderness, loss of muscle function, and usually a palpable defect in the joint. Roentgenograms are usually necessary as they can demonstrate soft-tissue swelling and an avulsion fracture at the tendinous attachment.

Treatment of strains focuses on decreasing the swelling and immobilizing the joint with the disrupted tissues approximated. It usually consists of elevating and resting the affected part, with cold compresses applied for 15 to 20 minutes 4 times a day for the first 24 hours. The vasoconstricting effect of the cold retards the extravasation of blood and lymph and reduces pain. Sometimes additional support is provided by temporary splinting or an elastic bandage. In third-degree strains, surgery may be required occasionally to suture the muscle and surrounding fascia. The joint is then immobilized until healing occurs.

SPRAINS

A sprain is an injury to the ligamentous structures surrounding a joint, caused by a wrench or a twist. Blood vessels are ruptured, resulting in rapid swelling due to the extravasation of blood within the tissues. Movement of the joint becomes painful. The function of a ligament is to maintain stability while permitting mobility, and a torn ligament causes the joint to lose functional stability.

Sprains are classified as first-degree or mild sprains, second-degree or moderate sprains, and third-degree or severe sprains. A mild sprain consists of a minor tearing of ligamentous fibers causing mild, focused tenderness, no abnormal motion, little or no swelling, minimal hemorrhage, and minimal functional loss. The principal complication is the recurrence of a mild sprain. A moderate sprain, the partial tearing of a ligament, involves focused tenderness, moderate loss of function, slight to moderate abnormal motion, swelling, and localized hemorrhage. Complications following a moderate sprain are a tendency toward recurrent sprains, persistent instability, and traumatic arthritis. A severe sprain, the complete tearing of a ligament, involves a loss of function, marked abnormal motion, possible deformity, tenderness, swelling, and hemorrhage. Stress roentgenograms, done when pain is adequately relieved, demonstrate a loss of joint stability. Complications following a severe sprain are the same as those following a moderate sprain.

The immediate treatment of sprains includes rest and elevation of the affected part and the use of intermittent cold compresses to retard the extravasation of blood and lymph and to reduce pain. After 24 hours, mild heat may be applied at 15- to 30-minute intervals 4 times a day to promote absorption. For mild or moderate sprains, additional support is usually provided by a temporary splint or an elastic bandage. If the sprain is severe, surgical repair or cast immobilization is necessary to restore joint stability. Ligaments are relatively avascular, so healing is slow. The larger ligaments must be protected until there is maturation of the scar, usually 8 to 16 weeks. (For further information on sprains, see Chapter 8 for the back, Chapter 10 for the knee, Chapter 11 for the ankle, and Chapter 12 for the wrist.)

DISLOCATIONS

A dislocation is when the articular surfaces of the bones forming a joint are out of anatomical position. Dislocations may be congenital (such as a congenital dislocated hip), pathological (i.e., due to a disease of the articular or periarticular structures), or traumatic (i.e., from an external force). Signs of a dislocation are pain, changes in the contour of the joint, changes in the length of an extremity, loss of mobility, and changes in the axis of the dislocated bones. (For a discussion of dislocations of the adult hip, see Chapter 9.)

Treatment involves the reduction of the dislocation (i.e., the return of the joint to anatomical alignment), which may be done without anesthesia, under a regional block, or under local or general anesthesia. The joint is then immobilized by bandages, splints, or a cast to keep it in a stable position until healing occurs.

FRACTURES

A fracture is a break in the continuity of a bone. Most fractures occur as the result of trauma. When sufficient force is applied to a bone, it breaks, dissipating the original force through nearby soft tissue and usually embedding small fragments of bone in adjacent muscles, small blood vessels, and nerves. A pathological fracture may occur during normal activity or following minimal injury when the bone is weakened by a disease process. A fatigue or stress fracture occurs in normal bone that has been subjected to repeated stresses, such as those arising from long and strenuous activities (Fig. 4–1).

Fractures are classified according to the mechanism of the injury and the type of bone discontinuity. Knowing how the fracture occurred, including whether it was caused by direct or indirect forces (Fig. 4–2), has therapeutic implications for the physician. A closed (or simple) fracture is one in which the skin over the injury site remains intact, with no connection between the bone and the skin surface. An open (or compound) fracture is one in which the skin over the injury site is broken. An open wound is caused either by the fracture fragments

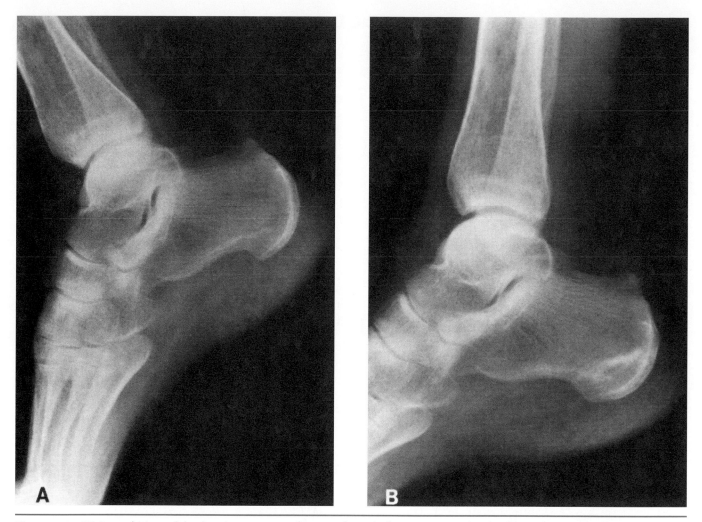

Figure 4–1 (A) Lateral view of the foot in a woman who complained of severe pain in her heel reveals no evidence of fracture. (B) Films taken one month later show a linear density of endosteal callus in the posterior of the os calcis, indicating a healing fatigue fracture. *(Rockwood, C.A., et al. (1996).* Rockwood & Green's Fractures in Adults. *4th ed. Philadelphia: Lippincott-Raven.)*

piercing the skin or by an outside force penetrating through the skin. An open fracture has a high risk of contamination that may lead to infection.

Fractures may be either complete or incomplete. In an incomplete fracture, only a portion of the bone is broken. A fracture is complete when there is a separation of the bone into two or more major parts. The part of the bone nearest the body is termed the proximal fragment, and the one most distant from the body is called the distal fragment. The proximal fragment is also called the uncontrollable fragment because its location and muscle attachments prevent it from being moved or manipulated during reduction of the fracture. The distal fragment is referred to as the controllable fragment because usually it can be moved and manipulated to bring it into alignment with the proximal fragment. Fractures in long bones are usually designated as being in the proximal, middle, or distal thirds of the bone. When the two major fragments remain in good alignment, the fracture is referred to as

a fracture without displacement, whereas if they are separated, it is a fracture with displacement.

Fractures may be classified into 12 major types. A *greenstick* fracture involves a break in only part of the thickness of a bone. It typically occurs in young children with soft bones. An *oblique* fracture has a fracture line at an oblique angle to the bone shaft (Fig. 4–3). A *transverse* fracture involves a break perpendicular to a bone's long axis (Fig. 4–4). In a *spiral* fracture, the fracture lines encircle the bone, spiraling or coiling toward the torso (Fig. 4–5). A *comminuted* fracture involves multiple bone fragments, usually several small pieces between two large ones. A *linear* or *longitudinal* fracture is a fracture along the long axis of a bone. An *impacted* (or telescoped) fracture occurs when the fracture fragments are forcibly pushed against and into one another. An *avulsion* fracture is when a fragment of bone connected to a ligament breaks off from the rest of the bone. A *compression* fracture is when a bone fracture occurs as a result of compression (Fig. 4–6). A *depression* fracture occurs when

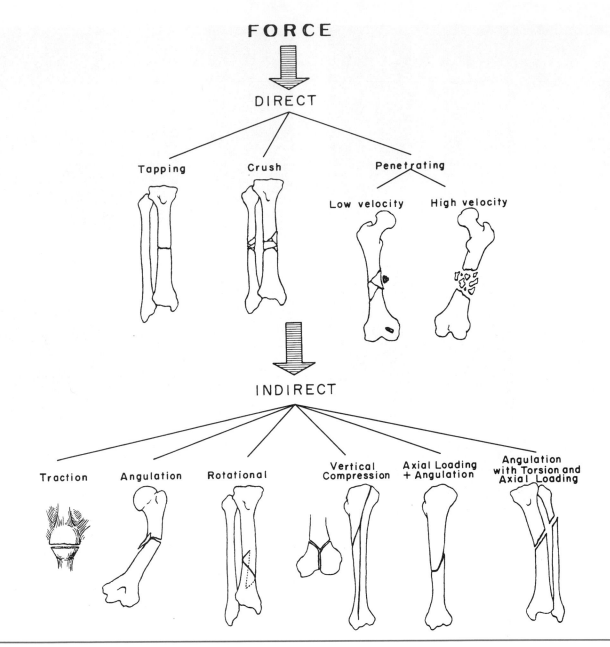

Figure 4–2   Classification of fractures according to the mechanism of injury.   *(Rockwood, C.A., et al. (1996).* Rockwood & Green's Fractures in Adults. *4th ed. Philadelphia: Lippincott-Raven.)*

bone fragments are forced below their normal level. It most commonly occurs in the skull. An *articular* fracture is a fracture involving an articulating surface of a bone (Fig. 4–7). A *segmental* fracture is a fracture of a small feature of a bone, typically a styloid process.

The signs and symptoms of fractures vary according to the type of fracture, the location of the fracture, the function of the involved bone, and the amount of related soft-tissue damage (Box 4–1). Fractures may occur without displacement, with little swelling, and with pain occurring only when direct pressure is applied. In most cases, however, the following signs and symptoms can be observed: (1) pain or tenderness at the site of the injury; (2) loss of function from pain, muscle spasm, or bone

instability; (3) deformity, such as a change in the alignment or contour of a bone or the appearance of soft-tissue swelling; (4) abnormal motility, particularly noticeable in long bones; (5) crepitus, a grating sensation that can be felt or heard, which is caused by bone fragments rubbing against each other; (6) ecchymosis; and (7) roentgenographic evidence of a fracture.

FIRST-AID MEASURES
The immediate management of a fracture may determine the patient's outcome and make the difference between complete recovery and disability or even death. Incorrectly moving an accident victim from one position to another may make a closed fracture an open one,

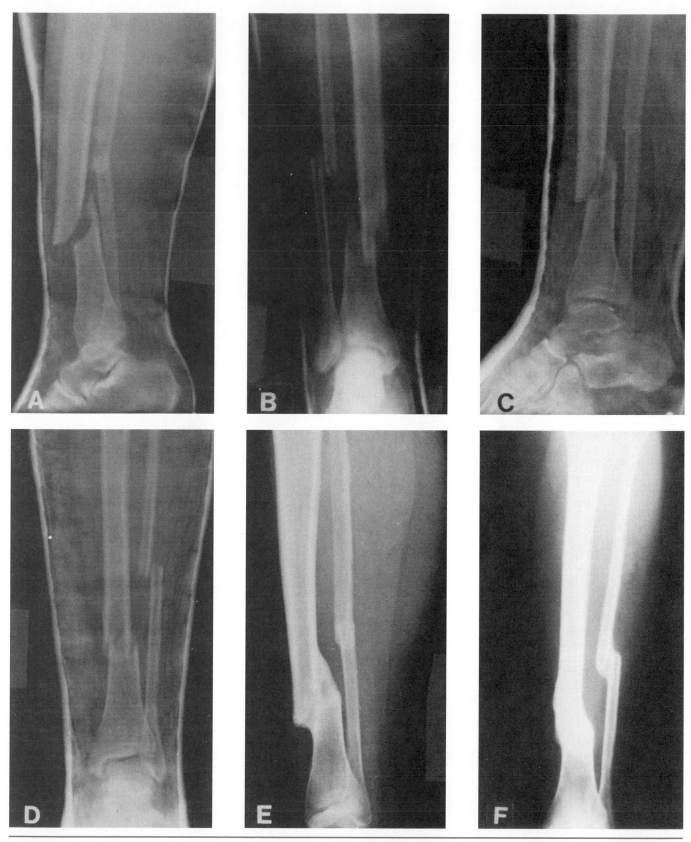

Figure 4–3   (A and B) Anteroposterior and lateral views of an oblique fracture. The proximal fragment is shaped like a trowel. This reduction, obtained by a tyro, is inadequate. Note the large air space at the upper end of the tibia where the cast has lost contact with the tibia. (C and D) After remanipulation and the application of three-point fixation, the proximal and distal fragments are parallel in both planes, and there is little or no shortening. (E and F) The fracture has united by periosteal callus. In spite of the offset, the cosmetic and functional results are excellent.   *(Rockwood, C.A., et al. (1996). Rockwood & Green's Fractures in Adults. 4th ed. Philadelphia: Lippincott-Raven.)*

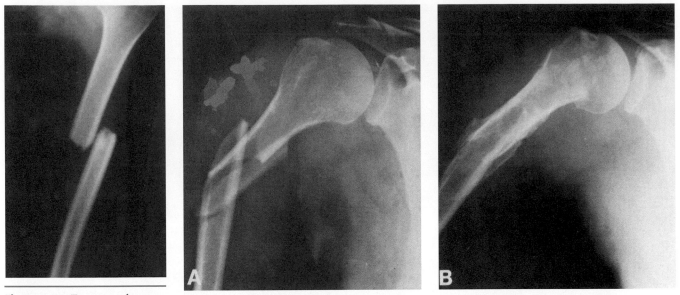

Figure 4–4   Transverse fracture of the humerus secondary to an angulation force.   *(Rockwood, C.A., et al. (1996). Rockwood & Green's Fractures in Adults. 4th ed. Philadelphia: Lippincott-Raven.)*

Figure 4–5   (A) Radiograph of a spiral fracture of the left humerus with a loose butterfly fragment in a 67-year-old man. (B) Ten years later the fracture seems to be well healed. After a subsequent fall, he sustained an impacted fracture of the humeral neck.   *(Rockwood, C.A., et al. (1996). Rockwood & Green's Fractures in Adults. 4th ed. Philadelphia: Lippincott-Raven.)*

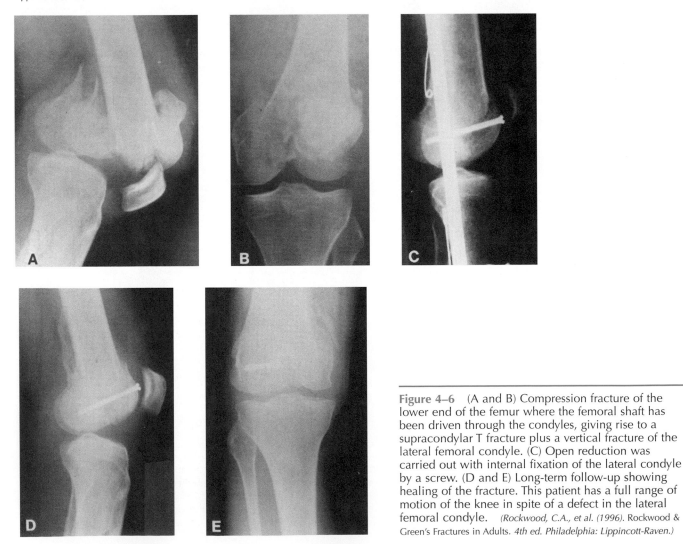

Figure 4–6   (A and B) Compression fracture of the lower end of the femur where the femoral shaft has been driven through the condyles, giving rise to a supracondylar T fracture plus a vertical fracture of the lateral femoral condyle. (C) Open reduction was carried out with internal fixation of the lateral condyle by a screw. (D and E) Long-term follow-up showing healing of the fracture. This patient has a full range of motion of the knee in spite of a defect in the lateral femoral condyle.   *(Rockwood, C.A., et al. (1996). Rockwood & Green's Fractures in Adults. 4th ed. Philadelphia: Lippincott-Raven.)*

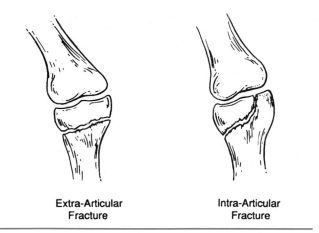

Extra-Articular   Intra-Articular
Fracture   Fracture

Figure 4–7   Extra- and intra-articular fracture patterns.
(Mallon, W.J., et al. (1990). Orthopaedics for the House Officer. Baltimore: Williams & Wilkins.)

Box 4–1
Signs of a Fracture

1. Pain
2. Loss of function
3. Deformity
4. Abnormal motility
5. Crepitus
6. Eccmymosis

---

puncture a lung, or sever the spinal cord or a major blood vessel. Look for fractures and dislocations in the extremities; check neurovascular status by palpating pulses distal to the injury (see Chapter 2); and look for the classic signs of arterial insufficiency—a decreased or absent pulse, pallor, paresthesia, pain, and paralysis. In examining for fractures, handle the limb gently and as little as possible. Keep in mind that the victim may have multiple fractures accompanied by head, chest, and other injuries.

Before a patient can be moved, the extent of the injuries must be assessed and all fractures immobilized by splints or backboards. Evaluate the patient for respiratory difficulties, take measures to control hemorrhage, and treat for shock. A conscious victim may be able to describe specific areas of pain. Pain over a bone or a joint should be treated as a fracture until proven otherwise, even if the victim can move the extremity. Inspect all fracture sites, relieve pain, improve circulation, minimize further tissue injury, and prevent a closed fracture from becoming an open one. Splints can be improvised using a variety of materials, including pillows, pieces of board, rolled-up newspapers, rifle barrels, golf clubs, and tennis rackets. If an open fracture is present, the wound should be covered by a clean cloth or dressing. Investigate any complaints of pain or pressure, and then transport the patient carefully and gently.

The following paragraphs discuss some general information on how trained personnel can move a victim with fractures of the spine, pelvis, hip, arm, and leg.

Fractures of the Spine. Any questionable injury to the neck or back, even in the absence of signs of paralysis, should be treated as a fracture of the spine. Check for paralysis by pinching or pricking the victim's toes and fingers with a pin or sharp object (see neurovascular assessment, Chapter 2). If the victim is lying flat, the vertebrae are examined by sliding a hand under the back without turning the victim. Observe for complications of spinal fractures, such as spinal cord damage, neurogenic shock, and interference with respiration.

If a cervical fracture is suspected, gentle traction may be applied to the neck and maintained until the neck can be supported by a cervical collar. A collar may be improvised by newspaper rolled up into a triangular bandage. The neck should not be flexed, twisted, or hyperextended. If no respiratory difficulties are present, the neck can be splinted in the position in which the victim was found. Some authorities say that the only first-aid reason to move a victim with an injured cervical spine is to improve an inadequate airway. To support the cervical spine during a move deemed necessary, place your hands on each side of the victim's head, cupping the victim's ears in your hands. The thumb should be in the temporal region, the index finger just below the zygoma, the third finger along the zygoma, and the fourth finger beneath the mandible. Keep the head in line with the victim's body. Slide the supine victim onto a flat, rigid surface, moving the entire body as a unit. Avoid twisting, turning, or pulling the spine. Watch for inadequate respiratory exchange due to paralysis of chest muscles or neurogenic shock. Once the victim is on a backboard, the victim's head can be additionally supported by placing sandbags, rolled towels, or rolled blankets on each side. A cravat can be placed through or around the backboard and over the forehead. In that way the victim's head, neck, and backboard will move as a unit.

If a lumbar fracture is suspected, the victim should be carefully placed on a flat, rigid surface such as a long backboard. Avoid flexion, extension, or rotation of the spine. The victim should be transported on a backboard as discussed in moving a victim with a cervical fracture.

Pelvic Fractures. An accident victim with a suspected pelvic fracture first must be turned carefully onto his or her back. Place padding between the victim's legs, splint them together to prevent unnecessary motion, and then turn the victim's body as a single unit. The supine victim should be placed on a firm, flat surface or stretcher. Immobilize the pelvis by binding a folded blanket around it.

Hip Fractures. A victim with a possible fractured hip must be splinted from the axilla to the ankle on the affected side. A board works very well, but if one is not available, bind the victim's legs together. If a half-ring traction is available, the half ring is slipped around the leg and placed at the groin and gluteal fold, and traction can be applied by means of a clove hitch around the victim's foot and ankle (see Chapter 5). The victim can then be transported on a stretcher or firm surface.

Leg Fractures. The leg of a victim with a femoral shift or knee fracture can be immobilized using a Thomas ring splint. The ring engages the ischial tuberosity for countertraction, and traction is applied to the end of the splint with an ankle hitch (see Chapter 5). If no ring splint is available, use boards or other devices to immobilize the victim's leg from the pelvis to the ankle.

A Jones compression splint can also be used for acute knee trauma and for ankle injuries. Alternatively, ankle injuries may be immobilized by tying the victim's lower legs, ankles, and feet together. If possible, transport the victim on a stretcher. The victim should not be allowed to bear weight on the affected leg.

Arm Fractures. For most fractures of the arm, place the victim's elbow at a right angle and apply a sling. The arm and sling should then be bound to the victim's body with a circular bandage or binder. Do not compromise the circulation in the antecubital area with the bandage. Check the radial pulse. Fractures of the clavicle may later be immobilized by a figure-of-eight clavicular strap; and shoulder dislocations, humeral fractures, and certain elbow fractures may later be immobilized by a Velpeau bandage. If the victim's injured elbow is in extension, bandage the extremity to the body in the position in which it is found. Always check the radial pulse in an elbow injury. Fractures below the elbow can be immobilized with a newspaper splint or with a commercial or inflatable air splint (see Chapter 5). The victim's arm is then placed in a sling with the elbow at a right angle. The air splint is closed over the extremity by its zipper and inflated by blowing air into the mouth tube. Skin maceration will occur if air splints are used for any extended period.

METHODS OF FRACTURE REPAIR

Objectives in the care and treatment of patients with a fracture include: (1) reduction of the fracture, (2) maintenance of the fragments in the correct position while healing takes place, (3) prevention of excessive loss of joint mobility and muscle tone, (4) prevention of complications, and (5) maintenance of good general health so that when the fracture heals the patient is restored to the preinjury level of health.

Reduction is the term used to designate the return of the bone fragments to their normal anatomical position. That may be accomplished by closed manipulation, traction, or open reduction. Closed manipulation is effected by the physician exerting a pulling force on the distal fragment while applying countertraction to the proximal fragment until the bone fragments engage or fall into their normal alignment. Pressure may also be applied over the site of the fracture to correct angulation or lateral displacement of a fragment. The fracture is then immobilized in a splint or cast. Closed manipulation is used to reduce closed fractures.

Traction, as a method of reduction, is accomplished by placing a continuous pull on the affected part for a period of hours, days, or even weeks to overcome muscle spasms and reduce the fracture (see Chapter 6). Skeletal traction is usually involved, and it may be a definitive method of treatment or a temporary method pending internal fixation. Skeletal traction is especially useful for fractures of the femur and severely displaced, unstable fractures of the humerus.

Open reduction is a method in which the fracture site is surgically opened and the fracture fragments replaced into correct anatomical position. The fractured bone is immobilized by the use of nails, rods, plates, screws, or pins, which hold the fragments together. Among the devices most commonly used for internal fixation are intramedullary nails, compression plates, and screws. Intramedullary nails are generally used in fractures of the middle two thirds of the femur, the humerus, and occasionally the tibia and the radius. They have the advantage of providing good fixation without damaging the periosteum, which is a major source of callus for the healing bone. Compression plates applied to the bone cortex provide rigid fixation, and, with proper techniques, substantial compression can be applied to the fracture site, which may speed healing. Compression plates are most suitable for fractures of the radius and the ulna and, less often, the humerus, the tibia, and the femur. Intra-articular fractures, for example, malleolar fractures of the ankle, are best fixed by screws. Certain hip fractures may require prosthetic replacement of the femoral head or, occasionally, a total joint replacement.

METHODS OF IMMOBILIZATION

The purpose of immobilization is to hold the reduced bone fragments in contact with each other until healing occurs. Any activity that involves the movement of the bone fragments must be restricted. Usually immobilization includes the joints immediately proximal to and distal to the fracture site. Bandages, adhesive tape, splints, casts (see Chapter 5), skeletal traction (see Chapter 6), internal fixation, and external fixation (see Chapter 7) are the most common methods of immobilization.

External fixation devices are used to hold fracture fragments in alignment when there is extensive soft-tissue damage in large, open fractures where inspection of soft tissues is essential, where vascular repair has been carried out in an open wound, and in burns with underlying fractures. Pins are surgically inserted through the skin and through the bone above and below the fracture. The pins are then clamped to the external framework that maintains the fracture fragments in correct alignment. In the upper extremity, the olecranon, the ulna, the distal third of the radius, and the second and third metacarpals are the usual sites for the insertion of pins. In the lower extremity, the supracondylar areas of the femur, the region of the tibial tubercle, the supramalleolar area of the tibia, and the os calcis are usually selected. For example, in a comminuted fracture of the tibia with a large, soft-tissue wound requiring debridement, fixation is secured by the insertion of two or more pins through the tibia in the area of the tibial tubercle, which are then connected with external fixation bars. When fixation is secure, the patient may be turned readily and the wounds inspected and dressed while alignment of the comminuted fracture is maintained.

FRACTURE HEALING

Fracture healing is a continuous process that begins immediately after a fracture (Fig. 4–8). The injury causes a hemorrhage into the fracture site from ruptured vessels within the bone, torn periosteum, and surrounding soft tissues. Within 24 hours, a hematoma is formed that fills the fracture site and the surrounding area. The coagulated blood of the hematoma gives rise to a loose fibrin mesh that seals off the fracture site and, at the same time, serves as a framework for the ingrowth of fibroblasts and capillary buds. During the first 24 to 48 hours following injury, the progressive disintegration of red blood cells provides a continuing inflammatory stimulus that results in significant edema, vascular congestion, and an infiltration of leukocytes, chiefly neutrophils. Two days after the injury, large numbers of macrophages begin the phagocytosis of the tissue and red cell debris. At the same time, fibroblasts and chondroblasts from the surrounding connective tissue, the periosteum, and the medullary cavity invade the

margins of the clot and begin to form a soft tissue callus in and about the fracture site (Fig. 4–9).

After the first few days, newly formed cartilage and bone matrix are evident in the fibrovascular response. By the end of the first week, well-developed new bone and cartilage are dispersed throughout the soft-tissue callus. During the following days, these bone spicules become sufficiently numerous and aggregated to create a large, fusiform, temporary bony union of the fracture fragments known as the provisional callus or procallus. By that time, the inflammatory reaction has mostly subsided and the repair is well under way.

The provisional callus is considerably wider than the normal diameter of the bone and extends up over the fractured ends to create a spindle-shaped, splint-like support (Fig. 4–10). In uncomplicated fractures, the provisional callus reaches its maximal size about 14 to 21 days after injury but continues to increase in strength from the precipitation of bone salts. At the same time, the procallus is remolded by osteoblastic and osteoclastic activity, which reacts to the muscle and weight-bearing stresses imposed upon the bone. If the fracture has been well aligned (with closed reduction the well-aligned fracture site will not be perfect with end-to-end fracture approximation) and weight-bearing stresses gradually restored, virtually perfect reconstruction of the bone is accomplished (Fig. 4–11). However, the repair may be impeded or prevented by many complications.

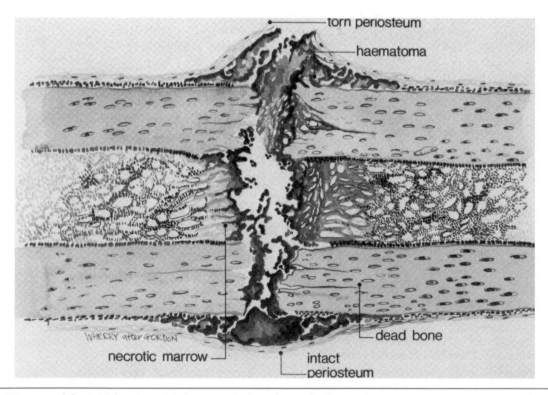

Figure 4–8   Diagram of the initial events after fracture of a long-bone diaphysis. The periosteum is torn opposite the point of impact and may remain intact on the other side. A hematoma accumulates beneath the periosteum and between the fracture ends. There is necrotic marrow and cortical bone close to the fracture line.   *(Developed by author.)*

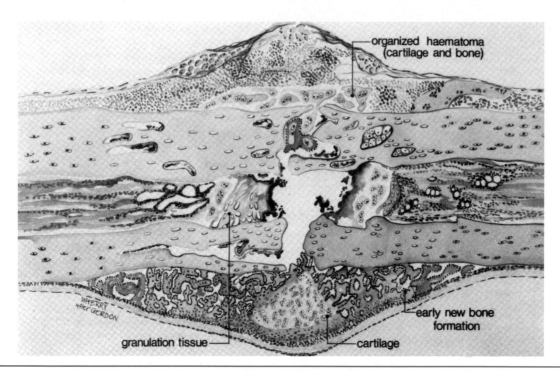

Figure 4–9 Diagram of early repair of a diaphyseal fracture of a long bone. There is organization of the hematoma, early woven bone formation in the subperiosteal regions, and cartilage formation in other areas. Periosteal cells contribute to healing of this type of injury. If the fracture is rigidly immobilized or if it occurs primarily through cancellous bone and the cancellous surfaces lie in close apposition, there will be little evidence of fracture callus. *(Rockwood, C.A., et al. (1996).* Rockwood & Green's Fractures in Adults. *4th ed. Philadelphia: Lippincott-Raven.)*

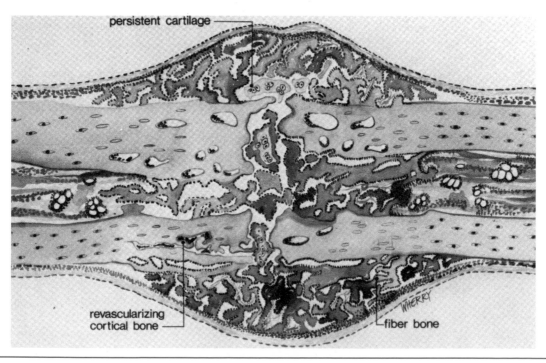

Figure 4–10 Diagram of a later stage in healing. Woven or fiber bone bridges the fracture gap. Cartilage remains in the regions most distant from ingrowing capillary buds. In many instances, the capillaries are surrounded by new bone. Vessels revascularize the cortical bone at the fracture site. *(Rockwood, C.A., et al. (1996).* Rockwood & Green's Fractures in Adults. *4th ed. Philadelphia: Lippincott-Raven.)*

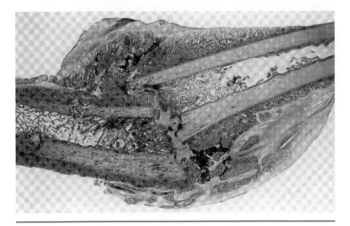

Figure 4–11 Light micrograph showing healing of a diaphyseal fracture. The fracture callus consisting primarily of woven bone surrounds and unites the two fracture fragments. As the callus matures, it progressively stabilizes the fracture. Note that the fracture callus contains areas of mineralized and unmineralized cartilage. *(Rockwood, C.A., et al. (1996).* Rockwood & Green's Fractures in Adults. *4th ed. Philadelphia: Lippincott-Raven.)*

COMPLICATIONS OF FRACTURES

The immediate complications following a fracture are (1) shock, which may be fatal in the first few hours after injury; (2) hemorrhage; (3) fat embolism; (4) pulmonary embolism; (5) compartmental syndrome; (6) neurological complications; and (7) infection. Late fracture complications, such as malunion, delayed union, nonunion, avascular necrosis, and chronic osteomyelitis, are primarily matters of orthopaedic reconstruction. Prevention of those complications, however, is best accomplished by avoiding errors in the early care of the injured patient.

Shock. Hypovolemic or traumatic shock resulting from hemorrhage (both external and internal) and loss of extracellular fluid into damaged tissues may occur in fractures of the extremities, thorax, pelvis, and spine. Because bone is very vascular, large quantities of blood may be lost as a result of bone trauma, especially in femoral and pelvic fractures. Treatment of shock consists of replacing depleted blood volume, relieving pain, providing adequate splinting of the fracture, and protecting the patient from further injury.

Hemorrhage. Hemorrhage is an excessive loss of blood. It is not an uncommon occurrence in orthopaedics for a patient to lose a substantial amount of blood following trauma or surgery (especially following repair of major fractures, joint replacements, or spinal surgery). Trauma patients lose an excessive amount of blood before surgery, and many have considerable blood loss during and after surgery. In addition to bones being vascular in nature, hemorrhages may occur from a blood vessel that was not sutured or cauterized during surgery or from a drainage/suction tube that has eroded a blood vessel. Hemorrhage may also occur as the result of abnormalities in the blood's ability to clot; these abnormalities may result from a pathologic condition, or they

may be a side effect of medications. Many orthopaedic patients are on anti-inflammatory medications before elective surgery, and those medications could play a role in the patient having an abnormal amount of bleeding during and after surgery.

The questions to be answered are, What is the cause of the blood loss? and Was it anticipated? If the patient has been on anticoagulant therapy before the surgery, one should anticipate that there will be more bleeding due to the increase in clotting time. What is the expected amount of drainage following a total knee replacement or posterior instrumentation of the back? Is the drainage exceeding that amount, is it occurring within the first 24 hours postsurgery, and what kind of drainage is occurring? Hemorrhage from a venous source is dark red, whereas an arterial hemorrhage is bright red.

If hemorrhage occurs, notify the patient's physician. Reinforce the patient's dressing with additional sterile gauze pads applied under pressure. Applying mechanical pressure with a gloved hand may be necessary for severe external bleeding. If indicated, prepare the patient, the patient's family, and significant others for emergency surgery in situations where the bleeding cannot be stopped.

Fat Embolism. Fat embolism syndrome is a major cause of morbidity and mortality in trauma patients (Karp & Freedman, 1998). It is fatal in 10% to 15% of the cases (Jaffe, Greco, & Wade, 1996). Fat emboli occur when fat in the blood, which is probably released into the blood from the bone marrow and tissue, becomes entrapped in the lung capillaries. There may also be occlusions of small vessels that supply the brain, kidneys, and other organs. The fat may originate at the fracture site and gain access to the venous circulation through ruptured marrow veins, or may be formed by an alteration of lipid stability in the blood caused by the stress of trauma. These fat droplets initially lodge in the pulmonary circulation; then platelets, red cells, and fibrin adhere to the plaques. Lipolysis results, leading to a chemical pneumonitis, with loss of surfactant activity that may eventually lead to the adult respiratory distress syndrome. If these emboli pass through the pulmonary circulation, they may go to the skin, causing petechiae changes, or to the cerebral circulation, causing central nervous system changes (Karp & Freedman, 1998). Occlusion of a large number of small vessels in the lungs causes pulmonary pressure to rise, possibly even resulting in acute right-sided heart failure. Edema and hemorrhage in the alveoli impair oxygen transport, leading to hypoxia.

Fat emboli are more likely to occur following comminuted fractures of long bones (especially the femur and the tibia) and the pelvis. The onset usually occurs 12 to 48 hours after injury or surgery. There may be no signs or symptoms despite pathologic evidence of fat emboli (tachycardia and tachypnea with blood gas levels showing hypoxia and hypocapnia). With progression to the central nervous system, symptoms may include abnormal behavioral changes varying from mild agitation and confusion (drowsiness, muscle weakness, spasticity, and rigidity) to delirium and coma, caused by the hypoxia. When personality changes occur following trauma or surgery, blood gas studies should be done to help confirm a diagnosis of fat emboli. Other symptoms are an increase in respiratory rate, sudden severe pericardial chest pain, dyspnea, pallor, exhaustion, and even collapse. With systemic embolization, by the second or third day petechiae can usually be detected in the buccal membranes and conjunctival sacs; on the hard palate; on the fundus of the eye; and over the chest, neck, shoulders, and anterior axillary folds. Other measures that may help to determine fat emboli are (1) a drop in the patient's hematocrit, (2) chest radiography may show unevenly distributed areas of pulmonary congestion, (3) arterial blood gas may reveal hypoxia and hypocapnia, (4) ECG may reveal myocardial ischemia and right ventricular strain, and (5) free fat may also be found in the urine when fat emboli affect the kidneys. Between the third and seventh day, the serum lipase level may rise.

Treatment of fat emboli syndrome begins with prevention (i.e., splinting and stabilizing long bone fractures as soon as possible). There is no specific treatment for systemic fat emboli. The primary objective of care is to support the respiratory system to avoid hyproxemia, which is usually accomplished by placing the patient in high Fowler's position and administering oxygen at high concentrations. Oxygen lowers the surface tension of the fat globules and reduces local anoxia. In many instances, controlled volume ventilation with positive end-expiratory pressure (PEEP) may be used to reach PAO2 of 60mm Hg and to assist in decreasing pulmonary edema. Hydrocortisone of 1.0 to 1.5 g/day for the first 2 days may help to reduce lung inflammation and help control cerebral edema. However, specific medications such as low molecular weight dextran, heparin, alcohol, and corticosteroids show no beneficial effect in treating fat emboli (Jaffe, Greco, & Wade, 1996).

Pulmonary Embolism. Pulmonary embolism (PE) is the most common cause of immediate postoperative death in patients who have had a reconstructive procedure on a lower extremity (Jaffe, Greco, & Wade, 1996). It also is a complication that frequently occurs following fractures of the pelvis, hip, and femur. It may occur as early as 2 to 3 days or as late as several weeks after injury. More than 70% of the patients who die from PE do not have the diagnosis considered before their death, and one third die within an hour of onset (Pellino, Polacek, Preston, Bell, & Evans, 1998).

The most common PE in orthopaedic patients is the obstruction of one or more pulmonary arteries by a thrombus (or thrombi), which originates somewhere in the venous system or the right side of the heart, becomes dislodged, and is carried to the lung. An infarction of lung tissue occurs due to the interruption of the lung's

blood supply. More than 95% of thrombi originate in the deep veins of the legs proximal to or at the popliteal vein (Karp & Freedman, 1998), but other sources include the pelvic veins and the right atrium of the heart. A stasis or slowing of the blood flow because of damage to the blood vessel wall (particularly the endothelial lining) and changes in the blood coagulation mechanism are conditions that can lead to the development of a thrombus.

The symptoms of PE are nonspecific and depend on the size of the thrombus, the number of emboli, and the degree and location of the occlusion. A massive embolism at the bifurcation of the pulmonary artery usually produces pronounced dyspnea, sudden substernal pain, rapid and weak pulse, shock, syncope, and even sudden death. If one or more branches of the right or left pulmonary arteries are obstructed, the patient usually experiences dyspnea, mild substernal pain, anxiety, weakness, and tachycardia from the pulmonary infarction. The patient may also have a fever, cough, and hemoptysis. When the terminal pulmonary arteries are occluded, a pleuritic type of pain, a cough, and hemoptysis develop. Multiple small emboli can lodge in the terminal pulmonary arterioles and produce multiple small infarctions, giving a clinical picture similar to bronchopneumonia. In some instances, however, the condition presents very few symptoms. However, probably the most common symptoms of PE are the sudden onset of unexplained dyspnea and pleuritic type chest pain. Diagnostic evaluation may include arterial blood gases, chest roentgenograms, electrocardiogram (ECG), pulmonary angiography, ventilation-perfusion scan, and tests for deep vein thrombosis.

The best treatment is prevention. Every effort should be directed toward preventing venous stasis by keeping the patient well hydrated, doing active and passive exercises, and beginning ambulation as early as possible. Patients may wear elastic stockings with graded pressure to increase blood flow to the deep leg veins, and intermittent external pneumatic compression leggings that intermittently inflate in an ankle-to-thigh pattern to promote venous return. Anticoagulation therapy (e.g., heparin, warfarin, low-molecular dextran, and aspirin) and thrombolytic therapy that has proven effective in myocardial infarctions (streptokinase and urokinase) may also be used. Treatment for patients who are unable to take anticoagulants or for whom anticoagulants are contraindicated may include such procedures as a pulmonary embolectomy (to extract emboli from the pulmonary artery) or the insertion of an inferior vena caval filter via the femoral vein (that traps emboli, preventing their traveling through the pulmonary circulation).

Posttraumatic Syndrome. Posttraumatic syndrome is a psychological reaction to trauma. Although it is not directly due to a fracture, it needs to be addressed as a fracture-related complication. Posttraumatic syndrome or posttraumatic stress disorder is the development of characteristic symptoms after a psychologically stressful event that is considered outside the range of normal human experience (Carpenito, 1993). Most commonly, the characteristic symptoms occur as the result of experiencing rape, combat, a motor vehicle crash, or a natural catastrophe. Symptoms that commonly occur with posttraumatic disorder include intrusive thoughts and dreams (in the hospital the patient may experience nightmares and try to deal with them by avoiding sleep), phobic avoidance reaction (avoidance of activities that arouse recollections of the traumatic event), heightened vigilance, exaggerated startle reaction, generalized anxiety, and societal withdrawal. In determining if the patient is suffering from posttraumatic disorder, the nursing assessment must also include an evaluation of the patient's pretrauma history, the trauma itself, and posttrauma functioning.

The goal for nursing care is to try to help the patient organize and begin to integrate the experience in order to return to their pretrauma level of functioning as soon as possible. There is a wide range of interventions that can be utilized. One method is to utilize crisis intervention strategies to help reduce the patient's stress and anxiety in order to begin to work on the problem. Another is establishing a trusting and sharing relationship so the patient can talk about what they are experiencing and about the accident/trauma. In order to develop this relationship, the nurse may need to share that some individuals who have experienced that same trauma as the patient develop a number of symptoms (and list a few you believe the patient is having). A third approach is to educate the patient and family about stress management. Patients must be assured that they are all right, that they are not losing their mind, and that their situation can be resolved. The patient, family, and significant other may be aware that posttraumatic stress disorder occurs with military personnel as the result of combat, but most are not aware that it can also occur as the result of experiencing any traumatic situation outside the range of normal human experience. Posttraumatic stress disorder may be acute, chronic, or delayed.

Compartmental Syndrome. One of the most devastating complications following an injury to an extremity is ischemic muscle necrosis and subsequent contractures. In 1881, Richard von Volkmann reported the first account of a posttraumatic muscle contracture of acute onset, with increasing deformity despite splinting and passive exercises (see Volkmann's Ischemic Contracture under the Care of a Patient with a Supracondylar Humeral Fracture and Side Arm Traction in Chapter 6). He argued that the paralysis and contracture of limbs "too tightly bandaged" resulted from ischemic changes of the muscles, which was later confirmed by Jepson with his research on laboratory animals. Since that time, physicians have become increasingly aware of the many varied circumstances in which increased

tissue pressure can compromise the microcirculation (Pellegrini, Reid, & Evarts, 1996).

Compartmental syndrome is defined as a condition in which the circulation or function of tissues within a closed space is compromised by increased pressure within that space. A compartmental syndrome is a condition in which high pressure within a closed fascial space (or muscle compartment) reduces capillary blood perfusion below the level necessary for tissue viability. Compartmental syndromes develop in skeletal muscles enclosed by relatively noncompliant osseofascial boundaries. A buildup of pressure within the muscle compartment is not easily dissipated because of the inelasticity of the fascia. If pressure remains high for several hours, normal muscle and nerve function is jeopardized, myoneural necrosis results, and permanent loss of function and limb contracture may occur. A prompt diagnosis of the condition and decompression of the compartment are essential to reinstate capillary perfusion and prevent irreversible sequellae. It is essential that the nurse look for the signs and symptoms of increased compartmental pressure: (1) pain, (2) pain on passive motion, (3) paresthesia, (4) paralysis, and (5) pulselessness. (For a more in-depth presentation of the symptoms and nursing care, see the Care of a Patient with a Fractured Tibia and a Long Leg Cast in Chapter 5.)

Although the clinical symptoms should be familiar to all clinicians, the clinical presentation of compartment syndrome is often indefinite and confusing, and delays in diagnosis occur even when health care providers are aware of the signs and symptoms. When compartmental syndrome is suspected, constricting casts or circular dressings must be removed immediately. Because the diagnosis of compartmental syndrome is often difficult based on clinical grounds alone, measures were developed to measure the intracompartmental tissue pressures. Whitesides and associates advocated the use of a simple pressure-measuring device, consisting of a needle and plastic tubing filled with saline solution and air, attached to a mercury manometer (Fig. 4–12); they also established tissue pressure measurement criteria as determinants of the need for a fasciotomy. Whitesides and associates believe that a fasciotomy usually is indicated when the tissue pressure rises to 40 to 45 mm Hg in a patient who has a diastolic blood pressure of 70 mm Hg and any signs or symptoms of a compartment syndrome (Pellegrini, Reid, & Evarts, 1996). Intracompartmental pressure monitors are also available from orthopaedic supply companies.

Early decompression of the intracompartmental spaces can be accomplished by a fasciotomy, which allows the muscles to swell out of their tight fascial enclosure. It is essential to decompress all tight compartments. The four compartments of the lower leg (superficial posterior, peroneal, anterior, and deep posterior compartments) are most frequently involved, but compartmental syndromes can occur in the forearm, hand, arm, shoulder, thigh, and buttocks (Fig. 4–13).

Figure 4–12   Mercury manometer for testing intracompartmental tissue pressures.   *(Rockwood, C.A., et al. (1996). Rockwood & Green's Fractures in Adults. 4th ed. Philadelphia: Lippincott-Raven.)*

Figure 4–13   Anatomy of the compartments of the thigh, lower leg, upper arm, and forearm.   *(Rockwood, C.A., et al. (1996). Rockwood & Green's Fractures in Adults. 4th ed. Philadelphia: Lippincott-Raven.)*

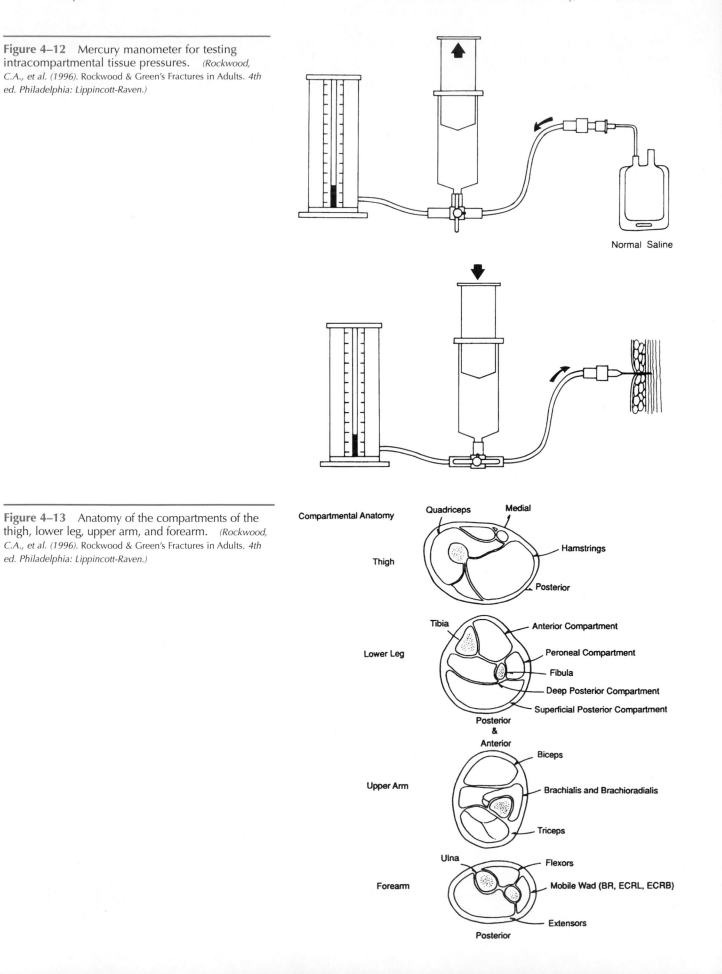

Normal Saline

Compartmental Anatomy

Thigh — Quadriceps — Medial — Hamstrings — Posterior

Lower Leg — Tibia — Anterior Compartment — Peroneal Compartment — Fibula — Deep Posterior Compartment — Superficial Posterior Compartment — Posterior & Anterior

Upper Arm — Biceps — Brachialis and Brachioradialis — Triceps

Forearm — Ulna — Flexors — Mobile Wad (BR, ECRL, ECRB) — Extensors — Posterior

Neurological Complications. A variety of neurological complications may occur, especially in long bone fractures. In general, satisfactory reduction of the fracture relieves the stress placed on nerves, because most nerve injuries following fractures are due to stress rather than laceration. Fractures of the humerus, particularly displaced fractures of the distal third, can compress the radial nerve. When nerve loss is complete and recovery has not occurred within a few weeks following fracture reduction, exploratory surgery may be necessary to try to relieve the symptoms. Lesions of the sciatic nerve, especially of the perineal branch, are associated with fracture dislocations of the hip in which a fracture fragment from the posterior acetabulum is driven into the sciatic nerve. Such fragments need to be surgically removed. Damage to the perineal branch of the sciatic nerve can also occur in fractures of the tibia and fibula, particularly proximal fractures of the fibula. The primary role of the nurse is to be alert to possible neurological abnormalities. For a discussion on how to assess neurological function, see Chapter 2.

Infections. An infection at a fracture site can cause poor fracture healing, nonunion, or malunion. Any fracture can become infected, but open fractures are particularly susceptible to infection. If an infection involves an internal fixation or prosthesis, the device may need to be removed, leaving a disability rather than a functional bone. Infections of the bone are extremely difficult to eradicate, so prevention must be the goal.

A patient with an open fracture is taken to the operating room where the wound is cleansed, debrided, and irrigated. Devitalized bone fragments are removed, the fracture is reduced, and internal or external fixation is used to stabilize the fracture. At the time of surgery, cultures are taken for sensitivity studies. Heavily contaminated wounds may be left open and later closed by suturing or by autogenous skin or flap grafts.

The most common infections are osteomyelitis, tetanus, and gas gangrene. (For more information on osteomyelitis, see Chapter 3.) Tetanus is caused by the bacillus *Clostridium tetani*, which is found in soil, especially where horses and cattle are present. The organism usually enters the body through penetrating or crush wounds. The symptoms usually occur 4 to 21 days after contamination, with an average of 10 days. Therapy usually consists of tetanus immune globulin (TIG) and penicillin G (or an alternative antibiotic). Prophylactic treatment is the debridement of the wound and the administration of a toxoid booster injection for patients previously immunized, or separate tetanus toxoid and TIG injections for nonimmunized patients. Gas gangrene is a severe infection caused by several species of gram-positive clostridia that may complicate trauma, open fractures, contusions, and lacerated wounds by producing exotoxins that destroy tissue. The organisms are anaerobic and spore forming and are found normally in soil and in the human intestinal tract. They grow primarily in deep wounds where the oxygen supply is reduced, a situation enhanced by the presence of foreign bodies or necrotic tissue. Those anaerobic bacilli are highly resistant to heat, cold, sunlight, drying, and many chemical agents. Because they normally inhabit the intestinal tract, they are likely to be the infecting organisms in thigh wounds and following amputations, especially when the patient is incontinent of feces.

Gas gangrene may be prevented if all devitalized and infected tissue is thoroughly debrided to render the wound unsuitable for the growth of *Clostridium*. Penicillin may be administered intravenously as a preventive measure. If gas gangrene develops, hyperbaric oxygen (i.e., oxygen administered under greater than atmospheric pressure in specially designed chambers) may be used. That increases the dissolved oxygen in the arterial system by increasing the partial pressure of oxygen inhaled by the patient and reduces toxin formation and microbial reproduction.

Malunion. Malunion is when union occurs with the fragments in a deformed or angulated position and is usually the result of inadequate reduction and immobilization. If malunion is severe, it may become necessary to manually or surgically manipulate the fracture site, realign the fragments, reimmobilize the fracture site, and allow the bone to recalcify.

Delayed Union. Delayed union (or delayed healing) is used to describe a fracture that is slow to heal but does demonstrate some calcification. Fractures heal at different rates depending on various factors (e.g., comminution, site, blood supply). Most fractures, however, unite by 4 to 6 months or show progressive healing on radiographs. Some reasons for delayed union are infection, inadequate immobilization or reduction that allows movement at the fracture site, inadequate blood supply, or metabolic disturbances that affect the protein and the vitamins available for bone healing. Treatment consists of discovering the cause and correcting the underlying problem. Some physicians may utilize a bone stimulator to stimulate calcification of the bone.

Nonunion. Nonunion (Fig. 4–14) is when there is an arrest of the fracture repair process and there is no further potential for fracture union after 9 months (Rosen & Koval, 1998). Nonunion may occur if (1) the space between the fracture fragments is too large for either callus or bone cells to bridge, (2) muscles or fascia are between the fracture fragments, (3) the callus is broken or torn by excessive activity, (4) an infection develops, (5) there is inadequate blood supply to the fracture site, and (6) there is marked dietary deficiency. Occasionally, nonunion occurs with no apparent reason.

With a nonunion, there is usually pain, tenderness, fracture motion, and increased heat at the fracture site. However, when a nonunion has been present for a long time and is hypertrophic, there may be little pain and no motion on physical examination. Treatment for nonunion includes surgical intervention to debride and revise the fracture ends and implant a bone graft (Fig. 4–15). In recent years, a noninvasive

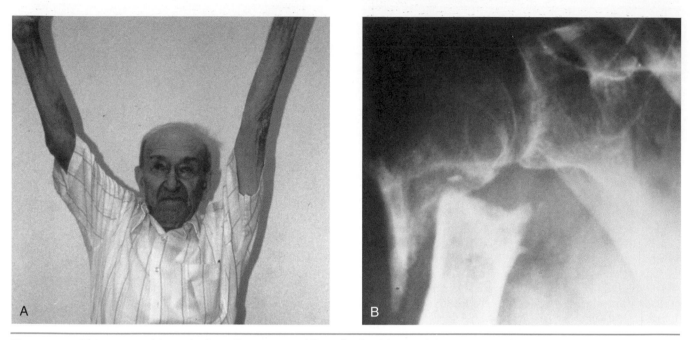

Figure 4–14   This 75-year-old man had excellent motion of the right shoulder (A), despite a proximal humeral nonunion (B).   *(Koval & Zuckerman (1998). Fractures in the Elderly. Lippincott-Raven.)*

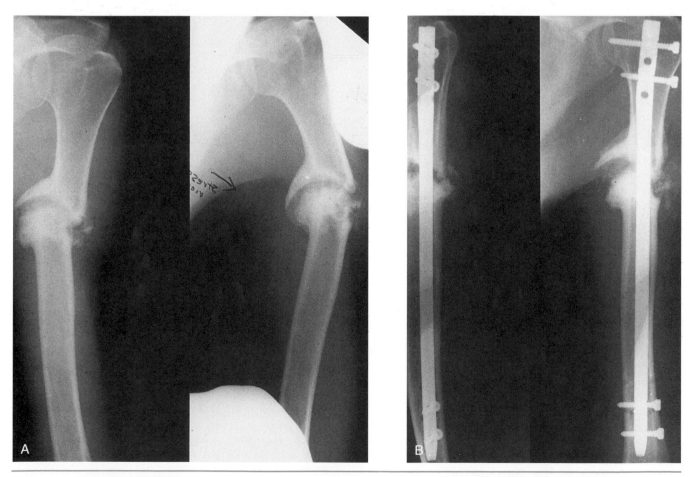

Figure 4–15   (A) Long-standing painful humeral nonunion with motion on stress testing. (B) Stabilization by locked intramedullary nailing and open bone grafting.   *(Koval & Zuckerman (1998). Fractures in the Elderly. Lippincott-Raven.)*

method, electrical stimulation, has proven very effective in treating nonunion (though not avascular nonunions). This method employs an electrode placed over the patient's skin or cast. Patients use the device 10 to 12 hours a day at home, usually while they sleep. The treatment may continue for 3 to 8 months.

Avascular Necrosis. Avascular necrosis may occur from infection or when bone loses its blood supply. It may be idiopathic or follow a fracture or dislocation. An interruption of blood supply may be an unpreventable complication that occurs at the time of injury. Healing can occur in the presence of avascular necrosis when dead bone is reabsorbed and replaced by new bone, but the patient usually develops a painful arthritis later.

Avascular necrosis is particularly common following fractures of the head and neck of the femur. The blood supply to the head and neck may be disrupted by an injury to the blood vessels, and bone death can result. To permit weight bearing, the head of the femur is removed and replaced by a prosthesis.

SYSTEMIC EFFECTS OF IMMOBILITY

RESPIRATORY COMPLICATIONS

Recumbency, drugs used for pain relief that depress respiration, a decrease in the body's need for oxygen, and the resistance of the bed against the chest wall are some of the factors that can lead to respiratory complications. Limited movement of the chest wall, collection of secretions, creation of dead spaces in the lung, and collapse of alveoli can lead to stasis pneumonia, pneumothorax, and oxygen–carbon-dioxide imbalance. Patients recovering from hip surgery may have added respiratory manifestations due to circulatory problems such as pulmonary embolism or fat embolism discussed earlier in this chapter.

The best method of treatment is prevention and quick observation of abnormalities. The procedures of turning, coughing, and doing deep-breathing exercises are essential to facilitate respiratory hygiene. Elevating the head of the bed assists the patient in coughing and doing deep-breathing exercises. When the patient turns to the side, give a vigorous back rub to stimulate circulation, including some clapping and vibration to loosen secretions if the patient's condition allows. Keeping the patient well hydrated assists in bringing up secretions. Other techniques to help inflate the lungs and promote gas exchange are incentive respiratory devices (e.g., spirometers) and intermittent positive pressure breathing (IPPB) machines.

CIRCULATORY COMPLICATIONS

The majority of adverse effects that occur within the circulatory system as the result of immobility include postural hypotension, increased risk of deep vein thrombus, and diminished workload capacity. If it is a surgical patient, there may also be circulatory overload from intravenous fluids. The body's first circulatory reaction to being placed on bed rest is to increase its circulating blood volume, which shifts extracellular fluid to the venous system. In turn, the increased venous volume stimulates volume receptors in the right atrium of the heart that normally inhibit antidiuretic hormone and aldosterone, leading to diuresis and a reduction in plasma volume over 2 to 4 weeks of immobilization.

POSTURAL HYPOTENSION
Postural hypotension (orthostatic hypotension or orthostatic intolerance) occurs when the patient is on prolonged bed rest and the muscles and blood vessels in the lower extremities lose their tone. The veins in the lower extremities will then accept a large volume of blood when the patient stands. That large amount of blood in the lower extremities deprives the other parts of the body, especially the brain, of an adequate blood supply and can cause the patient to become dizzy. Thus, getting the patient up after a period of immobility results in a significant increase in the heart rate (due to a reduction in cardiac output and stroke volume as a result of decreased circulating volume), and within a few minutes the patient will faint if maintained in the erect position. Additional symptoms that may occur include tachycardia, nausea, and diaphoresis.

In an effort to keep or develop good muscle tone and therefore more efficient vascular return, have the patient do active flexion of all muscle groups, particularly in the lower extremities (e.g., quadriceps and gluteal setting, ankle dorsiflexion, and plantarflexion [i.e., ankle pumps]). Other procedures to help reduce the effect are to have the patient sit on the side of the bed for a few minutes before ambulating, or to use a tilt table. Exercises in turning and lifting with the aid of the trapeze increase general circulation and should be encouraged.

VENOUS STASIS
When a patient is immobile, venous return is slowed, partly because of the decreased muscular activity in the lower extremities that would normally assist the return of blood from the legs back to the heart. When the walls of the vessels lose their tone, there may be stasis of some of the heavier components in the blood leading to inflammation of the veins and the formation of clots (thrombi). Thrombophlebitis, intravascular clotting in an inflamed vein, can easily occur in patients postoperatively. Thrombophlebitis and the formation of thrombi can lead to pulmonary emboli, which are discussed in further detail later in this section.

Measures used to help prevent venous stasis are leg movement, leg exercises, and assisting the patient in changing positions. Pneumatic or elastic stockings are usually utilized. They support the venous circulation and help to prevent dependent edema. The stockings must go from the toe to the groin and be the correct size, tight enough to assist with venous return but not so tight as to be constricting to the skin, nerves, and

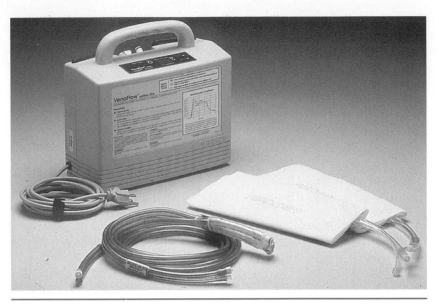

Figure 4–16   Sequintial pneumatic stocking.   *(Courtesy of Aircast, Inc.)*

vascular system. The stockings should be removed for one half to one hour mornings and evenings, and the legs, especially the heels, checked for any redness. The patient needs at least two pairs of stockings so they can be changed and cleansed.

Another measure employed is the use of anticoagulation therapy (e.g., heparin, warfarin, low-molecular dextran, and aspirin). With this treatment, the nurse should observe for signs of bleeding, especially around the site of the incision. That area should also be checked for edema, hardness, and increased temperature, which could indicate a hematoma. Keep the patient well hydrated, as patients with dehydration will have more problems with venous stasis.

DEEP VEIN THROMBOSIS

Deep vein thrombosis (DVT) is a common complication of orthopaedic surgery, occurring in 40% to 60% of patients not receiving prophylactic anticoagulants following hip fractures (Karp & Freedman, 1998). A DVT of the iliac, femoral, or popliteal veins is suggested by unilateral pedal edema, warmth, and erythema. In addition, there may be tenderness along the course of the vein, with a palpable chord. Diagnosis in the orthopaedic patient may be difficult, especially in patients who may have swelling secondary to the orthopaedic procedure. The gold standard of diagnosis is a venogram; however, in most instances, the diagnosis can be made by B-mode ultrasonography, impedance plethysmography, or phleborrheography (Pellino, Polacek, Preston, Bell & Evans, 1998).

Treatment of DVT is aimed at preventing further progression of the clot and possible pulmonary embolus. The patient should be placed on bed rest with the leg elevated to decrease swelling. Ensure that the affected leg is not rubbed or massaged, and apply heat as prescribed. Full course anticoagulation with heparin should be instituted, followed by oral warfarin for

about 3 to 6 months. (NSAIDs are not usually given along with anticoagulants, because doing so increases the anticoagulant effects.) The prothrombin time should be therapeutic for 4 to 5 days before stopping heparin, because the full anticoagulant effect of warfarin is delayed. Laboratory values need to be monitored for clotting times. Record bilateral calf or thigh circumferences every shift. Assess the color and temperature of the involved extremity every shift. The application of elastic stockings from toe to groin assists with venous return, but the stockings need to be removed for at least one-half hour twice a day. Sequential pneumatic compression devices (Fig. 4–16) are special pneumatic inflatable sleeves applied to the legs that provide for the cyclic emptying and refilling of leg veins.

Many methods are available for prophylaxis of DVT. These include the use of heparin, either minidose (5,000 units every 12 hours subcutaneously) or full dose (given either subcutaneously or intravenously in a dose sufficient to raise the partial thromboplastin time to 1.5 times control); aspirin; low-molecular-weight dextran; and warfarin. When using warfarin, 10 mg is given orally the night before surgery; dosing of warfarin is then determined nightly to maintain the prothrombin time at 1.5 times control until the patient is fully ambulatory.

CIRCULATORY OVERLOAD

Intravenous fluids ordered postoperatively provide a method to administer antibiotics and to keep the patient hydrated until oral fluid intake is adequate. The general rate of flow is usually 80 to 100 cc per hour. It may be advisable (based on the assessment of the patient) to run the intravenous fluids more slowly to prevent circulatory overload and strain on the heart, which may have a limited cardiac reserve. That is especially true in some elderly patients. Encourage oral fluids, in small portions, as soon as possible to reduce the need for IV fluids after the initial 24 to 48 hours.

GASTROINTESTINAL COMPLICATIONS

PARALYTIC ILEUS

Paralytic ileus is not an infrequent complication of immobility following surgery or trauma. It involves an absent or diminished peristalsis of the bowel due to the traumatic disturbance of the autonomic nervous system. However, there is no physical obstruction or interruption of blood supply to the intestines. Prophylactically, intravenous fluids and minimal oral fluids are utilized until peristalsis is established after surgery. To stimulate bowel sounds, abdominal setting exercises are done from the supine position. With hand on the abdomen, the neck and shoulder are raised far enough to tighten the stomach muscles. Depending on the patient's age and general musculature, the exercise can be made more vigorous by lifting the head and shoulders even farther. If no actual flexion of the spine is desired, the exercise can be done by only lifting the head and neck off the pillow just enough to tighten the stomach and abdominal muscles. An exercise that puts even less strain on the body involves tightening the abdominal muscles for a count of 3 and then relaxing for a count of 3. If a paralytic ileus should occur, the gastrointestinal tract is rested by allowing nothing by mouth and using intravenous fluids to prevent dehydration. A heating pad on the abdomen may be used to increase circulation in the area. A rectal tube may be used to help reduce distention, and a nasogastric tube may be necessary. The complication is usually resolved within 72 hours.

CONSTIPATION

Constipation is a potential problem for most surgical and immobile patients because of their decreased mobility and drug therapy (e.g., sedatives and pain medications). Elderly patients are at increased risk because the aging process slows bowel function. The usual preventive measures are increased fluid intake, a diet with increased roughage and fiber but fewer carbohydrates, exercises in bed, and ambulation as allowed. Stool softeners are usually ordered, but laxatives and enemas are almost invariably indicated.

GENITOURINARY COMPLICATIONS

Lower urinary tract infection is one of the most common problems of the aged, and immobile patients are potential candidates. Both men and women are susceptible. Older men usually have an enlarged prostate and an atonic decompensated bladder. Women may have interstitial cystitis and a contracted bladder. Older women may also have stress incontinency due to a prolapsed uterus or, when on prolonged bed rest, may have urine collect in their vagina.

To help prevent infection, give an acid-ash diet and encourage fluids, based as much as possible on preferences, to keep the urine acidic and to facilitate voiding. Assist with bedpan use on a schedule (even during the night) to prevent bladder distention and problems with overflow incontinence. Getting the patient out of bed to use a bedside commode or the bathroom facilitates a more complete emptying of the bladder. Every effort must be made to avoid having to use a catheter. If that is not possible, include a program for cleansing around the catheter and the meatus. The meatus area provides a good medium for bacterial invasion and subsequent infection.

MUSCULOSKELETAL COMPLICATIONS

A contracture, the inability to passively stretch a muscle, is a serious and permanent deformity that can easily develop in an inactive patient. The beginning stages of a contracture have been known to develop within 36 hours after injury. Keeping the patient in correct alignment, encouraging independent movement as much as possible, and doing exercises help to prevent contractures. Both active and passive exercises of all joints must be encouraged. There should be frequent changes of position with appropriate joint support and correct alignment. The feet should be supported with a footboard, flexion pillow, or some other support device, and there should be no pillow under the knees. Make sure the position of the hip, with the head of the bed elevated, differs from the position the hip is in when the patient is lying on a side. All contractures can be prevented.

INTEGUMENTARY COMPLICATIONS

Immobility, especially in older patients, can rapidly lead to pressure areas and skin breakdown. The skin over bony prominences is especially susceptible. It is essential that preventive measures be taken before pressure areas develop. Reposition the patient every 2 hours, using a written schedule for systematic turning and repositioning. Avoid placing the patient in the side-lying position directly on their trochanter. Use positioning devices such as pillows or foam wedges to protect bony prominences, and utilize devices to keep the pressure off the heels of totally immobile patients. Place patients at risk on pressure-reducing devices, such as foam, static air, alternating air, gel, or water mattresses. Discourage the patient from sitting all day with the head of the bed elevated, as this increases pressure on the coccyx. (Sitting on the side of the bed with feet on the floor or being in a chair does not have the same effect on the coccyx.) Encourage fluids and a well-balanced diet. Fluids keep the skin hydrated, and the balanced diet keeps the patient's tissues in a healthy state and thus less susceptible to breakdown from pressure.

ASSISTIVE DEVICES FOR AMBULATION

This section presents upper extremity exercises, measurement techniques, gaits, and maneuvering methods for using assistive devices such as crutches, canes, and walkers. In the treatment of various forms of arthritis, of most lower extremity fractures, after operations on the leg, and immediately following an amputation, assistive devices provide a practical way to get from one place to another. The use of crutches and other assistive devices must be taught, and the learning process should begin early. The patient's motivation to walk, which is influenced by the patient's age, interests, future intentions, and prognosis, is a crucial factor. It is also essential for the patient to develop power in the shoulder girdle and upper extremities to bear the necessary weight while walking.

UPPER EXTREMITY EXERCISES

Performing arm exercises (flexion and extension of the arms) strengthens the muscles in the shoulder girdle and upper extremities so that the patient can use an assistive device for walking. The use of a trapeze, which strengthens the biceps of the arms, is helpful, but the major muscle in the arm that needs strengthening is the triceps. This can be accomplished by the following two exercises. First, the patient, in a sitting position, takes a weight in each hand, flexes both arms, and then extends the hands above the head directly toward the ceiling. The second exercise uses sawed-off crutches or books placed on the bed on each side of the patient. The patient pushes down on the books or crutches and lifts the buttocks off the bed.

Good posture and balance are essential to crutch walking. Before the patient tries to use crutches, he or she should learn balance by standing next to a chair on the unaffected leg. The patient should also wear sturdy shoes (not bedroom slippers) to prevent falls.

AMBULATING WITH CRUTCHES

MEASUREMENT FOR CRUTCHES
Adjustable Wooden or Metal Crutches. Adjustable wooden or metal axillary crutches (Fig. 4–17) are practical because the disease may cause changes in the muscles and joints, or the patient may improve and progress to a different crutch base and gait. There are four ways to make approximate measurements of crutches. If the patient has to be measured for crutches while lying flat in bed, measure from the anterior fold of the axilla to the sole of the foot, and then add 5 cm (2 inches). Another method is to determine the height of the patient and subtract 40 cm (16 inches). If the patient is able to sit up in bed without a back support, have the patient sit up straight and abduct both arms straight out from the body. Ask the patient to flex one arm at the elbow, and then measure across the patient's back from the fingertip to the elbow. The back must not be bowed or hyperflexed. This method can also be utilized if the patient can stand. Another method for a standing patient is to measure 3.75 to 5.0 cm (1 1/2 to 2 inches) below the axillary fold to a point on the floor 10 cm (4 inches) in front of the patient and 15 cm (6 inches) laterally from the small toe. The handgrips should be adjusted to allow the elbows to be at 30 degrees of flexion when the patient is standing.

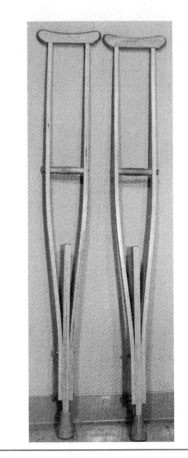

Figure 4–17   A pair of adjustable, wooden axillary crutches. *(Scully & Barnes (1989). Physical Therapy. J.B. Lippincott.)*

Forearm or Lofstrand Crutches. Forearm or Lofstrand crutches (Fig. 4–18) have no axillary bar but have a metal cuff that encloses the forearm and allows the patient to release the handgrip without dropping the crutch. These crutches are constructed of metal and are adjustable. Correct adjustment for the handgrips is the same as in the previous discussion. The cuff should fit comfortably around the forearm below the elbow. The distance between the handgrip and the top of the forearm cuff is determined by measuring from the patient's wrist to one inch above the elbow.

These crutches provide less stability but are less cumbersome and easier to use than axillary crutches, especially on stairs without a railing. They are more expensive than axillary crutches and are better suited for individuals with good to normal upper arm strength and good balance. Individuals using metal forearm or Lofstrand crutches use two- or four-point gaits as is discussed later in this chapter.

Forearm Crutches with Platforms. Platform crutches (Fig. 4–19) permit weight bearing to be distributed over the forearms rather than over the wrist and hands, while providing stability. While using the crutches, the elbows are kept at a constant 90-degree angle. The individual may need help in attaching the arm straps. A two- or four-point gait is used.

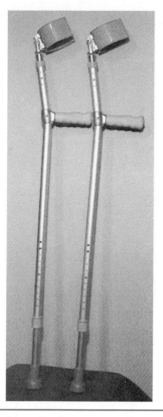

Figure 4–18   Lofstrand or lorearm crutches.   *(Scully & Barnes (1989). Physical Therapy. J.B. Lippincott.)*

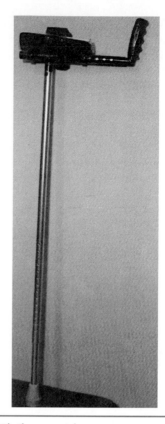

Figure 4–19   Platform crutch.   *(Scully & Barnes (1989). Physical Therapy. J.B. Lippincott.)*

CRUTCH WALKING

Learning crutch walking involves three different areas (Fig. 4–20). First is the stance or starting point from which the individual prepares to walk. Second is the crutch gait that is determined by the patient's general condition and the amount of weight bearing that is allowed on each leg. Third is the maneuvering techniques, where skills are developed to help the patient learn how to get in and out of a chair and to go up and down the stairs.

Stance. The tripod position is the basic crutch stance and gives the strongest and most balanced support. The three elements of the tripod are the patient and the two crutches (which are in front and to the sides of the patient). Because a greater height (or weight) requires a broader base, a taller (or heavier) patient needs a wider stance (with the crutches out farther from the body).

The patient should be taught to support his or her weight on the handpieces. If weight is borne on the axilla, pressure from the crutch can damage the brachial plexus nerves and produce "crutch paralysis." A foam rubber pad on the underarm piece of the crutch eases pressure on the upper arm and thoracic cage.

Crutch Gaits. The selection of a crutch gait depends on the type and severity of the disability, the patient's physical condition, the patient's arm and trunk strength, and the patient's body balance. The nurse must know how much (if any) weight can be placed on the affected side and whether the crutches are being used for balance or for support. Teach the patient two gaits (if possible) so he or she may change from one to the other. For example, a faster gait can be alternated with a slower one. Shifting crutch gaits relieves fatigue, because each gait requires the use of a different combination of muscles. If a muscle is forced to contract steadily without relaxing, the circulation of blood to that muscle is reduced.

All gaits (see Fig. 4–21) begin in the standing, tripod position. If the patient needs assistance or there is any question about safety in crutch walking, the nurse needs to utilize a gait belt and walk beside and slightly behind the patient as he or she ambulates. The more common gaits are

The Four-Point Gait

The four-point gait can be used when supported weight bearing is permitted for both legs. It is safe and gives maximal balance because there are always three points of contact with the floor. It is slow because it requires constant shifting of weight. The sequence is to advance the (1) right crutch, (2) left foot, (3) left crutch, and (4) right foot.

The Two-Point Gait

The two-point gait is faster, because there are only two points of contact at one time. The sequence is to advance (1) right crutch and left foot and (2) left crutch and right foot.

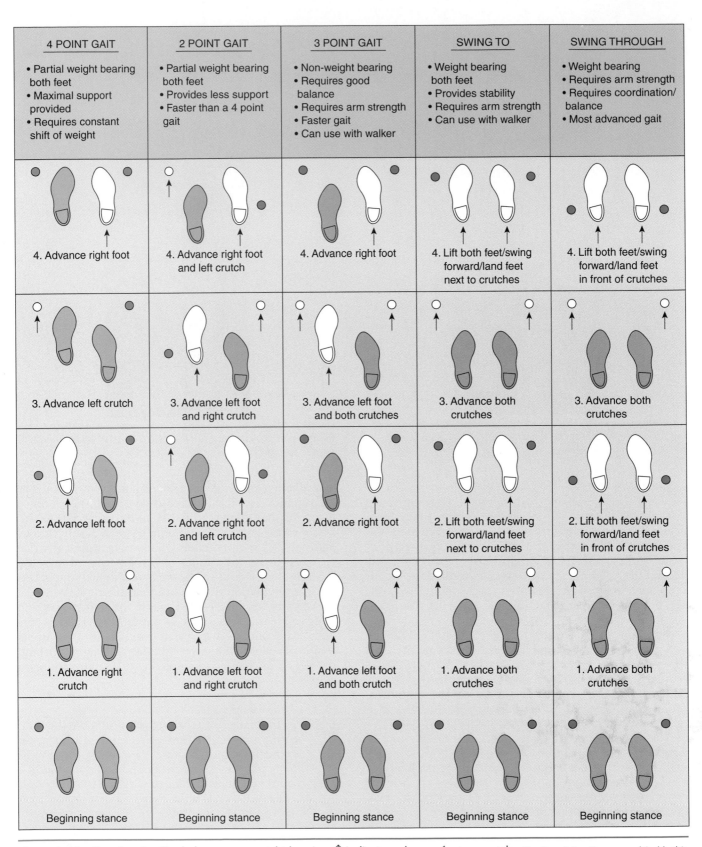

Figure 4–20 Crutch gaits. Shaded areas are weight bearing. ↑ indicates advance foot or crutch. *(Smeltzer & Bare Brunner and Suddarth's Textbook of Medical-Surgical Nursing. Lippincott.)*

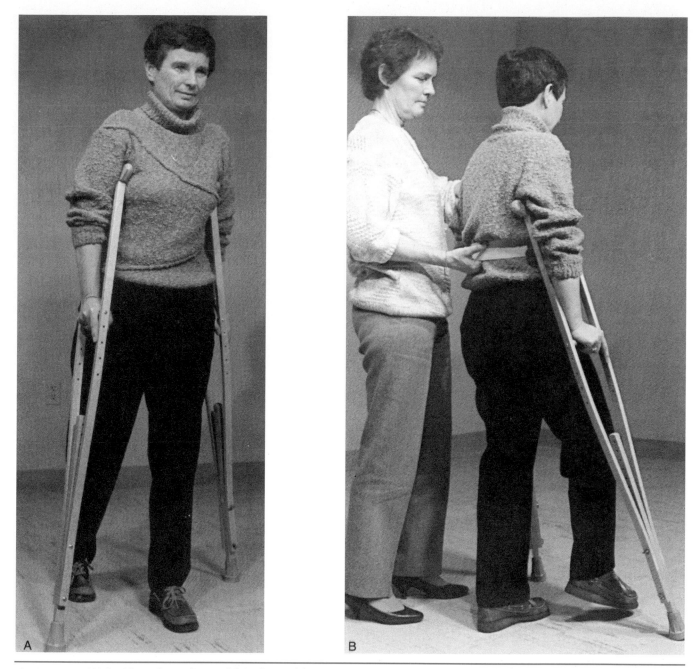

Figure 4–21   (A) Position of crutches and feet during four-point gait. (B) Position of crutches and the assistant during three-point non- or partial-weight-bearing gait.   *(Scully & Barnes (1989). Physical Therapy. J.B. Lippincott.)*

The Three-Point Gait

The three-point gait is a fast gait that requires the most strength and balance. Patients must be able to support their entire body weight on their arms. The sequence is to advance (1) the weaker leg and both crutches simultaneously and then (2) the stronger leg. The three-point gait is utilized when no weight bearing is allowed on one leg (Fig. 4–21).

The Swing-To and Swing-Through Gaits

The swing-to and swing-through gaits are usually employed when the patient's lower extremities are weak or paralyzed. The patient may or may not be wearing long leg braces. The starting position for both gaits is to have the crutches comfortably at the patient's side with the patient standing in a normal stance with feet together. The swing-to gait is used by patients who not only have weakened leg muscles but also have poor abdominal and back muscles, which make it more difficult to regain and maintain balance once they have moved forward. In the swing-to gait, the patient moves both crutches forward, lifts the body by transferring the weight to the crutches, and swings up to the crutches. The patient then straightens and stabilizes the body before once more placing the crutches forward. The swing-through gait is utilized by patients who are better able to stabilize themselves. The patient places the crutches forward, swings the body (with both feet together) past the crutches, and then straightens and balances the body before moving the crutches forward again.

Maneuvering Techniques. Maneuvering techniques are essential skills the patient must learn in order to ambulate safely. They involve going down and up stairs and getting in and out of a chair. These two skills can then be adapted for other needs the patient may have.

Going Down and Up Stairs

To go down stairs, the patient should begin by going to the forward edge of the top step. The patient should then advance the crutches and the weaker or affected leg to the next lower step by tilting the pelvis and bending the unaffected leg at the knee and hip. Once the crutches are safely placed on the lower step, the stronger or unaffected leg is advanced. In that way, the stronger or unaffected leg and the arms share the work of lowering the body's weight to the next step. If there is a handrail on the stairs, the patient places both of the crutches in one hand and grips the handrail with the other while going through the same sequence.

To go up stairs, the patient should walk forward to about a half-step width away from the lowest step. The patient should then place the weight on his or her hands and lift the stronger or unaffected leg up to the next step. Once that foot is safely on the next step, the affected or weaker leg and crutches are advanced. The arms need to be strong to support the patient's body weight during the move. If there is a handrail, the patient places both crutches in one hand, grasps the handrail, and then follows the same sequence.

There are a number of memory devices that can be used to help the patient remember which foot goes first. Two of them are "strong leg goes up first and comes down last," and "up with the good and down with the bad."

Getting In and Out of a Chair

Patients using crutches need to know how to get in and out of a chair, on and off the toilet, and in and out of a car. The technique used is essentially the same in all three cases. The patient using crutches should walk up to the chair, turn using their crutches (taking small steps), and back up until the back of the unaffected leg touches the seat. The patient should then grip both crutches by the handpieces using the hand on the unaffected side,

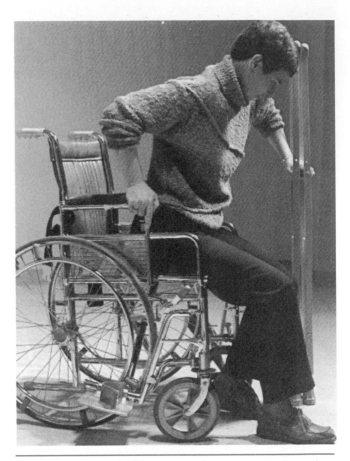

Figure 4–22   Crutch placement and position of patient when rising from the chair.   *(Scully & Barnes (1989). Physical Therapy. J.B. Lippincott.)*

bend at the waist, place the hand on the affected side on the seat, move the affected leg forward, and lower themselves onto the seat gradually. It is safer to place the crutches on the unaffected side because there is less chance that a casted, braced, or weakened leg will knock the crutches away while the patient is trying to sit. Holding the crutches on the unaffected side also assures the patient of ample room to sit, as he or she has made contact with the seat with both the unaffected leg and the hand on the affected side.

To rise from the seat, the patient should reverse the procedure, pushing off against the seat with the hand on the affected side, pulling upward with the other hand, which is holding both crutches, and bearing weight on the unaffected leg (Fig. 4–22). It is also acceptable for the patient to push off while each hand is grasping the handpiece of a crutch and to bear weight on the unaffected leg.

AMBULATING WITH A CANE

A cane is used to help the patient walk with greater balance and support and to relieve pressure on weight-

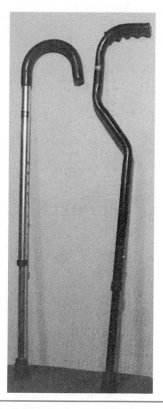

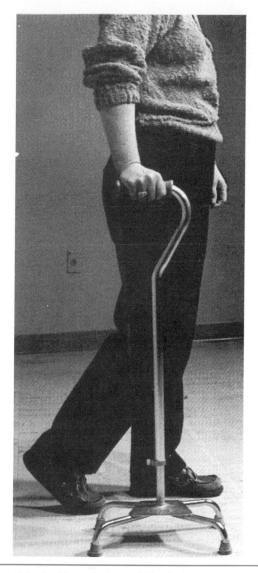

Figure 4–23 (*Left*) Standard cane with the point of support in front of the handle. (*Right*) Cane with the point of support directly below the handle. *(Scully & Barnes (1989). Physical Therapy. J.B. Lippincott.)*

bearing joints. However, canes are the least stable of the assistive devices for ambulation. There are many varieties of canes. A standard cane (Fig. 4–23) has a small base of support. By design, the point of support is in front of the hand, and thus the standard cane is appropriate only for those patients who have good balance and are not required to put a great deal of pressure onto the cane. The shafts of some canes are designed so that the shaft is offset in such a way that the point of support is directly below the hand (see Fig. 4–23). To fit the patient for a cane, flex the patient's elbow at a 25- to 30-degree angle and adjust the cane so that the handle is approximately level with the greater trochanter. An adjustable aluminum cane fitted with a rubber suction tip for traction gives optimum stability and helps the patient walk with greater speed and less fatigue.

Quad canes provides a wide base of support through four legs projecting from the base of the cane. They are available in a wide variety of styles and choices as to the point of support (Fig. 4–24). To fit the patient for a quad cane, use the same approach as with the standard cane.

Also available as an assistive device for ambulation is the Walkane. The Walkane provides greater stability than a quad cane and looks like a cross between a cane and a walker (Fig. 4–25). It is lighter and smaller than a walker, folds for storage, is more versatile than a hemi-

Figure 4–24 Position of cane and limb during gait. *(Scully & Barnes (1989). Physical Therapy. J.B. Lippincott.)*

walker, and is more stable than a cane. However, the base of the Walkane is too large to be used on stairs.

CANE-FOOT SEQUENCE
1. Hold the cane fairly close to the body on the unaffected side.
2. Advance the unaffected leg.
3. Advance the cane with the affected leg.

The patient can use two canes with the four-point and two-point gaits discussed under crutch gaits.

GOING UP AND DOWN STAIRS
1. Step up with the unaffected leg.
2. Then advance the cane and the affected leg.
3. Reverse this procedure for descending steps ("up with the good and down with the bad")

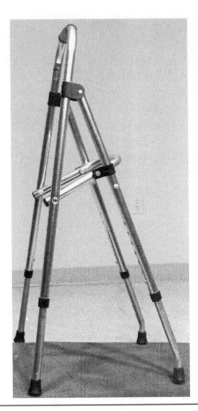

Figure 4–25   The Walkane allows for greater stability than a standard cane or a quad cane.   *(Scully & Barnes (1989). Physical Therapy. J.B. Lippincott.)*

AMBULATING WITH A WALKER

A walker provides more support and stability than a cane or crutches but does not permit a natural walking pattern and is less convenient. A walker is useful for patients who have poor balance or limited cardiovascular reserve or who cannot use crutches. The walker must be wide enough for the patient to walk into it. The height of the walker is adjusted to the patient. With the patient's arms resting on the walker's handgrips, the patient should exhibit 25 to 30 degrees of flexion at the elbows.

There are a variety of walkers. A stationary walker has four legs with rubber tips and no movable parts. There is a folding walker that has the same basic design as the standard walker except that it is hinged, allowing the sides to fold when not in use and the sides to swing out and lock into place when opened. Gliding walkers have metal plates on the tips instead of rubber and can be pushed or slid. Wheeled or rolling walkers have wheels on the front legs that lock when pressure is applied. Reciprocal walkers (Fig. 4–26) have a hinge mechanism allowing one side to be advanced ahead of the other. Some authorities believe it is more stable than a stationary walker. The hemiwalker is a modification designed for someone who has the use of only one arm. The handgrip is placed in the center front of the walker, which allows the person to maneuver the walker with one hand, using a step to gait.

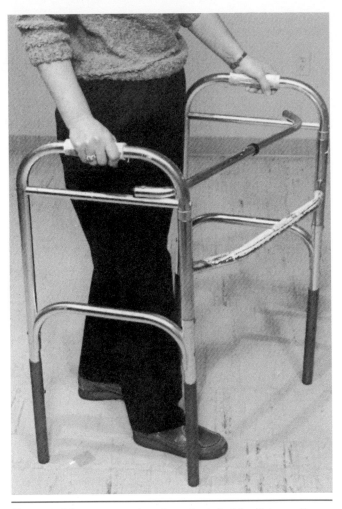

Figure 4–26   Reciprocal walker. The left side of the walker and the right leg move forward together.   *(Scully & Barnes (1989). Physical Therapy. J.B. Lippincott.)*

STATIONARY WALKER

The Four-Point Gait. The four-point gait is often used for patients with weak lower extremities or partial weight bearing on both legs. For safety, it may be necessary to have the nurse steady the walker while the patient is coming to a standing position from the bed or a chair, particularly when the patient is learning to use the walker. Once the patient is standing, the patient should:

1. Hold the walker on the handgrips for stability.
2. Stand straight, without putting all of the body's weight on the walker.
3. Advance the walker in front at arms' length.
4. Advance the right foot into the walker, supporting the body on the walker and left foot.
5. Advance the left foot into the walker, supporting the body on the right foot and walker.
6. Balance the body weight on both feet.
7. Continue by again advancing the walker at arms' length and repeating the foregoing sequence.

The Three-Point Gait. The three-point gait is used for a patient with no weight bearing on one leg:

1. Hold the walker on the handgrips for stability.
2. Stand straight, without putting all of the body's weight on the walker.
3. Placing weight only on the unaffected foot, advance the walker in front at arms' length.
4. Advance both feet while applying no weight on the affected foot.
5. Balance the body weight on the unaffected foot.
6. Lift the walker and place it in front at arms' length and continue.

RECIPROCAL WALKER

The Two-Point Gait. The two-point gait is used for patients with partial weight bearing or weak lower extremities:

1. Hold the walker on the handgrips for stability.
2. Stand with body weight evenly distributed between the walker and both feet.
3. Move the walker's right side forward with your right hand while moving your left foot forward.
4. Move the walker's left side forward with your left hand while moving your right foot forward.
5. Repeat the sequence.

The Four-Point Gait. The four-point gait is used for patients with partial weight bearing who need more stability:

1. Hold the walker on the handgrips for stability.
2. Stand with body weight evenly distributed between the walker and both feet.
3. Move the walker's right side forward with your right hand.
4. Advance your left foot forward.
5. Move the walker's left side forward with your left hand.
6. Advance your right foot forward.
7. Repeat the sequence.

Individuals using a walker can use the procedure described under crutch walking to get in and out of a chair (Fig. 4–27), on or off the toilet, or in and out of a car.

References

Addamo, S. M., & Clough, J. A. A. (1998). Modalities for mobilization. In A. B. Maher, S. W. Salmond, & T. A. Pellino (Eds.). *Orthopaedic nursing* (2nd ed., pp. 323–350). Philadelphia: W. B. Saunders.

Buckwalter, J. A., Einhorn, T. A., Bolander, M. E., & Cruess, R. L. (1996). Healing of the musculoskeletal tissues. In C. A. Rockwood, D. P. Green, R. W. Bucholz, & J. D. Heckman (Eds.). *Rockwood and Green's fractures in adults* (4th ed., pp. 261–304). Philadelphia: Lippincott-Raven.

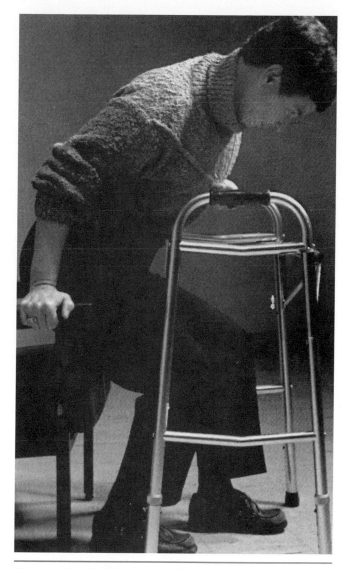

Figure 4–27   Coming to a standing position using a walker. *(Scully & Barnes (1989). Physical Therapy. J.B. Lippincott.)*

Carpenito, L. J. (1993). Nursing diagnosis: Application to clinical practice, Philadelphia: J. B. Lippincott.

Carroll, P. (1993). Deep venous thrombosis: Implications for orthopaedic nursing. *Orthopaedic Nursing, 12*(3), 33–42.

Childs, S. (1993). Avascular necrosis of the bone: The causes and the cures. *Orthopaedic Nursing, 12*(4), 29–34.

D'Eramo, A. L., Sedlack, C., Doheny, M. O., & Jenkins, M. (1994). Nutritional aspects of the orthopaedic trauma patient. *Orthopaedic Nursing, 13*(4), 13–20.

Evanovich, K. (1993). Hypothermia and trauma. *Orthopaedic Nursing, 12*(5), 33–37.

Hager, C. A., & Bencick, N. (1998). Fat embolism: A complication of orthopaedic trauma. *Orthopaedic Nursing, 17*(2), 41–46, 58.

Harkess, J. W., Ramsey, W. C., & Harkess, J. W. (1996). Principles of fractures and dislocations. In C. A. Rockwood, D. P. Green, R. W. Bucholz, & J. D. Heckman (Eds.). *Rockwood and Green's fractures in adults* (4th ed., pp. 1–120). Philadelphia: Lippincott-Raven.

Hefti, D. (1995). Complications of trauma: The nurse's role in prevention. *Orthopaedic Nursing, 14*(6), 9–14.

Karp, A. H., & Freedman, M. L. (1998). Postoperative complications. In K. J. Koval & J. D. Zuckerman. (Eds.). *Fractures in the elderly* (pp. 261–276). Philadelphia: Lippincott-Raven.

Jaffe, K., Greco, J., & Wade, J. (1996). Orthopaedic emergencies and infections. In V. R. Masear (Ed.). *Primary care orthopaedics* (pp. 35–50). Philadelphia: W. B. Saunders.

Lipp, E. J. (1998). Athletic physical injury in children and adolescents. *Orthopaedic Nursing, 17*(2), 17–22.

McCann, S., & Gruen, G. (1997). Fracture blisters: A review of the literature. *Orthopaedic Nursing, 16*(2), 17–22.

McDowell, J. H., McFarland, E. G., & Nalli, B. J. (1994). Use of cryotherapy for orthopaedic patients. *Orthopaedic Nursing, 13*(5), 21–30.

Morrison, R. A. (1994). Early identification of chronic posttraumatic stress disorder by nurse clinicians. *Orthopaedic Nursing, 13*(4), 22–24.

Murdock, M. A. (1994). Injury prevention: A nursing responsibility. *Orthopaedic Nursing, 13*(4), 7–11.

Pellegrini, V. D., Reid, S., & Evarts, C. M. (1996). Complications. In C. A. Rockwood, D. P. Green, R. W. Bucholz, & J. D. Heckman. *Rockwood and Green's fractures in adults* (4th ed., pp. 453–512). Philadelphia: Lippincott-Raven.

Pellino, T. A., Polacek, L. A., Preston, M. A. S., Bell, N. L., & Evans, R. L. (1998). Complications of orthopaedic disorders and orthopaedic surgery. In A. B. Maher, S. W. Salmond, & T. A. Pellino (Eds.). *Orthopaedic nursing* (2nd ed, pp. 212–260). Philadelphia: W. B. Saunders.

Proctor, M. C., Greenfield, L. J., & Marsh, E. E. (1997) Prophylaxis for thromboembolism in elective orthopaedic surgery. *Orthopaedic Nursing, 16*(5), 51–56.

Rosen, H., & Koval, K. J. (1998). Nonunion/malunion. In K. J. Koval & J. D. Zuckerman (Eds.). *Fractures in the elderly* (pp. 261–276). Philadelphia: Lippincott-Raven.

Ross, R. G. (1996). Chronic compartment syndrome. *Orthopaedic Nursing, 15*(3), 23–27.

Synder, P. E. (1998). Fractures. In A. B. Maher, S. W. Salmond, & T. A. Pellino (Eds.). *Orthopaedic nursing* (2nd ed., pp. 663–717). Philadelphia: W. B. Saunders

Thielman, G. T. (1996). Wrapping injuries for support. *Orthopaedic Nursing, 15*(3), 13–17.

Tom, J. (1989). Mobility and ambulatory aids. In R. M. Scully & M. R. Barners (Eds.). *Physical therapy* (pp. 1052–1072). Philadelphia: Lippincott.

Willliamson, M., Jr. (1994). Radiology review: Pediatric forearm fractures. *Orthopaedic Nursing, 13*(3), 65–68.

Wynd, C. A., Wallace, M., & Smith, K. M. (1996). Factors influencing postoperative urinary retention following orthopaedic surgical procedures. *Orthopaedic Nursing, 15*(1), 43–50.

Zavotsky, K. E., & Banavage, A. (1995). Management of the patient with complex orthopaedic fractures. *Orthopaedic Nursing, 14*(5), 53–57.

Chapter
5
Care of Patients with Casts and Splints

A cast is a rigid dressing that circumferentially encircles an extremity. It immobilizes an extremity to keep bone ends in apposition and fractures aligned until calcification occurs. A splint provides rigid support to an extremity while being held in place by a bandage that allows expansion from swelling to occur. Satisfactory immobilization and alignment may initially be obtained in the emergency setting with splinting. Splints are faster and easier to apply than casts, but they tend to loosen with time and require frequent adjustments. Casts provide more effective immobilization but require more skill and time to apply, and there is a higher risk of complications.

Splints and stiffened bandages have been used for immobilization for over two thousand years. Bandages soaked in gum were used by the ancient Egyptians for the immobilization of fractures; bandages stiffened with egg white were popular in the Middle Ages. The use of plaster of Paris as a splinting agent was mentioned in the writings of Rhazes, a ninth century Arabian physician. The advance to "walking plaster" came in 1887, when Krause described the results of 98 fractures of the lower limb treated by this method. However, the use of walking casts was not popular until Böhler, between 1910 and the 1930s, demonstrated their value (Naylor, 1948). Today, plaster of Paris is less frequently used in the application of casts and splints. Plaster casts are being replaced by fiberglass and other lighter and sturdier materials, and plaster splints are being replaced with prefabricated splints made of metal and other materials.

In contemporary practice, fewer patients with a cast or splint are hospitalized. That is due, in part, to new surgical procedures and instrumentations that allow successful reduction and fixation of fractures and consequent early discharge. Most hospitalized patients with a cast have sustained multiple injuries or other disabling conditions. A number of casts once fairly common (e.g., hyperextension body cast, hip spica cast, and shoulder spica cast) are now used rarely, if at all. When they are used, the patient is cared for in an extended care facility or at home with the assistance of home health nurses.

Today, most patients who require an open reduction for an open or closed fracture are admitted to the hospital for the surgical procedure and then discharged once they have recovered from the anesthesia. Immediate postoperative care and cast or splint care are accomplished at home. Patients with closed fractures who have a closed reduction and cast application in a physician's office, an outpatient clinic, or an emergency room are discharged to home. It is essential that nurses having contact with these patients know what to tell them about how to care for themselves and prevent complications.

CASTS

PURPOSE OF CASTS

The purpose of a cast is to immobilize the injured extremity for comfort and to maintain adequate alignment of fractures and/or ligamentous structures until healing occurs (Box 5–1). A cast secures the body part by applying uniform compression on soft tissues in order to (1) correct and prevent deformities, (2) improve function by stabilizing a joint, (3) maintain support and protect realigned bone, and (4) promote healing by allowing ambulation and weight bearing.

Box 5–1
Purpose of Cast

1. To hold bone fragments in reduction and alignment
2. To permit early ambulation and weight bearing
3. To improve function by stabilizing a joint
4. To correct and prevent deformities

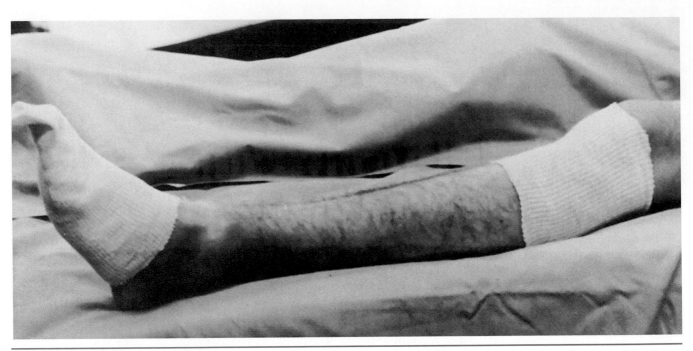

Figure 5–1   It is necessary to use stockinette only at the upper and lower ends of the cast. Not only is this economical, but it also prevents tension of the stockinette over bony prominences that may later give rise to burning pain and even pressure sores. *(Rockwood, C. A., et al. (1996). Rockwood & Green's Fractures in Adults. 4th ed. Philadelphia: Lippincott-Raven.)*

CAST MATERIALS, APPLICATION, AND DRYING

A cast, a temporary immobilizing device, is made of layers of plaster of Paris bandages or of synthetic materials, such as a polyester-cotton knit that is impregnated with polyurethane, fiberglass, or thermoplast. The following section on cast application and drying methods focuses on plaster of Paris casts first and then on fiberglass casts.

PLASTER OF PARIS

Plaster of Paris is an open-weave cotton roll or strip saturated with anhydrous calcium sulfate (a chalky white powder made from gypsum crystals). When moistened, heat is generated as a chemical reaction takes place between the water and the anhydrous calcium sulfate.

Application Method.   Preparation for the application of a cast begins with the psychological and physical preparation of the patient. Explain to the patient, the patient's family, and significant others the purpose and basic steps of cast application and the care of the patient with a cast. Answer questions as clearly and concisely as possible.

Position. Position the patient for the appropriate extremity to be casted. For the upper extremity, positioning usually involves having the patient lie supine. The shoulder is abducted to 90 degrees, the elbow is flexed 90 degrees, and the digits are held up toward the ceiling. Finger traps or an assistant may be used to hold the digits and keep the arm positioned appropriately. Lower-extremity positioning usually involves having the

patient sitting for a short leg cast and supine for either a long cast or a cylinder cast. For the application of the short leg and for some long leg casts, a footrest with a thin metal plate may be used to keep the ankle in neutral position while the cast is applied.

Stockinette. A stockinette is used to make the cast more comfortable and protect the patient from sharp edges of the cast. The stockinette may be applied only at the upper and lower ends (Fig. 5–1), or it may be applied over the entire length of the extremity. The stockinette expands its circumference but will stretch only minimally in length.

Padding. Padding. sometimes called sheet wadding or Webril, is a cotton material that is easily torn and stretched. Apply padding to the portion of the body to be casted after the stockinette and before the casting material. The appropriate width of padding is usually 4, 5, or 6 inches for the lower extremity and 2, 3, or 4 inches for the upper extremity. Apply the padding by rolling distally to proximally as much as possible. Tear the padding to go around joints and to advance up or down the extremity as necessary to obtain the needed coverage. The padding needs to be applied with approximately 50% overlap (Fig. 5–2). Apply an extra layer of padding over the heel or elbow and over the malleoli and other bony prominences to prevent pressure points. For additional protection, felt may be applied over the bony prominences of very slender patients. However, excessive padding causes the cast to fit too loosely, decreases the control over fracture immobilization, and

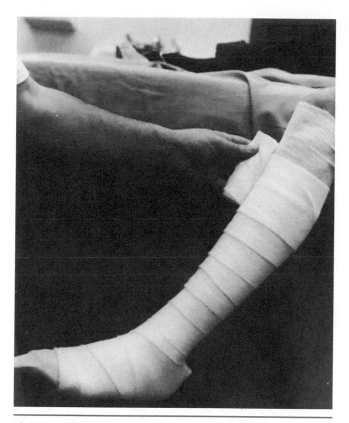

Figure 5–2   Padding should be applied from distal to proximal, taking care to apply the padding evenly. Each turn should be overlapped by 50% of the succeeding turn.
(Rockwood, C. A., et al. (1996). Rockwood & Green's Fractures in Adults. 4th ed. Philadelphia: Lippincott-Raven.)

increases the amount of movement possible within the cast. There is a recent trend toward using less padding. For example, Harkess, Ramsey, and Harkess (1996) state that "the thighs are so well padded by nature that we apply the plaster directly on the stockinette without any padding."

Water. Have a container of water at room temperature (or colder for extra-fast-setting plaster) available for wetting the cast materials. Water that is too warm will cause the plaster to set too rapidly and, more importantly, may burn the patient.

Plaster. Select an appropriate-sized plaster for the extremity to be casted. Usually 3- or 4-inch plaster is used for the upper extremity and 2-inch plaster if the thumb is included in the cast. Four- or 6-inch plaster (and sometimes both) is used for lower-extremity casts Posterior splints are sometimes needed to reinforce a cast.

Plaster Application. Prepare the plaster roll by unrolling the first 2 or 3 inches. Keeping hold of the end, immerse the plaster roll into the container of water until the bubbles stop. With one end in each hand, still keeping the end of the roll free, gently squeeze the water out of the plaster roll. Compress the

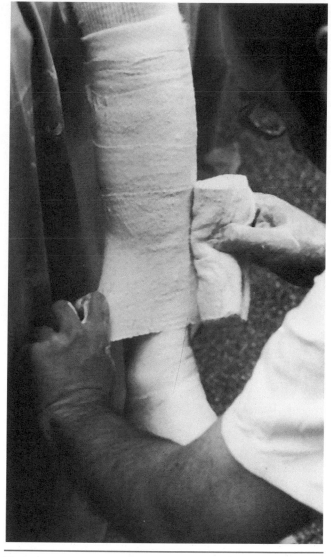

Figure 5–3   The plaster of Paris bandage should be applied in the same direction as the wadding. The roll should be applied with the fingertips and must never be removed from the extremity. To make the bandage conform to the varying circumferences of the arm or leg, tucks should be taken in it with the left hand.   *(Rockwood, C. A., et al. (1996). Rockwood & Green's Fractures in Adults. 4th ed. Philadelphia: Lippincott-Raven.)*

end into the middle until the desired consistency is achieved. Different individuals prefer different consistencies when applying plaster rolls. However, do not squeeze the roll too dry, or you will leave most of the plaster in the water. The plaster is then rolled on the extremity smoothly in a circular motion, beginning distally and proceeding proximally. Never reverse a plaster bandage during application. If one does so, the bandage runs against the grain and cannot be applied easily. The number of rolls depends on the extremity and the desired strength of the cast. Always keep the roll near the extremity to guard against stretching the plaster too tightly. Tucks are taken in the plaster to turn corners or to advance up the extremity (Fig. 5–3).

Plaster rolls overlap 50% of the width of the plaster roll as the application advances along the extremity. Smooth over the applied plaster after each roll is applied so that a strong laminate is formed between the layers (Fig. 5–4). To achieve maximum strength for the cast, rub the cast with wet hands. Avoid the tendency to place more plaster on the flexion surface of the ankle, knee, and elbow as the cast can become excessively thick in these regions. Such additional plaster also puts the patient at risk of thermal injury from the cast.

Add plaster splints to reinforce the extensor surface of the ankle, knee, and elbow if the cast appears too thin, instead of adding another roll of plaster as has been a common practice. Harkess, Ramsey, and Harkess (1996) propose to reinforce a lower-extremity cast with an anterior splint. Figure 5–5 shows a short leg cast that incorporates such a fin-shaped splint. It substantially increases the strength of the cast over the ankle, where the same amount of plaster applied posteriorly would have very little effect.

At the proximal and distal ends of the cast, pull back the stockinette and padding over the layers of plaster, and then roll a layer of plaster over the stockinette and padding to hold them in place. This makes a neat cast edge to help prevent discomfort or injury (Fig. 5–6). After the plaster is applied, trim the cast around the toes and digits (Fig. 5–7). Walking irons and rubber walking heels on weight-bearing leg casts have largely become supplanted by plaster boots or cast shoes.

Cleanse the patient's skin of any plaster. Wearing gloves during the application of a cast is optional. If gloves are not worn, plaster in the hair of the forearm can be more easily removed if sugar is applied to the hands when washing.

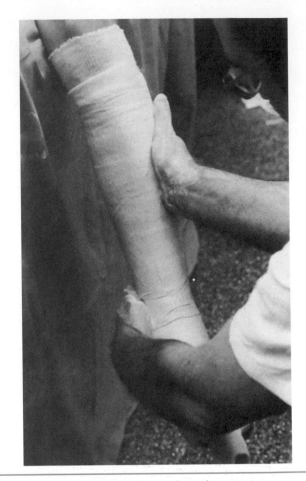

Figure 5–4   When manipulating through a wet cast or rubbing in the turns of the bandage, always use the palms of the hands and thenar eminences and never the fingertips. *(Rockwood, C. A., et al. (1996). Rockwood & Green's Fractures in Adults. 4th ed. Philadelphia: Lippincott-Raven.)*

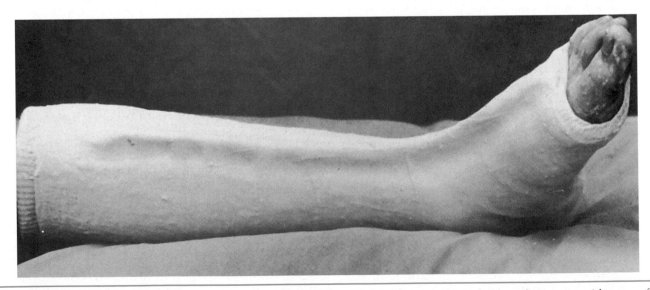

Figure 5–5   To reinforce the cast with a splint, it is much better to apply it in the concavity of an angulation, as an I-beam or fin, than to apply it over a convexity, such as a lamina. Such a fin substantially increases the strength of the ankle, whereas the same amount of plaster applied posteriorly would have very little effect.   *(Rockwood, C. A., et al. (1996). Rockwood & Green's Fractures in Adults. 4th ed. Philadelphia: Lippincott-Raven.)*

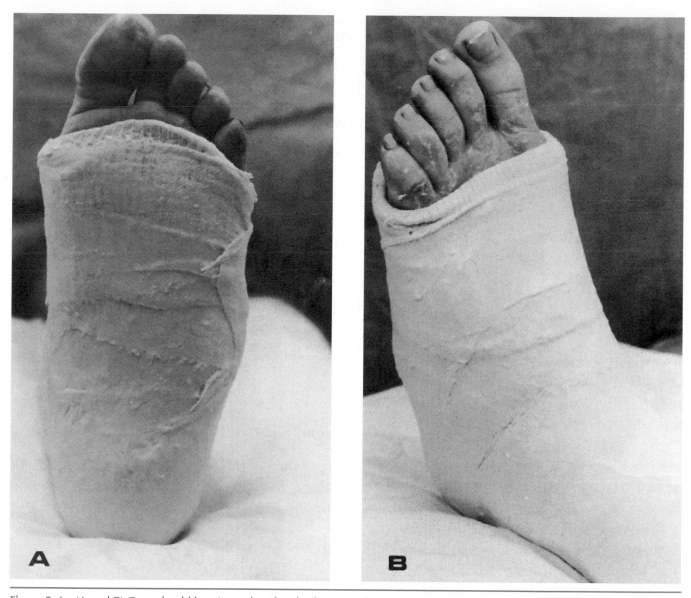

Figure 5–6   (A and B) Casts should be trimmed so that the fingers and toes are free to move. The stockinette is then folded over the edges of the cast and anchored with a plaster of Paris strip. Care should always be taken in make sure that the lateral border of the cast does not impinge on the fifth toe.   *(Rockwood, C. A., et al. (1996). Rockwood & Green's Fractures in Adults. 4th ed. Philadelphia: Lippincott-Raven.)*

Drying Method. A chemical reaction makes the cast warm to hot in the beginning, but the cast soon becomes cold and damp. Expose the cast to the air so it can "breathe" and dry. Do not cover the cast as that would interfere with the drying process. Turn the patient (or reposition the casted extremity) every 2 to 3 hours so the cast will dry evenly. If turning and repositioning do not occur, the cast can be wet on one side and dry on the other. Always move and handle the casted extremity with flat hands (palm of your hand and your fingers together) so that your fingers and thumbs do not cause indentations or pressure areas in the cast. If approved by the facility or the physician, the following methods may be utilized for cast drying. They are (1) a commercial dryer with the heat set at a very low temperature, (2) a heat cradle with a 25-watt bulb, (3) a hair dryer set on low, or (4) an electric fan to circulate the air (but not to blow directly on the cast). The major concern with these methods is that the cast will dry on the outside but not on the inside. Thus, you will have a weak cast that is soggy against the patient's skin and can lead to skin necrosis.

Drying Time. Drying times may differ, depending on the thickness of the cast. As a general rule, allow (1) up to 24 hours for a regular arm or leg cast, (2) 24 to 48 hours for weight-bearing casts, and (3) 36 to 72 hours for large body casts. A number of the newer forms of plaster of Paris may dry more quickly. A dry plaster of Paris cast should be white, shiny, and odorless; and the cast should be hard, firm, and resonant when tapped.

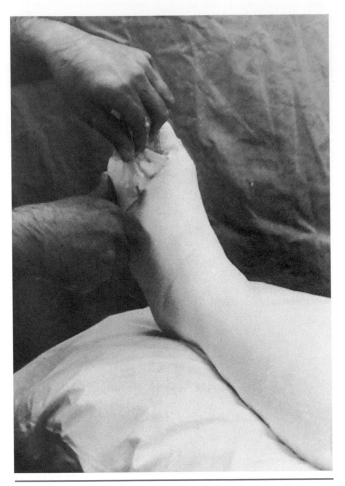

Figure 5–7   In trimming the extremities of plaster of Paris casts, a good method is to brace the thumb against the plaster and hold a sharp knife in the remaining four fingers. Tension is applied to the plaster to be removed by the other hand as the knife cuts.   *(Rockwood, C. A., et al. (1996).* Rockwood & Green's Fractures in Adults. *4th ed. Philadelphia: Lippincott-Raven.)*

Cleansing the Cast. The best approach is to avoid soiling the cast. Discuss ways to prevent soiling the cast with the patient, bearing in mind that this is not always realistic. The cast may be cleansed with a damp cloth and cleanser, but it should not become wet. Remember that the cast is made of plaster. Small stains that cannot be removed may be covered with white shoe polish if the patient does not have an incision or open lesion. Old bleeding through the cast can be covered by applying new casting material.

FIBERGLASS

A fiberglass cast is an open-weave fiberglass tape saturated with polyurethane prepolymer. When soaked in water, it cures to form a light, durable material that is radiolucent. The most popular bandage material is knitted fiberglass and typically has a ratio of 45% polyurethane resin to 55% fiberglass. The prepolymer is methylene bisphenyl di-isocyanate (MDI), which converts to a nontoxic polymeric urea substance. The advantage of the material is that it is strong, lightweight,

and waterproof. (However, most physicians do not recommend that their patients shower with a fiberglass cast on, because the stockinette and padding will take a long time to dry.) The major disadvantages of fiberglass are that it requires skill to handle, is more difficult to mold, and is significantly more expensive than plaster. It is best used for long-term casts and for patients who are particularly "hard" on casts, and it is less used in acute injury cases where frequent cast changes are required.

Application Method. The positioning and the preparation of the patient, both physically and psychologically, follow those discussed under plaster of Paris. The application procedures already described can be followed except (1) a nylon stockinette and padding should be used, (2) each roll of casting should only be opened immediately before using, and (3) gloves are mandatory for all who handle these bandages.

The application of the fiberglass differs from plaster of Paris in that you cannot easily make generous "tucks" in the bandage, so smaller-width bandages must be used (3- to 4-inch width for legs, 2-inch for hand, and 3- to 4-inch for forearm and arm). Fiberglass material conforms more easily if applied spirally, squaring the upper and lower ends by making horizontal turns. The bandage rolls can also be applied with a little more pressure. The cast needs to be applied so as to decrease the amount of trimming needed. Fiberglass casts cannot be cut by the cast knife. A "green" cast can be trimmed using Böhler scissors; when the cast is dry, a saw is usually needed.

Drying Method. An open-air drying method is needed, which takes approximately 7 minutes. However, no weight bearing is allowed for 20 minutes after application. Should a cured fiberglass cast become wet, the stockinette and padding can be dried by judicious use of a hair dryer.

RESHAPING/REMODELING THE CAST

To preserve the purpose of the cast and to maintain patient comfort and prevent injuries, the cast may need to be readjusted or changed. The following are some of the procedures involved.

PETALING THE EDGES

"Petaling the cast" is a method of making the edge of the cast smooth. Only casts without stockinette will usually need to be petaled. Inspect the skin for pressure areas and signs of irritation from rough edges on the cast. Trim the cast edges and smooth out the padding. To prevent irritation or abrasion, petal-shaped strips of adhesive tape or moleskin adhesive may be applied to the exterior surface and rough edges of the cast and anchored smoothly to the interior surface of the cast. To prepare the "petal," use a roll of adhesive tape, unroll a small portion of the tape, and fold the two non-adhesive sides together. For each petal, cut the tape at a 45-degree angle. When each segment of the tape is

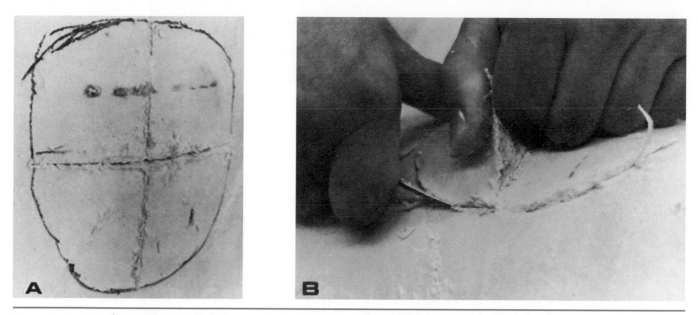

Figure 5–8   (A and B) Cutting a belly hole in a plaster jacket or spica can be tedious, especially when the plaster is hard. The easiest method is to outline the dimensions of the hole with a pencil and then divide the area into four quadrants with a reciprocating plaster saw. The circle is then outlined with a knife along the pencil marks, and the free edges of the quadrant can be pried upward and the periphery cut with the knife. It is always safer to brace the thumb against the cast to prevent the knife from slipping.   *(Rockwood, C. A., et al. (1996). Rockwood & Green's Fractures in Adults. 4th ed. Philadelphia: Lippincott-Raven.)*

unfolded, it will have a sharp point like the point of a petal. The point of the tape goes into the interior surface and reduces the likelihood of a wrinkle developing in the tape that could irritate the skin under the cast.

CUTTING A WINDOW
A window results from cutting out a portion of the cast, usually over a suture line or a pressure area. It is done to change a dressing, check on drainage, check on the skin over a bony prominence when a patient is complaining of pain, or relieve pressure over the abdomen of a patient in a body or spica cast (Fig. 5–8). If the window is removed and a dressing changed, the same amount of dressing must be replaced before the cast window is taped back into place. If the cast window is not to be replaced, felt, sponge rubber, or other materials the size of the hole are placed in the window and held snugly in place while an elastic bandage is applied to provide uniform compression. That is necessary to prevent unnecessary swelling and possible skin necrosis.

WEDGING
Wedging enables the physician to turn and realign the foot portion of a leg cast (though not to correct a lateral shift or rotation). After a closed reduction and cast application, there may be some varus or valgus angulation or posterior bow that needs to be corrected. If the deformity is small, a transverse cut is made, usually one half to two thirds of the way around the cast. The cut cast is then opened up until the angulation is adequately corrected. Once that is done, the cast edges are turned back and corks, blocks of wood, or sheet wadding are placed in the defect. After the wedge materials are

inserted, the cast is then repaired, using a new roll of plaster or fiberglass, while the extremity is held in the corrected position. For larger corrections, a combination of an opening wedge on the concave side and a closing wedge on the convex side is done. Sometimes it is best just to apply a new cast.

SPLITTING
A split is a cut in the cast to help relieve possible neurovascular impingement. When splitting a cast, try not to cut directly over a bony area where there is very little flesh (such as directly over the tibia). Once the cast has been split using a cast cutter, it is sometimes necessary to put something in the split to keep it open.

BIVALVING
Bivalving is when the cast is cut lengthwise into two equal parts. Bivalving a cast is usually done to facilitate care or when a rigid cast is not needed at all times but is used for support or turning. The cast is cut using the procedure that follows for cast removal.

CAST REMOVAL
Position the patient and explain the procedure before starting to remove the cast. Allow the patient time to ask questions. A cast saw (cutter) sounds and looks dangerous, even though it is quite safe because it cuts by vibration. Demonstrate the safety of the cutter by touching it to the palmar surface of your thumb, and then encourage the patient to test it the same way. The patient should be told that patients only feel heat and some pressure during the cutting process. However, if too much

pressure is applied for too long to an area after the cast has been penetrated, the patient can receive a burn.

Start the cast removal by first getting a grip on the cast saw and then applying it to the cast with an even amount of pressure. Placing your thumb on the cast and holding the cast saw with your fingers give you better control over the saw and the amount of pressure you apply. Gentle pressure and the vibrating cast blade allow the blade to penetrate the hard cast. Release the pressure once you feel the blade penetrate the cast. Move along the length of the cast (usually distally to proximally) by applying and releasing the pressure. Remember, avoid keeping pressure on for even a short time once the hard cast has been penetrated, as the patient will feel a hot sensation. Starting distally is usually more comfortable for the patient as the saw is further from the trunk of their body. First, bivalve the cast, usually by cutting along the lateral and medial sides. Try not to cut directly over a bony prominence.

Once the cast is bivalved, you can separate the cast with a cast spreader and cut through the stockinette and padding below with large scissors. Once you have completed cutting through the stockinette and padding, gently remove the anterior portion of the cast. Expect to see old, loose or semiattached skin, what appears to be a large amount of long hair on the extremity, and skin discoloration if there has been bleeding into the tissues. While supporting the joints of the extremity, gently remove the posterior portion of the cast.

The casted extremity may appear slightly smaller than the other extremity, especially if the cast was worn for a long period of time and no muscle-setting or other exercises were done. If another cast is to be applied, gently brush off the old skin, BUT DO NOT WASH THE CASTED EXTREMITY. Washing the extremity will lead to more itching and discomfort under the new cast. If another cast is not to be applied, carefully cleanse the skin. Do not try to remove all of the dead skin. Apply a little oil, and in a couple of days it can easily be washed away. After cast removal, some patients may need an elastic bandage to support the joint for a few days until their muscle strength returns.

GENERAL NURSING CARE FOR THE PATIENT IN A CAST

Nursing care for the patient in a cast should include the following:

1. Assessing neurovascular status
   a. Neurovascular compression
   b. Compartmental syndrome
   c. Volkmann's contracture
2. Assessing for and intervening to relieve pain and pressure
3. Assessing the amount of drainage into the cast
4. Assessing for signs and symptoms of tissue necrosis or infection
5. Turning the patient every 2 hours during the day and every 4 hours at night
6. Keeping the extremity elevated on pillows to prevent swelling
7. Keeping the casted extremity off a hard surface
8. Utilizing ice as needed to prevent or reduce swelling
9. Providing skin care to prevent irritation and dryness
10. Encouraging the patient to do as many activities of daily living as possible
11. Setting up an exercise program to prevent the effects of immobility
12. Setting up an exercise program for the affected extremity
13. Providing for patient self-care and home care activities
14. Determining the patient's emotional adjustment to wearing a cast

PATIENT TEACHING

The following list includes tasks that should be included in patient teaching:

1. Discuss the nature and purpose of the cast.
2. Explain exercises and positioning.
3. Discuss ways to maintain activities of daily living while in a cast.
4. Demonstrate the application and utilization of a sling for the upper extremity.
5. Demonstrate ambulation techniques.
   a. Weight-bearing cast with a plaster boot or cast shoe
   b. Three-point gait crutch walking for non-weight-bearing cast
   c. Four-point gait crutch walking for partial-weight-bearing cast
6. Discuss how to do cast care and maintain the integrity of the cast.

COMPLICATIONS OF CASTS

All casts are prone to some kind of complication. Prevention is the best treatment. Teach the patient about the signs and symptoms of potential complications for their specific cast.

IMPAIRED CIRCULATION AND NERVE DAMAGE

An orthopaedic patient who has sustained an injury causing soft-tissue trauma, a fracture, or a surgical procedure and is then placed in a cast is at risk for neurovascular compromise. The cast is rigid and will not expand, while the patient's extremity will have swelling that can lead to increased pressure within the cast. Another way neurovascular compromise can occur is for the cast to impinge on the flexion surfaces of the extremity. If undetected or ignored, neurovascular injuries can be catastrophic. They include Volkmann's ischemic contracture of the upper extremity (see care of a patient in side arm traction in Chapter 6) and the

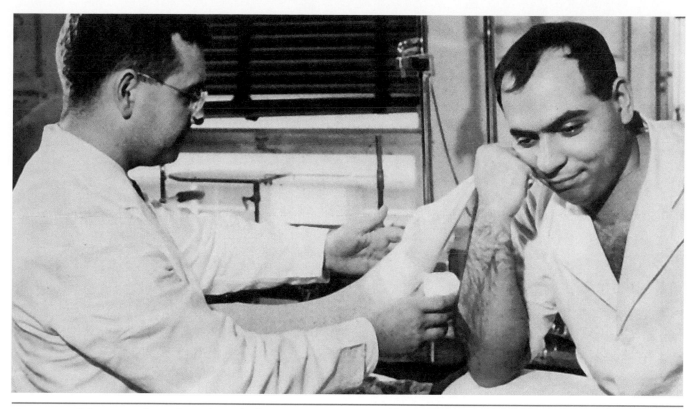

Figure 5–9 It is not good practice to have the lower extremity supported by an assistant holding the stockinette. This inevitably causes undue pressure of the stockinette over the heel, and it may cause burning pain or even a sore. The same effect can be produced by pulling too vigorously on the stockinette when holding it over the sharp edges of the cast.   *(Rockwood, C. A., et al. (1996). Rockwood & Green's Fractures in Adults. 4th ed. Philadelphia: Lippincott-Raven.)*

compartmental syndromes (see care of a patient in a long leg cast later in this chapter). In the postoperative or postreduction period, the neurovascular system must be carefully monitored (see Chapter 2).

Today, with many injuries, physicians do not admit the patient to the hospital for neurovascular monitoring unless the patient is at high risk (i.e., displaced supracondylar fractures, tibial shaft fractures, and knee dislocations). As an adult, the patient is instructed in the signs and symptoms of neurovascular compromise. It is essential that the nurse understand the seriousness of neurovascular complications, the signs and symptoms, and the importance of teaching the patient, the patient's family, and significant others how to assess for and thus prevent potential problems.

PRESSURE AREAS, TISSUE NECROSIS, AND IRRITATION

Pressure areas can develop on the patient's skin under the cast. The skin cannot withstand being compressed for an extended period of time without relief. When pressure is applied for as little as 2 hours, irreversible damage may occur. The skin and the underlying fat, which has a poor blood supply, may necrose, and a plaster sore (decubitus) can occur. An indentation in a cast can cause such pressure. If the patient complains of pain, it is usually best to check the skin over the area. Occasionally, patients will complain of pain for some time, which then subsides. If the pain is in response to an area

of pressure, this pain will be relieved only when the skin has necrosed in that area. This problem tends to occur more frequently in individuals who are immobilized in hip spica or long leg casts, and who keep the leg elevated for long periods of time with pressure on the heel.

Things that occur during the cast-application process that might cause skin irritation or necrosis are (1) having an assistant support the patient's lower extremity using an extension of the stockinette while the cast is being applied (Fig. 5–9), which may create pressure over the heel and burning pain; (2) pulling too vigorously on the stockinette or using stockinette that is too small, which may cause pressure on bony prominences; (3) handling the wet cast with the fingers instead of with the palms of the hands or at least with the fingers together, which may cause finger indentations that can produce pressure points in a cast (Fig. 5–10); (4) leaving rough or tight edges on the cast, which can be prevented by petaling or trimming (Fig. 5–11); and (5) having areas of skin excoriation due to pressure from the cast, especially at the folds of the buttocks in obese patients in long leg casts, which can be prevented by bending the upper edge of the cast so that it flares outward (a pair of pliers may be used).

After the cast is dry, make sure patients understand that they should not put anything between the cast and their skin, as that can cause pressure areas. They should not put anything into the cast to scratch an area that itches or insert tissues or other items to relieve discomfort

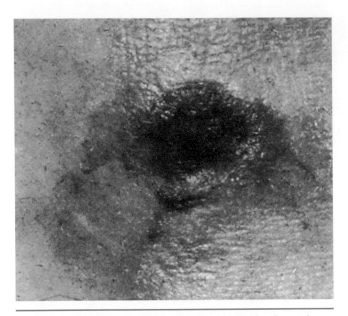

Figure 5–10   The surgeon in this case inadvertently made an indentation with his thumb while modeling the fractured ankle. The result was skin necrosis over the medial malleolus. *(Rockwood, C. A., et al. (1996). Rockwood & Green's Fractures in Adults. 4th ed. Philadelphia: Lippincott-Raven.)*

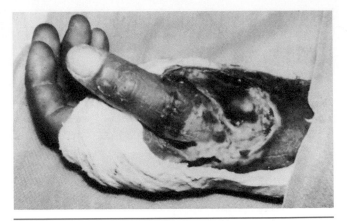

Figure 5–11   This is the end result of pressure exerted by an improperly applied cast over the thumb metacarpal. The patient had a large, full-thickness skin slough and lost the abductor and extensor tendons of his thumb in the bargain. The sharp edges of the thumb hole must always be everted, and undue pressure over the base of the thumb metacarpal must be avoided.   *(Rockwood, C. A., et al. (1996). Rockwood & Green's Fractures in Adults. 4th ed. Philadelphia: Lippincott-Raven.)*

they feel is caused by the cast. Using pencils or other such objects inside the cast can cause the padding and stockinette to wad up and cause a pressure area and excoriation to develop.

Severe maceration of the skin secondary to a wet cast can be a significant problem. If a cast has gotten wet and is made of plaster, there will probably be no satisfactory way of drying it. In most cases, a physician would probably remove and reapply the cast after checking the patient's skin. Even fiberglass casts can have serious problems with skin maceration even though the cast itself is not harmed by moisture. If the cast stockinette and padding are not thoroughly dried with warm air following exposure to or immersion in water, then significant skin problems can occur.

INFECTION

A wound infection due to casting materials and application is quite rare, but it has been reported. For patients with wounds, most physicians apply a sterile dressing and padding over the wound before cast application, and plaster buckets are cleansed after each use. However, the patient who swims with a fiberglass cast and dries the cast with hot air still runs a very high risk of skin maceration and wound infection. This discussion does not include wound infection from other causes, such as contamination during surgery or during dressing changes and systemic infections.

CAST SYNDROME

Cast syndrome is caused by an obstruction of the third portion of the duodenum resulting from constriction by the superior mesenteric vessels. In the past, individuals with compression fractures were treated with hyperextended body jackets. Occasionally, these patients developed pernicious vomiting and electrolyte imbalance, which in some instances led to death. Today, very few individuals with compression fractures are immobilized, and the position of hyperextension is avoided.

LACK OF FRACTURE IMMOBILIZATION

Lack of fracture immobilization occurs when the cast does not properly support the fracture site and prevent the bones at the fracture site from moving. This can occur if too much padding is applied. The padding flattens, and the cast may become too loose. A second way is if there is a large amount of swelling or edema in the extremity when the cast is applied. Once the swelling and edema recede, the cast becomes loose and allows the fracture site to move. A third possible source of movement occurs when the cast is not applied properly, that is, it is not molded to the extremity while the plaster is still wet. Movement at the fracture site can lead to delayed union or nonunion.

CAST CLAUSTROPHOBIA

Cast claustrophobia is a condition that affects a very small number of people when a cast is applied. These individuals find an extremity cast or a body cast unduly constricting. They may vomit or have a variety of psychosomatic complaints, leading to the need to remove the cast. The vomiting is rarely as severe and life threatening as in cast syndrome.

THERMAL EFFECTS OF PLASTER

As discussed in the section on cast application, when dehydrated gypsum becomes wet, an exothermic reaction occurs and the plaster becomes warm. How warm/hot a plaster of Paris cast becomes depends on the amount of plaster applied, the external environment, the amount of water in the plaster, and the temperature of the water used to moisten the plaster. In most instances, a patient having an application of a plaster of Paris cast will only have a nice warm feeling immediately after the application of the cast. However, it is possible for the patient to receive a thermal burn from a cast, especially from a thick splint. To avoid such potential problems, cold water should be used, and the thickness of the cast or splint limited to the least thickness that will accomplish satisfactory immobilization. If the patient states that the cast or splint is burning the skin, it should be removed immediately and the skin checked.

TIGHT CAST

Care should be taken when applying a cast to avoid making it tight. However, if swelling occurs, the cast can become tight. Pain is the first and most constant complaint of the patient with a tight cast, even if peripheral circulation appears unimpaired. The most prudent course of action is to split or even bivalve the cast. If the cast is split, the decompression should be continued until the symptoms are relieved. Decompression may mean that padding must also be split as bloodsoaked padding is as unyielding as plaster of Paris. Some physicians presently split casts at the time of application and spread them if there is any concern that significant swelling might occur (Harkess, Ramsey, & Harkess, 1996). Circular bandages of gauze or encircling adhesive tape should never be applied under a cast, because they may have the effect of acting as a tourniquet on the affected extremity. (For further discussion, see Volkmann's ischemic contracture in Chapter 6).

MAJOR TYPES OF CASTS

The basic rule of casting is to immobilize a joint above and below the level of a fracture and to do so in a position of function. This is necessary to give rotational stability to the fracture and facilitate restoration of function. Many joints will stiffen with prolonged immobilization despite appropriate exercises and rehabilitation after cast removal. For example, immobilization of the metacarpophalangeal joints in extension for as short as 3 weeks can result in loss of range of motion. So, if the metacarpophalangeal joints need to be immobilized for an extended period of time, physicians will immobilize them in 90 degrees of flexion if possible. Flexion maintains the length of the collateral ligaments and allows for recovery of range of motion after immobilization.

UPPER-EXTREMITY CASTS

Most upper-extremity casting can be divided into long and short arm casts. Short arm casts are used for metacarpal fractures, carpal fractures, and when it is necessary to protect a distal radial fracture in the later stage of healing. Long arm casts are used for fractures of the ulna, radius, and distal humerus. In addition, there are different types of short and long arm casts used less frequently, such as the thumb spica, hanging arm, and shoulder spica casts. This section presents information related to upper-extremity casts and a nursing process for each. Information related to cast materials, application, and drying that was presented earlier in the chapter is not repeated here.

THUMB SPICA CAST

The thumb spica is a short arm gauntlet cast, which extends from the proximal forearm (below the elbow) to the proximal palmar crease, including the distal joint of the thumb, with a spiral bandaging between the thumb and the hand. The arm is placed in a cast with the wrist at 20 to 45 degrees of dorsiflexion and at slight (20 degrees) radial deviation. The thumb is maintained in a functional position, and the fingers are left free to move distally from the metacarpophalangeal joints. The thumb spica is used for immobilization in the treatment of scaphoid or thumb fractures of the carpal navicular and the thumb metacarpal and phalanges, and in the treatment of ligamentous thumb joint injuries.

A fracture of the carpal scaphoid bone is the most common fracture of the carpus and also the most commonly undiagnosed fracture of the upper extremity. Fractures of the scaphoid are difficult to view on roentgenograms for the first 10 to 14 days after trauma. Scaphoid fractures occur in young teenagers to older adults, but most commonly in younger adult males. The fracture usually occurs as a result of a fall on an outstretched palm, which causes severe hyperextension and slight radial deviation of the wrist. Limitation of extremes of wrist motion is usually present because of pain and tenderness in the wrist near the styloid process of the radius. Immediate closed reduction and immobilization in a cast for 6 to 12 weeks is the preferred treatment. However, the patient may require an open reduction and insertion of Kirschner wire (see Chapter 12 for further discussion on scaphoid fractures).

NURSING PROCESS (Patient with a Fractured Scaphoid and Thumb Spica Cast)

To demonstrate nursing care, the following nursing process presents the care of a patient with a thumb spica cast for the treatment of a fractured scaphoid bone. The nursing process begins after the cast is applied.

ASSESSMENT

The initial step in the assessment of a patient with a cast following a reduction of a fractured scaphoid is a neurovascular assessment (see Chapter 2). The assessment of the thumb is difficult, as the thumb is enclosed in the cast. Assess the location, duration, and severity of the patient's pain. Check that the casted arm is properly elevated with the hand higher than the elbow and the elbow higher than the patient's heart. Check for the tightness of the cast. If the patient had an open reduction, look for any drainage into the cast. Check for any indentations and rough edges in the cast. Assess the dryness of the cast, especially if it is plaster of Paris (see section on cast materials and application for further information).

NURSING DIAGNOSIS

Based on all of the assessment data, the major nursing diagnoses for a typical patient with a thumb spica cast following a fractured scaphoid bone may include the following:

- Pain and discomfort related to trauma and immobility
- Impaired physical mobility related to instability of the thumb
- Potential altered nutrition: Less than body requirement related to eating with the nondominant hand
- Potential impaired skin integrity related to the cast
- Potential self-care deficit related to restricted use of the affected hand and arm
- Anxiety related to knowledge deficit about the injury, treatment method, and the rehabilitation process

COLLABORATIVE PROBLEMS

- Postcast stiffness of thumb and wrist
- Delayed or nonunion of the fracture
- Pressure areas
- Infection (patients with an open reduction)

GOAL FORMULATION AND PLANNING

The goals are to have the patient experience (1) a decrease in pain through cast, nursing interventions, and medications; (2) an increase in physical mobility of the thumb through the use of the thumb spica cast and exercises; (3) a nutritional intake that meets the body's daily requirement; (4) no break in skin integrity due to the cast; (5) ability to provide self-care with minimal assistance; (6) a decrease in anxiety through patient education about the trauma, treatment method, and the rehabilitation process; and (7) an absence of complications. Long-term goals are to have the patient free of pain and to have a return of hand function.

INTERVENTIONS

ALLEVIATE PAIN

Following a scaphoid fracture and the application of a thumb spica cast, the patient usually has pain and swelling of the affected thumb. Measures that help relieve the pain and swelling are to elevate the arm, put ice at the fracture site (along the side of the thumb but not on top of the thumb), and have the patient do finger exercises. The finger exercises help increase the circulation to the fracture site and the thumb even though the thumb is enclosed in the cast and is unable to move. Once these measures have been implemented and the neurovascular status of the affected hand is good (remember you may only be able to see or feel the tip of the thumb), give pain medications as needed.

INCREASE MOBILITY

Measures to increase mobility include correct positioning, exercises, and ambulation.

Position. Keep the patient's arm elevated while in bed, while sitting in a chair, and even while walking to reduce swelling and increase future mobility. Remember it is best to keep the hand above the elbow and the elbow above the heart. Patients with scaphoid fractures tend to have swelling. The thumb needs to be immobilized for fracture union to occur.

Exercises. Have the patient do finger exercises (Box 5–2), except approximating the tip of the thumb to each finger or exercising the thumb; elbow exercises (see dislocated lunate with short arm cast in this chapter); shoulder exercises (see Colles' fracture with long arm cast in this chapter) on the affected side; and active range of motion on all other unaffected joints.

Ambulation. The patient should have little to no problems with ambulation. If the patient happens to be elderly and needs to push down to get out of a chair, some adjustment may be needed. The patient must be encouraged to ambulate and get back to doing normal activities of daily living as soon as possible.

ADEQUATE NUTRITION

Having a cast on one hand and wrist, especially the dominant hand, can interfere with eating and food preparation. However, most young male adults would prefer to change their eating habits for a short time rather than ask someone to cut up their food. A family member may cut up the patient's food before bringing it to the table. By planning ahead, most patients can con-

---

Box 5–2
Finger Exercises

1. Fully extend the fingers and spread them into abduction.
2. Flex the fingers by touching the palm with the finger tips.
3. Flex the metacarpophalangeal joints by attempting to touch the front of the wrist.
4. Approximate the tip of the thumb to each finger in turn. The thumb must also be exercised.

sume adequate nutrition to maintain their daily needs. If the dominant hand is affected, select food that can be easily eaten with one hand. Assistance may be needed in opening cartons, putting butter on toast, and similar activities.

MAINTAIN SKIN INTEGRITY

Patients with a cast are at risk for a break in skin integrity due to the rough edges of the cast. Check the cast edges and petal as needed (see the section on remodeling and reshaping the cast earlier in this chapter). There can also be a break in skin integrity if there is excessive swelling in the patient's arm. Pressure on the skin from the cast can cause pressure points and skin breakdown. It may take only a couple of hours for skin irritation and necrosis to develop (see pressure areas under complications earlier in this chapter). Institute measures to prevent and/or reduce edema in the affected arm.

SELF-CARE

The patient may need some assistance in doing activities of daily living. For bathing, the patient's casted arm can be put in a plastic bag and then taped closed at the top to prevent water from getting on the cast. Assistance may be needed to help cleanse the unaffected arm. Minimal assistance may be needed for shaving (since this fracture often occurs in young males), even if an electric razor is used and the nondominant hand is casted. Open shirtsleeve seams on the affected arm as necessary. Assistance with buttoning shirts is usually needed. Discuss with the patient possible trousers/slacks/jogging pants to wear if the dominant hand is affected.

PATIENT TEACHING AND HOME CARE CONSIDERATIONS

The major tool for reducing a patient's anxiety is education about the trauma, treatment method, and the rehabilitation process. Patient teaching should include information on prevention of swelling, exercises, cast care, and techniques for accomplishing activities of daily living with a thumb spica cast (see the section earlier in this chapter).

The patient needs to continue with finger, elbow, and shoulder exercises and keep the casted arm elevated at all times to prevent swelling. If swelling should occur, the arm needs to be elevated immediately. If swelling continues, notify the physician.

MONITORING AND MANAGING POTENTIAL PROBLEMS

Complications following a closed or open reduction of a fractured scaphoid are potential stiffness of the thumb and the wrist following cast removal, delayed union or nonunion, impaired skin integrity, and, for open reductions, the additional risk of infection.

STIFFNESS OF THE THUMB AND WRIST

Stiffness of the thumb and wrist can be observed once the cast has been removed after 6 to 12 weeks of immobilization. In most instances, the patient will regain motion in the thumb and wrist after a period of rehabilitation and exercises. While the cast is place, maintaining the finger, elbow, and shoulder exercise regime helps to maintain muscle tone and prevent atrophy.

DELAYED UNION OR NONUNION

Delayed union (delayed healing) is used to describe a fracture that is slow to heal but does demonstrate some calcification, and nonunion is when the fracture fragments do not calcify together. Possible reasons why a scaphoid fracture may be delayed in healing are incomplete reduction and immobilization of the fracture that allows movement of the fracture site (or infection if there was an open reduction).

PRESSURE AREAS

Pressure points inside the cast can occur, especially over the styloid processes. The surface of the cast should be felt over areas where pain has been reported. If necrosis or infection is developing, the cast usually feels warm. Check the cast to make sure there are no indentations. Make sure the patient rests the casted arm on a soft or padded surface, as resting on a hard surface adds to pressure and discomfort. Implement measures to prevent swelling.

INFECTION

An infection at a fracture site can cause poor fracture healing, nonunion, or malunion. A scaphoid fracture with open reduction is more susceptible to infection because there has been a break in skin integrity. After a break in skin integrity, there is an opportunity for organisms to enter the body. Infections may result from a break of sterile technique during surgery, the sterile dressing becoming moist from wound drainage, the dressing becoming moist during cast application, or the cast becoming wet after application. Infection control measures need to be instituted before an infection occurs, and the patient, family, and significant others need to be aware of the signs and symptoms of infection.

EVALUATION/OUTCOMES

The patient should have a reduction in pain and swelling and no neurovascular impairment or infection. Patients should understand the rehabilitation process and feel comfortable in caring for themselves at home. The patient, the family, and significant others should be able to verbalize the signs and symptoms of potential complications, how to prevent them, and when to notify their physician.

SHORT ARM CAST (SAC)

The short arm cast extends from the proximal forearm (below the elbow) to the proximal palmar crease volarly and to the metacarpal heads dorsally (Fig. 5–12). Trim around the knuckles on the dorsum and obliquely across the proximal flexion crease of the palm on the volar side to allow unrestricted motion of the fingers. Make a cut around the thumb just large enough to allow unrestricted

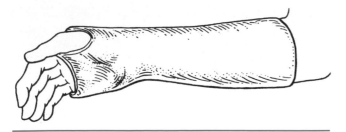

Figure 5–12   Short arm cast.   *(Mallon, W. J., et al. (1990).*
Orthopaedics for the House Officer. Baltimore: Williams and Wilkins.)

motion, and carefully evert the edges so there is no sharpness to cut the skin (see Fig. 5–11 for related complications). The cast should allow full flexion of the metacarpophalangeal (MCP) joints, to prevent the risk of stiffening due to immobilization. Extending the cast to the MCP joints dorsally will help control swelling and does not inhibit motion of the joints. The short arm cast is used in the treatment of stable fractures of the finger metacarpals, carpals, the distal radius, ulnar styloid fractures, and severe wrist sprains.

A dislocation of the lunate bone of the carpus is common and may be caused by a fall on the palm that forces the wrist into sudden extension. In some instances there may not be any other damage to the wrist, but in others it may dislocate anteriorly and proximally, tearing the capsule and coming to rest in the carpal tunnel. In that position, the lunate bone presses against the flexor tendons and causes the hand to be held with the wrist and the fingers in semiflexion. Motion of the wrist and the fingers is painful. The dislocated lunate bone may also press against the median nerve, causing a median neuritis characterized by pain, paresthesia, atrophy, and weakness or paralysis of the muscles of opposition. The injury may be difficult to detect on a roentgenogram. However, if the diagnosis is made early and a closed reduction is successful, the patient's wrist can be immobilized in a dorsal splint for 24 to 72 hours and the wrist then immobilized in a short arm cast for 4 to 6 weeks. For further discussion on carpal fractures, see Chapter 12.

NURSING PROCESS (Patient with a Dislocated Lunate and Short Arm Cast)

To demonstrate nursing care, the following nursing process presents the care of a patient with a short arm cast for a closed reduction of a dislocated lunate bone of the wrist. The nursing process begins after the cast is applied.

ASSESSMENT

The initial step in the assessment of a typical patient in a short arm cast following a closed reduction is a neurovascular assessment of the affected hand and arm and their comparison with the unaffected hand and arm (see Chapter 2). Be aware that there may have been neurological or circulatory impairment at the time of the injury. It will probably be impossible to assess the radial pulse because the wrist and the palm are covered by the cast. The cast may also impede a complete motor assessment of the arm.

Check the position of the arm. The affected arm must be elevated with the hand higher than the elbow. If there is swelling, keep the hand higher than the elbow and the elbow higher than the heart. Determine the location, duration, and severity of pain. Make sure the cast is cut out properly around the patient's thumb and little finger, so that it is not constricting or applying pressure on those areas. Check the plaster of Paris cast for drying (see section of cast materials and application earlier in this chapter).

NURSING DIAGNOSIS

Based on all of the assessment data, the major nursing diagnoses for a typical patient with a short arm cast following a dislocated lunate bone of the wrist may include the following:

- Pain and discomfort related to trauma and immobility
- Impaired physical mobility related to instability of the wrist and a short arm cast
- Potential self-care deficit related to the restricted use of the affected arm
- Potential impaired skin integrity related to the application of the cast
- Anxiety related to knowledge deficit about the injury, treatment method, and the rehabilitation process

COLLABORATIVE PROBLEMS

- Circulatory impediment
- Neurological deficit
- Necrosis or infection

GOAL FORMULATION AND PLANNING

The goals are to have the patient experience (1) a decrease in the amount of pain through immobilization, nursing measures, and prescribed medications; (2) an increase in mobility through the use of positioning and controlled exercises; (3) an ability to provide self-care with only minimal assistance; (4) no break in skin integrity related to the cast; (5) a decrease in anxiety through increased knowledge; and (6) an absence of complications. Long-term goals are to have the patient free of pain and to have a return of full arm function.

INTERVENTIONS

ALLEVIATE PAIN

Following a dislocated lunate bone in the wrist, the patient usually has pain and swelling of the affected wrist and hand. Some patients have their hand and forearm in a splint for the first 24 to 72 hours before cast application to prevent or reduce the amount of swelling in the fingers. Measures that help relieve pain and swelling are to elevate the arm, put ice along the side of the dislocation but not on it, and have the patient do finger exercises. To reduce the swelling, keep the hand and arm elevated above the heart; to prevent swelling, keep the hand above the elbow. Make sure the patient is not resting the casted hand and forearm on a hard surface, as this leads to discomfort and can cause a pressure area in a wet cast. Once these measures have been implemented and the neurovascular status of the affected arm is good, give pain medications as needed.

INCREASE MOBILITY

Interventions to increase the mobility of a patient with a short arm cast following a dislocated lunate bone in the wrist include correct positioning, exercises, and ambulation.

Position. The affected arm must be kept elevated to control swelling. One of the easiest ways to do that is to elevate the arm on one or more pillows. Another method is to use roller gauze or stockinette to encircle the cast at the patient's wrist and then to attach the casted arm to an intravenous pole. Make sure the gauze or stockinette does not cause an indentation in a plaster of Paris cast. If the cast is not completely dry, the stockinette may be pulled over the cast and then attached to the pole.

Exercises. Exercises of the fingers (see Box 5–2, thumb spica cast) and shoulder (Box 5–3) and active range of motion of the elbow are to be encouraged during the entire period of immobilization to minimize residual stiffness. Encourage the patient to return to normal activity. Activities that help to keep the elbow mobile utilize the affected arm as much as possible. Elbow flexion is accomplished through eating, hair combing, writing, and turning the pages of a book. Walking with the arm at one's side increases elbow extension (to be started after the problem of swelling has subsided).

Ambulation. The patient will be allowed to ambulate soon after the cast is applied. In the beginning, a sling may be used to help support the casted arm. Some older or frail individuals may require the use of a sling to support the cast at all times, except for periods of exercise and during activities of daily living. Assistance may be needed at the beginning because of the awkwardness of the cast.

SELF-CARE

Time with the patient, family, and significant others is needed to discuss potential problems in going home and doing activities of daily living, especially if the patient lives alone or is elderly. Discuss how the patient plans to prepare meals and do self-care, especially if the dominant hand is affected. How much assistance is needed

---

Box 5–3
Shoulder Exercises

RANGE-OF-MOTION EXERCISES
1. Use the unaffected arm for assistance.
2. Gently, without force, take the affected shoulder through range of motion.

PENDULUM EXERCISES
1. Have the patient bend forward.
2. Allow the affected arm to hang down and away from the body.
3. Slowly begin swinging the arm from side to side.
4. In the beginning, there will be very little swing, but it will gradually increase.

INTERNAL ROTATION EXERCISES
1. Have the patient place their hand behind their lower back.
2. Then have them gently reach upward toward the scapula as far as they can.

EXTERNAL ROTATION EXERCISES (WITH THE PATIENT LYING SUPINE OR STANDING WITH THE BACK TO A WALL)
1. With the arms parallel to the body, the palms are alternatively pronated and supinated.
2. With the hands clasped behind the head, the elbows are alternatively raised and flattened against the bed.
3. With the shoulders abducted to a right angle, the top of the bed is touched with each hand.
4. The patient reaches over the head to touch the opposite ear.

ELEVATION (WALL CLIMBING) EXERCISE
1. The patient stands sideways to a wall and gradually has his or her fingers "climb" up the wall as far as possible, thus extending and lifting the arm and abducting the shoulder.
2. It is encouraging for the patient to mark the level reached each time, so that the amount of progress can be observed.

---

for bathing? Using a shower and placing the casted hand and arm in a plastic bag, taping the top closed so water will not get in, seem to work best. Assistance may be needed in taping the bag. However, using a plastic bag over the cast to keep it clean and dry while preparing meals is unsafe and should not be practiced. If the patient's dominant hand is affected, some assistance may be needed in cooking and cutting foods. Customary ways of eating may need to be modified.

Clothing for the upper and lower portion of the body needs to be evaluated. Seams of sleeves can be released without destroying the garment. Buttons are difficult or at times impossible to fasten without assistance or at least an assistive device. Pullover garments may also be difficult to put on or take off, and it may be difficult to pull up and fasten pants or to tie shoes. Discuss possibilities with the patient, and they can usually come up with some good ideas on how to adapt the clothes they already own.

MAINTAIN SKIN INTEGRITY

Check the edges of the cast to make sure they are smooth and that the little finger and thumb do not have pressure from the cast. For further discussion, see the section on complications of casts earlier in the chapter.

The hand of the casted arm should be cleansed without getting the cast wet. Alcohol swabs may be used to cleanse between the fingers. The patient may need to apply lotion to the hand if the skin becomes too dry.

PATIENT TEACHING AND HOME CARE CONSIDERATIONS

Inform the patient that any increased discomfort that may occur in the form of tingling and numbness after cast application may be due to pressure on nerves or blood vessels and must be reported to the physician immediately. As compression on a nerve continues, it causes localized and constant pain, numbness of increasing depth, and, finally, loss of feeling and paralysis. Pressure that reduces the blood supply to an area leads to necrosis. Teach the patient, the family, and significant others how to check for possible neurovascular impairment (see Chapter 2).

Review the rehabilitation process and the use of exercises. Discuss cast care (see section on cast care earlier in this chapter), and reinforce the importance of not putting things in the cast.

MONITORING AND MANAGING POTENTIAL PROBLEMS

The major complications that may arise following a dislocated lunate bone are circulatory impediments, integumentary disruption, the recurrence of the prereduction deformity, and persistent pain. It is important that patients understand these potential complications, as in most instances the patient will not be admitted to the hospital and the teaching must be done in the clinic or outpatient setting. If they are admitted, patients are generally discharged when they are alert and have a satisfactory immobilization.

CIRCULATORY IMPEDIMENTS

Dislocated lunate bones of the wrist usually produce great swelling, which begins quickly and may involve the hand, the fingers, and part of the forearm. The swelling may be extensive before reduction. Once the reduction is accomplished and the cast applied, there may still be continued swelling. The patient is instructed to elevate the hand to help reduce swelling, to notify the physician if there is any neurovascular deficit or increase in pain, and to schedule appointments after discharge so that the swelling and the neurovascular status of the arm can be evaluated.

NEUROLOGICAL DEFICIT

The trauma of a dislocation of the lunate in a number of instances causes pressure against the median nerve. This may cause a median neuritis characterized by pain, paresthesia, atrophy, and weakness or paralysis of the muscles of opposition. Teach the patient to assess the neurovascular status of the affected hand.

MAINTAIN SKIN INTEGRITY

Patients in a cast are at risk of pressure points over bony prominences (e.g., the styloid processes). Unrelieved pressure can cause the development of necrosis and an infection. The patient usually will complain of pain in the area. Check the surface of the cast over areas where pain has been reported. If necrosis or infection is developing, the cast usually feels warm.

Severe edema often causes blisters and adds to the discomfort of patients in casts. That is particularly true over and around bony prominences where there is little tissue to absorb fluid. Check the skin around the cast edges and petal the cast as indicated (see petaling the cast edges earlier in this chapter).

EVALUATION/OUTCOMES

There should be a reduction in swelling from the application of ice, elevation of the arm, and finger exercises. If nerve or circulatory impairment should occur due to swelling, the cast should be split. There should be a reduction in the amount of pain with the immobilization of the dislocation. The patient should be able to demonstrate exercises for the fingers, the elbow, and the shoulder and verbalize an understanding of the rehabilitation process.

LONG ARM CAST (LAC)

The long arm cast extends from the upper level of the axillary fold to the proximal palmar crease with the elbow at a right angle (Fig. 5–13). Care needs to be taken that too much plaster is not placed into the elbow flexion crease. If the cast is thin over the extensor surface of the elbow, a few plaster splints may be used in this area and incorporated into the cast. Trim around the knuckles on the dorsum and obliquely across the proximal flexion crease of the palm on the

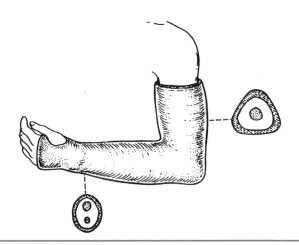

Figure 5–13   Long arm cast.   *(Mallon, W. J., et al. (1990). Orthopaedics for the House Officer. Baltimore: Williams and Wilkins.)*

volar side to allow unrestricted motion of the fingers. Cut an opening in the cast around the thumb just large enough to allow unrestricted motion, and carefully evert the edges so there is no sharpness to cut the skin (see Fig. 5–11 for related complications). The long arm cast is used for stable injuries of the elbow joint, stable fractures of the distal humerus, fractures of one or both bones of the forearm, unstable ligamentous injuries of the wrist joint, and unstable fractures of the carpal bones.

A Colles' fracture (often seen in elderly women) is a nonarticular fracture of the distal radius, with or without a fracture of the ulnar styloid, usually caused by a fall on an outstretched hand. There is a volar angulation of the radius and a dorsal displacement of the distal fragment. The arm and wrist of a patient with a Colles' fracture may be immobilized in a long arm cast, a short arm cast, or a forearm (sugar-tong) splint. In most patients, there is a closed reduction and immobilization in a long arm cast that includes the elbow and the distal half of the upper arm to help prevent rotation of the wrist. After 2 to 3 weeks for less severe fractures, and 3 to 4 weeks in more severe cases, the cast may be shortened to below the elbow. In patients with a closed reduction and percutaneous pinning with Kirschner wires through the radial styloids, the arm is immobilized in a long arm cast with the wrist in neutral position. For further discussion of Colles' fractures, see Chapter 12.

NURSING PROCESS (Patient with a COLLES' Fracture and Long Arm Cast)

To demonstrate nursing care, the following nursing process presents the care of a patient with a long arm cast for a closed reduction of a Colles' fracture. The nursing process begins after the cast is applied.

ASSESSMENT

The initial step in the assessment of a typical patient in a long arm cast following the closed reduction of a Colles' fracture is a neurovascular assessment of the affected hand and arm and a comparison with the unaffected hand and arm (see Chapter 2). It will probably be impossible to assess the radial pulse because the wrist and the palm are covered by the cast. The cast also impedes a complete motor assessment of the arm. Most patients have swelling at the fracture site, with edema and discoloration of the fingers and the thumb.

Check the position of the arm. The affected arm must be elevated with the hand higher than the elbow and, in most cases, the elbow must be higher than the patient's heart. Determine the location, duration, and severity of pain. Check the plaster of Paris cast for drying (see section on cast materials and application earlier in this chapter).

NURSING DIAGNOSIS

Based on all of the assessment data, the major nursing diagnoses for a typical patient with a long arm cast following a Colles' fracture of the wrist may include the following:

* Pain and discomfort related to trauma and immobility
* Impaired physical mobility related to instability of the radius and ulna
* Potential self-care deficit related to the inability to use the affected arm
* Potential impaired skin integrity related to the cast
* Anxiety related to knowledge deficit about the injury, treatment method, and the rehabilitation process

COLLABORATIVE PROBLEMS

* Circulatory impediments
* Neurological deficit
* Necrosis or infection
* Recurrence of deformity
* Persistent pain

GOAL FORMULATION AND PLANNING

The goals are to have the patient experience (1) a decrease in the amount of pain through immobilization, nursing measures, and prescribed medications; (2) an increase in mobility through the use of positioning and controlled exercises; (3) increased ability to do self-care; (4) no break in skin integrity; (5) a decrease in anxiety through increased knowledge; and (6) an absence of complications. Long-term goals are to have the patient free of pain and to have a return of full arm function.

INTERVENTIONS

ALLEVIATE PAIN
Following a dislocated Colles' fracture, the patient usually has pain and swelling of the affected wrist and hand. Some patients have their hand in a long arm cast immediately, whereas others have a pressure dressing over the hand for 24 to 48 hours to prevent or reduce swelling of the fingers. Measures that help relieve pain and swelling are to elevate the arm, put ice at the fracture site, and have the patient do finger exercises. Once these measures have been implemented and the neurovascular status of the affected arm is good, give pain medications as needed.

INCREASE MOBILITY
Interventions to increase the mobility of a patient with a long arm cast following a Colles' fracture include correct positioning, exercise, and ambulation.

Position. The affected arm must be kept elevated to control swelling. One of the easiest ways to do that is to elevate the arm on one or more pillows. Another method is to use roller gauze or stockinette to encircle the cast at the patient's wrist and then attach the casted arm to an intravenous pole. Make sure the gauze or stockinette does not cause an indentation in a plaster of Paris cast. If the cast is not completely dry, the stockinette may be pulled over the cast and then attached to the pole.

Exercises. Exercises of the fingers (see Box 5–2, thumb spica cast) and shoulder are to be encouraged during the entire period of immobilization to minimize residual stiffness. The most common shoulder exercises are range-of-motion, pendulum, internal rotation, external rotation, and elevation exercises (see Box 5–3). In the beginning, the unaffected arm may be used to assist the affected arm in doing these exercises.

Ambulation. The patient is allowed to ambulate soon after recovering from anesthesia (if given). Assistance is usually needed at the beginning because of the awkwardness of the cast. A sling (see Chapter 4) is used to help support the cast and distribute its weight.

SELF-CARE
Self-care follows some of the same issues as discussed during the care of a patient with a thumb spica and short arm cast. Here, there is the added problem of having a more restrictive cast, since the elbow is also enclosed and is at a right angle. Discuss potential problems with food preparation, eating, bathing, and dressing. A number of these patients are elderly women who are living alone. Some may need to have assistance in order to be able to continue to live at home. Others may live with friends or relatives for a short period of time, and still others may need to live in a rehabilitation or convalescent center for a while, depending on their overall health condition.

MAINTAIN SKIN INTEGRITY
Maintaining skin integrity with a cast in place follows what was discussed previously under thumb spica and short arm casts. However, since a number of the patients with Colles' fractures are elderly women, their skin is more fragile and more apt to develop problems related to the cast. Sometimes the patient will injure the skin on the unaffected arm by brushing the cast across the arm. Petal the edges of the cast, and teach the patient how to check the skin at the cast edges so any break in skin integrity can be detected early.

PATIENT TEACHING AND HOME CARE CONSIDERATIONS
Teach the patient that added discomfort in the form of tingling and numbness at any time after cast application may be due to pressure on nerves or blood vessels and must be reported to the physician immediately. As compression on a nerve continues, it causes localized and constant pain, numbness of increasing depth, and finally loss of feeling and paralysis. Teach the patient, the family, and significant others how to check for possible neurovascular impairment (see Chapter 2) and when to notify their physician.

Time is needed with the patient, family, and significant others to discuss problems in going home and doing activities of daily living, especially if the patient is elderly and lives alone. Discuss cast care, how to do personal care, and dressing. With the arm casted, it is especially important that the patient give attention to the hand of the casted arm, which should be cleansed without getting the cast wet. Alcohol swabs may be used to cleanse between the fingers. The patient may need to apply lotion to the hand if the skin becomes too dry.

MONITORING AND MANAGING POTENTIAL PROBLEMS
The major complications that may arise following a Colles' fracture are circulatory impediments, neurological impairment, integumentary disruption, the recurrence of the prereduction deformity, and persistent pain. It is important that patients understand these potential complications as their time in the hospital (if admitted) is very short. When admitted, patients are generally discharged when they have full active movement of the fingers and shoulder, minimal pain that is readily controlled with mild analgesics, and a satisfactory immobilization.

CIRCULATORY IMPEDIMENTS
Colles' fractures with displacement usually produce a large amount of bleeding and great swelling, which begins quickly and may involve the hand, the fingers, and the entire forearm. The swelling may be so extensive before reduction that the nature of the displacement is difficult to determine. Once the reduction is accomplished and the cast applied, the cast may need to be split (see splitting under cast reshaping and remodeling) to accommodate continued swelling. The patient is instructed to elevate the hand to help reduce swelling, to notify the physician if there is any neurovascular deficit or increase in pain, and to schedule appointments after discharge so that the swelling and the neurovascular status of the arm can be evaluated.

NEUROLOGICAL DEFICIT
The sensory branch of the radial nerve, which supplies the dorsum of the thumb and the radial side of the hand, may be stretched or even torn at the time of injury or reduction. Usually, the anesthesia and paresthesia that occur clear spontaneously within a few weeks. The median nerve is rarely injured, but a condition call Sudeck's atrophy may develop. This condition is suspected if the patient has unduly persistent pain after reduction and immobilization. In Sudeck's atrophy, the hand is typically warm, moist, and purplish in color from dilation of superficial blood vessels. The condition is apparently due to a hyperemia set up by nerve irritation, possibly from an injury to the median nerve in the carpal tunnel. The symptoms usually subside, but some patients may require anesthetic blockage of the inferior cervical or stellate ganglion, or small doses of deep x-ray therapy, to relieve the symptoms. The end result of

Sudeck's atrophy is usually a very stiff hand, and roentgenograms usually show evidence of bone destruction in the hand and the wrist.

NECROSIS AND INFECTION

Possible pressure points are over the styloid processes, the olecranon, and the epicondyles. The surface of the cast should be felt over areas where pain has been reported. If necrosis or infection is developing, the cast usually feels warm. Severe edema often causes blisters and adds to the discomfort of patients in casts. That is particularly true over and around bony prominences where there is little tissue to absorb the fluid. Check the skin around the cast edges and petal (see petaling the cast edges earlier in this chapter) as indicated.

RECURRENCE OF DEFORMITY

Despite a good initial alignment by closed reduction and an adequate plaster immobilization of a Colles' fracture, the prereduction deformity may recur if the cancellous bone of the distal fragment of the radius does not return to its normal location. In that event, muscle pulls tend to produce shortening and angulation in the distal fragment that produce a deformity resembling the initial injury. This complication is particularly common in the elderly. In spite of the deformity, the function of the hand may be quite good after healing is complete. In patients with considerable deformity and painful restriction of motion, excision of the distal ulna may not only afford relief of pain but also improve function and give a better cosmetic result.

PERSISTENT PAIN

Pain over the distal radioulnar joint on supination of the forearm is a common complaint after the cast is removed. The pain usually subsides gradually and disappears within 6 months. If the pain persists even after full return of function of the hand, excision of the distal ulna may be necessary.

EVALUATION/OUTCOMES

There should be a reduction in swelling from the application of ice, elevation of the arm, and finger exercises. If nerve or circulatory impairment should occur due to swelling, the cast should be split. There should be a reduction in the amount of pain with the immobilization of the fracture. The patient should be able to demonstrate exercises for the fingers and the shoulder and verbalize an understanding of the rehabilitation process.

HANGING ARM CAST

The hanging arm cast is a long arm cast with a loop on the radial surface between the wrist and the elbow, usually close to the wrist (Fig. 5–14). A strap is placed around the patient's neck and attached to the cast through the loop. The hanging arm cast is heavier than a normal cast because its purpose is to exert a pull on the upper arm to reduce and immobilize a fracture site.

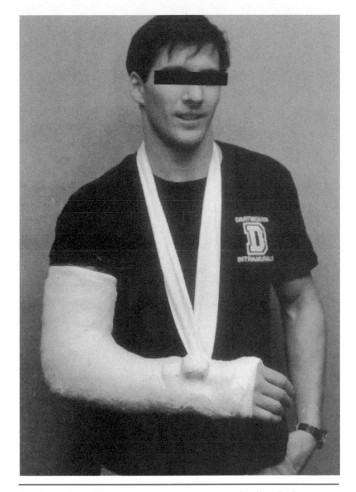

Figure 5–14   The hanging arm cast is applied with the elbow in 90° flexion and the forearm in neutral rotation. The supporting stockinette passes through one of three loops applied at the wrist.   *(Rockwood, C. A., et al. (1996).* Rockwood & Green's Fractures in Adults. *4th ed. Philadelphia: Lippincott-Raven.)*

It is used to treat some shoulder injuries, displaced fractures of the neck of the humerus, and spiral or comminuted fractures of the humerus. Because of the traction purpose of the hanging arm cast, see Chapter 6 for an in-depth discussion of the nursing care of a patient with a hanging arm cast.

SHOULDER SPICA CAST

The shoulder spica cast is a combination of a body jacket and a long arm cast with a spiral bandage between the trunk and the affected arm, the shoulder in abduction, and the elbow in a flexed position (Fig. 5–15). The casting material (usually plaster of Paris) is applied to the upper torso and may extend below the iliac crests. The cast envelops the upper trunk and one arm, although the wrist and the hand of that arm may or may not be included. The arm is held in a position of abduction and is supported by a strut from the body portion of the cast. Unless the patient is under anesthesia, a shoulder spica cast is applied with the patient standing or sitting on a stool. Padding is applied over bony prominences and

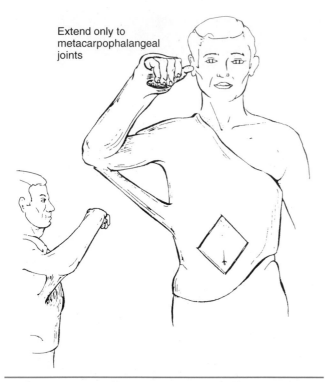

Extend only to metacarpophalangeal joints

Figure 5–15   The shoulder spica cast is made in a similar manner to the hip spica, in that a support is necessary, extending from the body of the cast to the arm. The position of the arm in the cast depends upon the condition being treated and upon the personal preference of the physician. *(Lewis, R. C. (1977). Handbood of Traction, Casting and Splinting Techniques. Baltimore: Williams and Wilkens. p 84.)*

under the breasts of female patients. After applying protective padding, the casting material is first applied in a circular fashion around the trunk of the body. It is then applied in a spiral reverse that goes between the arm and the upper torso, thereby immobilizing the shoulder joint.

The most usual position for an adult without a shoulder arthrodesis is 70 degrees of abduction, 40 degrees of flexion, and enough external rotation to allow the mouth to be reached by the fingers when the elbow is flexed. (If it is used following a shoulder arthrodesis, the position of the shoulder is determined by clinical signs; roentgenograms; and the patient's age, occupation, and surgical procedure). In all cases, the elbow is flexed at a right angle, the forearm is held in midrotation, and the wrist is dorsiflexed. In the past, the shoulder spica was used to immobilize the shoulder following a disease, injury, or surgery affecting the shoulder or the humerus. The most common of those conditions were unstable fractures of the shoulder girdle and humerus, postoperative shoulder fusions, unstable elbow joint injuries, and dislocations of the shoulder girdle.

Zuckerman and Koval (1996) write that today the indications for use of a shoulder spica cast are unclear. The primary indications may be when closed reduction of the fracture requires significant abduction and external rotation of the upper extremity. However, when this uncommon situation occurs, surgery is frequently

performed and, if needed, a different and more recently designed immobilizing device is used. The disadvantages of the shoulder spica cast include difficulty in application, cast weight and bulkiness, skin irritation, and patient discomfort. It should be avoided for patients with significant pulmonary problems. However, even with those disadvantages and the fact that it is a highly inefficient device for immobilizing the shoulder, it is still used in the treatment of some shoulder arthrodeses and proximal fractures of the humerus.

NURSING PROCESS (Patient with a Shoulder Arthrodesis and Shoulder Spica Cast)

To demonstrate nursing care, the following nursing process presents the care of a patient with a shoulder spica cast for the treatment of a shoulder arthrodesis. The nursing process begins after the cast is applied.

ASSESSMENT

The first step in the assessment of a typical patient following the reduction of a comminuted fracture of the proximal humerus and the application of a shoulder spica cast is to check the respiratory status. The rate, depth, and rhythm of breathing need to be assessed, as the cast may be constricting chest movements necessary for respiration. Make sure the patient is in correct alignment and that there are sufficient pillows to support the arm and the upper torso. Assess for possible nausea and potential vomiting from anesthesia (if given) and the possible tightness of the cast over a portion of the abdomen.

Check the neurovascular status of the involved arm and compare it to the uninvolved arm (see Chapter 2). As the cast may impinge on the ulnar nerve, assess the status of that nerve by asking the patient to abduct the fingers and respond to a pricking of the little finger. Note any swelling of the hand or the fingers. Check the cast over the incisional area and the posterior portion of the shoulder for bleeding into the cast (if the patient had an open reduction).

NURSING DIAGNOSIS

Based on all of the assessment data, the major nursing diagnoses for a typical patient with a shoulder spica cast following a shoulder arthrodesis may include the following:

- Pain and discomfort related to surgical trauma
- Impaired physical mobility related to bone stability and the shoulder spica cast
- Potential ineffective individual coping related to the surgery and immobilization
- Self-care deficit related to immobilization of the shoulder and the spica cast

- Potential impaired skin integrity related to the cast
- Anxiety related to knowledge deficit about the surgery, treatment method, and the rehabilitation process

COLLABORATIVE PROBLEMS

- Neurovascular deficit
- Circulatory impairment
- Respiratory infection

GOAL FORMULATION AND PLANNING

The goals are to have the patient experience (1) a decrease in the amount of shoulder pain through immobilization, nursing measures, and prescribed medications; (2) an increase in mobility and stability of the shoulder through the use of the cast and controlled exercises; (3) an effective method of coping with immobilization and the rehabilitation process; (4) no self-care deficit; (5) no break in skin integrity; (6) a decrease in anxiety through increased knowledge; and (7) an absence of complications. Long-term goals are to have the patient free of pain, have stability in the arm, and to have a return of function to the shoulder and arm.

INTERVENTIONS

ALLEVIATE PAIN

Immediately after the application of the shoulder spica cast, the patient may be restless and appear quite uncomfortable. This does not necessarily mean that the patient is having a lot of pain. It may be that the patient finds it difficult to get into a comfortable position with the heavy cast on and the arm in abduction. Help the patient change or readjust position. Correct alignment helps to relieve stress on the fracture site, the shoulder, and the arm.

Evaluate complaints of pain for possible neurovascular impairment. Specifically, there may be complaints of pain near bony prominences under the cast, especially the medial epicondyle and adjacent ulnar nerve. One way to help prevent or relieve that pressure is to encourage the patient to exercise their fingers and thumb frequently. The cast edges are also a potential source of pain and skin irritation. Petal the cast edges as a preventive measure. Sources of bone pain are the fracture site and discomfort from lying in the same position too long. Medicate the patient as needed.

INCREASE MOBILITY

Interventions to increase the mobility of a patient with a shoulder spica cast following a shoulder arthrodesis include correct positioning, exercises, and ambulation.

Position. When the patient is in bed, the head of the bed may be elevated or the patient's upper torso propped up with pillows. The amount of elevation of the head of the bed may be restricted by how far the cast extends down the trunk, and how much the patient can flex their

back. The patient needs pillows to support the casted arm. The patient will probably find the supine position the most comfortable when in bed. However, the patient may turn to the unaffected side. He or she will need help to do so and will need pillows to support the affected arm and torso to maintain the side-lying position. Turning is essential for comfort and for cast drying if the patient has a plaster of Paris cast.

Exercises. The patient needs to be encouraged to exercise. The recommended exercises include chest and abdominal exercises, active range-of-motion exercises for all unaffected joints, and finger and thumb exercises to stimulate circulation in the involved arm. Once the cast is removed, other exercises are begun.

Ambulation. At first, patients need assistance in getting out of bed. Once out of bed, some support is needed until they are able to adjust to the weight of the cast and strengthen their abdominal and back muscles. Maintaining balance with the heavy cast is very difficult for some patients in the beginning. The patient will also need assistance in learning how to sit and get out of a chair and how to go up and down stairs with the shoulder spica cast in place. Teach the patient to use their leg muscles to help raise and lower themselves. It is also important that the patient understand that they should not bend at the waist and try to pick something up from the floor. Many patients (especially at first) are unable to raise themselves once they have bent over.

SELF-CARE

Patients usually need assistance in food preparation. Although the dominant arm may be in a cast, most patients want to feed themselves. The patient needs to have suggestions on how to bathe and dress at home. Sponge baths are recommended as a safe method to prevent water getting on or under the cast. Some patients may need assistance in washing the lower portion of their body while sitting in a chair. All patients will need assistance in washing the unaffected arm and their hair. If it is difficult to have someone wash their hair at the sink, a plastic hair-washing board may be helpful at home.

Learning how to dress with a shoulder spica cast can be a challenge, and the patient needs some help. With the upper torso in a shoulder spica cast, the patient has one hand at the most to pull on clothing. What to wear on the lower extremity is influenced by the patient's ability to only use their unaffected arm and the level of the cast. For both men and women, wearing some kind of pants with an elastic waist is usually a good choice. Dressing the upper torso can be a problem, but does not need to be with some creative thinking and planning. A good approach is to open seams on the affected side of blouses or shirts and to use Velcro straps for closure, because once the cast is removed the seams can be repaired. Patients living in cold climates will probably be unable to wear a coat even if there is no strut supporting the arm. Wearing a poncho, cape, or large wool shawl is suggested. Discuss with the patient the availability of such items from family or friends before suggesting they buy them. Having someone tie the patient's shoes or wearing a good slip-on walking shoe is acceptable, as opposed to bedroom slippers that do not fit properly and can easily slip off the patient's feet or cause the patient to fall.

MAINTAIN SKIN INTEGRITY
Skin irritation and breakdown may develop at the cast edges and where the cast rubs on bony prominences. Make sure there are no pressure areas in the cast. Teach the patient not to lean back or put any part of the casted body on a hard surface for any period of time. Check the edges of the cast to make sure there are no rough or sharp edges. Petal cast edges (see earlier portion of this chapter) to prevent skin irritation. Even though the cast edges may be petalled, continue to assess. If the patient slouches or in any way lets the cast rest or put pressure on the skin, skin breakdown and infection may result. Make sure the patient knows that putting items under the cast can cause a break in skin integrity and possible infection. Doing muscle setting exercises or shifting the skin under the cast can help to relieve itching and feelings of discomfort. (For further discussion, see Pressure Areas, Tissue Necrosis, and Irritation earlier in this chapter.)

EFFECTIVE INDIVIDUAL COPING
Not infrequently, some patients become depressed at the prospect of living with a fused shoulder. Others have difficulty in adjusting to the temporary change in body image brought about by wearing the spica cast for 2 to 3 months. Spend time with the patients. Let them express their feelings and concerns. Be honest and realistic, and help the patient obtain answers to questions. For more in-depth discussion, see Chapter 2.

PATIENT TEACHING AND HOME CARE CONSIDERATIONS
Make sure the patient is able to do abdominal and respiratory breathing exercises and understands the rationale behind them. Go over range-of-motion exercises for all uninvolved joints and why they are necessary. Exercises for the fingers (see Box 5–2, thumb spica cast) are to be done 5 minutes every hour the patient is awake. If the patient awakens during the night, the finger exercises should be done then as well. The patient should continue all of these exercises until the cast is removed. A different set of exercises for the arm and the upper torso will then be prescribed so that the patient can regain as much function in the involved arm and shoulder as possible.

Instruct the patient on the proper ways to ambulate, get in and out of a chair, pick up items from the floor, and go up and down stairs while wearing a shoulder spica cast. Discuss possible problems that may arise in using public transportation (e.g., hitting somebody with the casted arm in a crowded bus). The patient should not attempt to drive a car even if the dominant arm is unaffected, because the casted arm may interfere with steering, shifting, and reacting to emergencies. If the right arm is affected, it is better to ride in the back seat behind the driver to allow space for the casted arm.

For a discussion on eating and dressing, see section on self-care. For ways to help the patient, the patient's family, or significant others should the patient become depressed or have difficulty coping, see Chapter 2.

MONITORING AND MANAGING POTENTIAL PROBLEMS

The most common complications following a humeral fracture and the application of a shoulder spica cast are circulatory, respiratory, and neurovascular impairments due to pressure from the cast at the medial epicondyle.

NEUROVASCULAR IMPAIRMENT
Neurovascular impairment can occur due to pressure from the cast at the medial epicondyle. An impairment of the ulnar nerve is indicated if the patient has decreased or no ability to abduct their fingers or feel pricking at the distal end of the fifth (little) finger. If that should occur, notify the patient's physician immediately. To help prevent nerve impairments, have the patient do finger and thumb exercises on a regular basis.

CIRCULATORY IMPAIRMENT
At times the patient may have decreased circulation to the affected hand because of a lack of activity and slow arterial flow caused by the elevated position of the arm. The decreased circulation may lead to numbness, whiteness, or coolness of the fingers, which should be relieved by finger exercises.

RESPIRATORY IMPAIRMENT
The cast may be too tight and prevent or decrease respiratory movement, which can lead to pneumonia. Have the patient turn, cough, and deep breathe. Incentive spirometry may also be used. Although the chances are small, be alert for the possibility of fat emboli (see Chapter 4).

EVALUATION/OUTCOMES

The patient should have good neurovascular status in the affected arm and no respiratory complications. There should be a decrease in the amount of pain and no side effects from pain medications. The patient should be able to demonstrate good balance and gait when ambulating, know how to safely get in and out of a bed or chair, and be able to go up and down stairs. He or she should be able to pick up objects from the floor with good body mechanics and no bending of the upper trunk (this may be difficult for some to accomplish). The patient should feel confident about their ability to perform activities of daily living and to move about and care for themselves when they go home. Exercises should be incorporated into a schedule for home care. The patient should accept the temporary restrictions imposed by the cast.

LOWER-EXTREMITY CASTS

Most lower-extremity casts are divided into two general types: short leg and long leg. Long leg casts and patellar-tendon, weight-bearing, short leg casts control lower leg rotation; other short leg casts protect the ankle but do not control rotation of the tibia. In addition, there are specific modifications of the short leg and long leg casts that are used, such as the walking, brace, cylinder, and hip spica casts. Information related to a specific cast and a nursing process that demonstrates the care of a patient in that cast are presented in this section. Information on cast materials, drying methods, and application of casts are discussed in an earlier section and are not repeated here.

SHORT LEG CAST (SLC)

The short leg cast generally extends from below the knee (above the level of the tibial tubercle anteriorly and short enough posteriorly to allow the knee to be flexed 90 degrees) to the base of the toes with the ankle in neutral position (Fig. 5–16). If the desire is to have a footplate under the toes, the cast padding needs to extend distally to the tip of the great toe, and if not, the cast padding can be stopped at the great toe metatarsophalangeal (MTP) joint. Extra splints are used to reinforce the bottom of the cast in the area over the heel since that area tends to be thin. Once the cast is applied, make sure that all five toes are visible dorsally; the plaster on the sole is left intact beneath the toes if a toeplate is desired. The short leg cast is used to treat fractures of the ankle and stable fractures of the distal tibia and fibula.

Bimalleolar or Pott's fractures can be reduced by either the open or closed methods. Closed reduction frequently can be accomplished once the swelling has been reduced, but often the anatomical position of the ankle is not maintained. In up to 20% of the bimalleolar fractures, intra-articular injuries to the talus and tibia are present and untreated when closed reduction

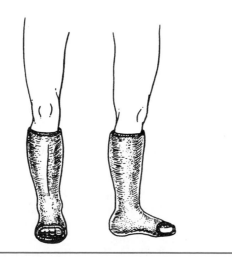

Figure 5–16 Short leg cast. *(Mallon, W. J., et al. (1990). Orthopaedics for the House Officer. Baltimore: Williams and Wilkins.)*

is utilized. For most displaced bimalleolar fractures, treatment by open reduction and internal fixation of both malleoli is essential to restore the ankle joint. To repair the joint, various methods are used, such as oblique pins, screws, Kirschner wires, or even a small plate.

If both malleoli have been securely fixed, the ankle is usually immobilized in a short leg cast from the toes to the tibial tuberosity to prevent rotation. In many instances, the distal portion of the front of the cast is removed as early as the third day so daily active dorsiflexion of the ankle may be carried out. The cast is then put back together and secured. That routine may be continued for 4 to 6 weeks, or until there is evidence of union. At that time, the cast is completely removed, and active range-of-motion exercises and protected weight bearing using crutches are begun. Those measures are continued until union is complete. If the lateral malleolus has not been securely fixed, the patient may be placed in a long leg cast (midthigh to toes with the knee flexed at 45 degrees and the foot in midplantar flexion and internal rotation). If a long leg cast is utilized, it is used for only 4 to 6 weeks and then a short leg cast is worn until union is achieved. As a rule, malleolar fractures require 10 to 12 weeks to unite.

NURSING PROCESS (Patient with a Pott's Fracture and Short Leg Cast)

To demonstrate the nursing care, the following nursing process presents the care of a patient with a short leg cast for an open reduction of a Pott's fracture. The nursing process begins after the cast is applied.

ASSESSMENT

Patients with a cast over the ankle following an open or closed reduction of a Pott's fracture must have the neurovascular status of the foot checked (see Chapter 2). There may be swelling due to the trauma or the surgery. In addition to possible discoloration of the skin from bleeding, there may be some discoloration from Betadine or other solutions used as preparation for surgery. Determine the amount of pain and whether the pain is due to nerve pressure or circulatory impairment.

For patients with an open reduction, determine the amount of bleeding. Note the size of any bloody area that appears on the cast. Be sure to check beneath the leg, especially on the lateral and medial sides of the ankle. Check frequently during the first 24 hours for any increase in the size of the bloody area. Bloody areas in the plaster cast retain their bright red color. Remember, bleeding into a wet plaster cast disperses the blood through the plaster, sometimes giving the impression that a lot more bleeding has occurred than actually has.

NURSING DIAGNOSIS

Based on all of the assessment data, the major nursing diagnoses for a typical patient with a short leg cast following a Pott's fracture of the ankle may include the following:

- Pain and discomfort related to trauma and immobility
- Impaired physical mobility related to instability of the ankle
- Potential impaired skin integrity related to the cast
- Anxiety related to knowledge deficit about the injury, treatment method, and the rehabilitation process

COLLABORATIVE PROBLEMS

- Incomplete reduction
- Nonunion
- Infection

GOAL FORMULATION AND PLANNING

The goals are to have the patient experience (1) a decrease in the amount of pain through immobilization, nursing measures, and prescribed medications; (2) an increase in mobility through the use of positioning, exercises, and ambulation with crutches; (3) no break in skin integrity; (4) a decrease in anxiety through increased knowledge; and (5) an absence of complications. Long-term goals are to have the patient free of pain and to have a return of full ankle function in approximately 12 weeks with no residual complications.

INTERVENTIONS

ALLEVIATE PAIN

The foot should be elevated on pillows with the "toes above the nose." The heel should be off the pillows to reduce pressure on the heel, while the elevation is helping to prevent or reduce swelling. If the elevation of the foot of the bed is sufficient, make sure the heel is off the end of the bed. To help prevent discomfort caused by swelling, ice bags may be placed along both sides of the ankle, but not at the site of the swollen toes. These bags should not be filled heavily with ice, and air should be eliminated before the bags are closed. The pressure of heavy ice bags on a swollen and painful ankle has been known to cause great discomfort to the patient and considerable interference with circulation.

Repositioning the patient's leg also helps to reduce discomfort. The best way to reposition the leg is to lift it by placing the palms of your hands under the cast (with your fingers close together to avoid making an indentation in the cast) and lifting the leg. Once the leg is elevated, flex the patient's knee a couple of times before bringing the leg to rest once more on the pillows. This maneuver helps to relax some of the tense muscles and increases blood circulation to the area. Medicate the patient as needed for pain after first assessing the complaints of pain to make sure it is from the surgery or trauma and not from nerve pressure or circulatory impairment.

INCREASE MOBILITY

Interventions to increase the mobility of a patient with a short leg cast following an open reduction of a Pott's fracture include correct positioning, exercise, and ambulation.

Position. The affected leg must be kept elevated to help control (or prevent) swelling. The general rule is that the leg should be higher than the heart; therefore, the patient may be asked not to have the head of the bed elevated more than a few degrees. The leg can be elevated using pillows, elevating the foot of the bed, or both. The patient can turn to either side while in bed as long as they keep the affected leg elevated.

If the patient needs a bedpan, keep the leg elevated on pillows while placing a fracture bedpan under the patient's buttocks from the side of the body opposite the cast. If the patient is able to assist, have him or her use the trapeze to lift their buttocks off the mattress while you slide the bedpan in place. Another approach is for the patient to use the trapeze to lift while at the same time pushing against the bed with the uninvolved leg. (For further discussion, see care of a patient with a fractured hip in Chapter 9.)

Exercises. Active and passive range-of-motion exercises for all unaffected extremities should be stressed. For the affected leg, start quadriceps- and gluteal-setting exercises (see the care of a patient with a total hip arthroplasty in Chapter 9) and flexion and extension of the knee on the first day after surgery. Dorsiflexion of the ankle should start on the third day if allowed by the patient's physician. As already discussed, the following procedure is followed: (1) remove the distal portion of the front of the cast (already prepared for removal by the patient's physician), (2) do daily gentle active dorsiflexion, and (3) replace the piece of the cast and secure in place. That routine may be continued for 4 to 6 weeks or until there is evidence of union. Once the cast is removed, active range-of-motion exercises are begun.

Ambulation. Depending on the amount of swelling, patients with an open reduction of a Pott's fracture may be able to ambulate on crutches shortly after surgery. Until there are signs of union, the patient is not allowed weight bearing; therefore, the patient will need to utilize a three-point crutch gait (see Chapter 4). Before getting the patient out of bed to walk with crutches, explain that there will be pain or throbbing in the affected foot when it is lowered to the floor and that the foot may become discolored. When the patient sits in a chair or returns to bed, the foot should once more be elevated, and the normal color will return. Teach the patient exercises to help build up strength in their arms so they can tolerate walking with crutches for longer periods of time. For further discussion on ambulation, see the care of a patient with a long leg cast that follows in this chapter.

MAINTAIN SKIN INTEGRITY

Skin complications can easily occur. Patients who have plaster of Paris casts following an open reduction may not have a stockinette under the plaster. Edges of the cast may be rough and need to be petaled when the cast is dry to protect the skin. (For discussion on how to petal a cast and care of a cast, see the section earlier in this chapter.) When a window is made in the cast to change a dressing or to remove sutures, make sure the cast window is replaced and secured with tape so there will not be swelling at the site of the window.

PATIENT TEACHING AND HOME CARE CONSIDERATIONS

The patient needs answers to questions concerning the postoperative course of treatment, the length of time before weight bearing, and the length of time of immobilization. The amount of time lost from work depends on the patient's condition, the type of work, and the health and safety policies of the patient's employer.

Once the patient is allowed to return home, make sure the patient, the family, and significant others understand cast care, how to detect complications related to the cast, and how to perform personal hygiene with a short leg cast on. The patient will need to have a covering over the cast to prevent water from getting on or under the cast. This can be accomplished by placing the patient's foot in a plastic garbage bag and then taping the top to prevent water from getting in, or by utilizing a plastic cast cover that is designed specifically for that purpose. Taking showers is preferable to a tub bath, since there is less chance of water getting on or under the cast. If a tub bath is taken, it is best to keep the plastic wrapped leg out of the tub as much as possible, because water will get through the tape and plastic wrap. Another thing some patients want to do is drive their car. Driving may not be feasible unless the patient's right leg is unaffected and the patient has a car with an automatic transmission.

A patient going home immediately after having a cast applied (following an open or closed reduction) must be knowledgeable about the cast. Teach the patient how to assess for neurovascular deficiencies. Have the patient contact their physician if any of the following occur (1) increasing pain; (2) pain unrelieved by prescribed medications; (3) swelling unrelieved by elevating the leg for at least an hour; (4) a change of sensation in the toes (e.g., numbness, tingling, or burning); (5) decreased movement or loss of movement in the toes; (6) a change in skin color above or below the cast; (7) a bad smell coming from inside the cast; (8) a warm area or fresh stain on the cast; (9) a foreign object dropped into or stuck in the cast; and (10) a weakened, cracked, loose, or tight cast.

Instruct the patient to keep the plaster cast elevated on two pillows and uncovered for at least 48 hours (or as ordered by the physician) as the cast dries. In addition, instruct the patient (family or significant other) to use the palms and not the fingertips to frequently change the position of the casted leg on the pillows. Remind the patient that all these measures promote even cast drying and help reduce swelling. Warn the patient that the wet cast will feel heavy, but reassure the patient that as the cast dries it will get lighter. Caution the patient against walking on the cast before weight bearing is allowed.

Discuss the observations necessary to ensure comfort and prevent complications. For example, show the patient how to move the toes to assess motion. Because the leg will be in the cast for some time, explain the importance of exercises in preventing complications. Also demonstrate how to perform any special exercises ordered. Emphasize cast care as discussed earlier in the chapter. Give the patient a copy of home care instructions.

MONITORING AND MANAGING POTENTIAL PROBLEMS

The major complications that may arise following a Pott's fracture of the ankle are incomplete reduction, nonunion, and infection at the fracture site. It is important that the patient understand the potential complications as the hospital stay is short (if the patient is admitted at all). Although these complications cannot necessarily be prevented by the patient, the alert patient can detect symptoms of such conditions so that appropriate action can be taken quickly.

INCOMPLETE REDUCTION

Incomplete reduction is less common in patients with open reductions. With an open reduction, the physician is able to see the fracture; complete the reduction; apply pins, screws, plates or other devices to maintain the reduction; and then apply a cast to maintain the reduction. With a closed reduction, the physician may believe the fracture is reduced when it is not, or the fracture may be reduced properly but reduction was lost as the cast was applied. Another possibility is that too much padding was applied, or the patient had a large amount of swelling when the cast was applied, and the cast became loose over time allowing the fracture site to move.

NONUNION

Nonunion is when the fracture fragments do not calcify together. Nonunion of a Pott's fracture may occur if (1) an infection develops following an open reduction, (2) there is inadequate blood supply to the fracture site, (3) muscles or fascia are between the fracture fragments, (4) the callus is broken or torn by excessive activity (e.g., weight bearing before a hard callus is formed), or (5) there is marked dietary deficiency. Patients should report any signs of infection or loosening of the cast.

INFECTION

A patient with an open reduction is at risk for infection. If there was an open fracture, the wound was contaminated and at risk for infection. There is also the possibility of contamination of the wound when there has been excessive bleeding into the dressing and cast. A number of physicians place their patients on an antibiotic for a short time following an open reduction as a precautionary measure. It is important to teach the patient the signs and symptoms of infection and that they should report them to their physician.

EVALUATION/OUTCOMES

Determine whether the patient has been provided with sufficient data to feel confident about going home with a short leg cast and ambulating on crutches. Ask specific questions to determine what the patient does not

understand, and explain it again. Postoperative pain should be reduced by nursing measures and medication. If not, observe for signs and symptoms of complications or consider the possibility of requesting a change in pain medications.

LONG LEG CAST (LLC)

The long leg cast (LLC) extends from the upper thigh (proximal to the greater trochanter on the lateral surface and to within about two finger breadths of the groin medially) to the base of the toes, with the ankle at a right angle and the foot in a neutral position (Fig. 5–17). Long leg casts may be applied with the knee flexed or

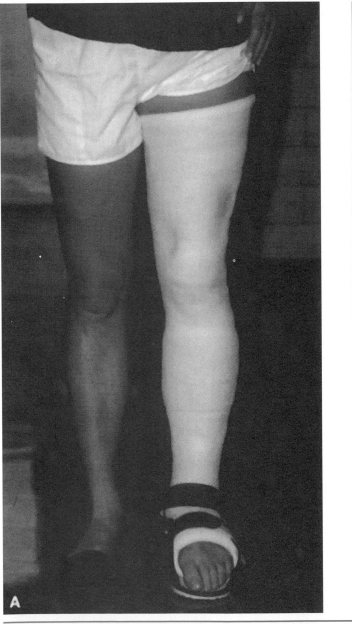
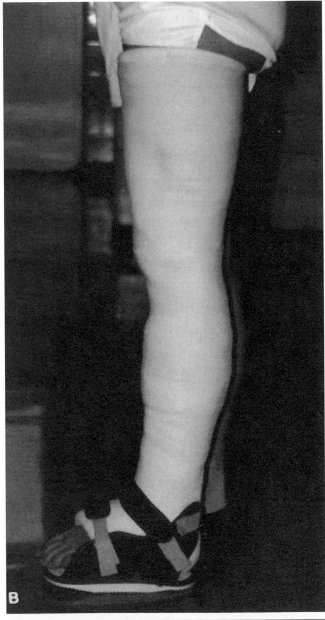

Figure 5–17   Correctly applied long leg cast; note suprapatellar molding resisting rotation, molding over medial tibia, position of knee in approximately 5° of flexion, and positions of foot and ankle in neutral.   *(Rockwood, C. A., et al. (1996). Rockwood & Green's Fractures in Adults. 4th ed. Philadelphia: Lippincott-Raven.)*

extended, but if weight bearing is to be allowed, the knee should be neutral or in 5 degrees of flexion. In many instances, the below-the-knee portion (like a short leg-cast) is applied first. The patient is then placed in a supine position and a leg holder placed under the short leg cast such that the knee is flexed to approximately 30 or 35 degrees, and the cast is applied to the proximal portion of the leg. Plaster layers are begun below the knee over the short leg cast and rolled proximally to incorporate the two sections. Failure to apply appropriate overlap layers of plaster between the leg and thigh sections of the cast will result in the cast being very weak about the knee, and it will eventually break at this point. Extra padding over the distal femoral condyles and patella may be necessary to avoid pressure points. Frequently, cast material splints incorporated across the knee to strengthen the cast in the region help to avoid the accumulation of excess plaster over the knee flexion crease. The cast is trimmed in line with the metatarsal heads on the plantar aspect and at the base of the toes dorsally. The fifth toe must be entirely free; this is a common site for a plaster sore (see Figure 5–7, plaster application). The long leg cast is used to treat stable injuries of the knee joint and distal femur and unstable fractures of the tibia, the fibula, and the ankle joint.

Tibial fractures may be repaired using a closed method of reduction followed by the application of a leg cast in two ways. One is to use a long leg cast until the bone calcifies, that is, for approximately 8 to 10 weeks. The second method is to apply a long leg cast for 2 to 4 weeks and then change to a below-knee, patellar-tendon, weight-bearing cast until calcification is complete. In instances of delayed union, calcification may take 4 months or longer.

NURSING PROCESS (Patient with a Fractured Tibia and Long Leg Cast)

To demonstrate the nursing care, the following nursing process presents the care of a patient with a long leg cast for a closed reduction of a fractured tibia. The nursing process begins after the cast is applied.

ASSESSMENT

Assessment of a patient following the application of a long leg cast for a fracture of the tibia includes a general assessment as well as an assessment of the affected extremity. Listen to the patient's complaints, as trauma or surgery affecting an extremity produces swelling from bleeding and edema. Check for unrelieved pain and increasing pain or swelling. Ask the patient to localize the exact site of the pain. Check for tingling, coldness, numbness, and the patient's ability to move the toes. Note any discoloration of the toes; the color should be pink. Pale and cold toes suggest an arterial obstruction, whereas blueness suggests a venous obstruction. Pinch

the nail beds to assess capillary filling in the involved leg; a rapid return of color should appear when the pressure is released (see Chapter 2). As the patient is in a long leg cast, only the femoral pulse is usually obtainable, and that is nondiagnostic as it is proximal to the injury. Always compare the uninjured leg with the injured leg.

The assessment of the cast depends on the type of material used for casting. Here, the emphasis is on the assessment of a patient with a long leg cast made of plaster of Paris. (For more information on fiberglass casts, see the section earlier in this chapter.) Observe the color of a freshly applied cast. A white, shiny cast is one that is dry. Assess the complete cast, turning the patient to the unaffected side to check the back. At the edges of the cast, check for tightness or any skin irritation. At the distal end of the cast, check to make sure that the little toe is able to move freely. The linen should be off the cast, exposing it to the air to dry; that also serves to keep the linen dry. The complete leg is elevated by raising the foot of the bed, placing the leg in a sling, or placing the cast leg on pillows. After several days, a postoperative assessment includes smelling both ends of the cast for signs of an infection under the cast.

NURSING DIAGNOSIS

Based on all of the assessment data, the major nursing diagnoses for a typical patient with a long leg cast following a fractured tibia may include the following:

- Pain and discomfort related to trauma and immobility
- Impaired physical mobility related to instability of the tibia
- Potential impaired skin integrity related to the cast
- Anxiety related to knowledge deficit about the injury, treatment method, and the rehabilitation process

COLLABORATIVE PROBLEMS

- Delayed union
- Compartmental syndrome

GOAL FORMULATION AND PLANNING

The goals are to have the patient experience (1) a decrease in the amount of pain through immobilization, nursing measures, and prescribed medications; (2) an increase in mobility through the use of positioning, exercises, and ambulation; (3) no break in skin integrity; (4) a decrease in anxiety through increased knowledge; and (5) an absence of complications. Long-term goals are to have the patient free of pain and to have a return of full leg function in approximately 10 to 12 weeks with no residual complications..

INTERVENTIONS

ALLEVIATE PAIN

Pain following a fractured tibia is usually severe for 3 to 7 days, but that varies depending on the type of fracture and the individual. Elevating the affected leg helps to reduce pain, but make sure that the patient is able to relax the leg in that position. Apply ice bags along the fracture site and refill as needed. Muscle-setting exercises also help to increase the blood flow to the area and reduce pain and swelling. Once the assessment determines the level of pain and that it is not due to circulatory and nerve impairment, offer analgesics on schedule.

INCREASE MOBILITY
Interventions to increase mobility of a patient with a long leg cast following a fractured tibia include correct positioning, turning, exercises, and ambulation.

Position. The patient with a fractured tibia and a long leg cast needs to be immobilized with the involved leg elevated until the cast is dry, usually 24 hours but sometimes longer, depending on the cast. Make sure that there is no pressure on the soft tissue at the proximal end of the cast or on the patient's low back area while they are lying.

Turning. Whether in the hospital or at home, most patients finding lying supine the most comfortable and would probably prefer to stay that way because they fear that moving will cause them pain. However, they must turn to their side to promote homeostasis, to relieve pressure on the coccyx, and to allow the posterior side of the cast to dry. The procedure for helping a patient turn is the same as the one discussed for a patient following a fractured hip (see Chapter 9). In most cases, the patient is able to use the overhead trapeze and side rails to move all of the body except the affected leg. In the beginning, someone will need to lift and support the affected leg during the turn and then reposition the leg on pillows once the turn is completed. The patient may turn to either side, but would probably prefer the unaffected side.

Exercises. Patients in a long leg cast need exercises if they are to maintain muscle strength and prevent the complications of immobility. General body exercises and self-care (as discussed for a patient following a fractured hip in Chapter 9) as well as more specific exercises for the leg are involved. Joints above and below the cast need to be exercised to prevent stiffness. Encourage flexion and extension movements of the toes and as much range of motion of the hip as possible.

Muscle-setting or isometric exercises are taught using the uninvolved leg so they can be done on the fractured leg while it is in the cast. Check with the physician on the specific exercises, when to start the exercises, and how much exercising should be done. The most frequently used exercises are quadriceps-setting and straight leg raises. For a discussion of these and other possible exercises, see the care of the patient following a total hip replacement in Chapter 9 and total knee replacement in Chapter 10. Start teaching the patient exercises to build up their arm muscles for crutch walking (see Chapter 4) as soon as possible. However, in the beginning, patients will tire very easily with only a short period of ambulation with crutches.

Ambulation. After the cast is dry, the patient is usually allowed up in a chair or wheelchair. Before attempting to get the patient up, explain every step of the procedure. Alert the patient to the likelihood of increased pain when the affected leg is lowered. Explain that the patient should arise slowly to prevent orthostatic hypotension. Tell the patient how he or she can be of help, and make sure the patient is informed about weight bearing on the affected leg. Do not rush or try to hurry the patient through the transfer.

If the patient is to be seated in a wheelchair, check that the wheelchair is locked and has a foot extension that can be elevated before beginning the procedure. Use the foot extension to elevate the leg, placing a pillow between the leg and the foot extension so that the casted leg will be more comfortable. Once in the wheelchair, the casted leg should be secured to the foot extension using a strap with a buckle, a towel and safety pins, or (preferably) wide adhesive tape. The tape holds the cast securely without damaging it, is easily removed, and can be used at home. A thin patient with a heavy long leg cast may be able to tip the wheelchair forward if they lean toward their foot. Discuss the problem with the patient, and consider adding sandbags to the back of the wheelchair. Because the foot extension does not elevate the leg relative to the body to the same degree as when the patient is in the bed, the patient may experience some pain and swelling.

The procedure to move the patient is to first move the patient so that the unaffected leg is at the side of the bed (getting out on the unaffected side is easier but either will work). Raise the head of the bed. Bring the patient to a sitting position on the edge of the bed. One person is supporting the casted leg and getting it positioned on the floor while the other helps the patient get to a sitting position. (If only one person is available, the patient can use the upper side rail and the trapeze to help themselves to sit on the side of the bed.) Talk to and reassure the patient during the activity. Let the patient sit there for a few minutes to prevent orthostatic hypotension. Next, pivot the patient into a chair, ensuring that there is no weight bearing on the affected leg. Let the patient assume a sitting position with their leg elevated on a soft surface. Encourage the patient to do exercises such as deep breathing, abdominal, gluteal, and quadriceps-setting exercises. If the chair has armrests, encourage the patient to periodically push down on the chair arms and raise their buttocks off the chair. The raising allows circulation to the buttocks and also helps build up muscles in the upper extremity for crutch walking.

Patients get out of bed to ambulate the same way as to pivot to a chair. Once they are sitting on the side of the bed, they can use the upper side rail (or if in a chair, the arms of the chair) to help them come to a standing position. Once standing, they can take their crutches (or walker, depending on the patient) and prepare for a non-weight-bearing gait. For a discussion of the steps for how to ambulate with a walker or crutches using a three-point gait, see Chapter 4. Crutches allow for more and easier mobility, and the patient should be encouraged to use them even if he or she feels less sure at first. Patients should also be taught how to get in and out of a chair and on and off the toilet, how to go up and down stairs with or without arm rails, and how to get in and out of a car with a long leg cast.

Patients who are allowed to ambulate while weight bearing will have a long leg cast but also wear a cast shoe or boot to assist them in ambulation. These patients would also be advised to wear a sturdy shoe with an elevation on the unaffected side to equalize leg length so that they can walk with a more normal gait.

MAINTAIN SKIN INTEGRITY

Attention should be given to the positioning and turning of a patient with a long leg cast. The bed is normally equipped with an overhead trapeze, and the patient should be encouraged to lift and change positions frequently. Use pillows under the casted leg to prevent flat spots and underlying pressure areas, especially on the heel and the posterior portion of the cast. Indentations in the cast can also occur when a flat hand is not used to handle a wet cast. Assess for pressure behind the knee in the popliteal area, at the proximal end of the fibula (on the lateral side of the leg, where the peroneal nerve transverses), at the Achilles tendon, and on the heel; and reposition the patient as indicated.

Utilize measures to prevent swelling of the toes that puts pressure on the skin at the cast edges. Note that the cast is not irritating the patient's skin around the top of the cast, especially at the fold of the buttocks in the back. Make sure the patient's skin is not pinched between the bedpan and the cast if the patient needs to utilize a bedpan.

PATIENT TEACHING AND HOME CARE CONSIDERATIONS

Some patients find that lying supine is the most comfortable position for their leg. Others find it difficult to sleep at night lying supine. Sleepless patients tend to be a bother to other patients and tend to worry excessively about their injury or other problems. The pain in the leg may also appear to become worse at night. Try therapeutic communication, back rubs, smoothing of the bedding, fluffing and repositioning pillows, and having the patient drink warm milk. Giving a second sedative or another pain medication should be done only after other methods fail. Patients who have difficulty sleeping at night frequently want to sleep late in the morning. They must understand that difficulties in sleeping should not be allowed to interfere with their rehabilitation program. In some instances, the exercises done in the rehabilitation program may actually help the patient sleep better.

Patients with a fractured tibia and a long leg cast need emotional support from the staff, the family, and significant others. They may remember seeing people on the street with a long leg cast, and wonder why they are still in the hospital. Patients need to understand the location of the fracture, how it was reduced, why the exercises are necessary, and the need for their continued hospitalization.

Before discharge, the patient, the family, and significant others need to know about cast care, personal hygiene with a long leg cast, and ambulation activities. If the hospital has a movie on cast care, make sure these patients have an opportunity to see it. Personal hygiene can present difficulties for the patient. Bathroom facilities should be convenient and allow the patient room to sit on the stool with the casted leg extended. Although patients often feel that sponge baths are inadequate, tub baths are difficult and inconvenient and risk getting the cast wet. Showering twice a week should be encouraged. To protect the cast in the shower, enclose the leg in a large plastic bag that is taped to the skin at the top (or use a commercial plastic cast cover). Initially, the patient needs assistance in getting the bag over the cast and in getting into and out of the shower.

At home, it is essential that the patient realize the importance of elevating the leg when sitting and of continuing with the exercise regime. In bed, if the casted leg is elevated on pillows, a chair may be placed next to the bed to prevent the casted leg from falling to the floor. Patients who share their bed with another should realize that the cast can scratch and irritate and is best placed on the side away from their bed partner. Patients in a long leg cast need not abstain from sexual activities, though they may have to adjust their positioning and wrap the casted leg with a sheet to prevent abrasions.

MONITORING AND MANAGING POTENTIAL PROBLEMS

The major complications that may arise following a fractured tibia and the application of a long leg cast are delayed union and compartmental syndrome.

DELAYED UNION

Delayed union (or delayed healing) is a term used to describe a fracture that is slow to heal but does demonstrate some calcification. Some reasons for delayed union are infection, inadequate immobilization or reduction that allows movement at the fracture site, inadequate blood supply, or metabolic disturbances that affect the protein and the vitamins available for bone healing. Treatment consists of discovering the cause and correcting the underlying problem.

COMPARTMENTAL SYNDROME

One circulatory complication of special concern is known as compartmental syndrome, a condition in which progressive pressure within a confined space compromises the circulation and the function of tissues within that space. A compartment is enveloped by tough, inelastic fascial tissue, and when swelling of the muscles occurs the fascia does not expand. In the lower leg, that can occur in the anterior, lateral, superficial posterior, or deep posterior compartments. Such an ischemic condition can occur after unusually strenuous activities, fractures (especially of the proximal tibia), or knee surgery. The onset of the symptoms can vary from as little as 2 hours to as much as 6 days after the trauma or surgery. If the pressure is not relieved within approximately 12 hours of the onset of the syndrome (i.e., from the onset of excessive intracompartmental pressure), irreversible nerve and tissue damage is likely to result, which can render the extremity useless because of contractures, paralysis, and loss of sensation, and can, in some cases, lead to amputation. (See Chapter 4).

The orthopaedic nurse plays an absolutely vital role in detecting compartmental syndrome. In assessing for compartmental syndrome, remember the so-called "five Ps":

*   *Pain,* specifically progressive intense pain. A "red flag" is burning pain.
*   *Pain on passive motion,* as severe pain on passive motion of a distal extremity is likely due to muscle ischemia. Two particularly significant signs are pain referred to the anterior compartment on passive plantar flexion of the toes, and acute calf pain on passive dorsiflexion of the foot (a positive Homan's sign).
*   *Paralysis,* as a decrease of the blood supply to the muscles leads to progressive paralysis of the active voluntary function. To assess whether a motor nerve has been rendered ischemic, check the voluntary ability of the patient to flex and extend the toes.
*   *Paresthesia,* because as the sensory component of the peripheral nerve becomes progressively ischemic, the patient will notice numbness and tingling in the nerve that transverses the involved compartment. The anterior compartment contains the deep peroneal branch, and its sensory area is the web space between the first and second toes. The posterior tibial nerve transverses the posterior compartment and supplies the plantar surface of the foot and toes.
*   *Pulselessness,* though it is the least important and least reliable of the signs. Peripheral pulses may remain intact in the presence of complete ischemia of a compartment. Capillary filling, pallor, and skin temperature are similarly of almost no help in making a timely diagnosis of compartmental syndrome. The physician may check the compartmental pressure by a variety of techniques.

Effective treatment for compartmental syndrome depends upon early observation. Loosen any tight dressing or cast material that may be adding to the problem. There is disagreement about whether elevating the leg reduces swelling or further impedes circulation. If the intracompartmental pressure does not subside, the patient is returned to surgery for a fasciotomy. The incision in the fascia allows the muscles freedom to expand, relieving the pressure. The fascia is not sutured closed until all signs of swelling have subsided. The patient returns from surgery with an open lesion covered by dressings. Further surgery (and in some cases skin grafts) is needed to close the wound. To prevent disability, the fasciotomy must be performed before the pressure damages the tissue.

EVALUATION/OUTCOMES

In evaluating the goal of alleviating pain in the knee, determine whether the individual is having any pain by verbal responses and by the patient's outward appearance, including facial grimacing during activities, the position assumed, and restlessness or sleeplessness. If pain still exists, determine the location, duration, and intensity of the pain; what aggravates and intensifies it; and what measures have been able to relieve the pain.

When evaluating care to increase mobility, determine the patient's compliance with the exercise routine and utilization of assistive devices such as the trapeze and crutches. Evaluate the steadiness of the crutch walking. Determine whether or not the patient, the family, and significant others have been able to follow the rehabilitation regime, how useful the discharge plan appears to be, and how well they understand what the patient can and cannot do. Regarding complications, look for skin breakdown, an elevated temperature, and other problem signs. Determine that the patient knows how to provide personal hygiene, dress, and do cast care.

WALKING CAST

A walking cast has been described as a short or long leg cast with a walking device implanted on the bottom. Today, the Böhler walking irons and rubber walking heels have largely become supplanted by plaster boots or cast shoes (Fig. 5–18). The boots or shoes have the advantage of being removable at bedtime,

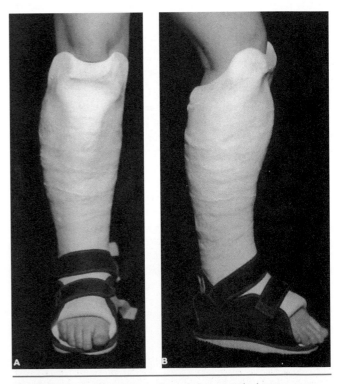

Figure 5–18   Sarmiento patellar-tendon–weight-bearing cast. Note that the cast shoe is removable.   *(Rockwood, C. A., et al. (1996). Rockwood & Green's Fractures in Adults. 4th ed. Philadelphia: Lippincott-Raven.)*

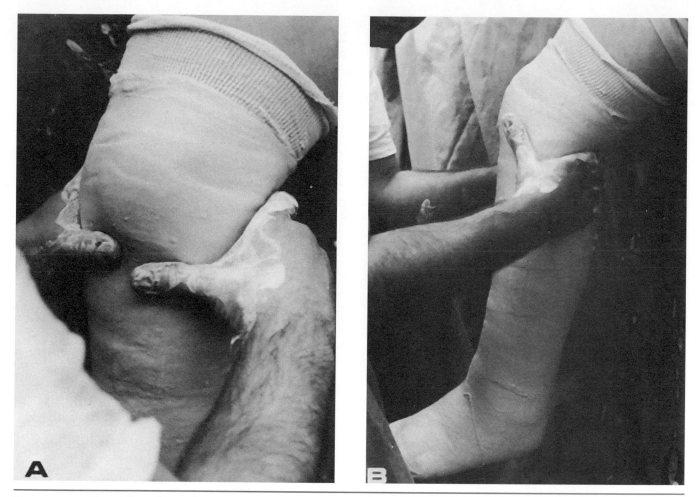

Figure 5–19 (A and B) In the application of a patellar-tendon–weight-bearing cast, indentation must be made over the patellar tendon, and the cast must be carefully molded around the patella. At the same time, the posterior calf must be molded to make a triangular cross section at the upper end of the leg. *(Rockwood, C. A., et al. (1996). Rockwood & Green's Fractures in Adults. 4th ed. Philadelphia: Lippincott-Raven.)*

and the patient walks with a better gait. The patient can strike down on their heel and then rock up on their toes for pushoff in a normal walking gait. The short or long leg cast is applied and the bottom or sole to the cast left flat. The plaster boot or cast shoe, which has an oval-shaped bottom to yield a rocking motion, is then put on.

PATELLAR-TENDON–WEIGHT-BEARING CAST

The patellar-tendon–weight-bearing cast is a special type of short leg weight-bearing cast that extends higher on the leg than the typical short leg cast and resembles a patellar-tendon–weight-bearing prosthesis (Fig. 5–19). In contrast to long leg casts, the patellar-tendon–weight-bearing cast allows flexion in the knee. The cast is usually applied very meticulously in segments over minimal padding. In applying the upper portion of the cast, the knee should be flexed to a right angle and the cast molded flat over the upper calf to develop a triangular cross section. The cast is molded anteriorly around the patella, an indentation is made over the patellar tendon, and then the cast is trimmed to look like the prosthesis

(Fig. 5–20). The patellar-tendon–weight-bearing cast is used in the treatment of unstable fractures of the tibia and fibula, especially tibial shaft fractures. Nursing care of a patient in a patellar-tendon–weight-bearing cast follows that of a patient in a short leg cast, as discussed earlier in this chapter. Special care needs to be taken at the proximal end of the cast to prevent skin irritation and breakdown.

LONG LEG CYLINDER CAST (LLCC)

A long leg cylinder cast is similar to a long leg cast except that the foot and ankle are not casted, and the cast may not extend as high on the upper leg. The LLCC extends from just proximal to the malleoli up to the greater trochanter, which leaves the foot and ankle free but immobilizes the knee. The application of the cast begins distally (above the level of the malleoli) with the rolling of six or more layers of sheet cotton padding. The plaster begins several centimeters proximal to the edge of the cotton padding at the distal end (approximately 3 cm should be left between the malleoli and the lower end of tibia cast to prevent irritation of

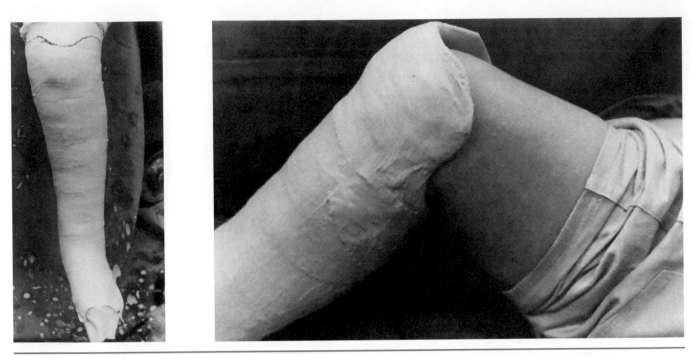

Figure 5–20   The patellar-tendon–weight-bearing cast should be cut out to resemble a patellar-tendon–weight-bearing prosthesis, and it is particularly important to trim the lateral portion like a wingback chair. When the knee is flexed, pressure is taken from the patellar tendon, but in full extension, pressure is exerted on the thick skin over the tendon.   *(Rockwood, C. A., et al. (1996). Rockwood & Green's Fractures in Adults. 4th ed. Philadelphia: Lippincott-Raven.)*

the malleoli from the cast). The knee is kept in 5 to 10 degrees of flexion as the cast material is rolled proximally to the greater trochanter on the lateral surface and as high as possible medially. While the cast is still malleable, use your hands to mold the cast around the supracondylar and suprapatellar areas to keep the cast from sliding down the leg. Irritation about the Achilles tendon and malleoli will be the primary problem caused by the cast. Make sure the cast has adequate padding in those areas and that the cast is kept well proximal to the malleoli. The long leg cylinder cast is used in the treatment of stable injuries of the distal femur, proximal tibia, and knee joint. Nursing care for a patient with a long leg cylinder cast follows that of a patient in a long leg cast, with special emphasis on preventing skin irritation at the ankle.

CAST BRACE

The cast brace is a combination of cast and brace made up of three components. First, there is a patellar weight-bearing cast on the lower leg, either as a short leg cast or a cylinder cast. Second, there is an ischial weight-bearing cast on the thigh, molded well around Scarpa's triangle, the ischial seat, and the greater trochanter. The thigh component is applied snugly to increase the hydrodynamic compressive effect of the thigh muscles and to immobilize the fracture fragments. Third, there are external polycentric knee hinges that connect the below-the-knee portion to the thigh portion and that allow 90 degrees of knee flexion. In the application of the cast brace, a long leg cast is applied over a long spandex stocking with the upper end molded to the

shape of a quadrilateral socket, or a plastic socket is incorporated in the cast. The knee is then cut out and hinged (Harkess, Ramsey, & Harkess, 1996). The cast brace allows for mobility of both hip and knee joints, which permits a fairly normal gait when ambulating. The cast brace is used in the treatment of midshaft or distal-shaft fractures of the femur, although it is not very popular today. For further information regarding the care of the patient with a cast brace, see Chapter 6.

HIP SPICA CAST

A hip spica cast extends from midtrunk (just below the nipple line) down the entire length of the affected leg with a spiral bandage from the trunk to the legs (Fig. 5–21). For a one-and-one-half spica, the affected leg will be casted to include the foot but leave out the toes, and the unaffected leg will be casted to just above the knee. A support (usually a wooden rod) will be casted from above the knee on the unaffected side to below the knee on the affected side. This rod will keep the legs in abduction and give support to the cast. The cast application is done with the patient on a fracture table, usually in the OR following a surgical procedure. The steps of padding, plaster preparation, and cast application follow those discussed earlier. The hip spica cast may also be a single or a double hip spica cast, depending on the need for immobilization of the affected hip. To reduce the weight of the cast and make the patient more comfortable (help prevent cast claustrophobia), a substantial window is cut out over the patient's abdomen. The hip spica cast is used in the treatment of a dislocated hip and to immobilize a hip following

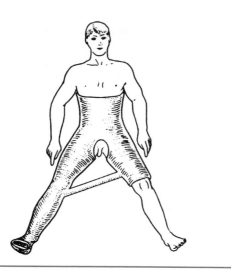

Figure 5–21   Hip spica cast.   *(Mallon, W. J., et al. (1990).* Orthopaedics for the House Officer. *Baltimore: Williams and Wilkins.)*

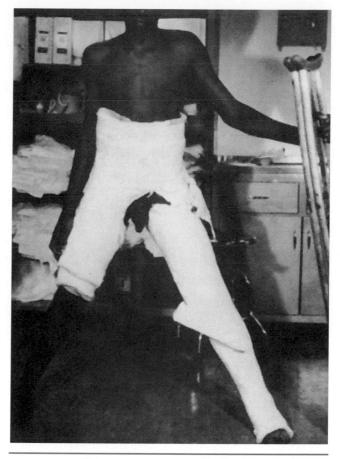

Figure 5–22   This sporting patient walked in his spica, which failed at its weakest point, the open section of the thigh at the "intern's angle."   *(Rockwood, C. A., et al. (1996).* Rockwood & Green's Fractures in Adults. *4th ed. Philadelphia: Lippincott-Raven.)*

reconstructive surgery or injury to the pelvis, the hip joint, or the femur. Because of the complications encountered with the hip spica, it is rarely used for adults.

A hip arthrodesis is the surgical fusion of a hip joint (see Chapter 9 for details). Its purpose is to halt the disease process, provide stability, and relieve pain. After surgical fusion with an internal fixation, some physicians (1) never apply a cast; (2) may or may not apply a cast if no femoral osteotomy was done; (3) apply no cast for 2 weeks, then apply a short spica cast, which allows knee motion for 8 to 10 weeks, and then gradually begin weight bearing after the removal of the cast; and (4) place the patient in a hip spica cast until union occurs. Partial weight bearing on crutches may be allowed a few days or weeks after surgery. Crutches must be used until the fusion is solid.

If the surgical procedure did not use an internal fixation, or a femoral osteotomy was also done, most patients will be in a one-and-one-half hip spica cast. The cast may be changed at 8-week intervals, but roentgenographic studies of the hip will determine the length of immobilization. When the fusion is far advanced, some physicians may apply a single spica walking cast (Fig. 5–22), which will usually be from the nipple line to above the ankle on the affected side. Partial weight bearing in the cast with crutches is then allowed to a limited extent. If the hip has not fused after 4 months, a short spica cast is applied until the fusion becomes solid.

NURSING PROCESS (Patient with a Hip Arthrodesis and Hip Spica Cast)

To demonstrate the nursing care, the following nursing process presents the care of a patient with a hip spica

cast following a hip arthrodesis. The nursing process begins after the cast is applied.

ASSESSMENT

Because most of the patients undergoing hip arthrodesis have a history of infection, look for systemic infection and for pain in the soft tissue and bone of the hip. Following a hip arthrodesis without an internal fixation device, or after an intertrochanteric or subtrochanteric osteotomy is done, the patient will be in a hip spica cast from the nipple line to the toes on the affected side and to just above the knee on the other side. Assess for physical discomfort from the cast and for emotional reactions such as feelings of claustrophobia, tightness, or being unable to breathe. Assessment of the respiratory and gastrointestinal systems is an ongoing need during the time the patient is in the cast. Check the neurovascular status of both legs. Check for any flat or potential pressure areas in the cast, and assess for any skin irritation at the cast edges. Check for bleeding into the cast at the surgical site and the area posterior to the surgical site and note the size of the bloodstained area.

NURSING DIAGNOSIS

Based on all of the assessment data, the major nursing diagnoses for a typical patient following a hip arthrodesis and the application of a hip spica cast may include the following:

- Pain and discomfort related to surgical trauma and immobility
- Impaired physical mobility related to instability of the hip and the hip spica cast
- Potential impaired skin integrity related to the cast
- Self-care deficit related to the instability of the hip and the hip spica cast
- Anxiety related to knowledge deficit about the surgery and rehabilitation process

COLLABORATIVE PROBLEMS

- Nonunion
- Fatigue fractures
- Disabilities related to immobilization
- Malpositioned femur
- Infection

GOAL FORMULATION AND PLANNING

The goals are to have the patient experience (1) a decrease in the amount of pain through immobilization, nursing measures, and prescribed medication; (2) an increase in the potential for ambulation by utilizing exercises and immobilization; (3) no break in skin integrity; (4) the ability to perform activities of daily living; (5) a decrease in anxiety through increased knowledge about the surgery and the rehabilitation process; and (6) the absence of complications. Long-term goals are to have the patient free of pain or with only minimal pain in the hip and to ultimately be able to ambulate without an assistive device.

INTERVENTIONS

ALLEVIATE PAIN
While talking with the patient, try physical measures such as turning the patient for pain relief; encourage diversions such as reading, watching television, and doing handicrafts; and provide prescribed medications. The hip spica cast prevents some discomfort by immobilizing the hip joint.

INCREASE MOBILITY
Interventions to increase the mobility of a patient with a hip spica cast following a hip arthrodesis include positioning, turning, and exercises.

Positioning. The cast prevents raising the head of the bed unless the entire bed is tilted using 4- to 8-inch blocks. If the bed is flat, some patients have a feeling that their head is actually lower than their body.

Turning. Turning is a primary concern following an arthrodesis of the hip. The schedule is every 2 to 3 hours during the day and every 4 hours at night. With the patient in a hip spica cast, the patient can lie supine, on the unaffected side, or prone. In turning the patient from the supine position, turn the patient to the unaffected side and then to the prone position. To turn the patient from the prone position to the supine position, reverse the procedure and turn the patient to the unaffected side and then to the supine position. While the patient is lying on their unaffected side, their casted (involved) leg can be supported by at least two slings connected to the overhead frame, and the patient's trunk can be supported with pillows.

To turn a medium-sized adult in a one-and-one-half hip spica cast, adequate help (usually three people) is needed. First, explain the procedure to the patient to allay their fears so that they understand and will not interfere with the turning process. With the patient supine and the bed in the low position, move the patient so that the trunk and affected hip are at the edge of the bed and the casted leg extends beyond the side of the bed. To do so, two persons should be on the affected side and one on the nonaffected side. One of the two persons on the affected side helps the patient move their trunk to the edge of the bed, while the other supports the affected leg as it extends beyond the side of the bed. With the patient on the edge of the bed, the patient's trunk and affected leg are then lifted and turned so the patient is placed on his or her unaffected side. The person on the affected side assists in turning the patient's trunk. The patient can have their hands crossed across the front of their chest to keep them out of the way, or the patient can help by utilizing the trapeze to lift and turn the upper part of the trunk. The hand placement and actual turn is very much like the procedure described in turning a patient with a hip fracture (see Chapter 9). The patient should be in the center of the bed on their side once the turn is complete. The person supporting and moving the affected leg continues to hold the leg in position until it has been securely supported in at least two slings, one above where the bar is attached to the cast and the other below the bar. Pillows need to be placed in front and in back of the patient's trunk to help the patient maintain a relaxed side-lying position.

To turn the patient from their side to the prone position, one person must support the affected leg while the slings are removed. It is sometimes easier to then move the patient (with the patient still in the side-lying position) toward the side of the bed. Make sure that the patient is positioned in bed so that their feet will be off the end of the mattress when the turn is complete. The person holding the patient's leg now moves so they can support the patient's affected leg as it is lowered onto the bed. When the turn is complete, the patient should be lying on their abdomen in the center of the bed with their toes off the end of the mattress. Most patients do not like this position and will only tolerate it for short periods. However, it is important that they are turned prone to relieve pressure on other parts of their body.

To turn the patient back to the supine position, the procedure must be reversed. That means the patient will first need to be moved to the edge of the bed and turned onto their unaffected hip. Care must be taken that someone always has a secure hold on the affected leg. DO NOT USE THE BAR IN THE CAST THAT CONNECTS THE TWO LEGS AND GIVES SUPPORT TO THE AFFECTED LEG FOR TURNING OR MOVING THE PATIENT.

Exercises. Bed exercises, such as muscle-setting exercises (i.e., quadriceps, gluteal, and abdominal), are encouraged. That will lessen atrophy in the muscles that are immobilized by the cast. Active range of motion to the unaffected lower joints and the upper extremities is important. Some patients may be able to use the trapeze, but most will have very restricted use of the trapeze because the cast begins at the nipple line.

PATIENT TEACHING AND HOME CARE CONSIDERATIONS

Allocate time for therapeutic communication with the patient, the family, and significant others. Special points of concern are most likely to be (1) the adjustment to the long period of immobility and what that means to the patient's personal, social, vocational, and economic status; and (2) whether the patient has to stay in the hospital during the recovery period, go to a nursing home, or return home with a hip spica cast and the assistance of a home health nurse and family members. Once out of the cast, the patient must be extremely careful about stumbling or falling, which could easily result in a fracture of the femur. In patients with internal fixation, such a fracture usually occurs just below the fixation device. Work closely with a social worker in making arrangements for accommodations, and with the family, significant others, and possibly public health workers or home health nurses concerning the specifics of care. Depending on where the patient will spend the time while they are in the hip spica cast, activities of daily living, cast care, and the prevention of complications need to be discussed.

MONITORING AND MANAGING POTENTIAL PROBLEMS

The patient has undergone a major surgical procedure and is immobilized; therefore, nursing measures must focus on preventing complications common to all surgical and immobilized patients. For a more detailed plan of care, see the nursing care of a patient following an internal fixation of the hip in Chapter 9. However, a special concern following an arthrodesis is infection, because most patients have a history of hip infection.

NONUNION

Nonunion is when the fracture fragments do not calcify together. A nonunion of a hip arthrodesis may occur as the result of (1) muscles or fascia between the bone fragments, (2) callus being broken or torn by excessive activity allowed by a loose or improperly fitting hip spica cast, (3) inadequate blood supply to the fusion site, and (4) marked dietary deficiency. Occasionally, nonunion occurs with no apparent cause.

FATIGUE FRACTURES

A number of physicians believe that a fatigue fracture occurs as the result of muscle fatigue. Normally, the muscles allow the body to shunt stress from the bones; this stress shielding is lost when muscle action is no longer optimal. Being in a hip spica cast for a long period of time reduces muscle mass and weakens the large muscles of the hip and leg so they become easily fatigued when they are used after the cast is removed. Care is needed to provide as much muscle activity as possible while the patient is in the cast. Once the cast is removed, it is essential that the patient progress slowly from nonweight bearing, to partial weight bearing, and finally to full weight bearing on the affected side.

DISABILITIES RELATED TO IMMOBILIZATION

These patients are at risk of all of the complications of surgery and immobility when they are placed in a hip spica cast following a hip arthrodesis. Potential complications as the result of the surgical procedure are fat and pulmonary embolism and infection. Potential complications from the cast are neurovascular impairment and the deleterious effects of immobility. Those effects are complications of the (1) respiratory tract, such as pneumonia from decreased respiration; (2) circulatory system, such as circulatory overload, orthostatic hypotension, and venous stasis; (3) gastrointestinal system, such as paralytic ileus and constipation; (4) genitourinary tract, such as lower urinary tract infection; (5) integumentary system, such as pressure areas and skin irritation; and (6) musculoskeletal system, such as weakened muscles. For more in-depth discussion of these complications, see Care of the Patient with a Fractured Hip in Chapter 9.

MALPOSITIONED HIP

A malpositioned hip is usually the result of the surgical procedure and the placement of the hip at the time of fusion and rarely the result of hip spica cast application.

INFECTION

An infection in the fused hip can occur as the result of a break in operating room sterile technique, an infection elsewhere in the patient's body, or an infection in the hip being fused. An infection can cause poor healing, nonunion, or malunion. If the infected hip arthrodesis involves an internal fixation, the device may need to be removed. Infections of the bone are extremely difficult to eradicate, so prevention must be the goal. Patients are usually placed on prophylactic antibiotic therapy following the fusion and sometimes preoperatively.

EVALUATION/OUTCOMES

For a typical patient with a hip arthrodesis and hip spica cast, the evaluation and outcome cover the following goals. For the goal of alleviating pain in the hip, determine whether the individual is having any pain by verbal response and by the patient's outward appearance, including facial grimacing during movement. Sympathoadrenal signs signifying pain might be changes in pulse, blood pressure, and respiration; diaphoresis; depression; and mood swings. If pain still exists, determine the location, duration, and intensity of the pain; what aggravates it; and what intensifies it.

Determine the patient's compliance with the exercise routine and their willingness to help with activities of daily living. Look for the absence of pressure areas and skin irritation due to the cast. Check for the absence of an elevated temperature, and other signs that complications are absent. Special emphasis should be given to evaluating the patient's response to long-term immobilization in the initial stage and ability to walk and sit in the later stage.

BODY CASTS

Body casts have been used to immobilize a patient's vertebral column in instances of fractures, degenerative conditions, and infections such as tuberculosis of the spine. Although the utilization of most body casts has been greatly reduced, the following section presents the most commonly used body casts (i.e., the hyperextension, body jacket, and minerva jacket casts) with a discussion of their use and the complications that have lead to their disuse. This section also presents a brief discussion of the halo cast, still in use today.

HYPEREXTENSION BODY CAST

This body cast is applied with the patient's vertebral column in a position of hyperextension. It extends from the symphysis pubis to the suprasternal notch in front, and from the tip of the coccyx to the scapulae behind, so as to prevent the smallest degree of forward flexion of the spine. In the past, it was used to treat compression fractures of the spine or following spinal surgery in specific cases. Today it has very limited, if any, usefulness.

BODY JACKET

The body jacket extends from the upper chest over the trunk to the pubis. The iliac crests are enclosed, but the buttocks and perineal areas are exposed. Some body jackets may include the thighs and pelvis or the cervical spine. In the past, body casts were used to immobilize the spine to relieve degenerative disorders and to promote healing of surgical fusions and unstable spinal injuries. Today, with more use of braces, there is less use of body jackets. For a discussion on the care of a patient in a body cast following a posterior spinal fusion with implementation, see Chapter 8.

MINERVA JACKET

The minerva jacket cast covers the frontal and occipital regions of the skull and extends over the neck, chest, back, abdomen, and iliac crest. The face, ears, buttocks, pubic areas, and extremities are exposed. Since this is a cast principally used in pediatrics, no further discussion is presented here.

HALO CAST

The body jacket portion of the halo cast is made of a casting material, and the halo cast is used to immobilize fractures of the cervical spine. Today, however, the halo brace is almost always used. For further discussion of the halo brace, see Chapter 6.

SPLINTING

Immediate splinting of injured extremities is an important principle of emergency care, as immediate immobilization can prevent further injury during transportation and triage. Splints may be used as initial emergency treatment for injuries prior to definitive treatment, and in some cases simple splinting may be appropriate as a definitive treatment. Splinting has a number of advantages over cast. A splint is faster and easier to apply and remove in order to check wounds or the condition of the skin. It is a less-constrictive and noncircumferential dressing, so it is more forgiving with regard to swelling and compartmental syndrome. Splints can be made of a variety of materials, including casting materials. Prefabricated splints and immobilizers are commercially available. Some specialized immobilizers provide a means of applying cold or intermittent pressure. A list of some common types of splints follows:

- *Basswood splints,* used for many years and still found in some first aid kits and hospitals, fall into the category of improvised splints.
- *Universal splints,* designed to fit the arms and legs of everyone, are really splints that fit no one.
- *Creamer wire splints* are splints that resemble miniature ladders with malleable metal uprights and wire rungs. These splints can be bent into appropriate shapes, padded, and bandaged to the extremities. They also do not interfere with roentgenograms.
- *Thomas splints,* first introduced in World War I by Sir Robert Jones, reduced the high mortality rate from fractures of the femur from 80% to 20%. They have a long and effective history in the emergency care of lower-extremity fractures and are now required by national standards as ambulance equipment. Traction can be accomplished by using a padded hitch over the patient's shoe with a Spanish windlass, and the leg is held firmly in place with Velcro fasteners.
- *Inflatable splints/air splints* are splints that consist of a double-walled polyvinyl jacket with a zip fastener that is placed around the injured limb. There is a valve on the outer wall that allows the jacket to be inflated, either by mouth or by a pump. In the past, these splints were endorsed as being easy to apply, comfortable, effective, and safe. They were said to control swelling and bleeding and were thought to be the splint of choice in fractured limbs where burns were involved. However, that enthusiasm has waned. Some physicians state that when the leg splint is applied to immobilize a fractured femur, it barely reaches the fracture site. Ambulance attendants may mistakenly believe they have splinted the fracture and proceed to move the patient. Inflatable splints also have the disadvantage of being

compressive to the injured extremity and may accentuate problems with compartmental syndrome. They should not be applied over clothing, because folds can cause high-pressure points and blistering.

- *Structural aluminum malleable (SAM) splints* are made by coating 0.016-inch-thick aluminum foil with low-density, closed-coil polyethlene foam. Cut into 34 by 4 1/2-inch strips, they can be rolled up like a bandage or packed flat, weigh 5 1/2 oz, take up very little room, and are easily carried by soldiers, ski patrols, and ambulances. When folded longitudinally, these floppy, malleable strips become rigid. A structural bend gives the splint a configuration like a slat from a Venetian blind (Harkess, Ramsey, & Harkess, 1996, p. 28). The SAM splints can be made into sugar-tong splints for the upper arm, a two-poster splint to stabilize the cervical spine, or a Liston splint to immobilize the femur. They are self-padded, are stain resistant, can be trimmed to size by scissors, conform to any contour, and present no impediment to roentgenography. The ideal splint should be efficient, light, inexpensive, easily applied to a variety of anatomical locations, easily stored or carried, and radiolucent. None of the splints meet all of these requirements, but the SAM splints come the closest.
- *Custom-made plaster splints* are available in continuous rolls of various sizes and contain 10 to 14 layers of plaster and a closed cell foam backing,

all encased in stockinette. One has only to cut off the appropriate length and dip the entire splint into water before applying it, which makes for a very quick and efficient customized splint. Custom plaster splints can also be made by rolling out strips of plaster and then applying sheets of cotton for padding. The sheet cotton may be applied either to the plaster splints themselves or to the extremity.

UPPER-EXTREMITY SPLINTS

Splinting is a useful method of immobilization in the acute injury period. In the upper extremity, excellent immobilization can be obtained with a splint while allowing for significant swelling. In this section, ulnar gutter, radial slab, long arm posterior, coaptation-type, sugar-tong, volar and dorsal forearm, elephant-ear, gauntlet-length wrist, and hand and digital splints are described.

ULNAR GUTTER SPLINTS

Fractures involving the ring or small fingers can be adequately immobilized with an ulnar gutter plaster splint, leaving the radial digits completely free. (A similar radial gutter splint, with a hole for the thumb, can be used for fractures of the index and long fingers.) The ulnar gutter splint consists of a single slab of plaster (5 to 8 thicknesses) applied over a lightly padded forearm and hand (Fig. 5–23). If the forearm and hand are heavily padded, the gutter will not encompass enough

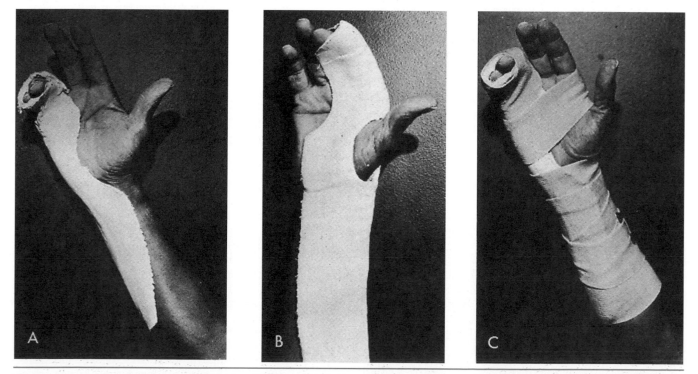

Figure 5–23 Gutter plaster. (A) Fractures involving the ring and small fingers can be adequately immobilized with an ulnar gutter splint, leaving the radial digits completely free. (B) A similar splint can be used on the radial side of the hand, cutting out a hole for the thumb. (C) The splint is held in place with an elastic bandage, wrapped securely but not tightly. We rarely use these now, preferring separate anterior and posterior splint. *(Rockwood, C. A., et al. (1996). Rockwood & Green's Fractures in Adults. 4th ed. Philadelphia: Lippincott-Raven.)*

of the ulna and hypothenar eminence to control motion and maintain a reduction. Care should be taken not to allow padding to gather in the folds of the fingers.

The splint begins at the proximal palmar crease and extends along the ulna to the elbow flexion crease (Green & Butler, 1996). If the injury being treated is distal to the wrist, the splint may be extended beyond the metacarpophalangeal (MCP) joints to include the fingers. The splint is molded to obtain immobilization and wrapped snugly with a bias-cut stockinette. Observe closely for loosening, as stockinette cut on the bias usually loosens within 24 hours. Ulnar gutter splints are useful for the treatment of nightstick fractures of the ulna and fractures of the neck of the fourth and fifth metacarpals (boxer's fractures).

RADIAL SLAB
The radial slab consists of 8 to 10 thicknesses of 6-inch plaster with a thumb hole cut in it. Stockinette, but not other padding, is applied, and then the wet plaster is applied to the radial side of the forearm overlapping the dorsal and volar surfaces of the wrist and forearm. The splint is then wrapped with a 2- or 3-inch wet gauze bandage and allowed to set. Because of the tendency for the hand to swell, some physicians apply a hand dressing of fluffs or absorbent cotton on top of the splint, with only the fingertips showing. The arm should be elevated.

LONG ARM POSTERIOR SPLINT
The long arm posterior splint extends from the axilla across the posterior surface of the elbow and along the ulna to the proximal palmar crease. The padding and splint application follow the steps for the ulnar gutter and radial slab already discussed.

COAPTATION-TYPE SPLINTS
The Coaptation-type splints are U-shaped plaster slabs that extend from around the humerus and over the shoulder (deltoid area) down the lateral aspect of the arm, around the elbow, and up the inner arm to the axilla (Fig. 5–24). They are used in conjunction with a sling or collar and cuff and are also sometimes called sugar-tong splints or U splints. They have the advantage of dependency traction with local splinting, especially for management in the first few weeks after injury. However, the disadvantages of this technique include (1) axillary irritation, (2) patient discomfort, and (3) the bulkiness of the splint. Not uncommonly, a plaster slab slips and requires reapplication. Because coaptation splints limit shoulder and elbow motion, replacing after 1 to 2 weeks with a functional brace is usually essential (see Chapter 6 for further discussion).

Coaptation-type splints are useful for the immobilization of fractures of the humerus. The patient's arm is padded from the shoulder to below the elbow. A single splint is again constructed from rolls of plaster to extend from above the acromion over the lateral aspect of the arm to the elbow, incorporate the elbow, and extend into the axilla. The splint thickness is 7 to 12 thicknesses of plaster that is applied over the padding

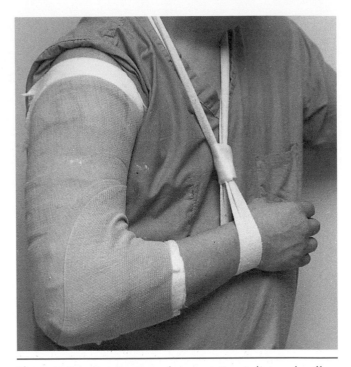

Figure 5–24 Application of a coaptation splint and cuff. *(Koval & Zuckerman (1998). Fractures in the Elderly. Philadelphia: Lippincott Raven.)*

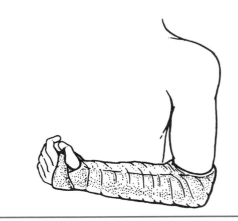

Figure 5–25 Sugar-tong splint. *(Mallon, W. J., et al. (1990). Orthopaedics for the House Officer. Baltimore: Williams and Wilkins.)*

and wrapped into place with a bias-cut stockinette. With this splint, the shoulder is placed into adduction and internal rotation. The forearm can be immobilized with a commercially available shoulder immobilizer or held to the trunk with a sling and swathe.

SUGAR-TONG SPLINTS
Sugar-tong splints extend from the MCP flexion crease along the volar forearm, wrap around the posterior surface of the elbow, continue onto the dorsal surface of the forearm, and then extend distally to the metacarpal heads (Fig. 5–25). They are often applied with an elastic bandage or bias-cut stockinette. This splint is commonly used to immobilize the entire fore-

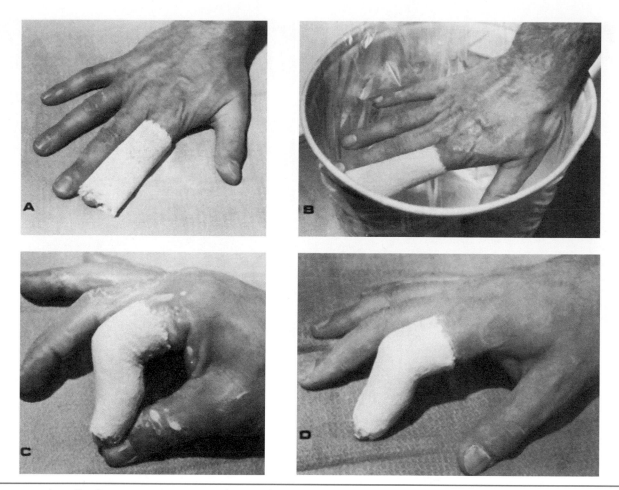

Figure 5–26   A mallet finger cast. (A) An 18-inch strip of 3- or 4-inch dry plaster is rolled into a tube and slipped over the end of the injured finger. No padding is used. (B) The patient dips his or her hand into a bucket of water, holding the tube of plaster in place over the finger. (C) The patient holds the finger in the correct position of immobilization while the physician smooths out the plaster. (D) The completed cast. Removal is facilitated by soaking the plaster. We virtually never use this technique, but it is a simple way to make a plaster cast for a single digit.   *(Rockwood, C. A., et al. (1996).* Rockwood & Green's Fractures in Adults. *4th ed. Philadelphia: Lippincott-Raven.)*

arm with respect to supination and pronation following a fracture of the wrist.

The arm is padded from the metacarpophalangeal joints to above the elbow. Unroll a 3- or 4-inch roll of plaster to make a single slab that will reach the distance described. Since the injured extremity is usually painful, measure the desired length by using the unaffected arm. To obtain the desired thickness (7 to 10 thicknesses), often two or three rolls of plaster are necessary. While the patient's arm is held in the desired position by an assistant, the plaster slab is dipped and applied to the extremity and held in place with an elastic bandage or bias-cut stockinette. The splint is molded to the extremity and held until it is set. Care should be taken to prevent contractures of the hand (especially extension contractures of the MCP joint, adduction contractures of the thumb, and flexion contractures of the wrist and PIP joint). Check for full motion of the hand after the cast is set. In distal radius (Colles') fractures, the sugar-tong splint may be extended onto the upper arm with an additional slab of plaster to minimize motion of the elbow.

VOLAR AND DORSAL FOREARM SPLINTS
Volar and dorsal forearm splints are usually used only on their respective surfaces and may be used to immobilize the wrist as well as the forearm while allowing elbow motion and supination and pronation.

ELEPHANT-EAR SPLINT
An elephant-ear splint extends from the wrist along the posterior aspect of the arm and over the shoulder to immobilize and support the humerus.

GAUNTLET-LENGTH WRIST SPLINT
Gauntlet-length wrist splints may be used to immobilize the wrist, leaving the forearm free.

HAND AND DIGITAL SPLINTS
Hand and digital splints may be stopped at either the MCP joint or over the palm, depending on the level of injury and desired degree of immobilization. Illustrations of possible methods are shown in Figure 5–26 and Figure 5–27.

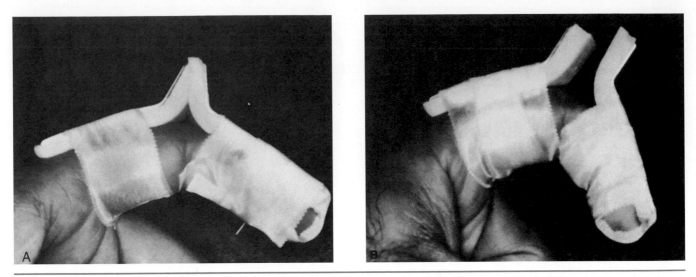

Figure 5–27   A simpler form of dorsal extension block splinting, made with two pieces of padded aluminum splint material bent to prevent extension at a predetermined level (A) and to allow flexion of the proximal interphalangeal (PIP) joint (B). This method should be used only in very reliable patients who understand the critical importance of not allowing the PIP joint to extend fully. *(Rockwood, C. A., et al. (1996). Rockwood & Green's Fractures in Adults. 4th ed. Philadelphia: Lippincott-Raven.)*

LOWER-EXTREMITY SPLINTS

In the lower extremity, splints may be used to immobilize most fractures distal to the middle portion of the femur. Medial and lateral slabs may be applied along the length of the lower extremity on the anteromedial and anterolateral surfaces of the leg and thigh to immobilize distal femur fractures, fractures about the knee, and proximal tibia fractures. The lower-extremity splints presented in this section are short leg posterior, long leg posterior, three-sided, and the U splint.

SHORT LEG POSTERIOR SPLINT

A posterior splint may be used to immobilize ankle and distal tibia fractures that do not require heavier and more stable splints. The short leg posterior splint is used for isolated fibula fractures, metatarsal fractures, and ankle sprains.

These splints can be applied without assistance if the patient is able to cooperate. The patient needs to be in the prone position with the knee flexed at 90 degrees. The lower extremity is padded from toe to knee with additional padding over the malleoli and the fibular head. In adults, the splint can be easily constructed from three sets of 5 by 30-inch splints (5 thicknesses for the medial and lateral slabs and 10 thicknesses for the posterior slab). These splints are then applied over the padding. The medial slab begins 2 to 4 cm below the medial joint line of the knee and extends distally to encompass the heel and lateral malleolus. The lateral slab is applied at the level of the fibular head and extends distally to overlap the medial slab at the heel. The splint is completed by bringing a third slab from just distal to the knee over the heel and out over the toes. Excess cast material is then folded back on itself to form a footplate. The splint is wrapped into place with

one or more bias-cut stockinettes (or elastic wrap or gauze). When wrapping, care should be taken not to allow the plaster to overlap on the anterior aspect of the leg. The splint is completed by molding the ankle into neutral position.

LONG LEG POSTERIOR SPLINT

This splint is useful for the treatment of ankle or tibia fractures where severe swelling is expected. Note that initially a long leg splint may be used in order to control rotation, but eventually the patient will require a long leg cast. The posterior splint is not as stable a construct as a bivalved or split cast, but it allows for greater swelling without the development of ischemic contractures. A long leg splint is initially applied in the same fashion as the short leg splint and is then extended above the knee using additional plaster slabs placed along the medial, lateral, and posterior aspects of the thigh. In addition to molding the splint at the malleolus, the splint can be molded at the thigh.

THREE-SIDED SPLINT

Three-sided splints are made by using a long posterior splint as a footplate that extends up the posterior surface of the leg to an appropriate height, depending on the level of the fracture. The other two sides of the three-sided splint are applied medially and laterally to add stability and strength, as discussed for the short leg posterior splint.

U SPLINT

A U splint is constructed by taking a long plaster splint down the lateral side of the leg, under the heel, and then back up the medial side. A second plaster splint is used as a footplate to control ankle dorsiflexion and plantar flexion. The splint is distal to the knee and is held in place with a bias-cut stockinette, elastic bandage, or gauze wrap.

References

Carpenito, L. J. (1993). *Nursing diagnosis: Application to clinical practice.* (5th ed.). Philadelphia: J. B. Lippincott.

Bryant, G. G. (1998). Modalities for immobilization. In A. B. Maher, S. W. Salmond, & T. A. Pellino (Eds.), *Orthopaedic nursing* (pp. 296–322). Philadelphia: W. B. Saunders.

Cornell, C. N., & Schneider, K. (1998). Proximal humerus. In K. J. Koval & J. D. Zuckerman (Eds.). *Fractures in the elderly* (pp. 85–92). Philadelphia: Lippincott-Raven.

Green, D. P., & Butler, T. E. (1996). Fractures and dislocations in the hand. In C. A. Rockwood, D. P. Green, R. W. Bucholz, & J. D. Heckman (Eds.). *Rockwood and Green's fractures in adults* (4th ed., pp. 607–744). Philadelphia: Lippincott-Raven.

DeLee, J. C. (1996). Fractures and dislocations of the hip. In C. A. Rockwood, D. P. Green, R. W. Bucholz, & J. D. Heckman (Eds.). *Rockwood and Green's fractures in adults* (4th ed., pp. 1659–1826). Philadelphia: Lippincott-Raven..

Dinowitz, M. I., Koval, K. J., & Meadows, S. (1998). Distal radius. In K. J. Koval & J. D. Zuckerman (Eds.). *Fractures in the elderly* (pp. 127–141). Philadelphia: Lippincott-Raven.

Dougherty, J. (1996). Same-day surgery: The nurse's role. *Orthopaedic Nursing, 15*(4), 15–18.

Georgiadis, G. R., & Behrens, F. F. (1998). Humeral shaft. In K. J. Koval & J. D. Zuckerman (Eds.). *Fractures in the elderly* (pp. 93–106). Philadelphia: Lippincott-Raven

Harkess, J. W., Ramsey, W. C., & Harkess, J. W. (1996). Principles of fractures and dislocations. In C. A. Rockwood, D. P. Green, R. W. Bucholz, & J. D. Heckman (Eds.). *Rockwood and Green's fractures in adults* (4th ed., pp. 3–120). Philadelphia: Lippincott-Raven.

Naylor, A. (1948). *Fractures and orthopaedic surgery for nurses and masseuses* (2nd ed.). Baltimore: Williams and Wilkins.

Mallon, W. J., McNarmara, M. J., & Urbaniak, J. R. (1990). *Orthopaedics for the house officer.* Baltimore: Williams and Wilkins.

Richards, R. R., & Corley, F. G. (1996). Fractures of the shafts of the radius and ulna. In C. A. Rockwood, D. P. Green, R. W. Bucholz, & J. D. Heckman (Eds.). *Rockwood and Green's fractures in adults* (4th ed. pp. 3–120). Philadelphia: Lippincott-Raven.

Savage, P. L., & Masear, V. R. (1996). Casting and splinting techniques. In V. R. Masear (Ed.). *Primary care orthopaedics* (pp. 337–347). Philadelphia: W. B. Saunders

Smeltzer, S. C., & Bare, B. G. (Eds.). (1996). *Brunner and Suddarth's textbook of medical surgical nursing* (8th ed.). Philadelphia: Lippincott.

Zuckerman, J. D., & Koval, K. J. (1996). Fractures of the shaft of the humerus. In C. A. Rockwood, D. P. Green, R. W. Bucholz, & J. D. Heckman (Eds.). *Rockwood and Green's fractures in adults* (4th ed., pp. 1025–1054). Philadelphia: Lippincott-Raven.

Chapter

6

Care of a Patient in Traction

Traction has been widely used as a medical treatment in orthopaedics for more than 3,000 years. The Aztecs and ancient Egyptians used manual traction and splints made of bark and tree branches. Hippocrates (460–377 B.C.) gave explicit instructions in his writings concerning the treatment of fractures and advocated the use of traction. For treatment of a fractured humerus, he said ". . . the best plan is to put round the arm a broad and soft skin, or broad shawl, and to hang some great weight on it, so as to produce moderate extension" (Naylor, 1998,1).

In contemporary practice, the prevalence of traction use is diminishing. That is due, in part, to new surgical procedures and instrumentations that allow successful reduction and fixation of fractures; this, in turn, allows early discharge for patients who would previously have undergone lengthy hospital stays in skin or skeletal traction. Many insurance companies and HMOs greatly curtail the use of traction as a treatment method when lengthy hospitalization is required. When the application of traction is essential in providing care for a patient, that patient is often acutely ill. Many cases involve patients with multiple traumas, preoperative and/or postoperative reduction, and chronic skeletal involvement. These patients are transferred as quickly as possible to subacute care, extended care, or home care. Thus, traction is being delegated more to outpatient and home care. It is imperative that nurses in the acute, subacute, extended care, and home health care areas develop the knowledge and skills necessary to provide care to patients in traction. They also need an understanding of the application, purposes, and principles underlying different types of traction to prevent complications and solve problems easily and quickly.

The skeleton is the bony framework of the body. Movements of its joints are kept under control by the balanced action of opposing groups of muscles; that balancing principle is the basis of all traction and suspension devices. Traction is the application of a pulling force to an injured or diseased part of the body or an extremity with countertraction, a pull in the opposite direction. The pulling force can be applied to the spine, the pelvis, and the long bones of the upper and lower

extremities and, as such, is an important form of orthopaedic immobilization. Traction can be applied as an alternative to surgery, is used to ensure proper positioning of an affected extremity, and can be used in the correction of deformities.

PURPOSES OF TRACTION

Traction has several purposes (Box 6–1): (1) to reduce a fracture and realign bone fragments by overcoming muscle spasms (This can be accomplished by applying manual traction for a very short time or by applying mechanical traction over a period of hours or days. Correct alignment is then maintained with traction or another type of immobilization device, (such as a cast or surgical fixation); (2) to maintain skeletal length and alignment (Fractures of extremities, especially the lower extremities, involve large muscular structures that help the body move and maintain different positions. When a bone is fractured, the traumatized muscles go into spasm as a protective mechanism, but one which can also cause deformities and shortening of an extremity. A reduced fracture cannot maintain bone stability on its own. A continual pull on the muscles is required to counteract the muscle spasms and maintain the affected extremity in correct alignment until calcification occurs); (3) to reduce and treat dislocations (Both manual and mechanical traction are used to reduce dislocations of the extremities. For example, with

---

Box 6–1
Purposes Of Traction

1. To reduce a fracture and realign bone fragments
2. To maintain skeletal length and alignment
3. To reduce and treat dislocations
4. To immobilize to prevent further soft-tissue damage
5. To prevent the development of contractures
6. To relieve muscle spasms
7. To lessen deformities
8. To rest a diseased joint

a dislocated hip [see Chapter 9], manual traction is utilized for reduction of the dislocation and the patient is then maintained in mechanical traction until the muscles regain their ability to maintain the joint in anatomical alignment); (4) to immobilize to prevent further soft-tissue damage (Once a fracture or dislocation occurs, there is soft-tissue damage around the fracture or dislocation site. If the bones at the fracture or dislocation site are not kept immobile, movement can allow additional soft-tissue—or even circulatory or nerve—damage beyond what occurred during the original trauma); (5) to prevent the development of contractures when there is a pathologic condition that causes the muscles to contract; (6) to relieve muscle spasms that occur as a reaction to musculoskeletal trauma in the absence of a fracture, such as cervical sprain or low back pain (see Chapter 8); (7) to lessen deformities, such as with arthritis and the curving spinal deformities of scoliosis; and (8) to rest a diseased joint.

CLASSIFICATION OF TRACTION

Traction is *static* in that it promotes or provides a form of immobilization, but it is also *dynamic* in that it also promotes movement. Traction can be continuous or intermittent. *Continuous traction* means that the traction is maintained at all times (e.g., traction on an unrepaired fracture). *Intermittent traction* refers to traction that is either applied for short periods of time (e.g., intermittent cervical traction) or traction that can be released for short periods of time (e.g., pelvic traction to relieve muscle spasms). Traction is used as running (or straight) traction or balanced suspension traction. *Running traction* is traction applied to a body part with a pull in one direction or along one plane. The only countertraction is the patient's body, and any movement made by the body changes the pull of the traction (e.g., Buck's, pelvic, and cervical traction). *Balanced suspension* traction applies traction while using a suspension apparatus to support a part of the body without pulling on that part; the patient's body provides countertraction. It can be used in conjunction with skin or skeletal traction and keeps the fracture site immobile when the patient moves. The affected extremity is held in place by balanced weights attached to an overhead bar.

Traction is commonly classified as manual or mechanical by the way it is applied to the patient's body. Mechanical traction is also divided into skin and skeletal traction. In addition, there are two other forms of traction—plaster and brace—that are also used in specific situations.

MANUAL TRACTION

Manual traction is traction that is accomplished by a person's hands exerting a pulling force. It is utilized to reduce fractures and dislocations and to apply a steady pull while mechanical traction is released for readjustment or while a cast is being applied. Manual traction must be done with a smooth, firm grip, as sudden jerky

motions of the extremity can cause severe pain. Never use manual traction without specific orders to do so.

SKIN TRACTION

Skin traction is attached directly to the patient's skin to immobilize a body part continuously or intermittently over a short or extended period. The direct application of a pulling force to the patient's skin and soft tissues may be accomplished by using adhesive or nonadhesive traction tape or other skin traction devices such as a cast, a boot, a belt, or a halter.

SKELETAL TRACTION

Skeletal traction is attached directly to the patient's skeletal system to immobilize a body part. The direct application of the pulling force to the patient's skeletal system may be accomplished by attaching pins, screws, wires, or tongs. Skeletal traction allows greater traction time and heavier weights than does skin traction.

PLASTER TRACTION

Plaster traction is skeletal traction applied by incorporating the ends of Steinmann pins or Kirschner wires in a cast that maintains a continuous pulling force. An example is when a short arm cast with skeletal traction on the thumb is used for correction of a first metacarpal fracture.

BRACE TRACTION

Brace traction employs a brace to exert a pull on a portion of the body, as in the case of hyperextension braces or long leg braces for correction of leg alignment deformities due to fractures of the distal portion of the femur.

OBSERVING THE PATIENT IN TRACTION

Learn to make routine observations each time nursing care is given until such observations become so habitual that they are no longer conscious. Learn to ask yourself these questions:

1. Are the circulation and nerve status of the extremity adequate?
2. Is the condition of the skin around the tape and straps satisfactory?
   a. Look for irritation, reddened areas, and maceration.
   b. Look for pimples, abrasions, and purulent discharge.
3. Are you using your nose as well as your eyes to detect signs of trouble, are there any distinctive odors of macerating soft tissue and infection?
4. Are the tapes slipping or is the wrapping coming loose?

5. Is there any pressure on the popliteal region?
6. Is the heel free of pressure?
7. Is there any pressure over the outer aspect of the head of the fibula (the lateral upper calf)?
8. Is there sufficient countertraction?
9. Is the angle of elevation of the heel enough or too much?
10. In balanced skeletal traction, is hip flexion 20 degrees or less (between the bed and the thigh)?
11. In arm traction, is there pressure on the dorsum of the hand, at the elbow, at the wrist, or in the axilla?
12. Is there any deformity at the fracture site?
13. Is the patient comfortable and warm?
14. Is the patient having an undue amount of pain?
15. Is the patient's body positioned correctly?
16. Are there complications due to prolonged bed rest and reduced activity?

PATIENT TEACHING

To reduce the patient's anxiety and to have a cooperative and informed patient, teach the patient about the following topics as they related to his or her traction setup:

1. The nature of the traction equipment
2. The purpose of the traction
3. Exercises and positioning to prevent effects of immobility and increase muscle strength
4. Maintaining activities of daily living while in traction
5. Possible diversional activities
6. The rehabilitation process

GENERAL PRINCIPLES ON THE CARE OF TRACTION EQUIPMENT

The following are general principles that apply to the care of all traction equipment to provide a safe environment for the patient in traction:

1. Check for weakness in the traction cord; never reuse a cord.
2. Tie knots properly and then secure knots with adhesive tape.
3. Check for correct poundage, apply weights in a slow manner, avoid any bumping or jerking of weights, and make sure weights hang free of any obstruction.
4. Make sure all parts of the traction equipment are working correctly.
   a. Never oil any pulley without notifying the patient's physician first.
   b. Apply manual traction if any piece of the equipment needs to be readjusted or replaced.

5. Check countertraction and ensure that the patient does not slide into the headboard, footboard, or side of the bed.
6. Check for obstructions that may interfere with the pull of the traction, such as knots pressing against the pulleys; traction pieces such as spreader bars, the footplate, or splints coming in contact with the bed frame; or bed linen on top of traction straps and ropes.
7. Check the line of pull and be certain that fracture fragments are in correct alignment.
8. In continuous traction, make sure the pull is maintained 24 hours a day.
9. Check the position of the patient for correct body alignment, comfort, support for all body parts, and undue stress or pull.

TRACTION TO THE UPPER EXTREMITY

Although traction as a treatment method for upper-extremity fractures is being replaced with new technology and surgical procedures, traction is still being used. In some instances, patients are treated with traction in a subacute unit, in an extended care facility, or at home. The purposes of traction to the upper extremity are (1) to reduce and immobilize fractures of the humerus or elbow; (2) to reduce and immobilize fractures or injuries involving the shoulder; (3) to reduce and immobilize fractures of the wrist and thumb; and (4) to hold the arm in either extension or flexion. The most common types of traction utilized for the upper extremity are side arm, overhead, Dunlop's (a temporary skin traction most often used for children), functional bracing, hanging arm cast, and plaster.

The most common complications related to upper-extremity traction are (1) potential circulatory or nerve impairment due to pressure; (2) skin breakdown from pressure of straps, cast, or bed rest; (3) infection due to skin breakdown or wounds at the pin sites; and (4) physical and psychological complications of enforced recumbency.

SIDE ARM SKIN TRACTION

TRACTION SETUP
Preparing the bed and setting up side arm traction (Fig. 6–1) involve the following steps (as adapted from Zimmer, 1996):

1. Slide a telescoping, under-mattress clamp between the bedspring and mattress and fasten with base clamps.
2. Attach one 36-inch single clamp bar vertically to the mattress clamp.
3. Attach one 27-inch plain bar with pulley to the top of the vertical single clamp bar.

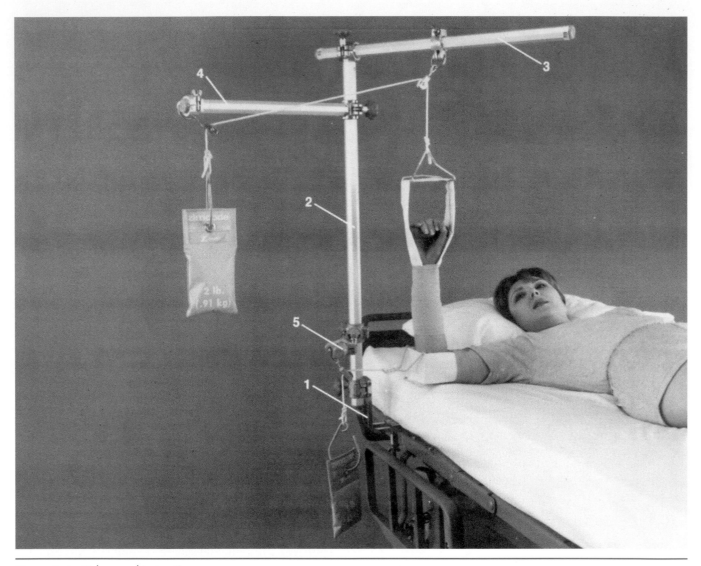

Figure 6–1   Side arm skin traction.

4. Attach one 18-inch clamp bar with pulley to the vertical single clamp bar approximately one quarter of the way from the top of the 18-inch clamp bar.
5. Attach a 9-inch single clamp bar with pulley to the bottom vertical single clamp bar.
6. Prepare the patient's arm as discussed in Traction Application (following).
7. Tie the traction cord (Fig. 6–2) to spreader blocks, thread through the pulleys, and then attach to the weight carriers.
8. Slip the spreader block under the traction straps, and then gently apply the weights.

TRACTION APPLICATION

Fractures of the humerus, with or without shoulder involvement, may be treated with traction attached to the skin or the skeleton, with an overhead or side arm pull, and with the arm in flexion or extension, depending on the location of the fracture and associated

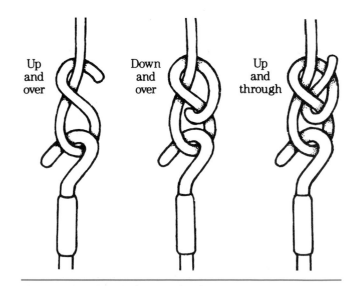

Figure 6–2   How to tie a traction knot.   *(Zimmer, Inc. (1996).* Zimmer Traction Handbook *Warsaw, IN: Zimmer, Inc.)*

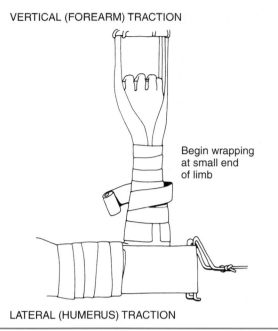

VERTICAL (FOREARM) TRACTION

Begin wrapping at small end of limb

LATERAL (HUMERUS) TRACTION

Figure 6–3 Applying traction tapes to the forearm. *(Zimmer, Inc. (1996). Zimmer Traction Handbook Warsaw, IN: Zimmer, Inc.)*

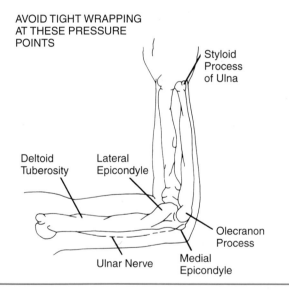

AVOID TIGHT WRAPPING AT THESE PRESSURE POINTS

Styloid Process of Ulna

Deltoid Tuberosity

Lateral Epicondyle

Ulnar Nerve

Medial Epicondyle

Olecranon Process

Figure 6–4 Pressure points on the arm. *(Zimmer, Inc. (1996). Zimmer Traction Handbook Warsaw, IN: Zimmer, Inc.)*

injuries. Utilize the patient's physician or the institution's method of skin preparation before applying the skin traction. Skin side arm traction is accomplished by the use of two sets of two traction tapes that are secured by an elastic bandage wrap (or SKIN TRAC and Orthopaedic Wraps) at separate sites on the arm (Fig. 6–3). Avoid wrapping the bandage too tightly over pressure points (Fig. 6–4).

One set of tapes is applied to the upper arm and extends past the elbow. It is attached to a spreader and pulley weight setup, and it exerts a horizontal (or outward) pull on the humerus. The weights are determined by the needs of the individual patient based on the size

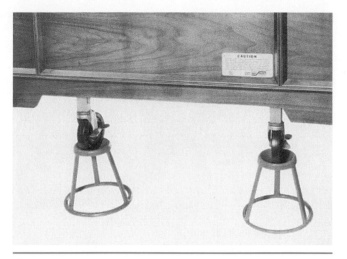

Figure 6–5 Shock blocks under the bed. *(Zimmer, Inc. (1996). Zimmer Traction Handbook Warsaw, IN: Zimmer, Inc.)*

and the age of the patient and the type of fracture, but they rarely exceed 6 pounds. The other set of tapes is applied to the forearm and extends beyond the hand where it is attached to a spreader (that can include a hand grip) and pulley weight setup. It exerts a lateral (or upward) pull to support and suspend the arm vertically. The weights rarely exceed 3 pounds. A suspended handle within the forearm apparatus allows the patient to flex and extend the fingers and exercise the wrist. The elbow is usually flexed, although some authors discuss side arm traction that uses a Thomas arm splint to hold the elbow in extension. Many physicians prefer not to place the elbow in extension, however, because immobilization in that position causes muscle strain and discomfort at the elbow.

Countertraction is provided by the patient's body. To provide additional resistance to the traction, the side of the bed on the affected side can be elevated. That can be accomplished in two ways. One is to place shock blocks under the legs of the bed on the side where the traction is attached (Fig. 6–5). However, that may cause the patient to slide too far away from the traction apparatus. The second method is to place a folded blanket between the mattress and the bed frame on the affected side.

SIDE ARM SKELETAL TRACTION

Side arm skeletal traction is accomplished by the same bed frame traction as discussed under side arm skin traction. Side arm skeletal traction is obtained by placing a pin through the olecranon process at the elbow and attaching weights that rarely exceed 12 pounds (Fig. 6–6). The forearm still has traction tapes, and the positioning of the forearm is the same as in side arm skin traction. Skeletal traction is utilized instead of skin traction when the traction is in place for a longer period of time or requires more weight, or when an elastic bandage wrap over the upper arm is inappropriate. An increase in countertraction can be accomplished as in side arm skin traction, already discussed.

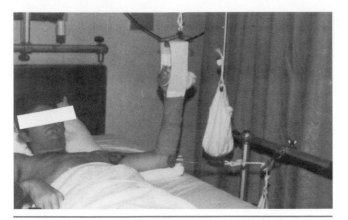

Figure 6–6 Olecranon traction is sometimes used in the treatment of fractures of the humerus, especially supracondylar fractures. The pin is inserted through the ulnar shaft immediately distal to the olecranon, taking care to avoid the ulnar nerve. The forearm and hand are supported by skin traction. *(Zimmer, Inc. (1996). Zimmer Traction Handbook Warsaw, IN: Zimmer, Inc.)*

OVERHEAD 90–90 TRACTION

TRACTION SETUP

Preparing the bed and setting up overhead 90-90 traction (Fig. 6–7) involves the following steps (as adapted from Zimmer, 1996):

1. Attach a basic frame (an overhead traction bar designed for retractable beds) to the bed.
2. Attach one 36-inch center clamp bar to the overhead bar above the patient's arm.
3. Attach one 36-inch center clamp bar to the overhead bar at the extreme foot end of the bed (a 9-inch single clamp bar may be placed on the upright bar at the foot of the bed to attach the 36-inch clamp bar to provide greater clearance for the weights).
4. Attach two pulleys to each center clamp bar, one on each side.
5. Prepare the patient's upper arm as discussed in Traction Application (following).

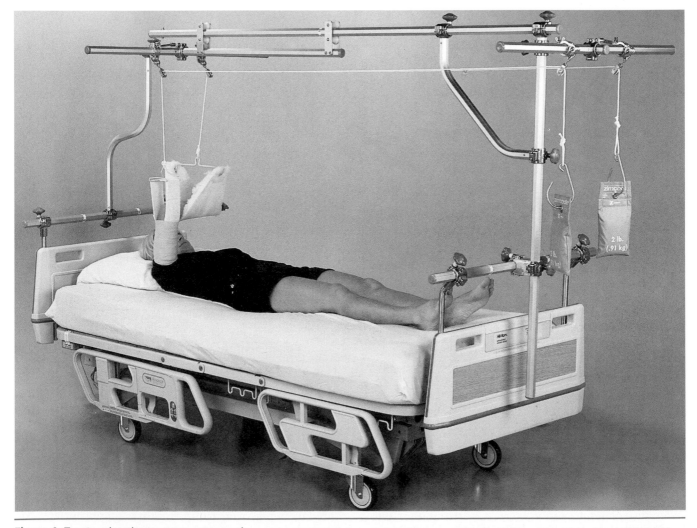

Figure 6–7 Overhead 90 = 90 traction to the arm. *(Rockwood, C. A., et al. (1996). Rockwood & Green's Fractures in Adults. 4th ed. Philadelphia: Lippincott-Raven.)*

6. Tie traction cord (see Fig. 6–2) to spreader block and pulley and attach weights to the carrier.
7. Place patient's forearm in sling and apply weights.

TRACTION APPLICATION

With overhead 90 90 traction, the shoulder and the elbow are in 90 degrees of flexion. The forearm is suspended over the patient's chest with the upper arm perpendicular to the body. The forearm is usually supported by a sling suspended from an overhead pulley, and the upper arm is prepared with traction tapes as discussed for side arm skin traction. Utilize the patient's physician's or institution's preference for skin preparation before the skin traction is applied.

Overhead 90-90 skin traction is possible but overhead skeletal traction with a pin or a Kirschner wire through the olecranon process is more common. Here the traction tapes to the upper arm are replaced by a pin or wire through the olecranon process, which is attached to weights, while the forearm is supported in a sling. In other cases, the sling and traction tapes may both be replaced with a long arm cast applied over the pin, with the pin attached to a loop and pulley. Overhead traction allows the patient more freedom than side arm traction, and less edema and fewer circulatory problems result. The weight of the patient's body provides sufficient countertraction.

NURSING PROCESS (Patient with Side Arm Traction)

The following nursing process presents the care of a patient in side arm traction for a supracondylar fracture of the arm. The nursing process begins after the traction is applied.

ASSESSMENT

The first step in the assessment of a typical patient in traction following a supracondylar fracture of the humerus is to determine the neurovascular status of the affected arm and hand and compare it with the unaffected side. Because of the potential for circulatory impairment, the radial pulse must be checked immediately after the application of traction and then at least every 3 to 4 hours while the patient is in traction. Check for any swelling at the shoulder, elbow, or hand; for cyanosis or pallor of the hands or fingers; and for numbness or decreased function of the fingers (see Chapter 2). Fingers that have good color, sensation, and movement may be cold because the hand is elevated and immobile.

Assess for pain. If the patient complains of pain under the traction tapes, you can run your fingers gently under the tapes and the wrapping to assess whether the pain is from skin breakdown or neurovascular impairment. To detect painful pressure points under the skin traction, palpate the area over the traction tapes at least daily. When skin traction is applied to the arm, check that the area around the elbow where the ulnar nerve is located is not wrapped too tightly. Check the areas near the shoulder, the anterior surface of the elbow joint, and the wrist for any irritation, reddened areas, skin breakdown, or macerations. Check for any slipping of the traction tapes or loosening of the wrapping, which can lead to skin problems. If the patient has skeletal traction, check the pin site for any signs of inflammation. With overhead 90-90 traction, check the sling or cast edges for possible skin irritation. Always follow up on patient complaints of pain. Check the patient's body alignment, and make sure that the pull of the traction is at the proper angle in relation to the patient's body. Check the traction for possible mechanical problems.

NURSING DIAGNOSIS

Based on all of the assessment data, the major nursing diagnoses for a typical patient in side arm traction following a supracondylar fracture of the humerus may include the following:

- Pain and discomfort related to trauma and immobility
- Impaired physical mobility related to instability of the humerus
- Risk of impaired skin integrity related to immobility and the traction device
- Potential individual ineffective coping related to trauma and immobilization
- Altered nutrition: less than body requirement related to eating in a supine position (and possibly having the dominant arm and hand immobilized)
- Anxiety related to knowledge deficit about the injury, treatment method(s), and the rehabilitation process

COLLABORATIVE PROBLEMS

- Inadequate or incomplete reduction of the fracture site
- Neurologic damage in the affected arm
- Circulatory impairment in the affected arm

GOAL FORMULATION AND PLANNING

The goals are to have the patient experience (1) a decrease in pain through traction, nursing measures, and prescribed medications; (2) an increase in physical mobility through the use of traction and controlled exercises; (3) no break in skin integrity as a result of turning and skin care measures; (4) effective individual coping through the use of one-to-one interactions about treatment and prognosis; (5) a nutritional intake that meets the body's daily requirement; (6) a decrease in anxiety through patient education about the trauma, treatment method(s), and the rehabilitation process; and (7) an absence of complications.

INTERVENTIONS

ALLEVIATE PAIN

The amount of pain the patient has is affected by the type of immobilization, the trauma, and the patient's adjustment to the trauma. Nursing measures to help reduce pain are to maintain the traction in correct alignment and to have the patient do gentle finger exercises to increase circulation. Other noninvasive measures for pain relief may be utilized (see Chapter 4). Nonetheless, the patient will almost certainly require prescribed medications for pain relief.

INCREASE MOBILITY

The two most important interventions to increase the patient's mobility are correct positioning and exercises.

Position. Arm traction is designed for a patient who is supine in bed. The bed is level or flat when the traction is applied. Any shift of the patient toward the head or foot of the bed changes the line of pull of the traction. A physician's order is necessary before the head of the patient's bed can be elevated. The head of the bed may be elevated *only* when the side arm traction pulley has been attached to the basic frame that clamps to the bed under the mattress, so that the traction apparatus moves with the head of the bed. This allows a change in the position of the head of the bed without disrupting the traction. If the head of the bed *cannot* be elevated, the knee gatch may be raised periodically to flex the patient's knees, which helps relieve strain on the patient's back.

The patient is able to use the overhead trapeze to stabilize their upper body and their feet to lift their buttocks to use the bedpan or for the changing of linen. Using two draw sheets for the linen for the bottom of the bed assists with linen change when only one portion of the bed is soiled. If the patient needs to turn for back care, turning to the affected side is best since the bed maintains support for the arm.

Exercises. Active range-of-motion finger exercises with the affected hand are to be done frequently as they increase circulation to the elevated hand and assist with arterial flow. This activity also helps prevent muscle atrophy that can occur during immobility. Breathing exercises and abdominal exercises should also be encouraged (see Chapter 4). Active range-of-motion exercises for all uninvolved joints should be stressed. The patient must do quadriceps- and gluteal-setting exercises, ankle pumps, and flexion and extension of the legs to maintain joint function (Box 6–2).

MAINTAIN SKIN INTEGRITY

Because the patient is unable to turn, there is a potential for skin breakdown on the patient's upper back. Problems with the lower trunk and extremities are much less frequent as patients are able to life their trunk and move

---

Box 6–2
Exercises for the Lower-Extremity

To begin *quadriceps-setting exercises,* the patient should be comfortable. Place your hand under the patient's knee and instruct them to press the knee down against your hand or have the patient pretend they are pushing their knee into the bed. A strong contraction of the quadriceps should occur when the patient presses. This tightening is followed by complete relaxation. The patient presses and holds for a slow count of 5 and then relaxes for a slow count of 5. Gradually build up until they can perform this 20 times an hour. This exercise helps to maintain the quadriceps femoris muscle that extends the leg and is necessary for walking.

Gluteal-setting exercises, which simply tighten and relax the gluteal muscles on a slow count of 3 help to increase circulation to the gluteal area and preserve muscle tone. Gluteal-setting exercises are isometric exercises that strengthen the muscles but do not move any joint.

Ankle pumps involve doing plantar and dorsiflexion exercises of the foot and ankle. The exercise maintains the range of motion of the ankle needed for walking and also increases the circulation in the calf muscles of the leg.

---

their legs. Measures to prevent skin breakdown are (1) keeping linens wrinkle free, dry, and free of food crumbs; (2) having two persons change the linen with care so as not to disrupt the traction (the bed is usually changed from head to foot); and (3) giving skin care to the back at least every 3 to 4 hours. Avoid use of lotions as they soften the skin and leave it sticky. Alcohol leaves the skin dry and also helps to toughen the skin and prevent further trauma. Gentle rubbing is essential to increase circulation to the area. Take care that the skin along the traction edges is kept dry, clean, and free of irritation. Make sure the affected hand has lotion applied to help prevent dryness, but apply alcohol rubs to the bony prominences of the wrist to toughen the skin where the traction tapes might rub. If the patient is in skeletal traction without a cast, do pin care as determined by the institution.

COPING MECHANISM

Depression occurs in the patient who lies in bed "with nothing to do" and is cared for like a baby; and the patient develops an unrealistic view of their condition and prognosis. To help prevent or reduce boredom and self-centeredness, find activities that the patient likes to do and still can do. Listening to music and reading are two examples. The nurse may need to obtain prism glasses and a device to hold a book or newspaper so that the patient can read comfortably in bed. The family may be able to get books and "talking books" from the local library. Other possible activities include playing games or cards. There are card holders available that allow the patient to play with one hand. Try to make the activities mentally stimulating as a change from the passive role of a television viewer. Occupational therapists, social workers, and hospital volunteers may be of assistance. Because the patient may be immobile for some time, a social support system can increase the patient's feelings of competence and self-worth.

MAINTAIN ADEQUATE NUTRITION

Patients who are immobilized in a supine position need a well-balanced diet high in fiber and with adequate fluids. Some patients may have decreased appetite or not want to eat because they are unable to feed themselves. Arrange a consultation from the dietitian for the patient to help identify likes and dislikes and to develop creative ways that food can be prepared so the patient can feed him-or herself as much as possible. According to Jagmin (1998), an immobilized adult needs one gram of protein per kilogram of body weight per day, and 1 to 1.5 grams of calcium to prevent hypoproteinemia and osteoporosis. Patients may need to have smaller and more frequent feedings in order to feed themselves and ensure that they are getting an adequate amount of fluids and nutrition. Explain the importance of fluid intake for elimination, even though they may have to use a bedpan. *Make sure patients are safe in feeding themselves so that they will not aspirate any food or fluids.* A safety precaution is to have suction available in the patient's room.

PATIENT TEACHING AND HOME CARE CONSIDERATIONS

The patient lying supine in traction because of a fractured humerus may have a feeling of helplessness because of an unrealistic appreciation of the severity of the injury and the potential for recovery. Once the initial pain is reduced, the patient should be encouraged to begin doing simple activities of daily living with assistance as needed from the nurse. How much the patient is able to do depends on whether the dominant arm was affected. Occupational therapy may be needed to help with assistive devices. Schedule self-help activities when the patient is not tired. Many patients fear that any motion, including self-care, will disturb the traction. Tell the patient what movements are allowed. The "can't do" activities should be discussed, but if too much emphasis is placed on them, the patient is less likely to engage in any activity.

Most patients benefit psychologically from understanding the rehabilitation program, especially

- when and whether they will get return of function in the arm,
- how long they will be in traction,
- whether they will need to be in a cast after the traction is removed,
- what kind of exercises they will need to do and when, and
- whether they will be able to return home when they leave the hospital.

Because the answers to those questions depend on the age of the patient, the location and type of fracture, the length and type of treatment (whether the traction is preoperative or the only treatment method), and the patient's response to that treatment, they must be answered by the physician. Help the patient obtain that information, for example, by suggesting that he or she prepare a list of questions to discuss with the physician.

MONITORING AND MANAGING POTENTIAL PROBLEMS

The major complications that may arise following a supracondylar fracture of the humerus are (1) inadequate or incomplete reduction of the fracture, (2) neurologic damage, and (3) circulatory impairment.

INADEQUATE REDUCTION

Inadequate or incomplete reduction of the humeral fracture can result in a permanent limitation of motion or an obvious physical deformity such as cubitus valgus or cubitus varus. Keep the patient's body in correct alignment, maintain the traction at all times, and evaluate the success of pain reduction with traction and prescribed medications.

NEUROLOGICAL DAMAGE

Stretching or contusion injuries to the median, the ulnar, or the deep muscular branch of the radial nerve have been reported in approximately 6% of patients sustaining a supracondylar fracture of the humerus. The nerve injury may be of varying degrees of severity: (1) a neurapraxia involves minimal damage to nerves, which recover spontaneously within a few weeks; (2) an axonotmesis involves peripheral nerve degeneration due to axon damage with spontaneous regeneration occurring after many months; and (3) a neurotmesis involves nerve destruction due to severing or scarring that is correctable only by excising the damaged section and anastomosing the ends. The nerve damage in most patients with supracondylar humeral fractures proves to be only temporary, but nurses should still be alert to the possibility of serious nerve damage.

CIRCULATORY IMPAIRMENT

The most dreaded complication of a supracondylar fracture is Volkmann's ischemic contracture, a severely deforming condition of the hand and arm. If present before reduction, this circulatory impairment is usually due to antecubital edema, impingement of a bone fragment against the brachial artery, or, rarely, a torn or lacerated brachial artery. If the impairment appears after reduction, it is probably due to a vascular obstruction secondary to tight bandages or to a position of acute or extreme flexion of the elbow. The absence of a radial pulse in the presence of a supracondylar fracture of the humerus demands immediate attention. If it is not corrected within a 4- to 8-hour period, Volkmann's ischemic contracture may result.

Volkmann's Ischemic Contracture. Volkmann's ischemic contracture (Fig. 6–8) is a deformity most common in supracondylar fractures of the humerus, dislocations of the elbow, or fractures of the proximal third of the

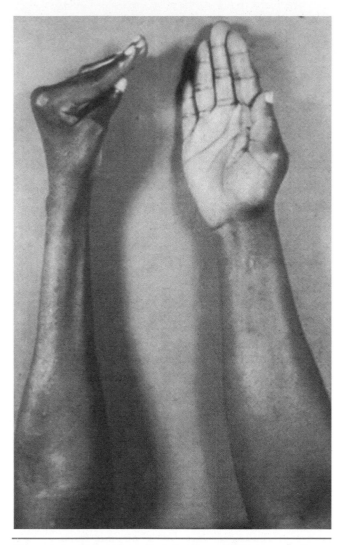

Figure 6–8   The end result of circular constriction may be Volkmann's ischemic contracture, which in this case involved the intrinsic muscles of the left hand. This is the "main d'accoucheur." When a patient complains of pain, all encircling dressings and casts must be split.   *(Zimmer, Inc. (1996). Zimmer Traction Handbook Warsaw, IN: Zimmer, Inc.)*

forearm. The ischemic contracture develops as a result of an irritation or injury to the brachial artery, which causes a reflex spasm of the main brachial artery and collateral vessels, severely diminishing the blood supply to the muscles of the arm. Volkmann's ischemic contracture may follow slight or severe injuries and may even be caused by constriction from a bandage, splint, cast, or tourniquet, or by compression of the artery by swelling from an immobilized flexed elbow. For that reason, patients with injuries to the elbow or the forearm are frequently kept in the hospital for observation until it is clear that circulation in the involved arm is unimpaired.

One of the first signs of an impending Volkmann's ischemic contracture is an absence of the radial pulse. The radial artery should be palpated before an immobilizing device is applied, at 15-minute intervals for 2

to 4 hours, and then hourly for the first 24 hours following application. Other neurovascular checks should also be done at those times (see Chapter 2). If ischemia develops, the fingers may become cool, swollen, and either cyanotic or pale; are held in slight flexion; and cannot be completely extended. Any attempt to passively straighten the fingers causes pain in the front of the forearm. Once ischemia develops, the patient may complain of severe burning pain in the forearm and the hand, but the onset is often painless. If the arterial spasm is not relieved within 6 to 8 hours, the muscles die and become matted, fibrosed, and contracted. Their functional ability is then permanently lost. The nerves of the arm and the hand degenerate, even if previously uninjured, and the fingers become anesthetic and fixed in a flexed position. A typical Volkmann's contracture includes a combined median and ulnar palsy, hyperextension of the MCP joints, flexion of the interphalangeal joints, and wasting of the intrinsic muscles of the hand and the thenar and hypothenar eminences.

Immediate measures to relieve the ischemia are essential. Inform the physician *at once* if any of the preceding signs are observed. Delay is dangerous. Keep the patient warm but do not attempt to warm the fingers by applying a hot water bottle or heating pad. Do not elevate the arm. If the arm is already elevated, reducing the elevation may help increase the arterial flow to the hand.

Treatment to relieve the ischemia consists of (1) removal of the front half of the cast or loosening of the encircling bandage, (2) further manipulation of any still unreduced fracture, (3) reducing the degree of flexion to less than 90 degrees, and (4) if those measures fail to relieve the symptoms promptly, doing a sympathetic nerve block or (5) exploratory surgery of the brachial artery to excise the damaged portion of the artery. After the arterial spasm is relieved, rehabilitation is aimed at improving the function of the arm by correcting any residual deformity and reeducating the muscles that remain functional.

Other Circulatory Complications. Other circulatory complications can occur because of immobility. The patient in traction for a supracondylar fracture has the potential for developing a thrombus or thrombophlebitis. Most patients should wear elastic stockings and do active range-of-motion exercises of all unaffected joints to increase circulation and help reduce that risk. Some patients may also be placed on a low dose of aspirin. Circulation can be impeded by blood vessel trauma, edema, or pressure from the immobilization device. In older patients, circulatory impairment may be a greater problem, because the blood flow to the extremities may be compromised by arteriosclerotic disease.

EVALUATION/OUTCOMES

Determine whether a patient's pain has been reduced by the application of traction, nursing measures, and pain medications. The patient should have normal neurovascular status with no circulatory impairment. The fingers and the hand should have good color, be warm, and have sensory and motor function.

There should be no signs of complications from bed rest or traction. Patients should be doing activities that stimulate their minds as well as their bodies. The exercise program should have become a routine part of their daily activities. They should have a good overall knowledge of the rehabilitation process and how they will regain function in their arm.

FUNCTIONAL BRACING

Despite its excellent fracture union rate (95%), the hanging arm cast (which is discussed later in this chapter) is largely being replaced by functional bracing (Fig. 6–9). Georgiadis and Behrens (1998) state that functional bracing is the preferred closed treatment method for humeral shaft fractures, as it is better tolerated by patients and is technically less demanding than the hanging arm cast. In functional bracing, a stockinette is slipped over the patient's upper arm and then a lightweight polyethylene plastic splint/sleeve is fastened around with patient's upper arm with Velcro straps (Fig. 6–10). A collar is then placed around the patient's neck and attached to a cuff around the wrist of the affected arm. The functional brace allows for gravity-induced traction (the weight of the patient's arm pulling downward on the fracture site) and also provides a circumferential molded sleeve that compresses the soft tissue of the upper arm. The brace does not provide rigid immobilization but allows for controlled motion at the fracture site, which is beneficial for healing. The union rate for functional bracing is 90% to 98%.

The advantage of functional bracing is that it facilitates early motion of the shoulder, elbow, and wrist joints and appears to avoid the loss of motion that can be associated with hanging arm casts. However, moderate edema does develop below the brace, which decreases with elevation and muscle exercises. Skin irritation or difficulties with satisfactory fitting of the humeral sleeve occasionally occur. The brace is worn continuously until bony union, but it can be removed briefly for personal hygiene, another advantage over the hanging arm cast. The collar and cuff are required in the beginning but later can be removed for active elbow motion. Bony union occurs usually within 7 to 10 weeks, with minor anatomic deformities not affecting function. The patients may not be admitted to an acute care institution but are cared for in an outpatient clinic, physician offices, and/or home care. If they are admitted, it is for a very short period of time.

HANGING ARM CAST TRACTION

Although functional fracture bracing has become the most common treatment for closed humeral shaft fractures, the hanging arm cast (Fig. 6–11) is still used in spe-

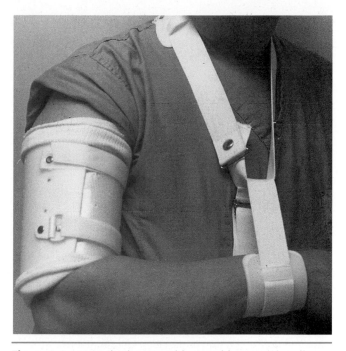

Figure 6–9   Use of a functional humeral brace with collar and cuff.   *(Rockwood, C. A., et al. (1996). Rockwood & Green's Fractures in Adults. 4th ed. Philadelphia: Lippincott-Raven.)*

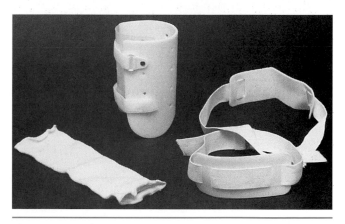

Figure 6–10   The components of a functional humeral brace, including the polyethylene sleeve, stockinette liner, and sling attachment.   *(Koval & Zuckerman (1998). Fractures in the Elderly. Philadelphia: Lippincott Raven.)*

cific cases. It is probably best used as an initial treatment for displaced spiral and oblique humeral shaft fractures with shortening, to be followed by functional bracing (Zuckerman & Koval, 1996). In rare instances, the hanging arm cast may still be the only method of treatment.

The hanging arm cast is a long arm cast (which extends from as high as the upper level of the axillary fold to the proximal palmar crease in the hand, with the elbow in a flexed position) that has a loop on the radial surface between the wrist and the elbow (Fig. 6–12), usually close to the wrist. A strap is placed around the patient's neck and attached to the cast through the loop. The strap is usually padded with felt, foam, or other substances that help relieve the pressure on the skin at

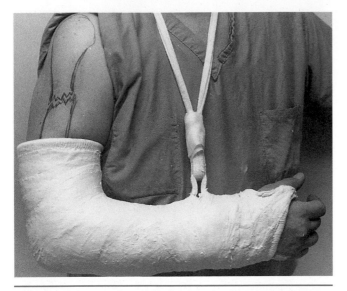

Figure 6–11   The classic gravity-assisted method for humeral shaft fractures is the hanging arm cast. Note that for many fractures, the cast does not immobilize the fracture circumferentially but rather provides for continuous ambulatory traction. Lengthening or shortening of the collar suspension corrects posterior or anterior angulation at the fractures site.   *(Koval & Zuckerman (1998). Fractures in the Elderly. Philadelphia: Lippincott Raven.)*

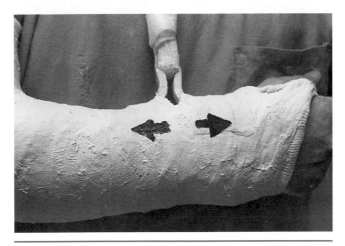

Figure 6–12   Moving the wrist loop toward the elbow or wrist on a hanging arm cast adjusts the traction force on the fracture.   *(Koval & Zuckerman (1998). Fractures in the Elderly. Philadelphia: Lippincott Raven.)*

the back of the neck. The hanging arm cast may actually be heavier than a normal long arm cast because its purpose is to exert traction. *Remember,* the hanging arm cast does not cover the fracture site and only immobilizes the fracture by the pulling force of its weight. If the cast is lifted or the pulling force of the cast on the upper arm is released, the traction is released and the fracture is no longer immobilized. A second loop may be attached just below the elbow on the ulnar side. If the patient is allowed to lie flat in bed, mechanical traction may be applied using the ulnar loop. A common practice is to use 5 pounds of weight.

NURSING PROCESS (Patient with a Hanging Arm Cast)

The following nursing process presents the care of a patient in a hanging arm cast for a fractured humerus. The nursing process begins after the cast is applied.

ASSESSMENT

The first step in the assessment of a patient with a hanging arm cast applied following a fractured humerus is to note the position of the affected arm in relation to the patient's body. The humerus should be in correct alignment. When the patient is in bed, the head of the bed must be elevated high enough so that the casted portion of the arm applies downward traction to the proximal humerus. The strap that is attached to the cast and goes around the patient's neck must support the distal portion of the cast but should not reduce the downward pull on the humerus.

Check the neurovascular status of the affected arm (see Chapter 2). Compare the involved arm with the uninvolved arm to check for deficiencies. Determine the amount, location, and severity of pain. Check the patient for the possibility of other injuries, especially skin abrasions and contusions. Remember that most patients will be older adults, as the fracture usually results from a fall.

NURSING DIAGNOSIS

Based on all of the assessment data, the major nursing diagnoses for a typical patient with a fractured humerus and a hanging arm cast include the following:

- Pain and discomfort related to trauma and the hanging arm cast
- Impaired physical mobility related to the instability of the humerus
- Risk of impaired skin integrity related to immobility and the cast
- Altered nutrition: less than body requirement related to immobilization of dominant arm
- Potential individual ineffective coping related to the trauma and the cast
- Anxiety related to knowledge deficit about the injury, treatment method(s), and the rehabilitation process

COLLABORATIVE PROBLEMS

- Radial nerve injury
- Decreased shoulder function
- Malunion of the fractures

GOAL FORMULATION AND PLANNING

The goals are to have the patient experience (1) a decrease in pain through traction, nursing measures, and prescribed medications; (2) an increase in physical mobility through positioning, traction, and exercises; (3) no break in skin integrity related to the cast; (4) nutritional intake appropriate for age; (5) effective individual coping through ability to do self-care; (6) a decrease in anxiety through patient education; and (7) an absence of complications.

INTERVENTIONS

ALLEVIATE PAIN
In the treatment of a patient with a fractured humerus and a hanging arm cast, pain relief may be the patient's most important goal. The hanging arm cast is a method of immobilizing a fracture by applying traction. The traction helps to realign the fracture and reduce muscle spasms, thus reducing the amount of pain in the arm. Do not place the casted arm on a pillow, as that reduces the pull, manipulates the fracture site, and increases muscle spasms.

The patient may hold the affected arm protectively against their body and be afraid to relax and let the hanging arm cast support the arm. In the beginning, the patient may keep the muscles of the arm so tense that they are actually working against the pull of the cast, thus increasing the pain in the arm. Spending time with the patient and explaining the purpose of the cast are the best nursing interventions.

Determine whether pain is from the fracture site or from neurovascular impairment. Administer prescribed pain medications as needed.

INCREASE MOBILITY
The three most important interventions to increase the patient's mobility are correct positioning, exercises, and ambulation.

Position. Immediately after the application of a hanging arm cast, the patient should be sitting upright in bed with the head of the bed elevated so that the casted arm pulls downward on the humerus (Fig. 6–13). That position is to be maintained at all times. Occasionally the patient's arm may drop back and move out of alignment. That may be due to kyphosis of the thorax, which does not allow the patient's shoulders to lie flat against the bed. In that event, a small towel or other support may be placed under the patient's arm along the chest to correct the alignment of the humerus. Usually, the patient cannot have the bed flat or turn to either side. Some patients may be allowed to have their bed flat, and, if so, traction must be applied to the cast using a pulley and weights at the foot of the bed.

Exercises. Exercises are needed to prevent stiffness of the joints, especially the shoulder. The location and type of fracture and the age and physical condition of the patient determine the kind of exercises and when they are to be started. Finger exercises (See Box 5–2) are usually started as soon as the cast is applied, however, and shoulder exercises are done as directed to prevent adhesions in the

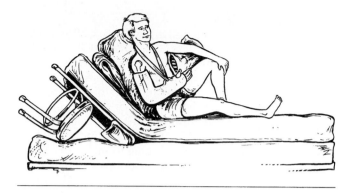

Figure 6–13 The patient is instructed to sleep in a semireclining position without the elbow supported. *(Koval & Zuckerman (1998).* Fractures in the Elderly. *Philadelphia: Lippincott Raven.)*

shoulder joint capsule. The most common shoulder exercises are pendulum, external rotation, elevation, and internal rotation exercises (See Box 5–3). In the beginning, these exercises to the unaffected arm may be used to assist the affected arm. A wall-climbing exercise, where the fingers "climb" up a wall, thus extending and lifting the arm and abducting the shoulder, may be used. After the cast is removed, a sling is applied and exercises of the shoulder, the elbow, and the wrist are begun.

Ambulation. At first, the patient needs assistance in getting out of bed. Do not support the patient on the affected side or apply pressure to the affected arm or shoulder. Patients may initially find it difficult to keep their balance with the heavy arm cast, so do not hurry them. The arm is usually properly positioned when the patient is standing or sitting in a straight back chair.

MAINTAIN SKIN INTEGRITY
Skin irritation is likely to develop in a patient with a hanging arm cast. Although the strap that goes around the patient's neck is padded, it is a source of pressure. The cast presses against the ribs and the chest. Women with large breasts may be particularly affected. The edges of the cast may be rough and irritating. Pad the axilla with a thick dressing, and petal the cast edges as needed (for plaster of Paris casts). All of those areas require observation and meticulous skin care, especially in the elderly.

MAINTAIN ADEQUATE NUTRITION
A patient with a hanging arm cast is able to sit up to eat. If their dominant hand is not affected, the patient may only need assistance with opening cartons, removing plastic covers from food, buttering their bread, or cutting their meat into bite size pieces. If the affected arm is their dominant arm, they may need more assistance. Consultation from the dietitian helps not only to identify likes and dislikes but also to identify ways the food can be prepared that makes it easier for the patient to eat with their nondominant hand. Most patients would prefer this to having someone feed them. Make sure the patient eats a well-balanced diet with adequate fluid intake.

COPING MECHANISMS

Depression can occur in patients with a hanging arm cast when they feel "helpless" and are unwilling to try to do anything for themselves. Keep the patient actively involved in their care, and emphasize the positive things they can do. Each day, try to include something new they can do for themselves, even if it is as simple as reading a paper by themselves. To help prevent or reduce boredom and self-centeredness, find activities that the patient likes to do. Listening to music or "talking books" and reading are some examples. Other possible activities include playing games or cards. There are card holders available that allow the patient to play with one hand. Try to make the activities mentally stimulating as a change from the passive role of a television viewer. The occupational therapy department can help with assistive devices and planning for home care.

PATIENT TEACHING AND HOME CARE CONSIDERATIONS

A patient with a fractured humerus treated by a hanging arm cast is not usually hospitalized for very long, so it is important that discharge planning start as soon as possible. Although having an arm immobilized is not necessarily disabling, the patient's ability to perform self-care will depend on his or her response to the trauma and whether the dominant arm was affected. Because many patients are elderly and live alone, they may be anxious about their ability to care for themselves or to continue to live independently. Some may need to stay with relatives or friends, whereas others may require a period of time in an extended care facility or the services of a home health professional. Not being able to return home may lead to a period of depression and a feeling of helplessness.

During the period of hospitalization, the focus is on the patient's strengths and their ability to do as many of the activities of daily living as possible. The nurse can help the patient make a start toward resolving some of the difficulties of home care by encouraging the patient to be as independent as possible in the hospital. Let the patient wash their face, comb their hair, and brush their teeth. Because the unaffected arm has to do the work of two arms, muscle fatigue may occur in that arm, and rest periods should be planned with the patient.

Discuss with the patient, the family, and significant others the best positions for sleeping, sitting, bathing, and dressing. Sitting is best done in a straight back chair. The patient needs to be aware of problems in sitting up and, more importantly, in getting out of a comfortable living room chair or couch. Patients are able to bathe themselves. Sponge baths are easiest. With a plaster of Paris cast, a plastic cast cover or even a garbage bag will protect the cast in the shower, but the strap will still get wet. Tub baths can be taken with minimal water in the tub and with someone to help the patient in and out. Hospital gowns are fine for day wear in the hospital, but clothing for home should be discussed, as wearing a gown at home may make the patient feel like an invalid. Make sure that the patient knows how to care for the cast (see Chapter 5), how to check for neurovas-

cular impairment (see Chapter 2), and do the exercises (see exercises under increased mobility).

MONITORING AND MANAGING POTENTIAL PROBLEMS

The major complications following a fractured humerus treated with a hanging arm cast are (1) radial nerve injury, (2) decreased shoulder function, and (3) malunion of the fracture.

RADIAL NERVE INJURY

There is the potential for damage to the radial nerve, which more or less wraps itself around the humerus. An injury or edema near the radial nerve may cause wrist drop. When a hanging arm cast is used, it immobilizes the wrist, making a complete motor assessment impossible. If the radial nerve has been injured, however, the thumb will not be able to offer resistance to pressure, nor will extension of the thumb be possible.

DECREASED SHOULDER FUNCTION

A stiff or "frozen" shoulder from a contracture is a real danger when motion in the shoulder is limited for a period of time. Shoulder exercises (exercises under increased mobility and Boxes 5–2 and 5–3 in chapter 5) can prevent that complication, and there is little danger of their displacing the fracture.

MALUNION OF THE FRACTURE

Malunion of the fractured humerus may also occur, but does not appear to be a severe problem. A satisfactory range of shoulder motion is usually regained even if the fragments heal in a moderately deformed position.

EVALUATION/OUTCOMES

Determine that the hanging arm cast is properly aligned and that the patient knows that the arm must not be elevated. Have the patient assess their neurovascular status to make sure they can perform the assessment correctly.

The patient should have a decrease in pain over time. When pain does occur, nursing measures and medications should relieve or at least reduce it. The patient should demonstrate the correct methods of doing the required exercises. The patient should show an absence of complications from the fracture and the traction.

TRACTION TO THE LOWER-EXTREMITY

In contemporary health care, lower-extremity traction is being replaced with new surgical techniques and instruments. This allows the patient early ambulation, shorter hospital stays, and reduced complications from immobility. Lower-extremity traction, when used, is usually for a much shorter period of time and is usually followed by surgery. The most common tractions to the lower extremity are Buck's, Russell's, Böhler Braun, and Balanced suspension traction.

BUCK'S TRACTION

TRACTION SETUP

Preparing the bed and setting up Buck's traction (Fig. 6–14) involves the following steps (as adapted from Zimmer, 1996; for another method, see the traction setup for cervical traction later in this chapter, which uses the Buck's extension apparatus without an overhead frame on the bed).

1. Attach a basic frame (overhead traction bar designed for retractable beds) to the bed.
2. Attach one 5-inch single clamp bar to the upright bar at the foot of the bed. (A 9-inch clamp may be used to gain greater clearance for the weights.)

3. Attach a 9-inch single clamp bar to the 5-inch single clamp bar.
4. Attach a pulley to the 9-inch single clamp bar (so the line of pull is a straight distal to proximal pull).
5. Apply the traction splint or tapes and wrap to the patient's leg.
6. Tie the traction cord (Fig. 6–2) to the splint or spreader block.
7. Thread the cord through the pulley and tie it to the weight carrier.
8. Gently lower the weights.

TRACTION APPLICATION

Buck's traction is a form of running (or straight) skin traction. The purposes of Buck's traction are (1) to immobilize a fractured hip or femur preoperatively; (2) to reduce muscle spasms after hip surgery; (3) to

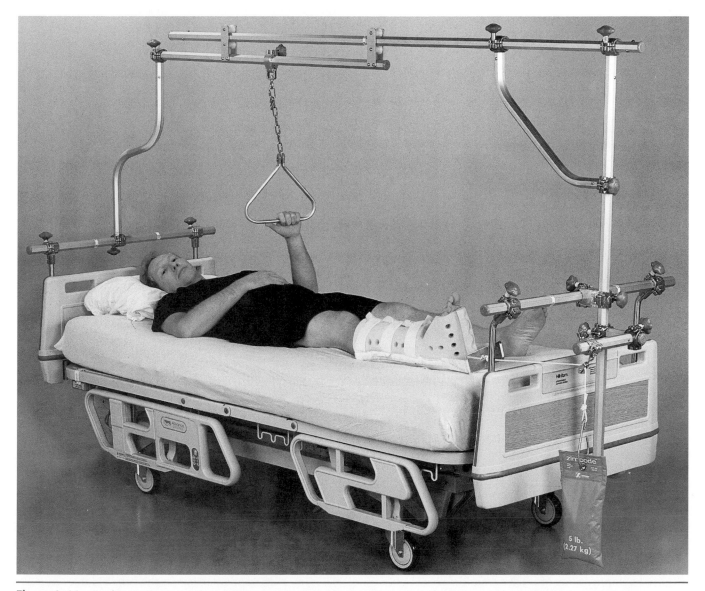

Figure 6–14   Buck's traction.   *(Rockwood, C. A., et al. (1996). Rockwood & Green's Fractures in Adults. 4th ed. Philadelphia: Lippincott-Raven.)*

Apply SKIN TRAC skin traction strip to limb allowing room for traction spreader block.

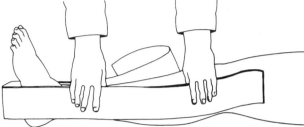

Begin wrapping at small end of limb. Avoid Achilles tendon.

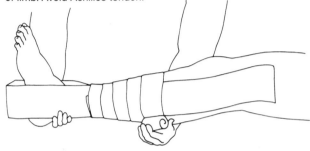

Application completed.

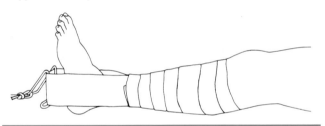

Figure 6–15   Applying traction tapes to the leg.   *(Zimmer, Inc. (1996). Zimmer Traction Handbook Warsaw, IN: Zimmer, Inc.)*

prevent hip flexion contractures; (4) to reduce low back spasms (when used bilaterally); (5) to reduce and immobilize injuries of the pelvis as an initial treatment; and (6) to reduce and/or immobilize a dislocated hip. Buck's traction is accomplished by the use of traction tapes on the lower leg(s) (distal to the fracture site) that are secured by an elastic bandage wrap (or SKIN TRAC and Orthopaedic Wraps) and then attached to a traction spreader block (Fig. 6–15). Make sure to avoid wrapping the bandage too tightly over pressure points (Fig. 6–16), and take care that the tapes do not overlap by leaving at least one inch between them. If SKIN TRAC is used, cover the area near the ankle with felt or sheet wadding to prevent the SKIN TRAC from sticking to the patient's foot and ankle. Another way to obtain Buck's traction is by applying a traction splint/boot to the patient's leg. In both instances, follow your institution's or physician's protocol for preparing the skin before traction application.

See Chapter 9 for the nursing care of a patient in Buck's traction to immobilize a fractured hip. The potential complications of Buck's traction are (1) potential neurovascular impairment (pressure on the peroneal

AVOID TIGHT WRAPPING AT THESE PRESSURE POINTS

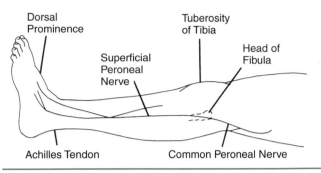

Figure 6–16   Pressure points on the leg.   *(Zimmer, Inc. (1996). Zimmer Traction Handbook Warsaw, IN: Zimmer, Inc.)*

nerve from the straps or splint); (2) foot drop from pressure on the Achilles tendon; (3) skin breakdown; (4) lack of immobilization of the fracture site causing trauma and pain; and (5) physical and psychological complications of enforced recumbency.

RUSSELL'S TRACTION

TRACTION SETUP
Preparing the bed and setting up Russell's traction (Fig. 6–17) involves the following steps (as adapted from Zimmer, 1996):

1. Attach an overhead traction bar (designed for retractable beds) on the patient's bed.
2. Attach one 9-inch single clamp bar to the upright bar at the foot of the bed.
3. Attach a pulley to the 9-inch single clamp bar.
4. Attach a 5-inch single clamp bar to the upright bar at the foot of the bed.
5. Attach a 9-inch single clamp bar to the 5-inch clamp bar.
6. Attach an 18-inch single clamp bar vertically to the 9-inch single clamp bar.
7. Attach two pulleys to the 18-inch single clamp bar so that they extend across the line of the injured leg.
8. Apply a traction splint to the leg or apply traction tapes and wrap to the patient's leg, attaching a footplate with a pulley to the bottom of the patient's foot.
9. Apply a knee sling under the patient's knee.
10. Tie the traction cord (see Fig. 6–2) as follows: (a) attach to the spreader bar for the knee sling; (b) thread the traction cord through the overhead pulley; (c) through the pulley attached to the 18-inch single clamp bar at the foot of the bed; (d) through the pulley on the footplate or traction splint; (e) and then through the lower pulley on the 18-inch single clamp bar at the foot of the bed; and (f) finally the traction cord is attached to the weight carrier.
11. Insert the spreader bar in the canvas knee sling.
12. Gently apply the weights.

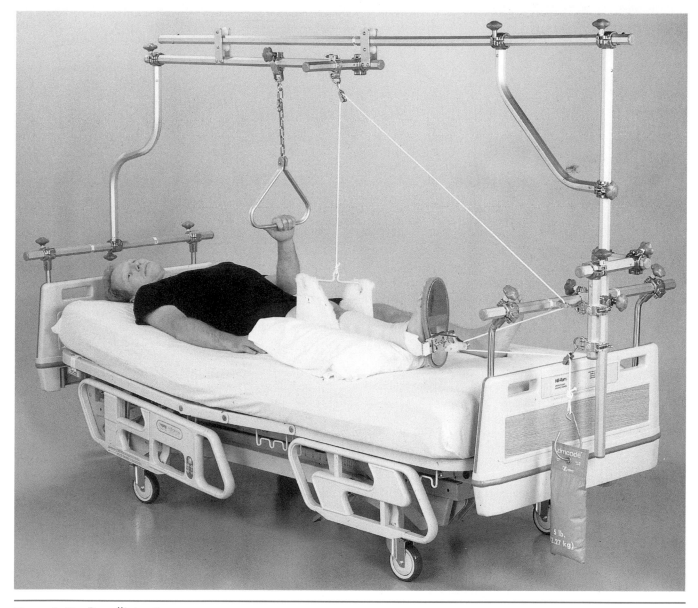

Figure 6–17   Russell's traction.   *(Zimmer, Inc. (1996). Zimmer Traction Handbook Warsaw, IN: Zimmer, Inc.)*

TRACTION APPLICATION

Russell's traction is a form of suspension skin traction to the leg consisting of a Buck's skin traction with a second, upward pull from a sling under the patient's leg just above the knee. The purposes of Russell's traction are (1) to reduce and immobilize preoperative hip fractures, (2) to reduce and immobilize fractures of the femur, and (3) to treat certain types of knee injuries. The application of the traction tapes and/or splint follows the procedure discussed under Buck's traction, with the addition of a sling placed under the patient's knee and a pillow under the lower leg.

Changes in countertraction can be obtained by elevating the foot of the bed or by gatching the bed at the knees with the patient supine. The patient is usually kept flat in bed; however, the head of the bed can be elevated if ordered by the physician. One thing to keep in mind when caring for a patient in this type of Russell's traction is that the pull on the foot is double the amount of weight applied (because of the vectors of force principle). For a patient in Russell's traction, the vectors of force are illustrated in Figure 6–18, which shows two pulling forces (A and B) on the footplate. Each has a pulling force of 5 pounds, and when combined they produce a resultant force (R) of 10 pounds. The vertical pull on the knee sling remains at 5 pounds and serves only to suspend the knee off the bed.

The nursing concerns for a patient in Russell's traction are the same as those in Buck's traction (discussed in Chapter 9) with a few additions. Make sure the knee sling is kept smooth and that the edges of the sling do not irritate the patient's skin and soft tissue. If the patient had a pillow under their lower leg when the traction was applied, make sure you keep the pillow there. If there was

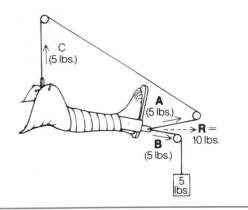

Figure 6–18 Vectors of force principle. *(Zimmer, Inc. (1996).* Zimmer Traction Handbook *Warsaw, IN: Zimmer, Inc.)*

no pillow under the patient's lower leg when the traction was applied, do not place one there unless discussed with and ordered by the patient's physician. Russell's traction affords the patient more movability than Buck's traction; the patient can utilize the overhead trapeze to change their position or to lift up for bedpan use, linen changes, and skin care. Include neurovascular checks and measures to prevent complications from immobility.

The potential complications with Russell's traction are (1) potential neurovascular impairment; (2) foot drop from pressure on the Achilles tendon; (3) skin breakdown; (4) lack of immobilization of the fracture site, causing trauma and pain; and (5) physical and psychological complications of enforced recumbency.

TRACTION USING BÖHLER-BRAUN FRAME

TRACTION SETUP

Preparing the bed and setting up a Böhler-Braun frame (Fig. 6–19) involves the following steps (as adapted from Zimmer, 1996):

1. Attach canvas slings to the Böhler-Braun frame.
2. Prepare the upper leg with traction tapes (including a spreader block), and wrap the lower leg with traction tapes (including a spreader block) or a traction splint for skin traction and a pin/wire through the tibia or femur for skeletal traction.
3. Lift the injured leg (usually done by the physician with assistance from others) and place the frame under the leg with the knee directly over the angle of the frame.
4. Adjust the slings so that any pressure points are eliminated (protect the heel and hamstring tendons).
5. Tie traction cords (Fig. 6–2) to the spreader block and footplate or splint, thread through the pulleys, and then tie to the weight carriers.
6. Gently apply weights as prescribed by the physician.

TRACTION APPLICATION

A Böhler-Braun frame is utilized to accomplish unilateral leg traction in the treatment of patients with

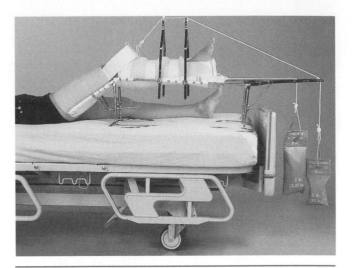

Figure 6–19 Böhler-Brown traction. *(Zimmer, Inc. (1996).* Zimmer Traction Handbook *Warsaw, IN: Zimmer, Inc.)*

(1) compound fractures of the tibia with severe soft-tissue damage, (2) markedly unstable fractures of the tibia and femur, and (3) comminuted fractures extending into the knee joint. Skeletal traction is accomplished by inserting a pin through the calcaneus, with the leg supported by the frame. With skin traction, the lower leg is placed in a traction splint and the leg is supported by the frame. The upper leg (and sometimes also the lower leg) has traction tapes applied to it. They are secured in place with an elastic bandage wrap (or SKIN TRAC and Orthopaedic Wraps) and are attached to a spreader block. Before applying the traction tapes, prepare the patient's skin, using the physician's or the institution's protocol for skin preparation.

Potential complications and nursing care are the same as those for the patient in balanced suspension skeletal traction (discussed later in this Chapter and in Chapter 4). It is important to remember that the slings should be placed so that there will be no pressure on the popliteal space, the Achilles tendon, or the heel. Keep the leg from externally rotating. Make sure the proximal portion of the frame does not press on the perineum. A large dressing or pieces of sheepskin can be used to pad this area and can be easily changed if they become soiled. To provide back care, have the patient tilt toward the affected side. Implement nursing measures to prevent the complications of immobility, neurovascular impairment, and infection (if skeletal traction is utilized).

BALANCED SUSPENSION SKELETAL TRACTION

TRACTION SETUP

Preparing the bed and setting up balanced suspension skeletal traction (Fig. 6–20) involve the following steps (adapted from Zimmer, 1996):

1. Attach a basic frame (an overhead traction bar designed for retractable beds) to the patient's bed.

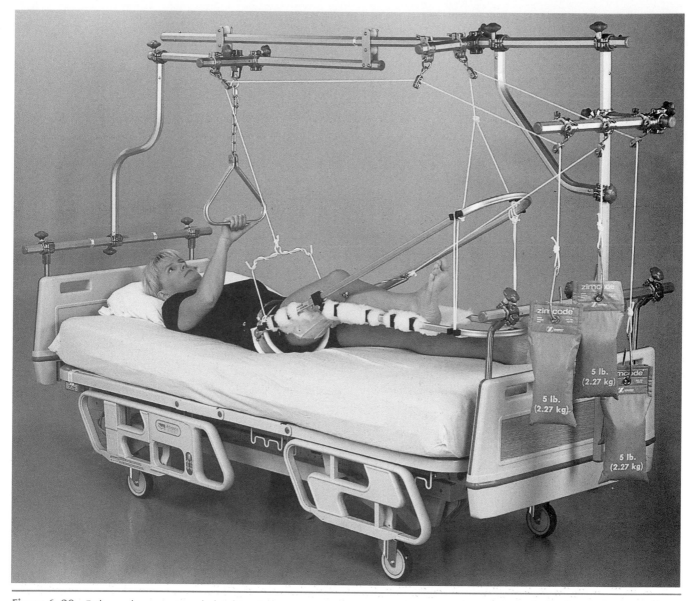

Figure 6–20 Balanced suspension skeletal traction.   *(Zimmer, Inc. (1996). Zimmer Traction Handbook Warsaw, IN: Zimmer, Inc.)*

2. Attach a 9-inch single clamp bar to the upright bar at the foot of the bed, with the bar extending beyond the bed.

3. Attach a 9-inch single clamp bar with pulley to the overhead bar above the patient's hip on the side of the injury.

4. Attach one 9-inch single clamp bar with two pulleys to the overhead bar near the foot of the bed, facing the side of the injury.

5. Attach one-18 inch single clamp bar with three pulleys to the 9-inch single clamp bar on the upright bar at the foot of the bed.

6. Attach the Pearson attachment to the Thomas or Brady leg splint with the point of attachment at the patient's knee joint.

7. Form a cradle for the patient's leg by attaching polyester pile slings to the splint (for supporting the upper leg) and to the Pearson attachment (for support of the lower leg).

8. Gently lift the leg (usually done by the physician with assistance from others) and move the splint with the Pearson attachment under the injured leg, with the ring of the splint resting loosely against the patient's ischial tuberosity.

9. Tie (Fig. 6–2) one end of the traction cord to the proximal lateral end of the splint, wrap the cord 3 times around the spreader bar, and then tie the cord to the medial side of the splint.

10. Tie another traction cord to the center of the spreader bar, thread through the pulley above the patient's hip, then through the top pulley at the foot of the bed, and then tie it to a weight carrier.

11. Thread another traction cord through the rope locators at the distal end of the splint (tie loose

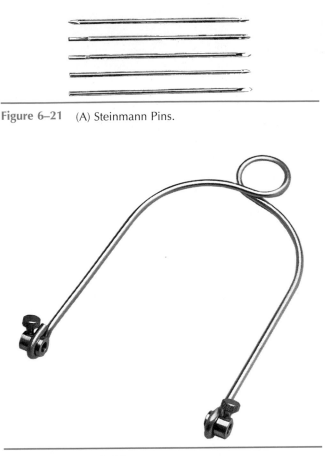

Figure 6–21 (A) Steinmann Pins.

(B) Steinmann pin holder. *(Zimmer, Inc. (1996). Zimmer Traction Handbook Warsaw, IN: Zimmer, Inc.)*

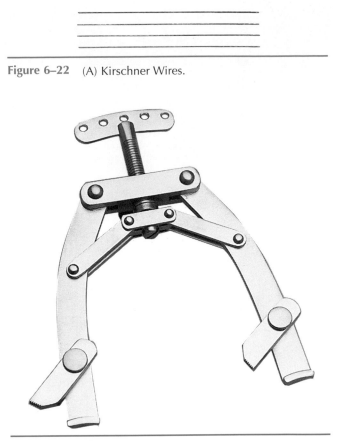

Figure 6–22 (A) Kirschner Wires.

(B) Kirschner wire tractor. *(Zimmer, Inc. (1996). Zimmer Traction Handbook Warsaw, IN: Zimmer, Inc.)*

ends of the traction cord back on themselves to form a triangle), thread the traction cord through the pulley on the 9-inch single clamp bar above the bed, then through the outside pulley on the 18-inch single clamp bar at the end of the bed, and, finally, tie the traction cord to a weight carrier.

12. Tie another cord to the end of the Pearson attachment, and tie it to the distal end of the splint.

13. Tie another traction cord to the pin holder or wire tractor, thread through the pulley on the high 9-inch single clamp bar beyond the bed, and then tie it to a weight carrier.

14. Gently apply the prescribed weights (weights are usually distributed through the various elements so that a delicate balance of traction and countertraction is maintained).

TRACTION APPLICATION

Although the more accepted treatment is surgical reduction and early ambulation of patients with femoral fractures, balanced suspension skeletal traction is still being used in specific cases. Traction can be utilized for patients with fractures of the femoral shaft,

fractures of the hip, fractures of the lower leg, or any combination of these. Balanced suspension skeletal traction is usually accomplished by inserting a Steinmann pin (Fig. 6–21) or Kirschner threaded or unthreaded wire (Fig. 6–22) into the skeletal system. Fractures of the femur and pelvis, unstable fractures of the acetabulum, and fractures of the acetabular rim with dislocations of the hip are usually treated by utilizing a Thomas or Brady splint. A pin is placed through the distal femur or proximal tibia, with the leg supported by a Thomas or Brady splint and a Pearson attachment.

NURSING PROCESS (Patient with Balanced Suspension Skeletal Traction)

To demonstrate the nursing care for a patient in balanced suspension skeletal traction, the following nursing process presents the care of a patient in traction for a femoral shaft fracture. The nursing process begins after the traction is applied.

ASSESSMENT

The patient admitted with a fracture of the femoral shaft and treated with balanced suspension skeletal traction often has multiple injuries to other systems of the body, because femoral shaft fractures frequently result from "high-energy" trauma. Because the femur is the longest bone and experiences a tremendous amount of stress, it is the strongest bone in the body. The powerful muscles that surround the femur provide it with a plentiful blood supply. When fractures occur, even closed fractures, they are associated with significant blood loss, especially during the first 12 hours. Assess for signs of shock, and look for other injuries, especially internal or head injuries, that may have occurred at the time of the accident. For further details on assessment, see Chapter 2 and, for details on trauma, see Chapter 4.

In the typical patient with a fractured femoral shaft, the leg tends to develop medial rotation of the lower fragment. The gluteus medius muscle has a tendency to pull the proximal fragment outward, and the strong pull of the adductor muscle group tends to cause outward bowing at the point of the fracture.

A neurovascular assessment is done to determine skin color, pulse, joint motion, and complaints of numbness, coldness, or swelling of the leg (see Chapter 2). If there is an open fracture, note the amount and color of drainage.

Observe the emotional reaction of the patient, the family, and significant others. Many times fractures of the femur occur to working-age adults during their leisure time activities, and the patient feels guilty about how the accident occurred and about missing work.

NURSING DIAGNOSIS

Based on all of the assessment data, the major nursing diagnoses for a typical patient in balanced suspension skeletal traction with a fractured femur are

- Pain and discomfort related to trauma and immobility
- Impaired physical mobility related to instability of the femur
- Risk of impaired skin integrity related to immobility and the traction device
- Constipation related to immobility and pain medications
- Altered nutrition: more than body requirements related to immobility
- Anxiety related to knowledge deficit about the treatment method(s) and rehabilitation

COLLABORATIVE PROBLEMS

- Deep vein thrombosis
- Pulmonary emboli
- Fat emboli
- Hypovolemic shock

GOAL FORMULATION AND PLANNING

The goals are to have the patient experience (1) a decrease in pain through traction application, positioning, nursing measures, and prescribed medications; (2) an increase in mobility through the stabilization of the femur and exercises; (3) skin free of abrasions; (4) normal bowel elimination; (5) normal nutritional intake without weight gain; (6) a decrease in anxiety through patient education; and (7) an absence of complications.

INTERVENTIONS

ALLEVIATE PAIN

In the beginning, patients placed in balanced suspension skeletal traction following a fractured femur have pain due to soft-tissue and bone trauma. Medications are ordered to help relieve the pain temporarily, and being in traction helps greatly in the long run. The traction helps to align the bone fragments, to counteract the muscle spasms that pull the bone out of alignment, and to maintain immobilization. Pain usually increases if the traction is readjusted, if someone disturbs the traction equipment, or if the patient moves the affected leg out of alignment.

INCREASE MOBILITY

The two most important interventions to increase the patient's mobility are correct positioning and exercises.

Position. The patient must be taught the correct body and leg positioning and the importance of staying in the proper position and not readjusting any part of the apparatus. Patients need to know how much movement is allowed, the ways in which they can help themselves, and the importance of reporting any pain, pressure, or discomfort that develops. Most patients with a fractured femur in balanced suspension skeletal traction lie supine. Some, depending on the level of the fracture and their general condition, may be able to tilt to the side, and most are able to move rather freely in bed. They may sit up with the use of the overhead trapeze or have the head of the bed elevated, generally at 30 degrees, with 45 degrees for meals. However, some patients may have restrictions on the amount of elevation allowed because it may reduce countertraction (i.e., the effective weight of the patient's body that balances the weight on the traction). To prevent hip flexion contractures, the head of the bed must be completely lowered several times daily. This provides for extension of the hip joints.

The position of the extremity in suspension traction is determined by the fracture, but usually the extremity is held in a neutral position or in a position of slight internal rotation. The amount of abduction may vary. The position the patient assumes in bed affects the amount of abduction maintained, and, if the patient lies diagonally, abduction is lost. A short footboard or small flexion pillow for the uninvolved foot helps the patient maintain the desired position. With suspension traction, the knee of the uninvolved leg should be at the same level as the fastening of the Pearson attachment onto the Thomas or Brady splint.

With the use of the suspension traction, the patient is able to pull on the trapeze, push down with the uninvolved leg, and lift their buttocks off the bed. This greatly helps in getting the patient on the bedpan, changing linen, and giving skin care to the coccyx area. (Two draw sheets instead of one bottom sheet may facilitate changing soiled linen with less stress to the patient.) When the patient raises himself or herself in the suspension apparatus, the line of traction pull remains unchanged. The suspension thus allows freedom for the body as a whole while maintaining efficient traction on the leg.

Exercises. Exercise increases circulation and maintains muscle tone and must be part of the care for a patient in skeletal traction. Muscle weakness and contractures occur from disuse. No unnecessary stiffness or atrophy should be allowed to occur because of the immobilization of the injured leg. Exercises for the uninvolved portions of the body should include flexion and extension of the hip and knee of the unaffected leg; ankle pumps and range of motion at the ankle; plantar and dorsiflexion of the foot; quadriceps- and gluteal-setting exercises; exercises to develop the extensors of the elbows and wrists (to facilitate future crutch walking); and breathing exercises. Encourage activities of self-care and the use of the trapeze if the patient's arms will allow.

Patients tend to guard joints near a fracture; therefore, explanations and encouragement are needed to promote the active and passive exercising of the foot and to prevent a contracture of the Achilles tendon of the affected leg. Quadriceps-setting and plantar and dorsiflexion exercises are also part of the exercise program for the affected leg (see Box 6–2, Exercises for the Patient in Side Arm Traction). Quadriceps muscles begin to atrophy in about one week if not used.

MAINTAIN SKIN INTEGRITY
In administering care, make sure that there is no pressure on the popliteal space, the lateral aspect of the leg over the head of the fibula, the heel, the ischial area, the groin, or the adductor muscles. Reposition the patient and/or slings to relieve any pressure. In the groin area, padding can be applied and then removed when soiled. There is a potential for infection from skin breakdown or at the pin site. There is no standard for pin care, and institutions differ greatly, so utilize whatever method your institution or physician prefers. Whatever the method, teach the patient to recognize the signs and symptoms of infection.

CONSTIPATION
The patient immobilized in traction has a potential to develop constipation because of immobilization, decreased muscle tone, inability to assume the normal position for elimination, reduced food and fluid intake, and a bland diet. Bowel elimination involves the smooth muscle, skeletal muscle activity, and complex visceral reflex patterns. The patient needs a well-balanced diet high in fiber with plenty of fruits and vegetables, complex carbohydrates, and adequate fluids.

Fluids are essential to keep the stool soft and moist to provide ease in elimination. Provide a variety of fluids the patient likes, but limit the amount of caffeine. Exercises that increase the patient's mobility also help to prevent constipation.

NUTRITIONAL INTAKE
A patient immobilized in traction needs a high-fiber diet with adequate fluids as already discussed in relation to elimination. According to Jagmin (1998), an immobilized adult also needs to consume one gram of protein per kilogram of body weight every day. For some individuals, this may be difficult. For others, the problem may be eating too much. The patient may be eating their "normal" diet, but since they are not as active as normal, that involves too much food. See Chapter 1 for a discussion on how to calculate the number of calories for a patient based on their sex, age, weight, height, and new sedentary lifestyle. Other patients may be overeating not because they are hungry but because they are bored or depressed (discussed under coping mechanisms).

PATIENT TEACHING AND HOME CARE CONSIDERATIONS
The accident was an emotional as well as physical shock to the patient, and being placed in balanced suspension skeletal traction can be a very fearful experience. Even though explanations are given when the traction is applied, most patients are unable to fully comprehend them. Once things have settled down, discuss the traction equipment and its purpose with the patient, the family, and significant others. Reinforcing what the different purposes of the traction are when you are working with it, or asking the patient to participate in their care, will also increase the patient's understanding.

Know what the physician has told the patient and what the plan of treatment will be. Will the patient be in the traction for only a few days before surgery, and, if they have surgery, what method will be used? Will the patient later be put in a cast brace, or is traction the only method of treatment? If traction is the only treatment, will the patient go home or to an extended care facility, since the patient may remain in the traction 3 months or more? If traction is not to be the only method of treatment, patient education should be started concerning follow-up care. Of course the answers need to be given with the clarifier that plans can change based on the patient's response to traction. Do not forget to make time to discuss with the patient the emotional reaction to the accident and what effect it has had on his or her life and the lives of others.

MONITORING AND MANAGING POTENTIAL PROBLEMS

The patient in balanced suspension skeletal traction is prone to all the complications of trauma and bed rest discussed previously in Chapter 4, especially deep vein thrombosis, pulmonary embolism, fat embolism, and hypovolemic shock.

CIRCULATORY

When a bone is fractured, surrounding soft tissue, blood vessels, and nerves are also injured, and there may be enough blood loss to cause shock. Generally, the patient is most vulnerable to shock during the first 12 hours.

EVALUATION/OUTCOMES

A patient in balanced suspension skeletal traction should feel reasonably comfortable, that is, free of any severe pain. A neurovascular evaluation of the affected extremity should find good nerve and vascular function. In evaluating whether traction is being maintained, note the alignment of the body and the leg. Evaluate whether the patient is complying with the exercise regime and rehabilitation program. The patient should be free of potential complications such as pressure areas, footdrop, hip flexion contractures, or other effects of immobility. If the goals have not been met, both the goals and plan of care must be reassessed and the nursing process begun again.

TRACTION TO THE SPINAL COLUMN

The forms of traction most commonly utilized in the care of patients with spinal column injuries include (1) cervical skin traction, (2) cervical skeletal traction, (3) halo skeletal traction, (4) Buck's bilateral traction for the treatment of low back pain (see Buck's unilateral traction earlier in this chapter), (5) pelvic traction, and (6) pelvic sling.

CERVICAL SKIN TRACTION

TRACTION SETUP

Preparing the bed and setting up cervical skin traction (Fig. 6–23) involves the following steps (adapted from Zimmer, 1996; this traction setup can be modified for home use):

1. Attach Buck's extension panel clamp to the headboard.
2. Attach a 27-inch single clamp bar vertically.
3. Attach a 9-inch single clamp bar with pulley perpendicular to the 17-inch single clamp bar.
4. Attach an 18-inch double pulley bar to the 9-inch single clamp bar.
5. Tie the traction cord (Fig. 6–23) to the spreader bar, thread through the pulleys, then tie to the weight carrier.
6. Apply head halter to the patient, attach spreader bar, and gently apply the weights.

An alternative setup (Fig. 6–24) is often used in the hospital setting. The steps (Zimmer, 1996) are as follows:

1. Attach a basic frame (an overhead traction bar for retractable beds) to the bed.
2. Attach an 18-inch single clamp with pulley to the upright bar of the setup at a 45-degree angle to the headboard.

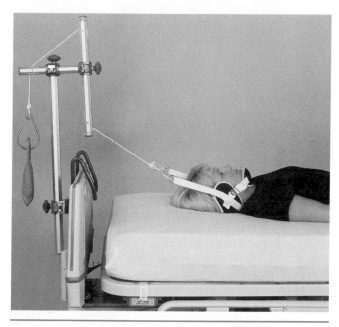

Figure 6–23 Cervical traction using Buck's apparatus. *(Zimmer, Inc. (1996). Zimmer Traction Handbook Warsaw, IN: Zimmer, Inc.)*

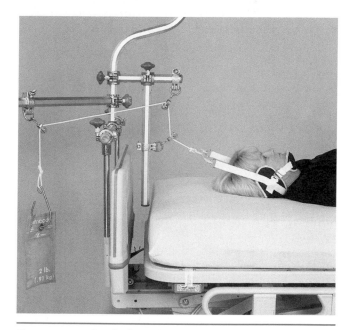

Figure 6–24 Cervical traction. *(Zimmer, Inc. (1996). Zimmer Traction Handbook Warsaw, IN: Zimmer, Inc.)*

3. Attach a 9-inch single clamp bar with pulley directly above the 18-inch bar perpendicular to the headboard.
4. Attach an 18-inch single clamp bar with pulley vertically to the 9-inch single clamp bar.
5. & 6. are the same as in the previous setup.

TRACTION APPLICATION

Cervical skin traction is accomplished by utilizing a head halter or two straps in a horizontal or vertical position to apply traction to the cervical spine. Continuous traction relieves muscle spasms with minimal weight, whereas intermittent traction stimulates blood flow and relieves muscle spasms with relatively heavy weights for short periods of time. Cervical skin traction is used (1) to relieve the pain of cervical arthritis with radiculitis, (2) to counteract muscle spasms associated with cervical disc syndrome, (3) to relieve static postural neck strain, and (4) to relieve symptoms of cervical sprain. Head halter skin traction may also be used at home by some patients for relief of cervical pain.

Cervical skin traction is applied to the patient's cervical spine by means of a head halter. Various types of head halters may be obtained from orthopaedic and surgical supply houses, including soft, disposable head halters; leather or canvas halters; and disposable, two-strap halters. Before applying the traction, explain to the patient the purpose of the traction and what it should do. Make sure the patient is comfortable and correctly positioned in bed.

Because cervical neck injuries cause muscle spasms and headaches, the patient should not be asked to hold the head up during the application of the traction. Support the patient's head by placing your left hand under the patient's head if you are on the patient's left or your right hand if you are on the patient's right. With your other hand, put the head halter over the patient's face and under the chin. You may have to bring the posterior portion of the halter down the back of the patient's head to get the halter completely under the chin. Adjust the posterior portion to the level of the occiput. For the halter with side adjustments, attach the side closures and adjust the straps so that the halter feels comfortable. The straps do not have to be tight, just secure enough to hold the halter in correct position. If the cervical traction is being applied with a disposable, two-strap halter, make sure the straps are in place and the ropes that connect them are applying equal pull. Connect the head halter to the spreader bar.

Apply a few pounds of pull manually to check the adjustment of the head halter before applying the weights. Put the correct amount of weight on the weight carrier and gradually, smoothly, let go of the traction. The direction of the pull of the traction must cause the chin to be tucked in toward the chest and not drawn upward or backward. The patient should be instructed to maintain proper body alignment. With cervical skin traction, countertraction is provided by the patient's body weight and position in bed.

NURSING PROCESS (Patient with Cervical Skin Traction)

To demonstrate the nursing care for a patient in cervical skin traction, the following nursing process presents the care of a patient in traction for a herniated cervical disc. The nursing process begins after the traction is applied.

ASSESSMENT

The nursing assessment of a typical patient with a herniated cervical disc who is in cervical traction includes a comprehensive assessment of the total patient with a focus on pain and the neurovascular status of the upper extremity. Neurovascular assessment of the upper extremity is described in Chapter 2. Assess the patient for any increased neck pain, pressure on the ears, and pain along the chin, jaw line, or ears. Assess for complaints of headaches as they could be an indication of venous pressure, venous stasis, or overpull on cervical muscles. Inspect the skin surfaces under the traction for possible irritation or pressure areas.

Determine that the patient is in correct alignment. The pull of the cervical traction should be equal on both sides and be evenly distributed between the chin and the occiput. Check that the patient's head is tilted slightly forward so that the pull is on a straight cervical spinal column. The patient may or may not require a small pillow to obtain the desired neck flexion. The direction of the traction pull must cause the chin to be tucked in toward the chest, not drawn upward or backward. Verify that the weights have the correct poundage and that the weights and the pulleys hang free of the wall, bed, or other obstructions. The weights are usually only 2 to 5 pounds, but may be more in some instances. Most authorities agree that the weights should not exceed 10 pounds.

NURSING DIAGNOSIS

Based on all of the assessment data, the major nursing diagnoses for a typical patient in cervical skin traction with a herniated cervical disc include the following:

- Pain and discomfort related to soft-tissue trauma of the cervical spine
- Impaired physical mobility related to neck and arm pain and muscle spasms
- Impaired adjustment related to immobility with traction application
- Anxiety related to knowledge deficit about the injury, treatment, and prognosis

COLLABORATIVE PROBLEMS

- Injury to the facial nerve
- Skin breakdown on the patient's chin
- Irritation and trauma to the temporomandibular joint
- Overpull of muscles of the neck

GOAL FORMULATION AND PLANNING

The goals are to have the patient experience (1) a decrease in pain through the use of traction, heat, and muscle relaxants; (2) an increase in mobility through traction; (3) an adjustment to the treatment method; (4) a decrease in anxiety through patient education; and (5) an absence of complications.

INTERVENTIONS

ALLEVIATE PAIN

The patient with a herniated cervical disc will have pain. If there is an increase in neck and head pain after the application of the traction, determine whether the traction has an even pull between the occiput and the chin. Too much pull on the occiput will interfere with circulation and cause increased pain in the neck and especially the head. Adjust by raising the chin and tilting the head backward. If the patient complains of jaw or ear discomfort, the pull may be too much on the chin, causing pressure on the temporomandibular joint, which in turn causes irritation and pain. Adjust by tilting the head forward. If there is pressure on the ears or discomfort along one side of the chin or jaw line, the traction may be pulling on that side more than the other. Correct the patient's positioning. Check to make sure the straps on the cervical traction are not pressing too tightly against the side of the patient's face, causing pressure on the facial nerve (cranial nerve VII). Such pressure on the patient's ears, jaw line, or glasses may be caused by a spreader bar that is too narrow. Replace the spreader bar with a wider one. Make sure the head halter is not pressing on the patient's ears, and have the patient remove any earrings that interfere with the traction.

For chin discomfort when the alignment is correct, look for redness or irritation. If they are present, some authorities feel that a soft pad should be placed between the halter and the patient's chin. Others disagree, saying that the padding only increases pressure on the chin, and advocate that the traction should be removed to relieve the pressure. Which method to follow depends on established procedures. If no inflammation is present, alcohol rubs may also be used to toughen the skin on the chin. If the patient has a beard, make sure the beard is brought down flat under the chin as the halter is applied. If the halter is readjusted, the beard needs to be smoothed again. Men who are prone to a "5 o'clock shadow" may have to shave twice a day to reduce discomfort from the head halter rubbing against their whiskers. Individuals with long hair and wearing the two-strap type of halter may need to keep their hair on the top of their head to reduce slipping of the posterior strap.

Heat application to the cervical area provides analgesic and muscle-relaxing properties and tends to improve circulation to the skin and the more superficial muscle layers. Having the patient recumbent during the heat applications further adds to muscle and psychic relaxation and pain relief. Massage also helps to increase circulation to the area and relax the muscles.

INCREASE MOBILITY

The two most important interventions, besides the traction, to increase the patient's mobility are correct positioning and ambulation.

Position. The patient in cervical skin traction should be in a comfortable supine position with the body in good alignment. The shoulders should be level and relaxed and the back flattened against the bed. No pillow is generally used, although if the patient needs an increase in forward flexion of the head, a cervical or other small pillow may be allowed. The patient must be down far enough in bed to allow room for the spreader bar when it is attached to the head halter. The traction equipment is attached to the head of the bed unless the headboard is too high. In that case, the head of the bed may be elevated or the patient's head and traction equipment may be placed at the foot of the bed. Today, with the variety of bed and traction equipment available, such adjustments are usually not necessary.

During the day, some patients may be able to have the traction reattached higher on the bed frame so they can be in a sitting position, or even have the traction equipment set up on a geri chair so they can sit in the chair. Many patients have problems sleeping, as lying on the back is not comfortable. If allowed, nursing measures can permit patients to sleep on the side. Fold a regular pillow and tape the pillow so that it stays folded. Disconnect the traction and allow the patient to turn to the side, placing the folded pillow under the head so that the cervical spinal column is still straight. Reattach the traction so the pull is correct, the patient is in correct alignment, and the spreader bar is free of the pillow.

Ambulation. Most patients are allowed out of cervical skin traction for activities of daily living, though they are encouraged to keep the traction on as much as possible. When patients have bathroom privileges, they will need assistance in getting out of bed as well as getting out of the traction. Many patients need to wear a cervical collar to help support the head during ambulation. If the patient has been on muscle relaxants, it is best to walk with the patient to ensure safety.

EMOTIONAL ADJUSTMENT

Some patients have difficulty in adjusting to staying in bed and keeping the traction on. Others become depressed and have an unrealistic view of the need for immobilization with traction, even for a short period. Nursing measures to help prevent those complications are one-to-one therapeutic discussions with the patient, giving the patient realistic information on the treatment and prognosis, and encouraging the patient to be as actively involved in self-care as physically possible.

PATIENT TEACHING AND HOME CARE CONSIDERATIONS

The patient must know the purpose of the traction and how it works to decrease their anxiety and fear of the equipment and to enable performance of self-care without undue stress. If home traction is indicated, explain its purpose, how it is to be set up, and how often it is to be used. Pictures are a great help. Most patients need to wear a cervical collar for a period of time. Tell them whether the collar is to be worn with the higher or lower portion in front (Fig. 6–25) and why. They should be told to report to their physician any increase in pain or pressure that may develop after they start to wear the collar.

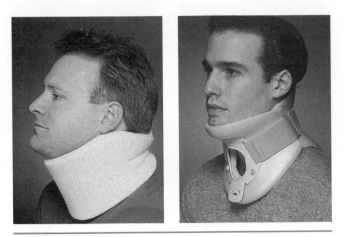

Figure 6–25   A. Cervical collar with neck in hyperextension or reversed for flexion. B. Philadelphia cervical collar.
(Zimmer, Inc. (1996). Zimmer Traction Handbook Warsaw, IN: Zimmer, Inc.)

Box 6–3
Neck Exercises

1. With the head held erect and face squarely forward, the patient places the base of the right palm (the part of the palm nearest he forearm)against the head, just above the right ear. The patient then pushes the head toward the right while resisting with the palm so there is no appreciable motion. The exercise is held for the count of ten.
2. The patient then repeats the same exercise on the left side.
3. With the patient's head held erect and face squarely forward, the patient places the right palm on the right side of the forehead and the left palm on the left side of the forehead with the hands touching each other. The patient then pushes their head in a forward direction while resisting with the palms so there is no appreciable motion. The exercise is held for the count of ten.
4. With the patient's head held erect and face squarely forward, the patient places the right palm on the right side of the back of the head and the left palm on the left side of the back of the head, intertwining the fingers. The patient then pushes their head in a backward direction while resisting with the palms so there is no appreciable motion. The exercise is held for the count of ten.

Most individuals with a cervical collar have no problem bathing, because they can remove the collar to shower.

At home, heat should be applied using an electric heating pad set on low or medium. (Be sure to remind the patient of safety factors, including not putting it on high and not going to sleep with the heating pad on.) After the traction is removed, the patient needs to begin an exercise program for the cervical area. *Isometric exercises* come first; they provide small changes of stress to the ligaments, bones, and joints to strengthen those structures as well as the muscles. Each set of exercises should be done approximately 15 minutes per day unless otherwise instructed. The amount of force the patient actually applies depends on a number of factors, including the patient's strength before the injury, level of pain, pain tolerance, and body build. Each repetition of the exercise should cause either slight discomfort or a pulling sensation. If the patient remains comfortable, the exercises are probably not beneficial. If they are painful, they will not be tolerated. The neck exercises (Box 6–3) can be done in a standing, sitting, or reclining position. They can be done all at once or spread out over the day. The number of times each exercise is repeated gradually increases, and active exercises are also added as the patient's condition improves.

Patients need to know how to prevent any undue stress or strain to the cervical area. "*Do nots*" include (1) sleeping with an arm under the face or over the head; (2) sleeping with a high pillow; (3) sleeping on their abdomen, as it forces the head to the side; (4) lying on the sofa while watching television; (5) lying in bed to read; and (6) sleeping in a chair. All of these can cause severe strain to the neck.

MONITORING AND MANAGING POTENTIAL PROBLEMS

The major potential complications for a patient with a herniated cervical disc being treated with cervical skin traction are (1) injury to the facial nerve, (2) break-down of skin on the patient's chin, (3) irritation and trauma to the temporomandibular joint, and (4) over-pull of muscles of the neck. Interventions to assess for and prevent those complications have already been discussed under how to alleviate pain and increase mobility.

EVALUATION/OUTCOMES

Determine whether the pain decreased in severity after traction and the administration of pain medications and muscle relaxants. Evaluate the effectiveness of the traction to relieve muscle spasms by how well the patient tolerates the traction and continues to utilize it. Check for any possible complications from the traction. To evaluate the status of the patient's facial nerve (cranial nerve VII), observe the patient's face for symmetry. Then ask the patient to raise and lower the eyebrows, again observing for symmetry. Next, ask the patient to close their eyes tightly while you try to raise the lids. Finally, ask the patient to smile, show their teeth, and puff out their cheeks so that you can assess facial muscle strength. If signs of decreased nerve function are observed, remove the traction and notify the physician. Evaluate how well the patient, family, or significant other understands home care by asking them to tell you how the patient should carry out the activities of a normal day. Have the patient explain to you the side effects of the prescribed medications.

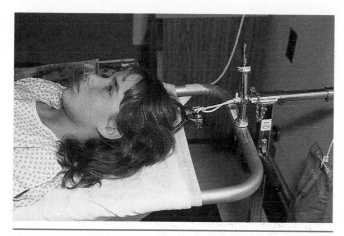

Figure 6–26   Traction for cervical fractures may be applied with tongs.   *(Zimmer, Inc. (1996). Zimmer Traction Handbook Warsaw, IN: Zimmer, Inc.)*

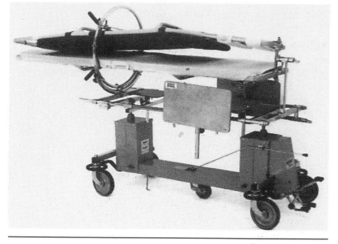

Figure 6–27   The Stryker wedge turning frame allows the patient to be turned from supine to prone without placing stress on the spine.

CERVICAL SKELETAL TRACTION

TRACTION SETUP

The patient in cervical skeletal traction (Fig. 6–26) is placed on a turning frame. Examples of these frames are the Stryker or Stryker wedge frame (Fig. 6–27), Foster frame, or the Circo-lectric bed. After the skeletal tongs are inserted, the patient is placed supine on a turning frame and prepared for the application of traction. Adequate room should be left at the head of the turning frame for the traction apparatus to hang free. A traction cord is attached to the skeletal tong apparatus, threaded through the hole in the center of the disc at the head of the frame, and laid over the pulley. The traction cord is then attached to the weight carrier, and all traction cord knots are taped. The weights should then be lowered gently to apply the traction to the cervical spine. The weights should be checked for correct poundage and hang free of the bed, wall, or other obstacles. The traction must be maintained without interruption until it is discontinued.

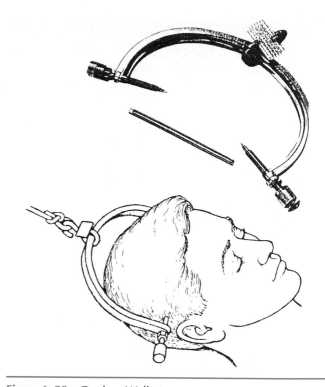

Figure 6–28   Gardner-Wells tongs.   *(Smelter & Bare (1996). Brunner and Suddath's Textbook of Medical-Surgical Nursing. 8th ed. Philadelphia: Lippincott-Raven.)*

TRACTION APPLICATION

The purposes of cervical skeletal traction are (1) to reduce fractures and dislocations of the cervical spine, (2) to immobilize cervical fractures, and (3) to reduce subluxations of the cervical spine. The application of cervical skeletal traction is accomplished by the use of skull tongs (Vinke, Crutchfield, Barton, or Gardner-Wells) with the patient positioned on a turning frame. Crutchfield tongs, for the most part, are being replaced by Gardner-Wells tongs (Fig. 6–28), which are easier to apply and have a self-contained tension device. The points of the Gardner-Wells tongs are needle sharp and need to be cleansed with an antiseptic before insertion. The hair and scalp are sprayed with an aerosol antiseptic and then rubbed at the temple ridges where the tongs will be inserted. A local anesthetic is injected at the site of the insertion, and the area is sprayed again. The tongs are then applied and tightened until the depth indicator shows a penetration of one mm. The tongs are checked and tightened over the next few hours as needed. Stability is usually achieved within 24 hours, after which the tongs usually need no further adjustment.

Although less frequently used, Crutchfield tongs are used to maintain cervical skeletal traction in a number of institutions. To apply Crutchfield tongs, the patient's head is shaved at the areas where the tongs are to be placed, and the points of contact are marked for the insertion of the tongs. The two areas are then injected with a local anesthetic, and an incision down to the skull just large enough to admit a drill is made in each

Table 6–1 Weights to Accomplish Cervical Vertebral Reduction	
Level of Fracture	**Pounds of Weight**
1st cervical vertebra	5 to 10
2nd cervical vertebra	6 to 10–12
3rd cervical vertebra	8 to 10–15
4th cervical vertebra	10 to 15–20
5th cervical vertebra	12 to 20–25
6th cervical vertebra	15 to 20–30
7th cervical vertebra	18 to 25–35

area. The drill penetrates only the outer portion of the skull, some 4 mm in adults. The points of the tongs are then fitted into the holes in the skull and held in position until the tongs have been locked in place. The tongs are checked daily to see that they are firmly in place and are tightened if necessary. Movements of the head result in local irritation, enlargement of the holes, and, eventually, disengagement of the tongs. On the other hand, excessive tightening of the tongs may result in a perforation into the inner skull.

Extension and flexion injuries to the neck cause dislocations and/or fractures with damage to the soft tissue in the cervical area, with or without neurologic damage. Whether or not neurologic damage is present, reduction of any displacement is essential and is accomplished with skull tongs. The amount of weight applied to the tongs depends on the patient's size and the degree of fracture displacement. The traction force is exerted along the longitudinal axis of the vertebral bodies with the patient's neck in neutral position. The amount of weight on the traction is gradually increased, usually in 2-pound increments, until the intervertebral space widens enough to let the fractured/dislocated vertebrae slip back into anatomical alignment (see Table 6–1). Once reduction is achieved, verified by neurologic examination and roentgenography, the weights are gradually removed until an appropriate amount of weight to maintain the alignment is obtained. After reduction is accomplished, the patient may be treated in a number of ways: (1) the traction may be utilized as a means of immobilization using the lighter weight for several days, (2) a halo brace with skull calipers may be used to immobilize the neck, or (3) the patient may go to surgery for surgical immobilization. Regardless of what additional treatment may be required, skeletal traction is usually applied promptly. (For further discussion, see Chapter 8 and references at the end of this chapter.)

NURSING PROCESS (Patient with Cervical Skeletal Traction)

The following nursing process presents the care of a patient in cervical skeletal traction for a cervical fracture. The nursing process begins after the traction is applied.

ASSESSMENT

The initial nursing assessment of a typical patient following a fracture of a cervical vertebra and the application of skull tong traction should include an in-depth neurologic assessment in addition to a general evaluation of the patient. The assessment should include monitoring for signs of increasing intracranial pressure, for any indication of cervical nerve impingement, and for vascular changes in the extremities. (For specific details on neurologic assessment, see Chapter 2 and the references at the end of this chapter.)

Observe the patient's body alignment with respect to the traction. Check the placement of the tongs and make sure there is an equal pull on both sides. Assess the tong sites for signs and symptoms of infection. Check for any friction or rubbing on the rope. The weights should have the correct poundage and hang free of all obstacles. Determine the level of discomfort and the effectiveness of the traction and nursing measures used to relieve discomfort. Note if the patient has any complaints of unusual pulling sensations. Determine the level of anxiety as evidenced by the patient's verbalization and cooperation with the plan of care. Assess the effectiveness of interactions between the patient and the family or significant others. Determine the status of the respiratory and gastrointestinal systems.

NURSING DIAGNOSIS

Based on all of the assessment data, the major nursing diagnoses for a typical patient in skeletal traction following a cervical fracture include the following:

- Pain and discomfort related to cervical spine trauma
- Impaired physical mobility related to instability in the cervical spine
- High risk for infection related to application of skeletal tongs
- Ineffective individual coping related to trauma and immobilization
- Ineffective breathing pattern related to immobility
- Altered nutrition: less than daily body requirement related to decreased intake
- Impaired skin integrity related to immobility and traction
- Anxiety related to knowledge deficit about the injury, the treatment method(s), and the rehabilitation process.

COLLABORATIVE PROBLEMS

- Decreased muscle tone
- Traction-induced cranial nerve lesion
- Paralytic ileus
- Lack of immobilization of the fracture site

GOAL FORMULATION AND PLANNING

The goals are to have the patient experience (1) a decrease in pain through immobilization, nursing measures, and prescribed medications; (2) an increase in mobility through controlled exercises and immobilization with skeletal traction; (3) a good appetite and adequate nutrition to meet daily requirements; (4) no infection at the tong site as a result of pin care; (5) a positive attitude and patient participation in self-care; (6) good oxygen exchange through normal breathing patterns; (7) a decrease in anxiety through increased knowledge; and (8) an absence of complications from decreased mobility and skeletal traction.

INTERVENTIONS

ALLEVIATE PAIN

If a patient in skeletal traction has the proper tong placement, the correct amount of force applied, and the correct body alignment, there will be a minimal amount of pain. For complaints of discomfort, analgesics are administered.

INCREASE MOBILITY

The most important interventions to increase physical mobility are correct positioning on a Stryker wedge turning frame, turning, and controlled exercises.

Position. The patient in continuous skeletal traction must be maintained in proper alignment when he or she is either supine or prone on a turning frame. A footboard is generally attached to prevent footdrop when the patient is in the supine position. When the patient is prone, the feet should hang over the end of the canvas in a flexed position. A sandbag or trochanter roll should be placed against the patient's hips to prevent external rotation at the hip. Armboards are attached to position the patient's arms to prevent adduction contractures of the shoulders and flexion contractures of the elbows. The armboards should be attached slightly below the level of the turning frame when the patient is in the prone position and level with the frame when the patient is in the supine position. In the supine position, the armboards may also be used as siderails.

Stryker wedge turning frame. Turning frames provide a way to safely turn a patient from supine to prone, or vice versa, without torsion or abnormal flexion-extension. They facilitate the movement and care of patients who should not or cannot move voluntarily. The turning frame may be a Foster bed, a Circo-lectric bed, a Stryker parallel frame, or a Stryker wedge frame. Today, most patients are placed on a Stryker wedge turning frame (see Fig. 6–27).

Stryker and Foster frames consist of an anterior and a posterior rectangular metal frame to which canvas covers are attached. Thin, sponge rubber mattresses covered with sheets are placed over the canvases. The frames are fastened to each other by a metal attachment with a knurled nut at both the head and the foot. Narrow forehead and chin straps are provided to support the head. The bed is also equipped with armboard and footboard attachments. Three restraining straps are placed around

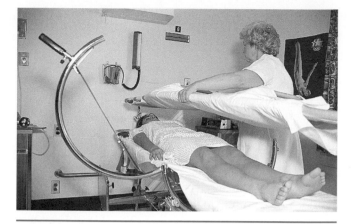

Figure 6–29 A patient on the Stryker frame is turned frequently to relieve pressure.   *(Smelter & Bare (1996).* Brunner and Suddath's Textbook of Medical-Surgical Nursing. *8th ed. Philadelphia: Lippincott-Raven.)*

both frames when turning the patient. They may also be fastened around the patient as a safety precaution either continuously or at night, because the bed is narrow. In the Striker wedge turning frame, which requires only one nurse to turn the patient, the anterior and posterior frames are not parallel to one another. Instead, the upper frame is angled toward the lower frame on the side toward which the frame will turn, preventing the patient from sliding out between the frames during the turn.

Turning. The patient in skeletal traction on a Stryker wedge frame is usually turned every 2 hours (Fig. 6–29). If the patient's condition permits, the patient is only turned every 4 hours at night. The turning schedule should accommodate meals and visiting hours. In preparation for turning, explain the procedure to the patient and ensure that the wheels of the turning frame are locked. When the patient is supine on the posterior frame, remove extra bed linen and place a sheepskin, pillow, or other comfort aid on top of the patient before applying the anterior frame. Be sure to place a pillow lengthwise over the lower legs and remove any armboards or footboards. Open the turning circle and put the head end of the anterior frame on the securing bolt and fasten it with the nut. Next, fasten the bolt at the foot end of the anterior frame, making sure that the patient's legs and feet are correctly positioned. The patient may then clasp their hands around the anterior frame, or the patient's arms may be placed at their side and a safety strap placed around the whole frame at the elbow level to constrain the patient's arms during the turn. Close the turning circle until it locks automatically, and pull out the bed turning lock at the head of the bed and the bed turning lock knob on the turning ring. Tell the patient you are about to make the turn, grasp the handle on the turning ring, and turn. The narrow side of the wedge (at the patient's right) will always turn down, and the frame will automatically lock when the bottom frame is horizontal. Push in the circular silver lock knob on the turning ring. Once the turn is complete, the turning circle can be opened and the knurled nuts unscrewed. The posterior (upper) frame can then be removed and the turning circle relocked for safety. To turn the patient on a Stryker wedge frame from prone to supine, reverse the procedure for turning from supine to prone. Remember that the narrow side of the wedge (on the patient's right) always turns down so the patient cannot slip out.

Exercises. Depending on the severity of the trauma, the patient may be started on passive range-of-motion exercises of the extremities within 48 hours after traction is applied. The goal of the exercises is to preserve joint motion and stimulate circulation. Toes, metatarsals, ankles, knees, and hips, as well as the joints of the upper extremities, should be put through full range of motion at least 4 and ideally 5 times daily. If the patient's condition permits, active range-of-motion exercises are also started.

INFECTION AT TONG SITES

With two pins inserted into the patient's skull, there is a chance of infection at the pin sites. Take the patient's temperature, and assess for pain, tenderness, heat, swelling, redness, and drainage at least once every shift. If there is drainage, send a culture to the laboratory and notify the patient's physician. To prevent or reduce pin site infections, do pin site care every shift.

COPING MECHANISMS

Patients in a cervical skeletal traction commonly have periods of anxiety and depression. Look for decreased concentration, fatigue, increased restlessness, increased complaints, or withdrawal from staff and others. Measures that help to reduce anxiety and depression are to listen to the patient express feelings, to educate the patient about the traction, and to encourage activities that distract the patient's focus from themselves. Encourage the patient and family to verbalize questions. Allow the patient (and the patient's family and significant others) to participate in planning daily activities.

EFFECTIVE BREATHING

The combination of recumbency, medications used for pain relief that depress respiration, a decrease in the body's need for oxygen due to inactivity, and the resistance of the bed against the patient's chest wall can lead to respiratory complications. Nursing measures are needed to prevent respiratory complications (see Chapter 4). However, having the patient cough or causing the patient to sneeze tends to jar the apparatus, which causes the patient discomfort and can manipulate the fracture site.

ADEQUATE NUTRITION

Because of the position and immobilization of the head and the neck, the patient may find that just getting a glass of water takes some effort. Make sure the turns are scheduled so the patient can eat. Patients who are able to feed themselves will want to eat while they are prone. Since they are lying on their stomach while they are eating, they may find that eating small amounts more frequently is a lot easier than eating three regular meals. The patient will need to be kept well hydrated. Offer fluids when they are supine, but make sure fluids are in easy reach when the patient is prone and can drink without assistance. Patients who are unable to feed themselves will need to be supine at meal time. Make sure the nurse or family member feeding the patient does not rush the patient and that the food is cut into small enough pieces to chew. *Make sure the patient does not choke on food or fluids.* (A safety measure is to keep a suction in the patient's room.) The patient needs a well-balanced diet with plenty of fluids. Special care should be taken to prevent the gastrointestinal problems that can occur with decreased mobility (i.e., constipation).

SKIN INTEGRITY

Skin breakdown can develop in less than 6 hours. Because the patient is immobilized, areas of local tissue ischemia develop where there is continuous pressure, and that may be compounded by inadequate peripheral circulation due to spinal shock. Turning every 2 hours aids in the prevention of pressure areas and prevents the pooling of blood and tissue fluid in the dependent areas. Every few hours, the patient's skin should be washed with a mild soap, rinsed well, and blotted dry. The sacrum, trochanter, ischia, iliac spine, knees, heels, scapula, and shoulders are especially susceptible to pressure. Those areas should be kept soft and well lubricated with an emollient lotion. Massage should be done gently with a circular motion. Linen under the patient should be kept dry.

PATIENT TEACHING AND HOME CARE CONSIDERATIONS

To help reduce anxiety, let the patient express fears and concerns. Carefully answer all questions in a way the patient can understand. Explain the purpose of the turning frame and how it works. Make sure the patient is informed before doing any procedure. Explain to the patient the potential problems and what nursing assessments and interventions are needed to prevent them. Let the patient participate in scheduling the daily activities, for example, procedures that can be done when the patient is either supine or prone.

The amount and kind of activities the patient can do depend on the amount and level of the trauma. Try to help the patient develop activities that are enjoyable and that stimulate an interest in the world outside the hospital. When the patient is prone, reading may be possible; and when supine, listening to music or to a "talking book" may be possibilities. Prism glasses can help the patient watch television. At other times, the patient may be able to do some kind of handicraft, especially while lying prone.

After a period of immobilization with tongs and traction, the duration of which depends on the severity and mechanism of the injury, the patient may be allowed to gradually assume an erect position. The patient usually requires a neck brace to reduce movement of the cervical spine and to allow continued bone healing. The commonly used orthoses (braces) are (1) a two-poster firm brace with chest extension, which gives support under the patient's chin and subocciput; and (2) a four-poster cervical brace with chest extension. (For patients without neurologic deficit, reduction in traction followed by rigid immobilization for approximately 16 weeks usually restores skeletal function.)

MONITORING AND MANAGING POTENTIAL PROBLEMS

Complications of skull tong traction include (1) decreased muscle tone, (2) traction-induced cranial nerve lesion, (3) paralytic ileus, and (4) lack of immobilization of the fracture site.

DECREASED MUSCLE TONE

Because of decreased mobility, patients in cervical skeletal traction may develop decreased muscle tone. A program of exercise within the patient's allowed activities is essential. Encourage active range-of-motion exercises and assist with passive range-of-motion exercises as indicated by the patient's condition and allowed by his or her physician.

TRACTION-INDUCED CRANIAL NERVE LESIONS

Stretching or kinking of cranial nerves can result from the traction force applied by the skull tongs to immobilize the head and the neck and reduce the cervical fracture. Those lesions are most likely to occur immediately after the skull tongs are inserted and traction is applied. A stretching lesion, referred to as a neurapraxia, is a temporary injury that causes palsy or paralysis of the innervated area with anatomical degeneration. Damage may be caused by overextension, nerve fiber compression, or disruption of the nerve's blood supply. Similarly, cranial nerve deficits may be caused by a kinking of the cranial nerve root at the base of the brain. The most important principle is prevention or, should dysfunction occur, immediate detection. The prognosis for complete recovery is good, but the time it takes to recover is directly related to the amount of time the nerve was kinked or overextended. When the skeletal traction is initially applied, do cranial nerve checks every 15 minutes for the first hour. If the patient has any subjective complaints that may indicate cranial nerve deficit, do an assessment immediately and notify the physician. The only effective treatment for traction-induced cranial neurapraxia or kinking is a prompt and substantial decrease in the force of distraction.

PARALYTIC ILEUS

The patient immobilized by a cervical fracture is prone to develop a paralytic ileus. Paralytic ileus involves an absent or diminished peristalsis of the bowel due to the traumatic disturbance of the autonomic nervous system. However, there is no physical obstruction or interruption of blood supply to the intestines. Prophylactically, intravenous fluids and minimal oral fluids are utilized until peristalsis is established after the trauma from the accident. Bed exercises and turning the patient increase circulation and muscle tone. If allowed, the patient can do mild abdominal exercises that involve tightening their abdominal muscles for a count of 3 and then relaxing for a count of 3.

If a paralytic ileus should occur, the gastrointestinal tract is rested by allowing nothing by mouth and using intravenous fluids to prevent dehydration. A heating pad on the abdomen may be used to increase circulation in the area. A rectal tube may be used to help reduce distention, and a nasogastric tube may be necessary. The complication usually is resolved within 72 hours.

FRACTURE INSTABILITY

Fracture instability may occur when (1) the traction is not being maintained as continuous traction, (2) the traction is frequently being jarred and manipulating the fracture site, (3) the amount of poundage is incorrect, or (4) the patient's body is not in correct alignment for the traction.

EVALUATION/OUTCOMES

Ensure that the patient is always in correct alignment and free of pain. During turns, verify that the patient's body is held firmly between the frames and that traction is maintained. If the patient experiences an increase in pain during the turn, have the patient describe the pain in detail, assess the patient's neurologic status and compare it to the preturn status, and consider the possibility of a psychological component to the pain. Notify the patient's physician if the pain persists or if there is a change in neurologic status. Evaluate the condition of the patient's skin. Verify that there are no wrinkles in the pads, canvas, or linen. Verify that the turning schedule is appropriate and that the patient does not remain in one position too long.

Evaluate the patient's understanding of the turning frame and the procedures performed. Observe for possible anxiety during interactions between the patient and the family or significant others.

HALO SKELETAL TRACTION

Skeletal fixation by halo skeletal traction (Fig. 6–30) is achieved with a stainless steel "halo ring" that fits around the patient's head and is attached to the skull by four pins. The sharp-pointed pins are placed approximately 0.5 mm deep into the outer portion of the skull. To prevent pin migration, bone erosion, and penetration of the dura, the pins are inserted in the frontal bones one cm above each eyebrow and in the

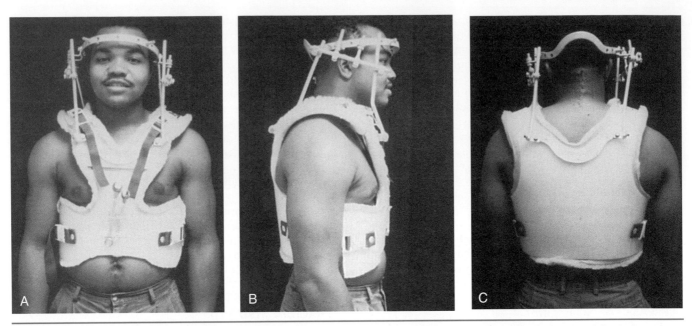

Figure 6–30   (A) Patient in a halo vest, anterior view. (B) Lateral view. (C) Posterior view. The posterior aspect of the halo ring allows access to the upper cervical spine.   *(Bridwell & DeWald (1997). The Textbook of Spinal Surgery. Philadelphia: Lippincott-Raven.)*

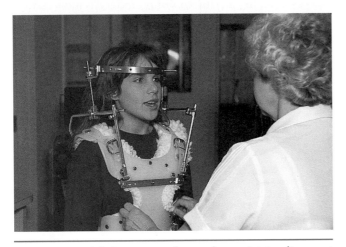

Figure 6–31   A halo vest may be used to maintain alignment in cervical injuries.   *(Bridwell & DeWald (1997). The Textbook of Spinal Surgery. Philadelphia: Lippincott-Raven.)*

temporal bones one cm above and behind the top of the ears. The insertion of the pins may be done under general anesthesia but is usually done with local anesthesia at the pin sites. Traction on the skeletal system is maintained by threaded steel uprights that are attached to the halo ring and to the body jacket (or brace). Although halo traction vests may look a little different (Fig. 6–31), they serve the same purpose.

A halo device may be used initially with traction, or it may be utilized as an immobilization device after the tongs are removed. The halo apparatus, first used for the traction and immobilization of a cervical fracture in 1959, is now used for a number of severe cervical and upper-thoracic spinal instabilities, including fractures that could cause spinal cord or nerve root damage, cervical fusions, tumors of the head or neck, and rheumatoid arthritis.

NURSING PROCESS (Patient with Halo Skeletal Traction)

The following nursing process presents the care of a patient in halo skeletal traction for a cervical fracture. The nursing process begins after the halo apparatus is applied.

ASSESSMENT

The initial nursing assessment of a typical patient following a fracture of a cervical vertebra and the application of a halo apparatus should focus on the patient's neurologic well-being. The patient's neurologic status is usually assessed every 15 minutes for the first hour after application, then every hour for the next 8 hours, and then every 4 hours for the next 2 days. (See Chapter 2 for neurovascular assessment of upper and lower extremities.) If there are no complications, the neurologic checks can then be done every shift. That assessment should include monitoring for signs of increasing intracranial pressure, any indication of cervical nerve impingement, and for vascular changes in the extremities.

The neurologic assessment for increased intracranial pressure should include (1) vital signs (temperature, pulse, respiration, and blood pressure); (2) the patient's level of consciousness; (3) orientation; (4) speech quality; (5) strength of the grip in both hands; (6) the patient's ability to raise their arms above their head; (7) the presence of any numbness or tingling in the upper extremities or difficulties with jaw movements, such as an inability to bite down, open their mouth wide, or stick out their tongue; (8) extraocular movement and pupil reaction; (9) peripheral vision checks; and (10) checks for any visual difficulties, such as blurred vision, double vision, or nystagmus. Minor nystagmus is normal in the extreme lateral gaze, but all other nystagmus findings should be considered abnormal. If one of the patient's eyes deviates nasally, record the movement as esotropic (ET); if there is a deviation toward the temple, record it as extropic (XT); and record any upward deviation as hypertropic (HT). Readers are referred to the neurologic nursing references in the bibliography at the end of this chapter for further details on neurologic checks for increased intracranial pressure.

Observe the patient's body alignment, and correct the positioning of the halo apparatus. Check for any loosening of pins or screws, and note if the patient has any complaints of an unusual pulling sensation on the head or scalp. Check for any friction or wearing where the halo is attached to the rest of the apparatus. Determine the level of discomfort and the effectiveness of nursing measures and medications to relieve discomfort. Determine the level of anxiety as evidenced by the patient's verbalization and cooperation with the plan of care. Assess the effectiveness of interactions between the patient and the family or significant others. Assess pin sites for signs and symptoms of infection such as redness, edema, drainage, increased temperature, or pain. Assess the function of the respiratory and gastrointestinal systems by auscultating the chest and the abdomen.

NURSING DIAGNOSIS

Based on all of the assessment data, the major nursing diagnoses for a typical patient in a halo apparatus with a fractured cervical vertebra are:

- Pain and discomfort related to cervical trauma
- Impaired physical mobility related to instability in the cervical spine
- Ineffective individual coping related to the trauma and immobilization device
- Ineffective breathing pattern related to the immobilization device
- Altered nutrition: less than daily body requirements related to the immobilization device
- Self-care deficit: bathing/hygiene related to the immobilization device
- Anxiety related to knowledge deficit about the injury, treatment method(s), and rehabilitation process

COLLABORATIVE PROBLEMS

- Pin site infections
- Loosening of screws
- Decreased muscle tone

- Cranial nerve lesions
- Paralytic ileus

GOAL FORMULATION AND PLANNING

The goals are to have the patient experience (1) a decrease in the amount of pain through nursing measures and prescribed medications; (2) an increase in mobility through the use of the halo apparatus, exercises, and ambulation; (3) effective coping with one-to-one interactions about the trauma and prognosis; (4) effective breathing pattern maintained with correct positioning; (5) an adequate intake of food and fluids; (6) an ability to maintain adequate hygiene with the assistance of others; (7) a decrease in anxiety through increased knowledge; and (8) an absence of complications from the fracture and the halo apparatus.

INTERVENTIONS

ALLEVIATE PAIN

If a patient in a halo apparatus has proper pin placement with a correct amount of force applied, there should be minimal to no cutaneous discomfort. For patients complaining of pain, first assess for the severity, duration, and location of the pain. Verify that the patient is in correct alignment and that there is no pull or stress on the halo apparatus. For complaints of minor discomfort, analgesics are administered.

Careful placement of the pins is important to avoid the risk of cranial nerve damage. If the anterior pins are placed too far medially on the frontal bone, severe pain can result from supraorbital nerve irritation. Similarly, if the posterior pins are placed too far forward on the temporal bone, the patient will have pain when chewing or speaking as a result of impingement on a branch of the trigeminal nerve, which controls jaw muscle motion and sensation. If the patient complains of undue discomfort related to the sensory motor pathways of the face or scalp, the physician must be notified. Depending on the severity of the symptoms, pin removal and replacement may be necessary.

INCREASE MOBILITY

Interventions to increase mobility include correct positioning, exercises, and ambulation.

Position. The patient in a halo apparatus following a cervical fracture will find that the only comfortable position in bed is lying supine. To help reduce the stress on the back, some patients use a pillow under the knees.

Exercises. The patient in a halo apparatus has no movement of the cervical spine and the head and will feel that the apparatus inhibits movement in the rest of the body. A program of active range-of-motion exercises is encouraged. If necessary, a program of passive range-of-motion exercises of the upper extremities should be done twice a day. For the lower extremities, the patient may be started on an exercise program utilizing a stationary bicycle twice a day for 15 to 20 minutes each time. The goal of the exercise program is to retain range of motion in the joints and to prevent decrease in muscle tone and strength.

Ambulation. It is important for the patient in a halo apparatus to understand the need for safety. The patient should become as independent as possible but realize that the field of vision is restricted, which could result in a fall or jars to the halo. The patient needs to learn to turn the body instead of the head to look to the side and realize that it will become easier as peripheral vision improves. The patient will need assistance in learning how to get out of bed with the added weight of an approximately 7-pound apparatus. If the patient holds onto the steel uprights when getting up or lying down, he or she is usually able to move better with the apparatus. Once out of bed, the patient may have trouble with balance and stability and initially will need to walk with someone. The patient must then learn how to get in and out of a chair and go up and down stairs. Going upstairs usually poses minimal difficulties, but going downstairs is more difficult because of the inability to look down to see the next step.

COPING MECHANISMS
Patients in a halo apparatus commonly have periods of anxiety and depression. Look for decreased concentration, fatigue, increased restlessness, increased complaints, or withdrawal from staff and others. Measures that help to reduce anxiety and depression are to listen to the patient express feelings and to educate the patient about the apparatus and how to live with it. Encourage the patient and family to verbalize questions, and introduce the patient to others who are wearing or have worn a halo. Allow the patient to participate in planning daily activities.

EFFECTIVE BREATHING
The combination of recumbency, the drugs used for pain relief that depress respirations, a decrease in the body's need for oxygen due to inactivity, and the resistance of the bed and halo apparatus against the patient's chest wall can lead to respiratory complications. Nursing measures are needed to prevent respiratory complications (see Chapter 4), but having the patient cough or causing the patient to sneeze tends to jar the apparatus, which causes the patient discomfort and leads to a loosening of the screws.

In the event of the need for cardiopulmonary resuscitation, the anterior chest plate is fabricated to allow easy access to the chest. The necessary wrenches to remove the halo vest should be taped to the vest, and the patient should be instructed that these must be available at all times.

ADEQUATE NUTRITION
Because of the position and immobilization of the head and the neck, the patient may find that just getting a glass of water takes some effort. Once the glass is filled, the patient must learn to get the water to the lips and drink without tilting the head. Using a straw helps. With eating, there are problems getting the food from the plate to the mouth. A mirror attached to the overhead bed frame can improve the patient's visual field and help self-feeding. The patient needs a well-balanced diet. Emphasis must be placed on preventing the patient from gaining weight as the halo apparatus does not allow for an increase in trunk size. Special care should be taken to prevent gastrointestinal problems that occur with decreased mobility.

HYGIENE
The skin under the vest needs at least daily cleansing. To accomplish this task, use a thin, soft cloth that has been saturated in rubbing alcohol, and then wring out any excess. Place the cloth under the halo brace and gently rub the skin. Alcohol is used instead of soap and water because alcohol does not leave a film, unlike soap and water, and the alcohol leaves a clean, cool feel to the skin and also helps to toughen the skin.

There may come a time when changing the lining of the vest may become necessary because of excessive perspiration, extended use of the halo apparatus, or the presence of wounds that drain and soil the liner. Changing the lining of the vest is done following the patient's physician's order. *(Under no circumstances should the patient remove any portion of the vest.)* The posterior liner can be changed safely by the following steps:

1. Have the patient lie prone on a firm bed with a pillow under the chest and a pillow under the head to support and maintain alignment.
2. Remove the lower two bolts on the vest. If the crossbar snaps out of alignment, the patient is not balanced on the pillows evenly; resecure the bolts, readjust the pillows, and then proceed.
3. Release the side straps and the shoulder straps. Check that the neck is maintained in correct alignment.
4. Remove the posterior section of the vest and liner.
5. Cleanse the patient's back, and dry well.
6. Replace the liner, which is held in place with Velcro.
7. Replace the posterior section and resecure.

To change the anterior liner safely, the following steps are required:

1. Have the patient lie supine with a small pillow behind the head.
2. Release the two bolts and four straps.
3. Remove the anterior section of the vest and liner.
4. Cleanse the patient's chest area, and dry well.
5. Attach a new liner, and replace the anterior section.
6. Refasten the straps, and then replace the two bolts.

The total time for changing the liners and cleansing the patient's chest and back is usually about 15 minutes (Ace Orthopedics).

PATIENT TEACHING AND HOME CARE CONSIDERATIONS
In most instances, there is very little time for the patient to learn about the halo apparatus before it is applied. Thus, the patient must learn how to live with the apparatus and how to perform self-care while wearing it. Help the patient adjust by always explaining what you are going to do, how you are going to do it, and why it is necessary. Learning to eat and to ambulate are some of the first activities a patient must learn. Others are how to bathe the body, shampoo the hair, sleep, dress, and ride in a car.

In bathing, sponge baths are easiest, but occasionally a tub bath is desired. Even though approximately 4 inches of water is allowed in the tub, a nonskid mat is recommended to prevent slipping. Someone may be able to assist the patient in cleansing under the brace with a damp (not wet) cloth and no soap. If permitted by the patient's physician, a family member or significant other can be taught to change the liner as discussed under hygiene.

Shampooing the patient's hair may not be done every day, but can be accomplished with little effort. One way is to have the patient kneel over the edge of a bathtub (or sink if the patient is tall enough) with a towel for padding at the tub edge. The patient will need to hold the side bars of the apparatus and brace his or her elbows on the tub. The helper is then able to gently wash and rinse the patient's hair. A hose spray attached to the shower is a great help in moistening and rinsing. If this is not available, water can be poured from a plastic container. Three things to remember in washing a patient's hair are: (1) place a towel around the patient's neck to prevent water getting under the vest; (2) be very gentle in cleansing and rinsing; and (3) make sure all of the soap is rinsed out. Short hair is easier to care for than long hair, so the patient may choose to have the hair cut. Changes in hair color are not recommended, as the patient has skin openings at the pin sites.

Getting into a comfortable position to sleep is a problem for most patients, because they must sleep on their back. Some ways to help the patient are to put a pillow under their knees (if allowed by the patient's physician) to reduce the stress on the back and to use a triangular pillow for a headrest. Most patients require more sleep than normal while they are wearing the halo apparatus, so plan for rest periods and naps during the day.

Learning what to wear and how to dress does not need to present a big problem. The patient will need clothing several sizes larger in the chest with a large neck opening to allow for the bars of the halo apparatus. The clothing could be a loose-fitting shirt or blouse or, for women, a large dress with a front zipper or buttons, or even a muumuu. The only real requirement is the large neck opening. Slacks or skirts can be worn as the apparatus does not extend below the waist. How-

ever, the patient needs to bend to put on shoes, socks, and stockings. Shoes should give support to the feet and help stabilize the patient during walking.

Traveling can be a problem, and getting into a car requires some thought. The easiest way is probably to have the patient ride in the front passenger seat. The patient can back up against the side of the seat, bend at the hips, and sit down. The patient can then bring the head inside the car, making sure that it clears the car frame, and then turn to the correct position. Reverse the procedure in getting out of the car. The patient can turn and lead out with the head. While riding, the patient should be advised to hold on to the side bars to prevent the jarring of the apparatus, especially when riding over railroad tracks or on bumpy roads. The use of seat belts is strongly recommended.

Patients must realize that other people will stare at them because of the apparatus. They should also recognize that the apparatus is only temporary and allows them to function while their fracture is healing.

MONITORING AND MANAGING POTENTIAL PROBLEMS
Complications that can occur with a halo apparatus include (1) infection of pin sites, (2) loosening of pins or screws, (3) decreased muscle tone, (4) traction-induced cranial nerve lesions, and (5) paralytic ileus.

PIN SITE INFECTIONS
With four pins inserted into the patient's skull, there is a chance of infection at the pin sites. Take the patient's temperature and assess for pain, headaches, dizziness, tenderness, heat, swelling, redness, and drainage at least once every shift. If there is drainage, send a culture to the laboratory and notify the patient's physician. Measures that help to prevent or reduce pin site infections are washing the patient's hair on a regular basis and doing pin site care every shift. Instruct the patient on the signs and symptoms of infection so that they will know to notify their physician should signs occur after the patient goes home.

Most agree that daily cleansing of the pin sites is necessary; however, controversy remains as to the best procedure. Daily cleansing to remove any encrusted drainage or ointments is needed in order to properly view the pin site. Cleansing is also needed before any new ointment is applied. Some prefer cleansing the sites every 8 hours with hydrogen peroxide followed by sterile saline and then reapplying an antibiotic ointment. Others prefer applying a Betadine wrap to the pin site, letting it dry, and then removing the wrap as a way of debriding around the pin site. Whatever the patient's physician prefers, always check the site for signs of infection and the loosening of screws.

LOOSENING OF SCREWS
The screws can be loosened by jars to the apparatus, getting the apparatus caught on clothing while dressing, roughness in washing the patient's hair, and by the

patient's coughing and sneezing. Loose screws need to be tightened or, in some instances, replaced. During pin care, check the pins and the screws for loosening. Listen for any complaints of an unusual pulling sensation on the head or scalp. Check the apparatus for any friction or wearing at the sites of contact. Notify the patient's physician if there is any loosening of pins, and keep a wrench at the bedside. For outpatients, make sure the patient understands the importance of notifying their physician immediately if they feel any motion of the apparatus or have headaches.

DECREASED MUSCLE TONE
Because of decreased mobility, patients with a halo apparatus may develop decreased muscle tone. A program of exercise is essential (see Exercise under Increase Mobility). Encourage active range-of-motion exercises and assist with passive range-of-motion exercises as indicated by the patient's condition.

CRANIAL NERVE LESIONS
Stretching or kinking of cranial nerves can result from the traction force applied by the halo to immobilize the head and the neck and reduce the cervical fracture. Those lesions are most likely to occur immediately after the halo is applied and attached to the extension bars. A stretching lesion, referred to as a neurapraxia, is a temporary injury that causes palsy or paralysis of the innervated area accompanied by anatomical degeneration. Damage may be caused by overextension, nerve fiber compression, or disruption of the nerve's blood supply. Similarly, cranial nerve deficits may be caused by a kinking of the cranial nerve root at the base of the brain. The most important principle is prevention or, should dysfunction occur, immediate detection. The prognosis for complete recovery is good, but the time it takes to recover is directly related to the amount of time the nerve was kinked or overextended. When the halo is initially applied, do cranial nerve checks every 15 minutes for the first hour. If the patient has any subjective complaints that may indicate cranial nerve deficit, do an assessment immediately and notify the physician. The only effective treatment for traction-induced cranial neurapraxia or kinking is a prompt and substantial decrease in the force of distraction.

PARALYTIC ILEUS
The patient immobilized by a cervical fracture is prone to develop a paralytic ileus. (For further discussion, see Patient with Cervical Skeletal Traction and Chapter 4.)

EVALUATION/OUTCOMES
Determine that the patient is free of pain and has only occasional headaches that are relieved by analgesics. Make sure the patient knows whom to contact if additional pain should occur after the patient is at home. Discuss with the patient the signs and symptoms of potential complications and what should be done if any

occur. Observe the patient closely to make sure that he or she knows how to get in and out of bed and is able to move about safely. Have the patient demonstrate going up and down stairs.

Go over the procedure for pin care with the patient and the person who will be helping the patient at home. Ask the person who will be helping the patient to demonstrate pin site care in the hospital before the patient is discharged. Allow the family or significant other to help with washing the patient's hair. Discuss with the patient the type of clothing to wear, and, if possible, have some clothing brought to the hospital so he or she can learn to dress.

PELVIC TRACTION
Most patients requiring pelvic traction are not hospitalized or, if they are, remain inpatients for a very short period of time. The patient may be placed in traction at home. In that case it would be better to utilize the Buck's extension apparatus to apply the traction device because it does not require an overhead frame. (See discussion under Cervical Skin Traction.)

TRACTION SETUP
For the standard hospital traction, preparing the patient's hospital bed and setting up pelvic traction (Fig. 6–32) involve the following steps (as adapted from Zimmer, 1996):

1. Attach a basic frame (overhead traction bar designed for retractable beds) onto the bed.
2. Attach a 9-inch single clamp bar to the upright bar at the foot of the bed.
3. Attach a pulley to the 9-inch single clamp bar.
4. Apply the pelvic traction belt to the patient.
5. Place a 22-inch spreader bar through the rings on the pelvic belt.
6. Tie the traction cord (Fig. 6–2) to the center of the spreader bar, thread through the pulley, and tie to the weight carrier.
7. Gently apply the weights.

Pelvic traction can also be accomplished in two other ways. One is to utilize the Zimcode Buck's extension apparatus as already discussed for home use. The other is to not use the spreader bar and to attach each pelvic strap to a separate set of weights. This can be accomplished by using numbers 1 and 2 of the preceding procedure and then adding the following:

3. Attach a 36-inch center clamp bar to the 9-inch single clamp bar.
4. Attach two pulleys to the 36-inch center clamp bar.
5. Apply the pelvic traction belt to the patient.
6. Attach a traction cord to the rings at the end of each strap of the pelvic belt, thread through the pulleys, and then tie to the weight carriers.
7. Gently apply the weights.

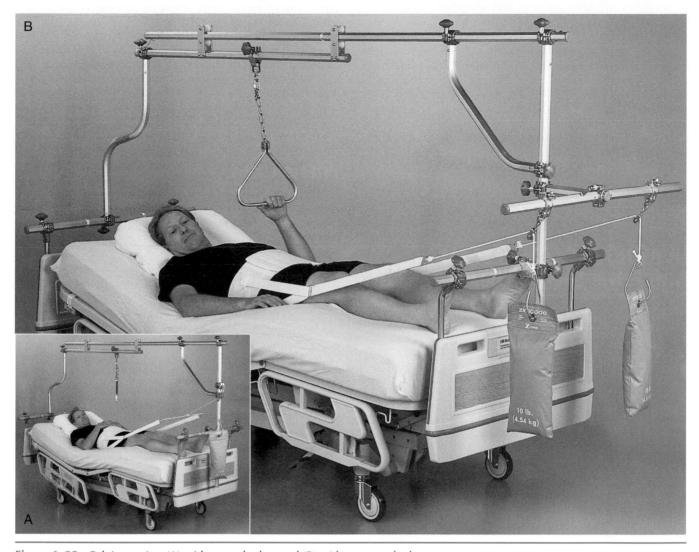

Figure 6–32   Pelvic traction (A) with spreader bar and (B) without spreader bar.   *(Smelter & Bare (1996). Brunner and Suddath's Textbook of Medical-Surgical Nursing. 8th ed. Philadelphia: Lippincott-Raven.)*

TRACTION APPLICATION

Pelvic traction is a form of running skin traction accomplished by a belt around the pelvis. Traction can be continuous or intermittent. Pelvic traction is used primarily in conservative management of low back pain. The purposes of the traction are (1) to relieve muscle spasms of the lower back, (2) to reduce pressure on spinal nerve roots, (3) to treat minor fractures of the lower spine, and (4) to immobilize the patient.

Pelvic traction is applied to the lower back by using a wide lumbar belt or a lumbar band that resembles an oversized garter belt with straps on each side (or at the center back). Those straps extend toward the foot of the bed and are attached to a spreader bar and weights (or just to weights). Pelvic belts are adjustable and come in several sizes or one universal size, depending on the manufacturer. Before applying traction, explain to the patient the purpose of the traction, what you are going to do, and the patient's role in maintaining the effectiveness of the treatment. If the pelvic belt comes in more

than one size, measure the patient's hips at the pelvis to obtain the correct size. It is necessary to measure because most patients do not know the size of their pelvis.

To apply the traction, have the patient lie flat in bed in correct alignment. Help the patient log-roll or turn the patient like you would roll a log by keeping their trunk and legs straight to one side (see Chapter 8 for specific steps on log-roll turning a patient). With the patient facing away, fold the pelvic belt in half and place the division line of the belt along the patient's spinal column. Holding the belt in place, fan fold the lower portion of the belt and tuck it under the patient's lower hip, as is done when changing the bottom sheet of an occupied bed. This method helps ensure that when the patient log-rolls back, the traction will be symmetrical about the spinal column.

Secure the pelvic belt across the patient's lower abdomen, making sure it is on the pelvis and that it does not go above the iliac crest or umbilicus. Do not pull the pelvic belt so tight that it interferes with comfort. With the patient supine, put the bed in contour or

Williams' position (i.e., 15 to 20 degrees of elevation of the knees or foot of the bed, and 30 to 45 degrees of elevation at the head of the bed). This position tilts the patient's pelvis, reduces the lordotic curve, and allows the pull to be applied to a straight lumbar spinal column. The straps from the belt should be attached to the spreader bar, and a rope from the center of the spreader bar should be threaded through the pulley and tied to the weight carrier. Apply manual traction to the spreader bar to check the pull before applying the weights. Connect the traction equipment to the spreader bar, apply the correct amount of weight to the carrier (probably 15 to 40 pounds), and release the traction smoothly.

NURSING PROCESS (Patient with Pelvic Skin Traction)

To demonstrate the nursing care for a patient with pelvic skin traction, the following nursing process presents the care of a patient in traction for low back pain. The nursing process begins after the traction is applied.

ASSESSMENT

The initial assessment of the typical patient with low back pain being treated by pelvic traction emphasizes the correct positioning and pull of the traction. Determine that the pull is correct, that is, equal on both sides if the belt has two straps or in the center of the back if there is one strap. Check that the weights are of the correct poundage and that they hang free. Observe the patient's body for correct alignment, and verify that the patient is in Williams or contour position. Note any increased pain or discomfort, any tightness of the pelvic belt over the pelvis or bladder area, and any pain or discomfort over any bony prominences.

NURSING DIAGNOSIS

Based on all assessment data, the major nursing diagnoses for a typical patient in pelvic traction with low back pain are

- Pain and discomfort related to soft-tissue trauma in the low back
- Impaired physical mobility related to muscle spasms in the low back
- Impaired skin integrity related to immobility and traction
- Anxiety related to knowledge deficit about the injury and prognosis

COLLABORATIVE PROBLEMS

- Orthostatic hypotension
- Venous stasis
- Muscle weakness

GOAL FORMULATION AND PLANNING

The goals are to have the patient experience (1) a decrease in the amount of pain through nursing measures, traction, and prescribed medications; (2) an increase in mobility through the use of traction and controlled exercises; (3) no break in skin integrity through nursing measures; (4) a decrease in anxiety through increased knowledge; and (5) an absence of complications from bed rest and traction.

INTERVENTIONS

ALLEVIATE PAIN

The patient with low back pain should gain relief from muscle spasms with correct positioning and the application of traction. The correct position in bed helps relax the sciatic nerve and relieve sciatic nerve pain. Analgesics and muscle relaxants are also administered to relieve discomfort.

Tightness of the traction over the pelvis and the bladder may make the patient feel the need to void when he or she only has a small amount of urine in the bladder. This can be corrected by adjusting the tightness of the pelvic belt. The belt need only be tight enough to keep it from moving or slipping, which can cause skin irritation and reduce the traction pull.

INCREASE MOBILITY

The major nursing interventions to increase mobility are correct positioning, exercises, and maintaining the traction.

Position. The correct position for a patient in pelvic skin traction is supine with the bed in contour or Williams' position. The patient needs to stay in that position at all times, including while asleep.

Turning. The patient in pelvic traction is not allowed to turn or to lie on their side or abdomen. However, if the patient needs to use the fracture bedpan, the bed may be flattened and the patient log-rolled to the side.

Exercises. The patient is encouraged to do back exercises (Box 6–4) while in traction. Exercises should be tailored to the patient's condition and should minimize painful exertion. Initially, supervision is needed to ensure that the exercises are performed properly, but patients must be encouraged to continue the activity program on their own. Low back exercises are designed to increase abdominal strength and endurance, stretch the low back, and develop and maintain the correct pelvic tilt. Back exercises should be done twice a day for the first 3 months and once a day thereafter. Each exercise should be done every day, as it builds on the day before to increase strength and endurance. The number of repetitions of each exercise depends on the patient's condition.

Ambulation. If the patient is allowed bathroom privileges, remove the weights and then the pelvic belt. Stay with the patient while he or she walks to the bathroom,

---

Box 6–4
Low Back Exercises

1. *Pelvic tilt.* Lying supine, the patient tightens the stomach muscles and then rocks the pelvis, flattening the low back. The position is held for the count of 5.
2. *Sit-up.* Lying supine with the abdominal muscles tightened, the patient raises their head and shoulders and reaches toward the knees, holding the position for a count of 5. As the patient's muscles become stronger, the patient may fold their arms across their chest and even advance to putting their hands behind the head.
3. *Knee-Chest.* Lying supine with the abdominal muscles tightened, the patient raises their head and shoulders and brings one knee up toward the nose, holding the position for a count of 5.
4. *Double Knee.* The same as (3), except that the patient brings both knees up at the same time.
5. *Straight Leg Raise.* The patient lies supine with one knee bent and held to their chest with their hands. The patient then lifts the other leg, keeping the knee straight and the ankle flexed.

---

as some patients may become dizzy, especially if they are receiving pain medications or muscle relaxants. The pelvic belt should be removed so that the patient does not trip or fall, and the patient should not reapply their own traction, as that will apply stress to the injured back.

SKIN INTEGRITY

The pelvic skin traction should be applied directly to the skin to be most effective. Some patients object because they feel exposed, because the top linen cannot come over the traction apparatus. However, the linen can be brought up between the two traction straps and then carefully spread over the patient. If the patient still insists on clothing, women may be allowed to wear cotton panties, and men may wear cotton shorts. Gowns and pajamas of silk, rayon, or blended fabrics should not be worn as they allow the traction to slide and thus reduce the amount of pull.

Sometimes a patient will develop pressure areas over the iliac crests or coccyx. Special padding helps relieve the pressure. To prevent skin breakdown, alcohol rubs can be used to toughen the skin.

PATIENT TEACHING AND HOME CARE CONSIDERATIONS

Patient teaching is an important, sometimes the most important, part of the treatment for the patient with low back pain. Patient education needs to focus on the mechanisms of injury, methods to prevent further injury, and how those methods work. (For a discussion of the mechanism of injury and methods of treatment, see Chapter 8.)

Exercise and good body mechanics are the keys to preventing further injury. Teach the patient the goals and the purposes of the exercise program. Make sure the patient does the complete program correctly, and

help the patient work out a routine he or she can use at home. A warm or hot shower before exercising may help relax the back muscles and make exercising easier and more effective.

Instruct the patient on proper body mechanics. The patient must learn to keep their back straight and use the leg muscles, not the back muscles, when picking up something from the floor or lifting a heavy object. When standing for any period of time (e.g., at the sink doing dishes), he or she should use a small stool or other means to elevate one foot in order to take stress off the back. The best and easiest position for sleeping is to lie on one side with knees and hips slightly flexed. Persons with back pain should not sleep prone. If the patient sleeps supine, the knees need to be elevated. Some patients place a couple of pillows under their knees, while others use a box that has been padded and covered. The box should be of sufficient size so the patient can flex their hips and knees and have the lower portion of the leg horizontal on top of the padded box.

While sitting, the patient must keep their knees higher than their hips, even when driving a car. If necessary the patient should pull the car seat forward to raise and flex the knees.

For some patients, sexual intercourse increases back discomfort. In particular, the standard "missionary" position with its basic to-and-fro pelvic thrusts may aggravate a compromised spine. Coitus is generally not advisable for persons requiring substantial pain medications or who cannot walk without considerable pain. For others, a change of position may be enough to reduce or prevent pain and enable the patient to obtain sexual satisfaction. Patients should avoid lying prone, lying supine with hips extended, or bending forward with their knees straight.

For the man or woman in more acute stages of low back pain, the "side-lie position" is likely to minimize discomfort. In the side-lie position, the sexual partners lie on their sides with their hips and knees flexed, and with the man facing the woman's back. In that position each person only supports their own body weight, not that of their partner, and the psoas muscle is not stressed. If the woman has chronic back pain, two possible positions are (1) the woman supine with hips flexed, upper torso supported by pillows, and thighs supported by the man's thighs and arms, as he is on his knees facing her; and (2) the man supine and the woman astride. The latter position is also appropriate when the man has low back pain, though in that case the man's upper torso should be slightly raised on pillows. A number of other coital positions, as well as noncoital activities, can be explored if care is taken to avoid stressful positions. As many patients are reluctant to ask questions about sexual matters, nurses should not hesitate to volunteer information on the subject.

MONITORING AND MANAGING POTENTIAL PROBLEMS

The most frequent complications are related to bed rest, e.g., orthostatic hypotension, venous stasis, and muscle weakness. For nursing interventions, see Chapter 4 for a discussion of the effects of immobility.

MUSCLE WEAKNESS

Muscle weakness and even atrophy can develop if the patient does not follow the prescribed exercise program. The importance of the exercises should be emphasized, and they should be continued after the traction is no longer needed.

EVALUATION/OUTCOMES

Evaluate the effectiveness of medications, positioning, and traction in relieving pain. Evaluate how well the patient tolerates the traction and cooperates in maintaining it. Observe the patient exercising, evaluate the patient's compliance with the exercise program, and note whether the patient utilizes proper body mechanics. Ask the patient how they will incorporate the exercise program into their daily activities.

PELVIC SLING

The pelvic sling (Fig. 6–33), a form of continuous skin traction, is a large canvas sling that fits under the patient's buttocks to support the entire pelvis. Crossbars are inserted into the sling on each side and attached to weights that provide an upward pull. The purpose of the pelvic sling is to stabilize and immobilize fractures of the pelvis, to suspend patients with pelvic fractures, to suspend and compress the pelvic girdle, and to treat separations of the anterior pelvic ring.

Potential complications of the pelvic sling are (1) lack of immobilization of the fracture site from too much lifting and turning, causing trauma and pain; (2) skin breakdown (back, sacral, and buttocks); (3) difficulty in voiding (especially for women); (4) perineal irritation because of difficulty in cleansing (especially in women);

(5) foot drop; and (6) physical and psychological complications of enforced recumbency.

References

Carpenito, L. J. (1993). *Nursing diagnosis: Application to clinical practice* (5th ed.). Philadelphia: J. B. Lippincott.

Cornell, C. N., & Schneider, K. (1998). Proximal humerus. In K. J. Koval & J. D. Zuckerman (Eds.), *Fractures in the Elderly.* (pp. 85–92). Philadelphia: Lippincott-Raven.

Folcik, M. A. (1998). Traction for lower-extremity fractures. In V. C. Williams (Ed.), *Management of lower-extremity fractures.* Pitman, NJ: National Association of Orthopaedic Nurses.

Folcik, M. A., Carini-Garcia, G. K., & Birmingham, J. J. (1994). *Traction: Assessment and management.* St. Louis: Mosby Year Book.

Georgiadis, G. M. & Behrens, F. F. (1998). Humeral shaft. In K. J. Koval & J. D. Zuckerman (Eds.), *Fractures in the Elderly* (pp. 93–106). Philadelphia: Lippincott-Raven.

Houston, M. S. (1996). Care of the school-aged child in 90-90 traction. *Orthopaedic Nursing, 15*(2), 57–62.

Jagmin, M. J. (1998). Assessment and management of immobility. In A. B. Maher, S. W. Salmond, & T. A. Pellino (Eds.), *Orthopaedic nursing* (2nd ed., pp. 92–114) Philadelphia: W. B. Saunders.

Johnson, J., Anderson, C., Barrett, A., Duke, K., & Sharp, D. (1995). Roller traction: Mobilizing patients with acetabular fractures. *Orthopaedic Nursing, 14*(1), 21–24.

Jones-Walton, P. (1991). Clinical standards in skeletal traction pin site care. *Orthopaedic Nursing, 10*(2), 12–16.

Koval, K. J. & Zuckerman, J. D. (Eds.) (1998). Fractures in the elderly. Philadelphia: Lippincott-Raven

Naylor, A. (1948). Fractures and orthopaedic surgery for nurses and masseuses. Baltimore. MD: The Williams and Wilkins Company

Rodts, M. F. (1997). Perioperative and postoperative nursing care for the spinal surgery patient. In K. H. Bridwell & R. L. DeWald (Eds.), *The textbook of spinal surgery* (2nd ed., pp. 11–30). Philadelphia: Lippincott-Raven.

Rodts, M. F. (1998). Disorders of the spine. In A. B. Maher, S. W. Salmond, & T. A. Pellino (Eds.), *Orthopaedic nursing* (2nd ed., pp. 545–585). Philadelphia: W. B. Saunders.

Smeltzer, S. C., & Bare, B. G. (Eds.). (1996). *Brunner and Suddarth's textbook of medical-surgical nursing* (8th. ed.). Philadelphia: Lippincott.

Styrcula, L. (1994a). Traction basics: Part I. *Orthopaedic Nursing, 13*(2), 71–74.

Styrcula, L. (1994b). Traction basics: Part II: Traction equiipment. *Orthopaedic Nursing, 13*(3), 55–59.

Styrcula, L. (1994c). Traction basics: Part III: Types of traction. *Orthopaedic Nursing, 13*(4), 34–44.

Styrcula, L. (1994d). Traction basics: Part IV: Traction for lower extremities. *Orthopaedic Nursing, 13*(5), 59–68.

Walsh, C. R., & McBryde, A. M., Jr. (1997). Cost-effectiveness of the orthopaedic advanced practice nurse: A joint protocol for home skeletal traction. *Orthopaedic Nursing, 16*(3), 28–33.

Zimmer, Inc. (1996). *Zimmer traction handbook* (6th ed.). Warsaw, IN Zimmer Inc.

Zuckerman, J. D., & Koval, K. J. (1996). Fractures of the shaft of the humerus. In C. A. Rockwood, D. P. Green, R. W. Buckholz, & J. D. Heckman (Eds.). *Rockwood and Green's fractures in adults* (4th ed., pp. 1025–1054). Philadelphia: Lippincott-Raven.

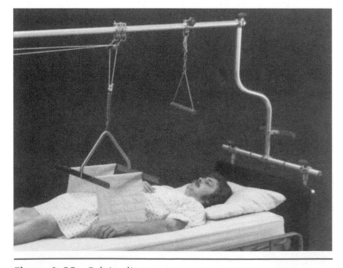

Figure 6–33 Pelvic sling. *(Zimmer, Inc. (1996). Zimmer Traction Handbook Warsaw, IN: Zimmer, Inc.)*

Chapter

7

Care of the Patient with an External Fixation Device

EXTERNAL FIXATORS

External fixators allow stabilization of a fracture at a distance from the fracture site without increasing soft-tissue damage. Utilizing a fixator to treat a fracture allows for (1) the length and alignment of a fractured extremity to be maintained without casting; (2) ease in the inspection and treatment of soft-tissue wounds incurred at the time of the fracture; and (3) early mobilization and activity based on the stability of the fracture. External fixation is particularly useful in the treatment of open fractures of the tibia, but it has also been used successfully, under certain circumstances, in fractures of the femur, the pelvis, the humerus, and other bones.

The use of external fixation devices to treat fractures is not a recent development but is new in comparison to other treatments like traction or casts. Alvin Lambotte has generally been given credit for introducing, in 1907, the use of transfixing pins attached to an external device to treat fractures, and the European use of external fixation is based on his work. In the United States, Roger Anderson is credited with devising, in 1934, a frame with transfixion pins used to line up difficult tibial fractures and then applying a cast that incorporated the pins. In cases of severe soft-tissue damage, the fixation device was used alone. In 1937, Otto Stader, a veterinarian, used the technique to treat animals. The Hoffmann apparatus, described in 1939, was modified by Vidal and Ardrey; and surgeons in France, Switzerland, and elsewhere achieved excellent results with that modified device. That revived interest worldwide, and the use of external fixation devices is now quite common.

External fixation is utilized when other means of fixation are inappropriate. In the United States, the most common reason for using external fixators is for fractures associated with extensive soft-tissue injuries. This allows free access to the wound and does not impede free tissue transfer, cancellous grafting, or hydrotherapy. External fixators may also be used to treat (1) grossly comminuted, unstable fractures; (2) fractures where there is bone deficit; (3) fractures associated with burns; (4) the preliminary fixation of pelvic fractures; and (5) patients with massive trauma (Harkess, Ramsey, & Harkess, 1996).

TYPES OF EXTERNAL FIXATORS

Today there are many different types of fixators; the major types are simple pin, clamp, and ring fixators. However, research and development in this area continue. An example of a newer and more innovative type of external fixator is the AO/ASIF external fixator (the pinless external fixator), which is attached to the tibia by clamps that are inserted through the soft tissue. Other new devices utilize a combined internal and external fixation.

SIMPLE PIN FIXATORS

Simple pin fixators provide great latitude in pin placement, both in the separation or spread of the pins and the angle of approach to the bone; and that enhances the rigidity of the frame. The major defect of simple pin fixators is that they allow very little adjustment after application without replacing the pins; thus, the fracture must be reduced before the frame is applied (Harkess, Ramsey, & Harkess, 1996). Examples of simple pin fixators are (1) the Roger-Anderson system, (2) the Wagner apparatus, (3) the Orthofix fixator (dynamic axial fixator), and (4) the AO/ASIF fixator (unilateral frame, bilateral frame, and triangulated assembly).

The Roger-Anderson System. In the Roger-Anderson system (Fig. 7–1), multiple pins can be inserted either as transfixion pins or as half pins. Each pin is connected to a clamp that also has a connection for an

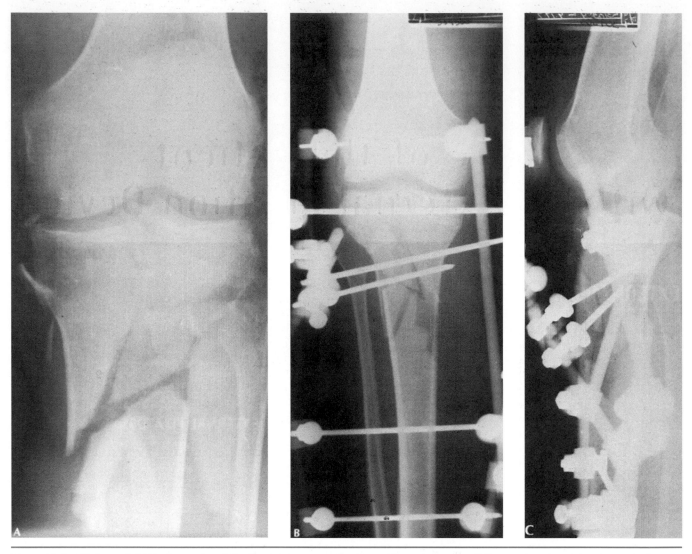

Figure 7–1   (A through E) Radiographs of the knee in a man who drove his motorcycle off the road and sustained a severely comminuted fracture of the proximal end of the tibia with disruption of the ligamentum patellae and the pes anserinus. (A) The comminuted fracture. (B and C) The tibia after application of a Roger-Anderson external fixator. Note that the patella has also been included in the assembly. This allowed immediate mobilization of the knee, even in the presence of a repaired ligamentum patellae. During movements of the knee, the patella was maintained in its proper relationship to the tibia by the external fixator. *(continued)*

aluminum rod. However, the frame also has double connectors for the aluminum rods so the physician can build a more extensive individualized system based on the patient's trauma (Harkess, Ramsey, & Harkess, 1996).

The Wagner Apparatus. Most U.S. physicians do not recommend external fixators for femoral fractures, stating that the procedure is tedious and inherently dangerous and that external fixators have received mixed results. Presently, external fixators are most often used to treat femoral fractures in high-energy

injuries in which rapid, rigid fracture stabilization is required because of the patient's associated injuries. Harkess, Ramsey, and Harkess (1996) state that such fractures need to be placed in correct alignment by traction first and then by inserting two Schanz screws proximally and distally to the fracture. The leg is then placed in the Wagner apparatus (Fig. 7–2). Alignment can be adjusted at the ends of the apparatus and the fracture distracted or compressed by turning the screws. Harkess et al. state that they have also found the Wagner apparatus useful when internal fixation is not an option.

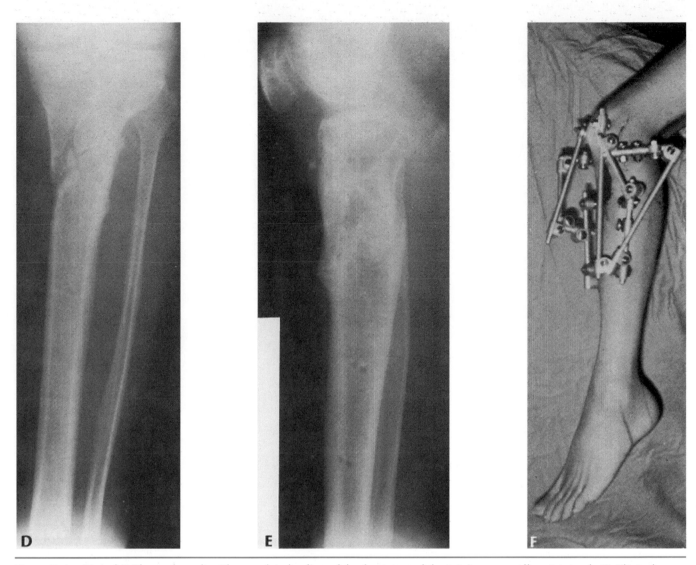

Figure 7–1 (D and E) The end result with complete healing of the fracture and the joint space well maintained. (F) Clinical photograph of a similar patient showing the external fixator with transfixion of the patella. *(Rockwood, C.A., et al. (1996). Rockwood & Green's Fractures in Adults. 4th ed. Philadelphia: Lippincott-Raven.)*

Unilateral/Bilateral Frames. The unilateral frame (Fig. 7–3) is good for the humerus and forearm where other fixators are inappropriate. They have been used for femoral fractures and for a large number of tibial fractures. A Schanz screw is placed in each fragment in the metaphysis close to the joint. Four or six clamps are then placed on a tube of appropriate length that is fixed to the Schanz screws. A closed reduction of the fracture is then accomplished, and the clamps are tightened. With the bilateral frame (Fig. 7–4), there is a tube on each side; the bilateral AO/ASIF configuration is used primarily for fractures of the tibia.

CLAMP FIXATORS

Clamp fixators allow for final reduction of the fracture after application of the device, with adjustments made by loosening the articulations of the clamps. Once the articulations are released, however, there is an inherent danger of losing the reduction. The pin spread and the direction of the pins with clamp fixators are dictated by the clamps. An example of clamp fixators is the Hoffmann frame (Fig. 7–5), which is attached with transfixing Steinmann pins by Bakelite clamps, which dictate the placement of the pins that were all inserted in the same plane.

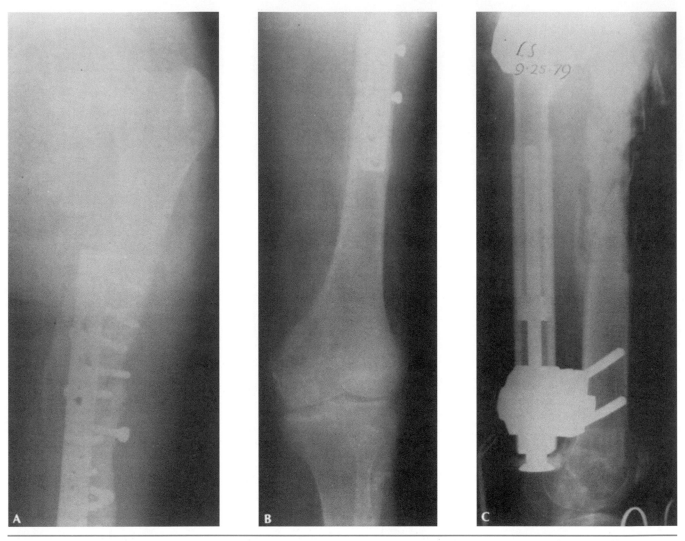

Figure 7–2   Radiographs of the leg in a 16-year-old boy who sustained a femoral shaft fracture that was treated by the application of a plate. (A and B) Anteroposterior and lateral films of the femur show that the plate has been applied to the anterior aspect of the femur instead of the lateral side, and the fracture at this point is infected with loose internal fixation and broken screws. (C) Because the internal fixation was performing no useful function, it was removed and a Wagner external fixator applied. Cancellous bone grafting was performed during the operation. *(continued)*

RING FIXATORS

Ring fixators allow for gradual and precise correction of angulatory and rotational deformity, however, unlike pin fixators, they tend to limit access for wound care to the extremity and make free tissue transfer difficult or impossible. The Monticelli Spinelli fixator, the Ace-Fischer fixator, and the Ilizarov frame are examples of ring fixators. The Ace-Fischer is a ring fixator in which the rings are connected by rods that have universal joints at each end and are capable of either compression or distraction by rotating a compression wheel. The fixation of the rings to the bone is accomplished by transfixion pins, half-pins, or Kirschner wires. The Ilizarov frame (Fig. 7–6), also a ring fixator, utilizes wires of small diameter (less than 2 mm) that are passed through the bone, secured to circumferential rings, and placed under tension of about 220 pounds. The smaller wires

cause less skin irritation and reduce pin tract infections. However, the bulk of the frame and the lack of access for soft-tissue care are drawbacks.

APPLICATION OF THE EXTERNAL FIXATOR

Regardless of type, application of the external fixator utilizes the following principles (Chapman & Olsen, 1996):

- Irrigation and débridement of open fractures and wound management
- Obtaining as anatomical a reduction as possible with maximum contact between bone fragments
- Predrilling for the fixation pins using a water-cooled sharp drill point to avoid bone necrosis
- Inserting the fixation pins by hand

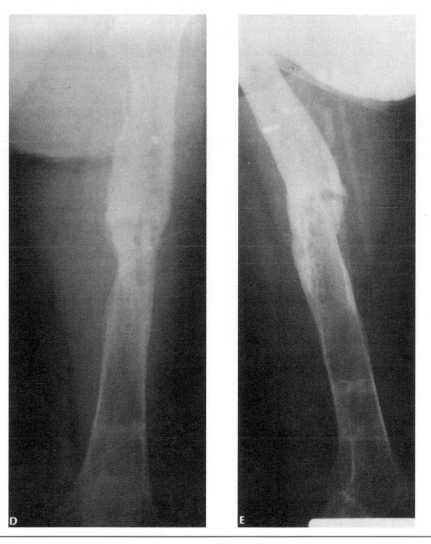

Figure 7–2   (D and E) The end result 16 months later, after having been maintained in the Wagner apparatus for 13 months. *(Rockwood, C.A., et al. (1996).* Rockwood & Green's Fractures in Adults. *4th ed. Philadelphia: Lippincott-Raven.)*

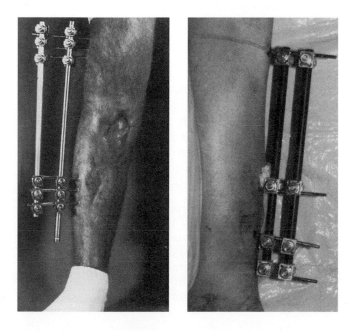

Figure 7–3   (A) The AO/ASIF external fixator, type I unilateral frame with double bar. Note that the upper pins are in the distal femur to reduce a comminuted plateau fracture by ligamentotaxis and to stabilize a comminuted fracture of the shaft. (B) Immobilization of a tibial fracture by an anterior unilateral frame with double bars (Trauma Fix). Note that these bars are made of a radiolucent fiber composite. *(Rockwood, C.A., et al. (1996).* Rockwood & Green's Fractures in Adults. *4th ed. Philadelphia: Lippincott-Raven.)*

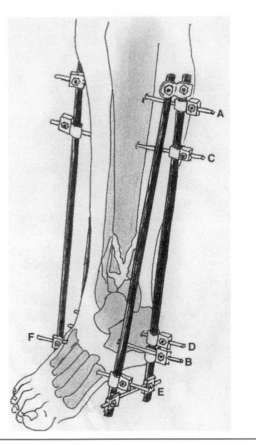

Figure 7–4   Double delta external fixator for open comminuted pilon fractures of the distal tibia and fibula. These are through-and-through centrally threaded pins. The fracture is aligned and then pins A and B are inserted. Half pins E and F can be used in the base of the metatarsals to support the forefoot when required. The medial or lateral half of the fixator can be removed for surgical procedures while maintaining stability of the limb.   *(Rockwood, C.A., et al. (1996). Rockwood & Green's Fractures in Adults. 4th ed. Philadelphia: Lippincott-Raven.)*

- Placing the pins to avoid injury to the neurovascular structures and restricting the musculotendon units
- Maintaining the stability of the fracture–external fixation frame construct by use of correct pin size, pin placement, and placement of the bar connecting the pins as close to the extremity as practical

COMPLICATIONS OF EXTERNAL FIXATION

The major complications that occur as the result of an external fixator are (1) pin tract infection, (2) pin loosening and breakage, (3) limitation of joint motion, (4) neurovascular damage and compartmental syndrome, (5) malalignment and malunion, and (6) delayed union or nonunion.

INFECTIONS
External fixations have a long history of pin tract infections, which greatly reduced their use in the past. Plac-

ing pins through soft tissue predisposes to infection. However, infections of the pin tract are infrequent with the use of the Ilizarov frame (and when they occur are usually only serous drainage [Grade I] infections). Many believe this is because of the small diameter of the Ilizarov transfixion pins/wires.

Pin tract infections may be classified as follows: (1) Grade I (inordinate serous or seropurulent drainage). All pin sites drain, but normal drainage should be minimal on the underside of the bandage, and free-flowing drainage or any degree of purulence is pathologic, requiring a broad spectrum antibiotic. (2) Grade II (superficial cellulitis). A halo of cutaneous erythema that develops and expands from the pin site usually indicates a soft-tissue infection, requiring oral antibiotics and increased pin site care. (3) Grade III (deep infection). Characterized by deep-seated infection along the entire pin site tract; it can be differentiated from superficial pin site cellulitis by purulent drainage and swelling and severe cellulitis encompassing more than one of the pins in a cluster, requiring intravenous antibiotics. (4) Grade IV (osteomyelitis). Uncontrolled deep infection, which can lead to bone infection and pin loosening; it requires intravenous antibiotics and surgical débridement (Nepola, 1996).

With the high risk of infection, prophylaxis is needed. It was once assumed that exposed screw threads increased the rate of pin site infections, but today most physicians disagree with that theory (Nepola, 1996). The most appropriate measures to prevent pin site infections are for the physician to ensure that the pin incisions are adequate and for caretakers to provide excellent pin site care. Meticulous cleansing of the pin sites with soap and water and cotton swabs is usually preferred. However, some institutions/physicians use providone-iodine or KISS (keep it simple with saline).

If infection does occur, the treatment usually involves therapy with antibiotics and the enlargement of the wound to allow for free drainage. If these measures are ineffective, the next course of action is usually the removal of the pins, the curettage of the pin tracts, and the reinsertion of new pins at different locations in the bone.

Although not a pin site infection, an infection in an open wound fracture can impact the calcification of the bone and undermine the effectiveness of the external fixation. Most open wounds are cleansed and débrided, and a number of physicians also insert antibiotic beads (Fig. 7–7) to prevent or control infection.

PIN LOOSENING AND BREAKAGE

Most authorities agree that pin loosening is inevitable if external fixators are on for long periods. Making sure that the pins are anchored securely is essential, since a loose pin is nonfunctional and contributes to a potential pin tract infection (Chapman & Olsen, 1996). How well the pin is anchored also depends somewhat on the quality of the bone. Physicians prefer cortical bone to metaphyseal bone as the former provides a better

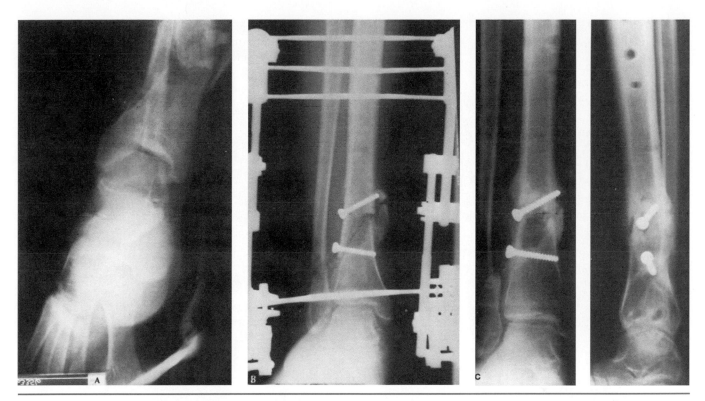

Figure 7–5 Combination of external and internal fixation used to treat an open tibial fractured incurred in a motorcycle accident. (A) Preoperative fracture. (B) Hoffman fixator and loose butterfly fragment fixed by two screws. (C) Healing after removal of fixator. *(Rockwood, C.A., et al. (1996). Rockwood & Green's Fractures in Adults. 4th ed. Philadelphia: Lippincott-Raven.)*

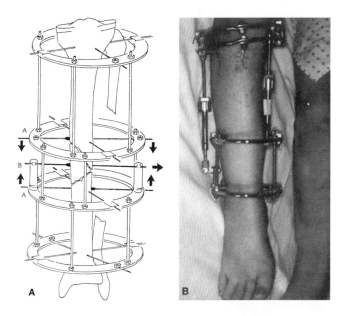

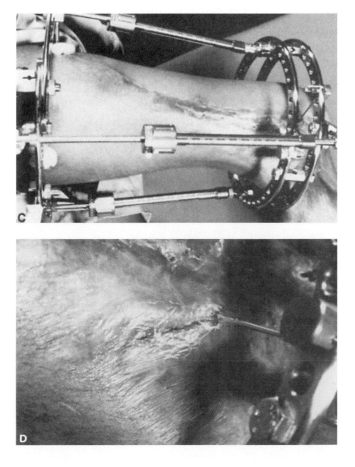

Figure 7–6 The Ilizarov apparatus. (A) The frame for a fractured tibia. (B) Lengthening of the tibia after angular correction. (C) Lengthening of the femur. (D) During lengthening, the wire cuts through skin with immediate healing as the wire progresses. *(Rockwood, C.A., et al. (1996). Rockwood & Green's Fractures in Adults. 4th ed. Philadelphia: Lippincott-Raven.)*

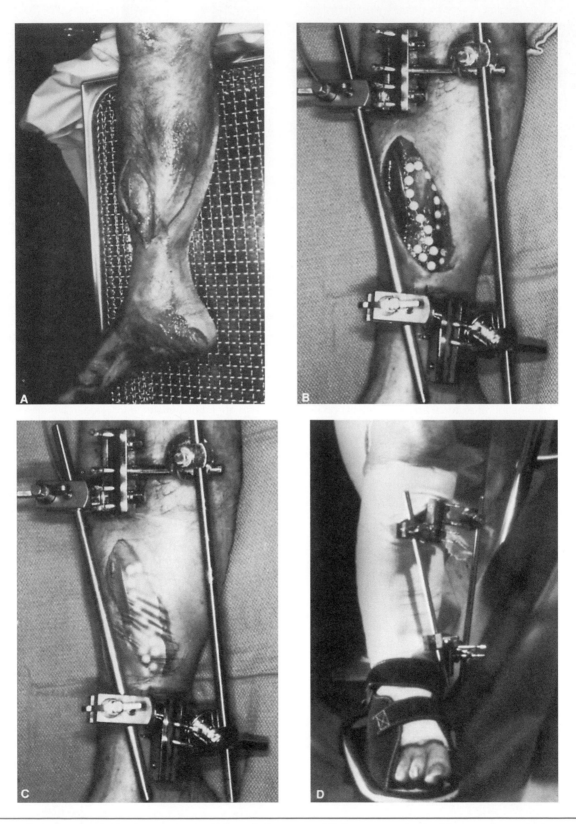

Figure 7–7   Clinical and radiographic views of a fractured tibia in an elderly woman who had been inebriated when injured, was unattended until the following morning, and did not remember how she was hurt. (A) Condition of the leg on admission. (B) After wound débridement and insertion of tobtamycin beads and fixation by a one-plane, double-bat, Hoffman fixator. (C) Bead pouch. (D) Cast supplementation of fixator. *(continued)*

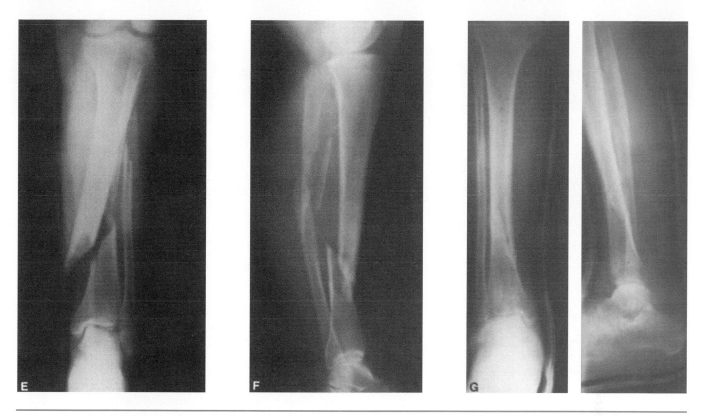

Figure 7–7 (E and F) Initial radiographs. (G) Early healing after 4 months. *(Rockwood, C.A., et al. (1996). Rockwood & Green's Fractures in Adults. 4th ed. Philadelphia: Lippincott-Raven.)*

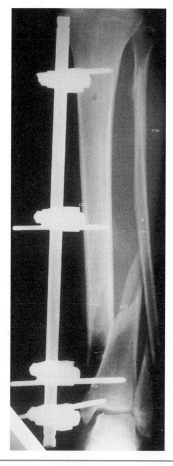

Figure 7–8 Loss of metaphyseal fixation in a 70-year-old woman with a distal tibia fracture treated with a unilateral half pin external fixator. *(Koval & Zuckerman (1998). Fractures in the Elderly. Philadelphia: Lippincott-Raven.)*

anchor (Fig. 7–8), and young healthy bone is better than osteoporotic bone. Proper pin insertion and the selection of pins that are appropriate for the type of fracture and the type of bone are essential to help prevent loosening. Harkess, Ramsey, and Harkess (1996) present a clinical classification of pin loosening (see Box 7–1). An infection can also allow the pins to loosen.

Breakage poses another problem, although rare. Nepola (1996) states that a 5.2% incidence of pin breakage has been reported with the use of 4-mm diameter half pins. However, today the current screws/pins that are normally utilized are of 5-mm or 6-mm diameter, and breakage of these is quite rare. External fixator frame breakage or bending is also rare.

LIMITATION OF JOINT MOTION

The percutaneous transfixion of soft tissue is a concern when an external fixator is inserted through muscle. When muscles or tendons are restricted by an implant,

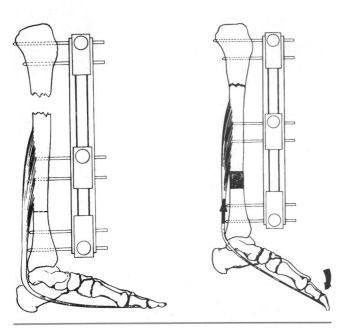

Figure 7–9   Distal-to-proximal transport in the tibia may be associated with tethering of muscle groups and attendant equinus deformity.   *(Rockwood, C.A., et al. (1996). Rockwood & Green's Fractures in Adults. 4th ed. Philadelphia: Lippincott-Raven.)*

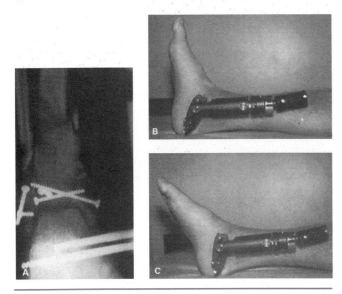

Figure 7–10   (A) A high-energy tibial plafond fracture treated with articulated external fixation. Lows limited (B) and (C) dorsiflexion plantar flexion of the ankle while maintaining reduction.   *(Rockwood, C.A., et al. (1996). Rockwood & Green's Fractures in Adults. 4th ed. Philadelphia: Lippincott-Raven.)*

a tenodesis or myodesis-like effect restricts the motion of the joint crossed by that motor unit (Fig. 7–9). Having the external fixator in place for an extended period may cause scarring to occur, requiring prolonged rehabilitation to regain joint motion. There is also a very slight chance that function will not return. That is more common in adults than children (Chapman & Olsen, 1996).

Another cause of limitation of joint motion is when external fixator pins or wires extend across joints. For example, when a quadrilateral frame is applied to the tibia, the foot is dorsiflexed to the neutral position and knee flexion may be compromised by supracondylar pins. Figure 7–10 shows an external fixator that allows limited dorsiflexion and plantar flexion of the ankle while maintaining reduction. With rehabilitation, joint function normally returns.

NEUROVASCULAR DAMAGE AND COMPARTMENTAL SYNDROME

Safe pin placement is crucial during the insertion of an external fixator to prevent neurovascular damage and the development of compartmental syndrome. For example, to avoid damage to the posterior tibial neurovascular bundle, the physician flexes the patient's knee when placing an anteroposterior pin in the proximal tibia. Harkess, Ramsey, and Harkess (1996) state it is crucial that attention be given to excessive bleeding from the pin holes and to the signs of compartmental syndrome and distal ischemia. A pin inserted through the anterolateral compartment of a leg that has been severely contused by a closed injury may initiate enough bleeding to produce a compartmental syndrome. A number of physicians believe it is safer to use half pins instead of transfixing pins when possible, but half pins are also not without risk. For further information on compartmental syndrome, see Chapter 4.

MALALIGNMENT AND MALUNION

Malalignment and malunion can occur even if the initial reduction and application of the external fixator were perfect. Pin loosening (discussed earlier) and weight bearing may allow angular deformities to occur, especially in unstable fractures. To prevent such an occurrence, the alignment needs to be checked clinically and radiologically throughout the healing period. One thing to remember: always investigate the patient's complaints as they are living with the device 24 hours a day and are the most sensitive resource for monitoring the hardware.

DELAYED UNION OR NONUNION

Delayed unions and nonunions are common among patients treated with external fixators. Some physicians believe that the external fixator keeps the fracture distracted and have advocated replacing the fixator with a cast after 6 weeks. However, Harkess, Ramsey and Harkess (1996) state that it is widely accepted that micromovement in the axial plane of the fixator enhances bone formation and healing in externally fixed fractures. To achieve axial micromotion, the frame may be destabilized by removal of pins, moving the longitudinal bars farther away from the

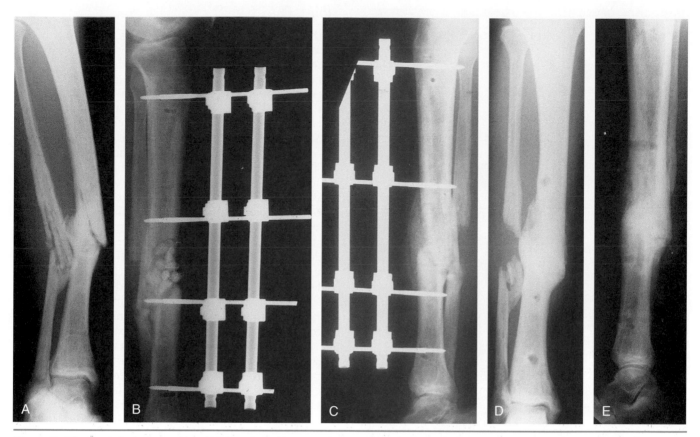

Figure 7–11   (A) Infected nonunion of the tibia in a 68-year-old woman. (B) The tibia was debrided with placement of antibiotic beads and stabilized with an external fixator. (C) After several debridement procedures, the tibia was bone grafted. (D, E) Anteroposterior and lateral radiographs at 2 years follow-up.   *(Koval & Zuckerman (1998).* Fractures in the Elderly. *Philadelphia: Lippincott-Raven.)*

bone, removing supplementary frames, or allowing the frame to telescope. However, the exact prescriptions for stress and strain magnitude have yet to be determined. Infection is another source for nonunion (Fig. 7–11).

EXTERNAL FIXATORS FOR SPECIFIC FRACTURES

The following section presents the nursing care of patients with different types of external fixators used for repair/immobilization of fractures in different parts of the body. Today, external fixation is most often indicated for open fractures of the tibia and fibula and in open fractures of the pelvis. The introduction of ring fixators using highly tensioned Kirschner wires and the half-pin or hybrid ring fixators has expanded the usefulness of external fixators (Chapman & Olsen, 1996).

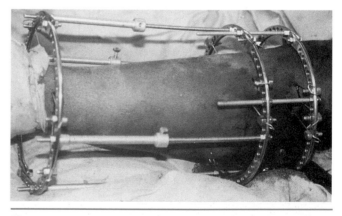

Figure 7–12   Use of a thin wire circular fixator to stabilize a proximal tibia fracture.   *(Koval & Zuckerman (1998).* Fractures in the Elderly. *Philadelphia: Lippincott-Raven.)*

TIBIAL FRACTURES

With the emergence of half-pin frames, external fixators have become the fracture stabilization method of choice for the treatment of most open fractures of long bones where there is marked soft-tissue damage and skin loss. There are many different external fixation devices available and utilized, each offering its own advantages and features.

Many different types of external fixators are utilized to treat fractures of the tibia and fibula, depending on the fracture site and type of fracture. Figure 7–12 shows the utilization of wires and a ring fixator to stabilize a proximal tibial fracture, while Figure 7–13 shows a bicondylar tibial plateau fracture that is being treated by an open reduction and a hybrid external fixator. In the treatment of distal tibia fractures, there is also a variety of devices, as shown in Figure 7–14, Figure 7–15 shows an external fixator for tibial-calcaneal distraction.

For open fractures of the tibia and the fibula, there are normally two or more heavy Steinmann pins inserted proximal to the fracture and two distal to the fracture, which are held in place by an external device such as a Hoffmann or Wagner device. With the use of a single or double frame mounting and universal joint clamps, segmental fracture fragments can be aligned. In open fractures needing that type of repair, it is common to see instability, malalignment, and soft-tissue complications with skin necrosis and deep infection. In many instances, these patients may return many times for skin grafts.

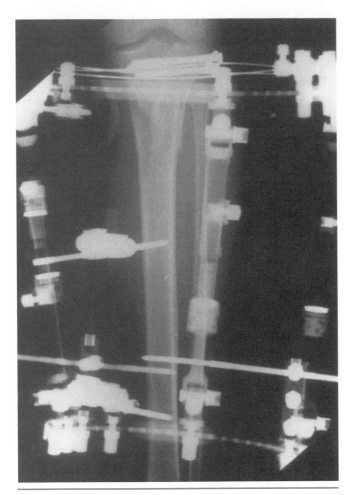

Figure 7–13   Bicondylar tibial plateau fracture treated with limited open reduction and placement of a hybrid external fixator. *(Koval & Zuckerman (1998). Fractures in the Elderly. Philadelphia: Lippincott-Raven.)*

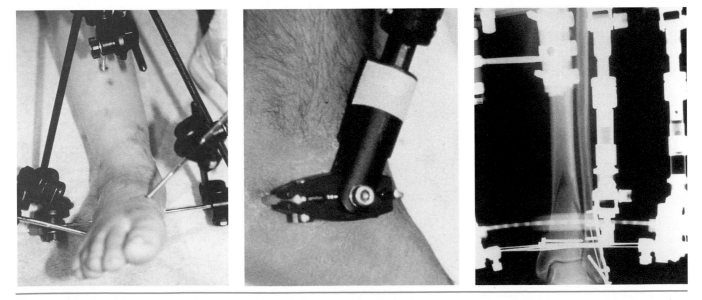

Figure 7–14   A number of distal tibia external fixator designs are available. They fall into three basic categories: (A) joint-spanning rigid, (B) joint-spanning articulated, and (C) non–joint-spanning. *(Koval & Zuckerman (1998). Fractures in the Elderly. Philadelphia: Lippincott-Raven.)*

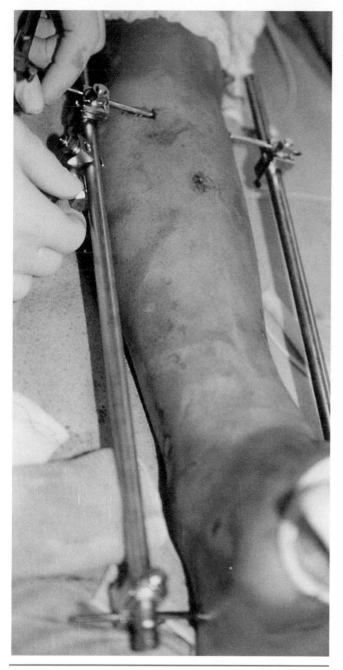

Figure 7–15   Use of external fixator to apply tibial-calcaneal distraction.   *(Koval & Zuckerman (1998). Fractures in the Elderly. Philadelphia: Lippincott-Raven.)*

NURSING PROCESS (Patient with an External Fixator for a Fractured Tibia and Fibula)

The following nursing process demonstrates the nursing care of a patient following the application of an external fixator in the treatment of an open fracture

(Fig. 7–16). The nursing process begins after the external fixator is applied.

ASSESSMENT

Patients treated with an external fixation device often have multiple injuries to other systems of the body and need an in-depth neurologic and cardiovascular assessment. Assess for signs of shock and look for other injuries, especially internal or head injuries, which may have occurred at the time of the accident. If there is a potential for head injury, monitor for signs of increasing intracranial pressure or any indication of nerve impingement in the cervical area. A neurovascular assessment is done to determine skin color; joint motion; and complaints of numbness, coldness, or swelling of the leg (Chapter 2). Check for a pulse in the affected leg, starting at the most distal pulse, and compare with the unaffected leg. Assess the open skin area for obvious bleeding, and check the dressing if one has been applied. Make sure the posterior area of the leg is assessed for bleeding or drainage. Check for correct positioning of the affected extremity and that the linen is not interfering with the external fixation device.

Determine the patient's level of anxiety and observe the emotional reactions of the patient, the family, and significant others to the open fracture site and the external fixation device. The injured leg and the external fixation device can be disturbing to many. Assess the effectiveness of the interactions between the patient and the family or significant others.

Assess the patient for pain in the affected extremity, or elsewhere, and the effectiveness of any pain medications. Continuous assessment includes assessing the patient for pain and the pin sites for signs or symptoms of infection or loosening of the pins.

NURSING DIAGNOSIS

Based on all of the assessment data, the nursing diagnoses for a typical patient with an external fixator in the treatment of an open fractured tibia and fibula include the following:

- Pain and discomfort related to bone and soft-tissue trauma
- Impaired physical mobility related to instability of the tibia and fibula
- Increased anxiety related to knowledge deficit about the external device and the rehabilitation process

COLLABORATIVE PROBLEMS

- Pin loosening
- Limitation of ankle motion
- Malunion
- Delayed union or nonunion
- Infection
- Compartmental syndrome

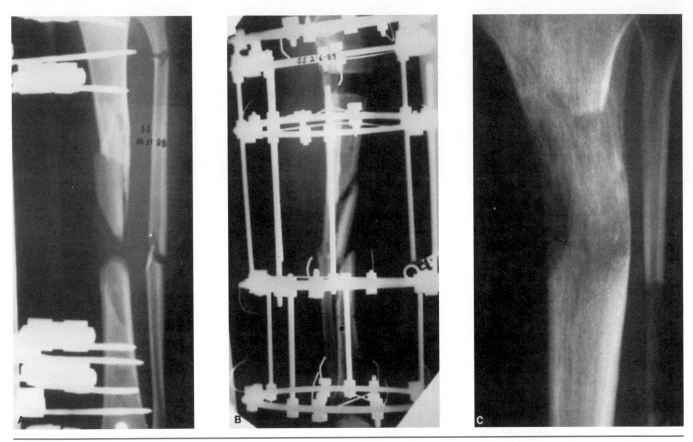

Figure 7–16   (A) Open fracture of the tibia with major segmental bone loss stabilized initially in a uniplanar external fixation. (B) Appearance after application of a ring fixator and proximal corticectomy for segment transport to close the defect. (C) Regenerate bone forming in the distraction zone.   *(Rockwood, C.A., et al. (1996). Rockwood & Green's Fractures in Adults. 4th ed. Philadelphia: Lippincott-Raven.)*

GOAL FORMULATION AND PLANNING

The goals are to have the patient experience (1) a decrease in pain through nursing measures and prescribed medications; (2) an increase in mobility through exercise, positioning, and the use of immobilizing devices; (3) a decreased anxiety through increased knowledge about the injury and the rehabilitation process; and (4) an absence of complications. Long-term goals are to have the patient free of pain and able to walk without an assistive device.

INTERVENTIONS

ALLEVIATE PAIN

The patient requiring an external fixation for the treatment of a fracture is likely to have multiple problems; hence, the complaints of discomfort may not be all bone related. Elevate the extremity, as prescribed by the patient's physician, to help prevent swelling and pain, and make sure the leg is safely and securely positioned. With an open lesion, the patient is likely to have had the external fixation device applied with very little explanation. Take time to have therapeutic communication with the patient, the family, and significant others. It

promotes relaxation and can be very effective in reducing pain.

INCREASE MOBILITY

Nursing interventions to increase mobility focus on correct positioning, exercises, and ambulation.

Position. Immediately after surgery, the leg with the external fixation device is elevated. The general rule is that the leg should be higher than the heart; therefore, the patient may be asked to not have the head of the bed elevated more than a few degrees. The leg can be elevated using pillows (depending on the external fixator) or balanced suspension traction or by securing ropes to the fixation device. Elevation is usually required until there is no longer concern about swelling.

Know how to move a patient in the external fixation device before moving the patient's leg. If it is a Hoffmann or Wagner device (with bilateral connectors), the best way to reposition the affected leg may be to help lift the leg by taking hold of the external fixation device. However, a large number of physicians/institutions require that the physician give specific directions to determine if the frame itself can be used to move the affected extremity. The leg and the external fixator must be moved as a unit, and the amount of support required by the nurse is determined by the patient's ability to control the leg during the move. During the move, the patient should be using the overhead trapeze to assist with body position changes and should be assisting with leg movement as much as possible. With short hospital stays, it is essential that the nurse take the opportunity to teach the patient, the family, and significant others whenever possible. It is essential that the family know how to assist the patient. Do not place your hands under the fracture site to assist with the movement as this may cause you to apply stress and even slightly manipulate the fracture site, depending on the external fixation device.

Exercises. Active and passive range-of-motion exercises for all unaffected extremities should be stressed. For the affected leg, quadriceps- and gluteal-setting exercises, plantar and dorsiflexion exercises (if allowed by the placement of the fixator), straight leg raises, and range-of-motion exercises for the ankle should be done, though they may not be allowed immediately. Teach the patient these exercises using the unaffected leg. Teach the patient exercises to increase their upper extremity strength for crutch walking (see Chapter 4).

Ambulation. Know the weight-bearing status of the patient before trying to get the patient up. Crutch walking with no weight bearing or partial weight bearing is usually allowed, using a three-point gait (see Chapter 4). Make sure the patient understands the steps involved in the crutch gait and that there will be an additional weight on the affected leg due to the external fixator. It is not really difficult to walk while the external device is attached to the leg, but it does require a psychological adjustment on the part of the patient in addition to learning how to crutch walk. Reassure patients that they will succeed with time, practice, and patience. Teach the patient how to get in and out of a chair and how to go up and down the stairs, all with no weight bearing on the affected leg.

PATIENT TEACHING AND HOME CARE CONSIDERATIONS
Emotional support is needed to help the patient accept what has happened, the method of treatment, the potential for skin grafts if necessary, and the potential for a longer than normal rehabilitation process for a fractured tibia and fibula. Hospital stays for these patients have shortened dramatically over the last few years. Today, once the patient's general condition is stabilized (considering other injuries) and the patient's fractured tibia and fibula are stable in the external fixator, the patient will go home for rehabilitation.

Educate the patient about the location and type of fracture and the method of repair. The patient should realize that the external fixation device stabilizes the fracture, allowing time for the bone and soft tissue to heal and enabling the leg to be moved freely without injury. Allow time for an open discussion of the prognosis with the physician and the patient. A social worker may be of help if the patient is concerned about

the costs of hospitalization, problems in returning to work, and home care needs if the fracture site is open.

Patients with open lesions go home with the external fixation device in place. Therefore, the patient, the family, or significant others will need to be instructed on how to do pin site care and how to cleanse the skin under the device. Some physicians believe that washing with soap and water during the daily shower (but no tub baths) is best for closed fractures. Patients with open fracture sites will need to sponge bathe. The patient must also know how to detect a possible infection (i.e., to look for redness, pain, heat, tenderness, hardness, or drainage). An easy plan is to write out the steps of care and the signs and symptoms of infection for the patient to take home and use as a reference.

Dressing at home is similar to the situation of a patient with a cast (see Chapter 5). If slacks are desired, the side seams can be split and Velcro straps attached to partially close the openings. Make sure the patient has appropriate shoes—not bedroom slippers—for crutch walking.

MONITORING AND MANAGING POTENTIAL PROBLEMS
General nursing measures to prevent complications of immobility are discussed in Chapter 4. Only concerns specific to patients with an external fixation device are dealt with here. Those concerns are pin loosening due to stress and strain or infection, limitation of joint motion in the ankle due to restriction of muscles and tendons as the result of pin insertions, malunion due to the initial reduction or limited movement allowed by the external fixator, or delayed union or nonunion related to infection and/or movement of the fracture site due to malfunctioning of the fixation device. For further discussion of these potential complications, see earlier sections in this chapter. The major complications for the focus of nursing attention are infection and compartmental syndrome.

INFECTION
Patients with an open fracture and an external fixation device are at risk for infection from two sources. The first is the contamination of the fracture site and the second is pin site infection. Thus, utilizing measures to control and/or prevent infection is essential. The patient may be receiving oral antibiotics, or antibiotics may have been placed in the wound, but special care is still needed at the fracture site and pin sites.

For an open contaminated wound, the fracture site is irrigated and débrided before the external fixator is applied. Some physicians may even prescribe wound irrigations as a sterile procedure following device application. Care should be taken to keep the upper leg and trunk dry by utilizing disposable pads. If the skin from an open fracture has been closed and if the patient's physician allows it, the use of bathing soap during a shower is helpful in keeping the wound clean.

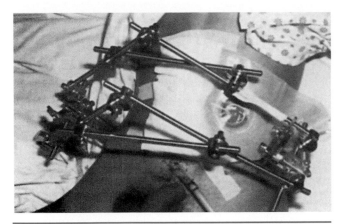

Figure 7–17   External fixation of an open pelvic fracture. Note colostomy and suprapubic catheter. Internal fixation was not used because of risk of infection in this open fracture.   *(Rockwood, C.A., et al. (1996). Rockwood & Green's Fractures in Adults. 4th ed. Philadelphia: Lippincott-Raven.)*

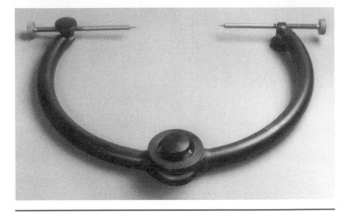

Figure 7–18   A large pelvic clamp for emergent temporary fixation in hemodynamically unstable patients with pelvic fractures is shown here.   *(Rockwood, C.A., et al. (1996). Rockwood & Green's Fractures in Adults. 4th ed. Philadelphia: Lippincott-Raven.)*

Care is needed to prevent pin site infection. The number one way to prevent this infection from occurring is meticulous pin site care at least once a day. Physicians/institutions have their own preferences for pin care, from soap and water to providone-iodine, hydrogen peroxide, and the application of Neosporin ointment. However, the simplest and the most effective seems to be soap and water and utilizing cotton swabs around the pin site to cleanse and keep the skin from adhering to the pin. If the skin around the pin sites is left unattended and becomes taut, it can cause the patient discomfort and the physician may then need to treat the problem by incising the skin around the pin. With signs or symptoms of infection at the pin site, the cleansing may be increased from once a day to 3 times a day.

COMPARTMENTAL SYNDROME

Compartmental syndrome can occur as the result of inserting a pin through or into a compartment. To assist in its identification and correction, note any excessive bleeding from the pin holes and signs of compartmental syndrome (see Chapter 5, Care of a Patient with a Fractured Tibia and Long Leg Cast) or distal ischemia.

EVALUATION/OUTCOMES

For a typical patient recovering from an open fracture of the tibia with soft-tissue damage and an external fixation device, the evaluation is essentially the same as that described for a patient who has had a total knee replacement. Be sure to check the patient's compliance with the exercises and rehabilitation regimes. Special emphasis must be given to determine the patient's responses to the injury and the method of treatment. Continue to evaluate the responses of the patient, the family, and significant others to long-term immobilization of the involved leg (usually months and even longer

with skin grafts) and the possibility of future hospitalization and surgery, bearing in mind the stages of adjustment discussed in Chapter 1. Regarding complications, look for pressure areas and decubiti, an elevated temperature, increasing pain, and other problem signs.

CERVICAL FRACTURES

The halo brace is a form of external fixation device utilized to stabilize and treat fractures of the cervical spine. The halo brace and the nursing care of patients in a halo brace are discussed in Chapter 6 and are not presented here. Some of the same concerns for external fixators discussed in this chapter also apply to the halo brace. Two major similarities are the potential for infection and pin loosening.

PELVIC FRACTURES

Chapman and Olsen (1996) state that one of the strongest indications for external fixation is an open fracture of the pelvis where stability is essential to control hemorrhage, management of the soft tissues is crucial, and early mobilization is a priority (Fig. 7–17). Because the perineal wounds and ruptured viscus that occur in open fractures of the pelvis add to the risk of infection, external fixation is generally the best choice for the acute management of these fractures. Nepola (1996) states that fixators work well for controlling the open-book pelvic injury but are inadequate for the stabilization of pelvic ring fractures with vertical instability. Exotic and complicated frames have not proven to be satisfactory for pelvic ring fractures with vertical instability. However, simple frames using two pins, one on each iliac crest, are usually sufficient for most injuries of the pelvic ring (Fig. 7–18). Those with vertical instability usually require supplemental skeletal traction or delayed posterior internal fixation.

NURSING PROCESS (Patient with an External Fixator for a Pelvic Fracture)

The following nursing process demonstrates the nursing care of a typical patient following the application of an external fixator for a pelvic fracture. The nursing process begins after the external fixator is in place and the patient returns to the nursing unit.

ASSESSMENT

The assessment (which may take place in the intensive care unit) involves an in-depth assessment of the patient's cardiovascular, respiratory, gastrointestinal, and genitourinary systems. Assess the patient's level of consciousness and orientation, and look for other injuries the patient may have sustained. Auscultate the patient's chest for clearness of their lungs, and determine if there are any heart abnormalities. Have the patient cough and deep breathe. Assess the patient for signs of shock or hemorrhage, and note if there is any drainage on the abdominal dressing if the fracture site is closed. Determine blood loss before and during the application procedure. Note the kind and amount of intravenous fluids. Do a neurovascular assessment of the lower extremities, and compare the two legs. Note the position of the patient's lower extremities in relation to the patient's trunk. Verify that the patient's nasogastric tube is connected to suction, and determine if a colostomy was also performed. Verify that the patient has a Foley catheter that it is connected to drainage, and observe the color and amount of the urine. Assess the type, severity, and location of pain and determine whether the patient received pain medications in the operating room.

Frequent assessments of the patient should be made during the postoperative period. These include the auscultation of the patient's chest, assessment of the neurovascular status of the lower extremities, evaluation of the amount of intake and output of fluids, and assessment for the presence of bowel sounds. Note any signs or symptoms of shock, pulmonary emboli, deep vein thrombosis, or infection.

NURSING DIAGNOSIS

Based on all of the assessment data, the major nursing diagnoses for a typical patient with pelvic fractures and an external fixator may include the following:

- Pain and discomfort related to bone and soft-tissue trauma
- Impaired physical mobility related to instability of the pelvis
- Potential impaired bowel/bladder function related to trauma
- Ineffective individual coping related to the trauma and the rehabilitation process
- Increased anxiety related to knowledge deficit about the procedure and the rehabilitation process

COLLABORATIVE PROBLEMS

- Deep vein thrombosis
- Pulmonary emboli
- Hypovolemic shock
- Infection
- Loosening of pins

GOAL FORMULATION AND PLANNING

The goals are to have the patient experience (1) a decrease in pain through nursing measures and medications, (2) an increase in mobility with the use of external fixators and crutches, (3) nonimpaired bowel function, (4) effective individual coping, (5) a decrease in anxiety through increased knowledge about the treatment method and rehabilitation process, and (6) the absence of complications.

INTERVENTIONS

ALLEVIATE PAIN

Pain management is essential for a patient following a pelvic fracture. Patient-controlled analgesia with morphine is usually used for the first 24 to 48 hours or until the patient is able to take fluids. The patient will then be placed on oral narcotics.

Assess the patient's pain for severity and location. Note whether any of the complaints of pain are related to any potential complications. Check to see what nursing interventions help to alleviate some of the patient's pain. Teach the patient relaxation techniques, and utilize activities as a means of distraction to help relieve the patient's feelings of pain. For further discussion of pain management, see Chapter 2.

INCREASE MOBILITY

Methods to increase the patient's mobility focus on correct positioning, exercises, and ambulation.

Position. While the patient is in bed, they should be repositioned and tilted (usually no more than 45 degrees) on to their sides every 2 hours. If the fracture and external fixator are only on one side, the patient may be turned from their back to the unaffected side (still only 45 degrees). Utilize log-rolling when turning the patient (see Chapter 8, Care of a Patient Following a Posterior Fusion with Instrumentation).

Exercises. Most patients will start muscle-setting exercises also immediately; however, it will depend on the patient's general condition, type of fracture, and the physician's preference. Exercises for most patients will be quadriceps- and gluteal-setting exercises, ankle pumps, and range-of-motion to ankle. Some physicians order continuous passive motion exercises, depending on the type of fracture, to prevent loss of range of motion in the hip (see Chapter 10, Total Knee Replacement). All patients will need to do exercises to increase the strength in their upper extremities for crutch walking (see Chapter 4).

Ambulation. One of the goals in the utilization of an external fixator is early ambulation, but the patient's general condition and other injuries also determine when the patient will be allowed to ambulate. A large number of patients are able to ambulate the first day after application of the external fixator. When the patient is allowed to ambulate, first assist them to the side of the bed. Next get them sitting on the side of the bed. Helping these patients learn to move will take time because of the restrictions placed on moving by the fracture and the additional encumberance of the external fixator. Patients with associated bilateral pelvic fractures are usually not allowed weight bearing and must transfer to a chair using a sliding board. Patients with unilateral posterior injuries are usually permitted early weight bearing on the noninjuried side, and non-weight bearing or toe touch on the injured side 8 to 12 weeks (or sometimes longer) after fracture. The extent and timing of weight bearing are determined by the type of fracture.

BOWEL AND BLADDER FUNCTION
Patients with pelvic fractures (especially open fractures) are at risk of trauma and lacerations to their bowel, bladder, and perineal area. Some patients may have a temporary or permanent colostomy. Others may have their bladder ruptured or lacerated. The bladder is more apt to be injured if the bladder was full of urine at the time of the trauma. Patients with pelvic fractures will have a catheter in place even if there is no damage to the bladder. Care for these injuries will not be covered here; please see the medical/surgical text listed in the references.

COPING MECHANISMS
Patient's with external fixators in place sometimes look at the device and develop their own ideas of how "sick" they are. How can they possibly do anything for themselves with that apparatus in place? Will they ever be able to walk again? They may be afraid that if they try walking with the apparatus in place, they will break something else. They develop a hopeless/helpless feeling and are unwilling to do the things they can for themselves. Look for decreased concentration, fatigue, increased restlessness, increased complaints, or withdrawal from staff and others.

Encourage the patient and family to verbalize questions. Keep the patient actively involved in their care and involved in any decisions that need to be made. To help prevent or reduce boredom and self-centeredness, find activities that can occupy the patient's time and that they like to do. Try to make the activities mentally stimulating as a change from the passive role of the tel-

evision viewer. Get the family and significant other involved. Get assistance from the occupational therapy department or any volunteers that come to the hospital. Get the patient involved in planning home care.

PATIENT TEACHING AND HOME CARE CONSIDERATIONS
Patient teaching focuses on the exercise and rehabilitation regime. The accident was both a physical and emotional shock to the patient, and the nurse needs to be aware that the patient may be suffering from anxiety and stress related to the trauma. Most of the activities of the doctors, nurses, and family members have focused on the patient's physical well-being; it is now time to let the patient talk about the accident and what occurred. The patient may also have symptoms related to posttraumatic stress syndrome (see Chapter 4). See Chapter 1 for a discussion of how patients adjust to a possible debilitating injury or long rehabilitation process.

Know what the physician has told the patient and what the plan of treatment will be. Reinforce these objectives and help the patient plan a realistic home rehabilitation program that involves exercises and ambulation. Make sure the patient understands the purpose of the exercises, how they are to be done, how often they are to be done, and what to do should pain or swelling develop after exercising. Make sure the patient is safe in non-weight-bearing transfers (if appropriate) or ambulating with nonweight bearing or partial weight bearing. If the patient is doing crutch walking, make sure they are performing safely and know how to go up and down stairs and how to get in and out of a car before going home (see Chapter 4).

Discuss with the patient home care issues such as activities of daily living, food preparation, and the best way to dress. Pin site and wound care are also reinforced as well as the signs and symptoms of infection. Make sure home care instructions are provided for any other injuries the patient may have received.

MONITORING AND MANAGING POTENTIAL PROBLEMS

The major complications that may arise following a pelvic fracture that is reduced by external fixation are (1) deep vein thrombosis, (2) pulmonary emboli, (3) hypovolemic shock, (4) infection, and (5) pin loosening.

DEEP VEIN THROMBOSIS
Patients with pelvic fractures are at risk for deep vein thrombosis for two reasons. One is the fracture itself, and the second is the immobilization imposed by the fracture. For those reasons, most patients are started immediately on prophylactic measures to prevent the condition from developing. Unless precluded by the patient's general physical condition, some physicians/institutions use a combination of pneumatic sequential compression stockings, elastic stockings, and low-dose heparin or Coumadin as prophylaxis against thromboembolism. For more information, see Chapter 4.

PULMONARY EMBOLISM

A pulmonary embolism is the obstruction of one or more pulmonary arteries by a thrombus that originated somewhere in the venous system or the right side of the heart became dislodged, and was carried to the lung. The most important treatment is prevention. Keep the patient well hydrated, have them do active and passive exercises, and move and ambulate as tolerated. Pharmacologic prophylactic measures and physical measures as already discussed are usually implemented. For further discussion, see Chapter 4.

HYPOVOLEMIC SHOCK

Hypovolemic shock is the result of hemorrhage and loss of extracellular fluid into damaged tissues. Due to the trauma, the patient has had a relatively large amount of blood loss before and during the application of the external fixators. Make sure adequate intake and output records are maintained, and assess the balance between them. Make sure vital signs are checked on time and an accurate record is maintained. Note any discomfort related to possible bleeding, and follow-up with an in-depth assessment. See Chapter 4 for further discussion.

INFECTION

Check that any dressing is dry and intact. Reinforce the dressing, and notify the physician if there is excess bleeding in the abdominal area. Utilize standard wound management, and implement meticulous pin care. These patients are at high risk for infection from pin sites, open wounds, and lacerations of the perineal area (if present). These patients are on antibiotics but still need to be observed for signs and symptoms of infection. See the discussion on infection earlier in this chapter.

PIN LOOSENING

There is always a risk that the external fixator pins will loosen. For further information, see the discussion earlier in this chapter.

EVALUATION/OUTCOMES

Some patients recovering from a pelvic fracture will have external fixation as their definitive method of treatment, while others initially treated by external fixation will return to surgery for an open reduction internal fixation. Pain and future ambulation are the primary concerns for all patients. Pain is controlled using nursing interventions and medications. With a unilateral fracture, the patient is usually able to ambulate safely using a three-point gait with non-weight bearing (or toe touch) on the injured side. Before going home, the patient is able to demonstrate compliance in doing exercises and going up and down stairs safely with crutches. If the patient received a bilateral injury, they are able to transfer safely to a chair using a sliding board. The patient will verbalize

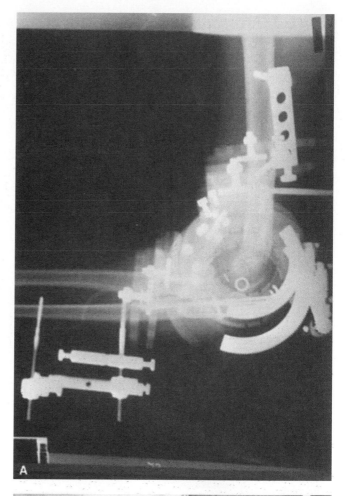

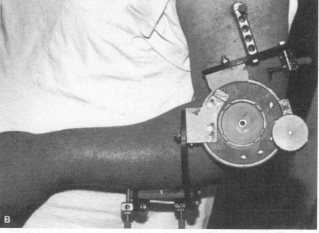

Figure 7–19   (A and B) This compass hinge fixator for the elbow maintains stability and congruity of the joint with controlled motion possible. *(Koval & Zuckerman (1998). Fractures in the Elderly. Philadelphia: Lippincott-Raven.)*

an understanding of the goals and objectives of rehabilitation and their role in achieving them. The patient will be free of complications.

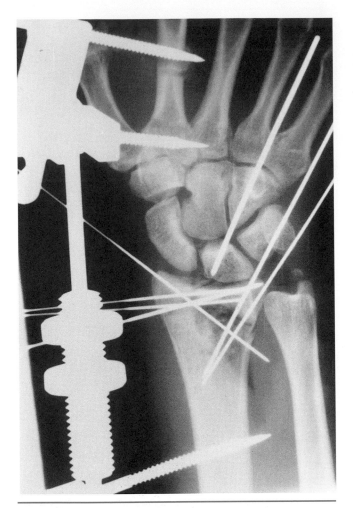

Figure 7–20   Comminuted intra-articular distal radius fracture in a 65-year-old man, depicting use of precutaneous pins in conjunction with external fixation.   *(Koval & Zuckerman (1998). Fractures in the Elderly. Philadelphia: Lippincott-Raven.)*

ELBOW FRACTURES

Chapman and Olsen (1996) state that external fixation is one of the best methods of treatment of a severe open fracture of the elbow joint where there is soft-tissue injury, bone loss, and gross instability. The half-pin frame bridges the humerus and ulna, and early motion is obtained with a compass hinge external fixator (Fig. 7–19).

Nursing care focuses on the prevention of infection with pin site care using soap and water and meticulous cleansing with a cotton swab. When the patient is at home, assistance may be needed with this task. When the patient is allowed to shower, they can cleanse the pin sites while showering. The patient must know the signs and symptoms of infection.

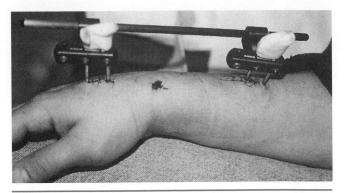

Figure 7–21   Clinical photograph demonstrating one type of external fixator. Note that the proximal pins were placed through a 3- to 4-cm incision.   *Koval & Zuckerman (1998). Fractures in the Elderly. Philadelphia: Lippincott-Raven.*

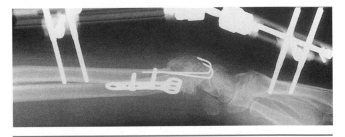

Figure 7–22   Use of open reduction and volar plating in conjunction with external fixation and percutaneous pinning to stabilize a comminuted distal radius fracture with an associated volar lip fragment.   *(Koval & Zuckerman (1998). Fractures in the Elderly. Philadelphia: Lippincott-Raven.)*

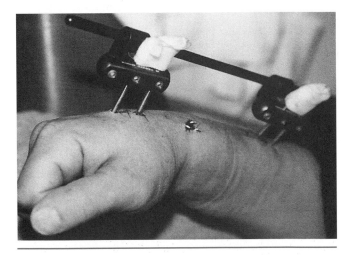

Figure 7–23   It is essential that the patient perform aggressive finger and hand range-of-motion exercises during fixator use.   *(Koval & Zuckerman (1998). Fractures in the Elderly. Philadelphia: Lippincott-Raven.)*

The other major concern is to regain mobility in the elbow. The compass hinge external fixator allows for movement and exercise. Prescribed exercises must be followed, or maximal functional ability in the elbow will not be regained. Make sure the patient knows that pins may loosen, so that they will be aware of any movement and notify their physician should this occur.

RADIAL FRACTURES

For the best stabilization, external fixation is often the method of choice in the treatment of radial fractures in the elderly due to the high incidence of fracture comminution and associated osteopenia. The use of external fixation in the treatment of radial fractures is most often indicated for unstable, open, comminuted, intra-articular fractures of the distal radius (Fig. 7–20). Application of the external fixator is performed on a fluoroscopic hand table, and pins are placed through two small incisions (distal and proximal). The fixator is assembled, the fracture is manually reduced, and the connector bar is applied to complete the apparatus. External fixation from the dorsolateral radius to the second or third metacarpal usually works very well (Fig. 7–21). Sometimes the external fixator is used in combination with an open reduction and plating (Fig. 7–22).

Nursing focuses on the prevention of infection (discussed previously) and exercises. Aggressive hand therapy (Fig. 7–23) is usually initiated during hospitalization and continued at home in order to prevent soft tissue contractures. The fixator is usually removed after about 6 weeks.

References

Bartlett, C. S., & Weiner, L. W. (1998). Tibia and pylon. In K. J. Koval & J. D. Zuckerman (Eds.), *Fractures in the elderly* (pp. 217–232). Philadelphia: Lippincott-Raven.

Behrens, F. F., Schenk, R., & Koval, K. J. (1998) Tibial plateau. In K. J. Koval & J. D. Zuckerman (Eds.), *Fractures in the elderly* (pp. 203–216). Philadelphia: Lippincott-Raven.

Belinsky, J. D. (1993). Acetabular fractures: ORIF. *Orthopaedic Nursing, 12* (1), 42–50.

Borrelli, J., Koval, K. J., & Helfet, D. L. (1998). Pelvis and acetabulum. In K. J. Koval & J. D. Zuckerman (Eds.), *Fractures in the elderly* (pp. 159–174). Philadelphia: Lippincott-Raven.

Bryant, G. G. (1998). Modalities for immobilization. In A. B. Maher, S. W. Salmond, & T. A. Pellino (Eds.), *Orthopaedic nursing* (2nd ed, pp. 296–322). Philadelphia: W. B. Saunders.

Carpenito, L. J. (1993). *Nursing diagnosis: Application to clinical practice* (5th ed.). Philadelphia: J. B. Lippincott Company.

Chapman, M. W., & Olsen, S. A. (1996). Open fractures. In C. A. Rockwood, D. P. Green, R. W. Buckholz, & J. D. Heckman (Eds.), *Rockwood and Green's fractures in adults* (4th ed., pp. 305–352). Philadelphia: Lippincott-Raven.

Childs, S. (1998). Management of the open fracture. In V. C. Williamson (Ed.), *Management of lower-extremity fractures* (pp. 55–59). Pitman, NJ: National Association of Orthopaedic Nurses.

DeGeorge, P., & Dunwoody, C. (1995). Transfer techniques of the lower extremity with an external fixator. *Orthopaedic Nursing, 14*(6), 17–21.

Dinowitz, M. I., Koval, K. J., & Meadows, S. (1998). Distal radius. In K. J. Koval & J. D. Zuckerman (Eds.), *Fractures in the elderly* (pp. 127–143). Philadelphia: Lippincott-Raven.

Dunwoody, C. (1994). External fixation. In A. B. Maher, S. W. Salmond, & T. A. Pellino (Eds.), *Orthopaedic nursing* (pp. 298–310). Philadelphia: W. B. Saunders.

Green, D. P., & Butler, T. E. (1996). Fractures and dislocations in the hand. In C. A. Rockwood, D. P. Green, R. W. Buckholz, & J. D. Heckman (Eds.), *Rockwood and Green's fractures in adults* (4th ed., pp. 607–744). Philadelphia: Lippincott-Raven.

Harkess, J. W., Ramsey, W. C., & Harkess, J. W. (1996). Principles of fractures and dislocations. In C. A. Rockwood, D. P. Green, R. W. Buckholz, & J. D. Heckman (Eds.), *Rockwood and Green's fractures in adults* (4th ed., pp. 3–120). Philadelphia: Lippincott-Raven.

Nepola, J. V. (1996). External fixation. In C. A. Rockwood, D. P. Green, R. W. Buckholz, & J. D. Heckman (Eds.), *Rockwood and Green's fractures in adults* (4th ed., pp. 229–260). Philadelphia: Lippincott-Raven.

Richards, R. R., & Corley, G. G. (1996). Fractures of the shafts of the radius and ulna. In C. A. Rockwood, D. P. Green, R. W. Buckholz, & J. D. Heckman (Eds.), *Rockwood and Green's fractures in adults* (4th ed., pp. 869–929). Philadelphia: Lippincott-Raven.

Rosen, H., & Koval, K. J. (1998). Nonunion/malunion. In K. J. Koval & J. D. Zuckerman (Eds.), *Fractures in the elderly* (pp. 261–276). Philadelphia: Lippincott-Raven

Salmond, S. W., Mooney, N. E., & Verdisco, L. A. (1996). *NAON: Core curriculum for orthopaedic nursing*. Pitman, NJ: National Association of Orthopaedic Nurses.

Smeltzer, S. C. & Bare, B. G. (1996). *Brunner and Suddarth's textbook of medical-surgical nursing* (8th ed.). Philadelphia: Lippincott.

Chapter

8

Care of Patients with Spinal and Pelvic Injuries

Chapter 8 discusses the nursing care of patients with traumatic and pathologic conditions of the spine, the thorax, and the pelvis. The spinal column is divided into five separate sections—the cervical, the thoracic, the lumbar, the sacral, and the coccygeal—and the chapter starts with a brief review of anatomy to help the nurse understand the rationale underlying nursing care. The emphasis is on orthopaedics, and there will be no discussion of paraplegia or quadriplegia.

ANATOMY

BONES

The bones of the spine and pelvis include the 26 vertebral bones of the spine; the 24 ribs and the sternum of the thorax; and the pubic, ilium, and ischium of the pelvis.

SPINAL COLUMN

The spine or vertebral column is a strong, flexible column that supports the head, provides a base for the ribs, and encloses the spinal cord. The 26 bones that comprise the adult spinal column are called the vertebrae and are divided into five regions. The cervical region has 7 vertebrae, the thoracic 12, the lumbar 5, the sacral one, and the coccygeal one. A lateral view of the vertebral column shows four curves, alternately convex and concave ventrally.

The vertebrae differ from one another in size and shape (Fig. 8–1, Fig. 8–2, & Fig. 8–3) but in general show a uniform structure. A vertebra is composed of (1) a weight-bearing portion, the body; (2) a part that protects the spinal cord, the neural foramen; (3) three projections on which muscles pull, the spinous process and the right and left transverse processes; and (4) four projections, the two superior and the two inferior articular processes, which restrict vertebral movements.

The body of the vertebra is the central mass of bone that forms its anterior part. The arch is composed of

two bony pedicles, which extend backward from the body, and two bony laminae, which complete the arch. The body and the neural arch enclose the spinal foramen, through which the spinal cord passes. The spinous process extends backward from the point of union of the two laminae. The transverse processes project laterally from each side at the junction of a lamina and a pedicle. The articular processes arise near the junction of a pedicle and a lamina. The superior articular processes project upward, and the inferior project downward, with the inferior articular processes of the

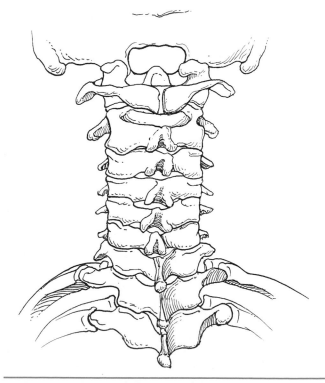

Figure 8–1 Drawing of the entire cervical and proximal thoracic posterior bony skeleton. *(Bridwell & DeWald (1997). The Textbook of Spinal Surgery. Philadelphia: Lippincott-Raven.)*

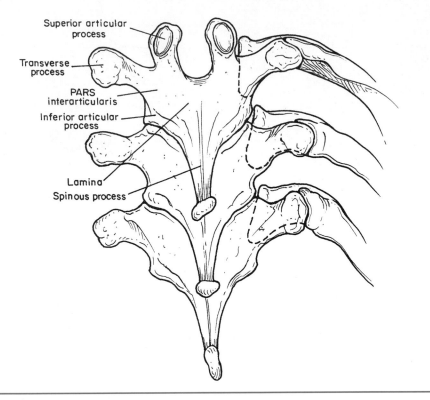

Figure 8–2   Thoracic spine bony anatomy.   *(Bridwell & DeWald (1997). The Textbook of Spinal Surgery. Philadelphia: Lippincott-Raven.)*

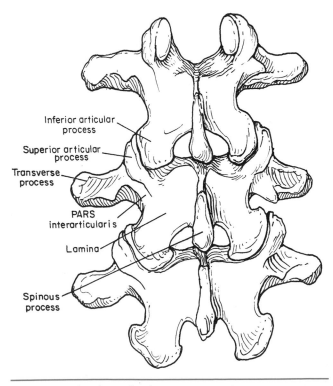

Figure 8–3   Lumbar spine bony anatomy.   *(Bridwell & DeWald (1997). The Textbook of Spinal Surgery. Philadelphia: Lippincott-Raven.)*

vertebra above fitting into the superior articular processes of the vertebra below. These are true joints, as their contact allows movement but prevents forward displacement of one vertebra with respect to another.

The vertebrae of the cervical region have foramina (openings) in the transverse processes. In the first six vertebrae, those foramina transmit the vertebral arteries. The spinous processes of the cervical vertebrae (Fig. 8–4) are short, with the third, fourth, and fifth vertebrae having bifurcated spinous processes. The seventh cervical vertebra has an unusually long spinous process, which can be felt as a prominence at the back of the neck. In general, the bodies of the cervical vertebrae are small, and the vertebral foramina are large and somewhat triangular. The first cervical vertebra (Fig. 8–5), called the atlas, has no body but is composed of an anterior and a posterior arch and two lateral masses. The second cervical vertebra (Fig. 8–6 & Fig. 8–7), the axis, has a process (the odontoid process) on the upper surface of its body that forms a pivot on which the atlas rotates. The thoracic vertebrae have facets for articulation with the ribs. All of the processes in the thoracic region (see Fig. 8–2) are larger and heavier than those in the cervical region, and the spinous processes are directed downward at a sharper angle. The vertebral foramen of the thoracic vertebrae are nearly circular. The lumbar vertebrae (see Fig. 8–3) have bodies that are larger and heavier than other vertebrae. The adult sacrum is composed of

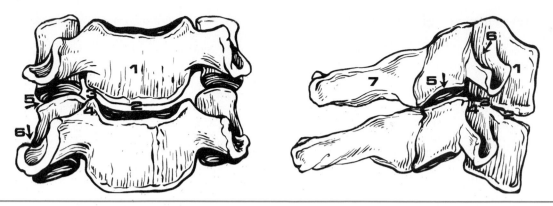

Figure 8–4   Anterior *(left)* and lateral *(right)* views of the midcervical vertebrae (C4 and C5). *(1)* Vertebral body, *(2)* disc, *(3)* uncovertebral joint, *(4)* uncinate process, *(5)* facet joint, *(6)* nerve root canal, and *(7)* spinous process.   *(Rockwood, C. A., et al. (1996). Rockwood & Green's Fractures in Adults. 4th ed. Philadelphia: Lippincott-Raven.)*

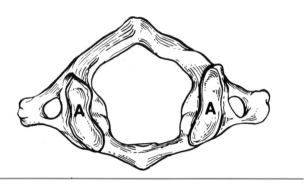

Figure 8–5   Superior view of the first cervical vertebra (atlas). The superior articular facets *(A)* provide support and flexion-extension motion of the occiput.   *(Rockwood, C. A., et al. (1996). Rockwood & Green's Fractures in Adults. 4th ed. Philadelphia: Lippincott-Raven.)*

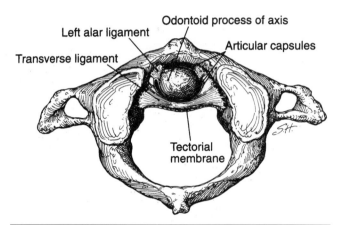

Figure 8–7   The thick transverse ligament is well positioned to prevent posterior displacement of the dens.   *(Rockwood, C. A., et al. (1996). Rockwood & Green's Fractures in Adults. 4th ed. Philadelphia: Lippincott-Raven.)*

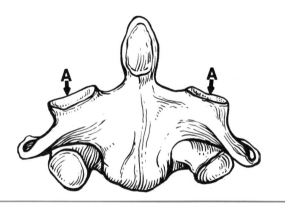

Figure 8–6   The second cervical vertebra (axis) superior articular facets *(A)* provide rotatory motion of C1 and C2. *(Rockwood, C. A., et al. (1996). Rockwood & Green's Fractures in Adults. 4th ed. Philadelphia: Lippincott-Raven.)*

five fused preadult sacral vertebrae. It is triangular in shape and fits like a wedge between the two halves of the pelvis. The coccyx is the terminal bone in the vertebral column. It is composed of four or five nodular pieces representing bodies of the preadult coccygeal vertebrae. The coccyx is triangular in shape, with its base attached to the sacrum.

THORAX

The thorax is a bony, cartilaginous cage whose walls are formed at the back by the thoracic vertebrae, at the sides by the ribs, and in front by the costal cartilages and the sternum. The 24 ribs, 12 on a side, are long, flat bones that both curve and twist. The first seven pairs, which are attached directly to the sternum by costal cartilages, are called "true" ribs. The next five pairs are called "false" ribs. The eighth, ninth, and tenth ribs are attached to the sternum through the costal cartilages of the rib immediately above. The eleventh and twelfth ribs are unattached and have been termed "floating" ribs. The sternum or breast bone is composed of the manubrium or handle, the body or blade, and the xiphoid process.

PELVIS

Pelvis is a Latin word meaning basin, and the pelvis can be seen as a basin formed by the right and left innominate bones, the sacrum, and the coccyx. The innominate bones, which constitute the pelvic girdle, are built for stability and are firmly united to the vertebral column. The pelvic girdle serves to link the legs to the spinal column. Each innominate bone is a large irregular bone. In children, the innominate bone is composed of three separate bones (the ilium, the pubis, and the ischium), all of which come together at the acetabulum.

The *ilium*, the upper portion of the innominate bone, has a broad and expanded prominence, the iliac crest. A projection of the anterior tip of the crest forms the anterior superior spine of the ilium. The anterior inferior spine is immediately below. There are the posterior superior and the posterior inferior iliac spines on the posterior crest. Beneath the posterior inferior iliac spine is the greater sciatic notch.

The *pubic* bone comprises the anterior part of the innominate bone and forms a joint at the body's midline known as the symphysis pubis. The pubic bone is composed of a body and two arms, or rami. The body of the pubic bone comprises about one fifth of the acetabulum. The upper, superior ramus is a rough ridge, the pubic crest. The inferior ramus passes downward and outward to meet the ischium. The pubic arch is formed by the inferior rami of both pubic bones, which converge at the symphysis.

The *ischium* forms the lower and back part of the innominate bone. It consists of a body and a ramus. The body of the ischium comprises a little over two fifths of the acetabulum. The lower portion of the ischium is a large, rough process, the ischial tuberosity, which supports the body in a sitting position. The sharp projection above the tuberosity is the spine of the ischium. The ramus of the ischium passes upward to join the inferior ramus of the pubis. The ischium and the pubis combine to form a large aperture, the obturator foramen.

JOINTS OF THE VERTEBRAL COLUMN AND THORAX

The vertebrae from the second cervical to the first sacral articulate with one another by a series of cartilaginous joints between the vertebral bodies and through a series of synovial joints between the vertebral arches. The vertebral bodies are united by an anterior and a posterior longitudinal ligament and by intervertebral discs of fibrocartilage known as symphyses. The anterior longitudinal ligament is a strong band that extends along the anterior surfaces of the vertebral bodies. The posterior longitudinal ligament is inside the vertebral canal on the posterior surfaces of the bodies of the vertebrae and extends from the axis to the sacrum.

INTERVERTEBRAL DISCS

An intervertebral disc is interposed between the adjacent surfaces of vertebral bodies from the axis to the sacrum. The shape of the disc corresponds to that of the adjacent vertebral bodies, and its thickness varies from anterior to posterior and by region of the column. The fronts of the discs are thicker than the backs in the cervical and lumbar regions and thus contribute to the anterior convexities of those levels. In the thoracic area, each disc is nearly uniform in thickness.

The discs are thinnest in the thoracic region and thickest in the lumbar region.

For the most part, discs are avascular in adults and are supported by diffusion through the spongy bone of the adjacent surfaces of the vertebrae. Each disc consists of an outer laminated portion, the annulus fibrosus, and an inner core, the nucleus pulposus. In teenagers, the intervertebral discs are so strong that when stress is applied to the vertebral column the bones ordinarily give way before the discs. After age 20, however, trauma may produce degenerative changes in the discs, leading to necrosis or sequestration of the nucleus pulposus and to softening and weakening of the annulus fibrosus. After such trauma, a comparatively minor strain may cause either an internal derangement of the disc with an eccentric displacement or bulging of the nucleus pulposus, or the nucleus pulposus may actually burst through the annulus fibrosus, usually in a posterolateral direction. In the former case, the unequal tension within the vertebral joint is responsible for muscle spasm and acute low back pain. In the latter case, the projecting nucleus pulposus may press upon and irritate the adjacent spinal nerve roots, causing referred pain, such as sciatica. Derangements of that kind may occur at any level but are most common in the lower lumbar region, especially at the lumbosacral joint and at the level of the fifth to seventh cervical vertebrae. Motor effects, with loss of power and reflexes, may also ensue.

VERTEBRAL ARCHES

The joints between the articular processes of the vertebrae are of two kinds, synovial and plain. Each joint has a thin, loose articular capsule attached just outside the margins of the articular facets of the adjacent articulating processes. They are longer and looser in the cervical region than in the thoracic and lumbar regions.

The laminae of adjacent vertebrae are connected by broad thin ligaments, the *ligaments flava*. They permit separation of the laminae in flexion and help to control movement. The ligaments flava also assist in restoring the vertebral column to the erect position after flexion and in protecting the vertebral discs from injury. The transverse processes are connected by the *intertransverse ligaments*.

In the cervical region (Fig. 8–8), the intertransverse ligaments consist of a few irregular, scattered fibers and are largely replaced by intertransverse muscles; in the thoracic region, they are rounded cords intimately connected with the deep muscles of the back; in the lumbar region (Fig. 8–9), they are thin and membranous. The spinous processes are connected by the *nuchal ligaments* from the occiput to the seventh cervical vertebra. From the seventh cervical vertebra to the sacrum, they are connected by the *supraspinal ligaments*. Adjacent spinous processes are connected by *interspinal ligaments* that extend from the root to the apex of each process and meet the ligaments flava in front and the supraspinal ligaments behind. The nuchal ligament is a fibroelastic membrane (or intermuscular septum) that, in the neck, is homologous to the supraspinous and interspinous ligaments of other levels. It extends from

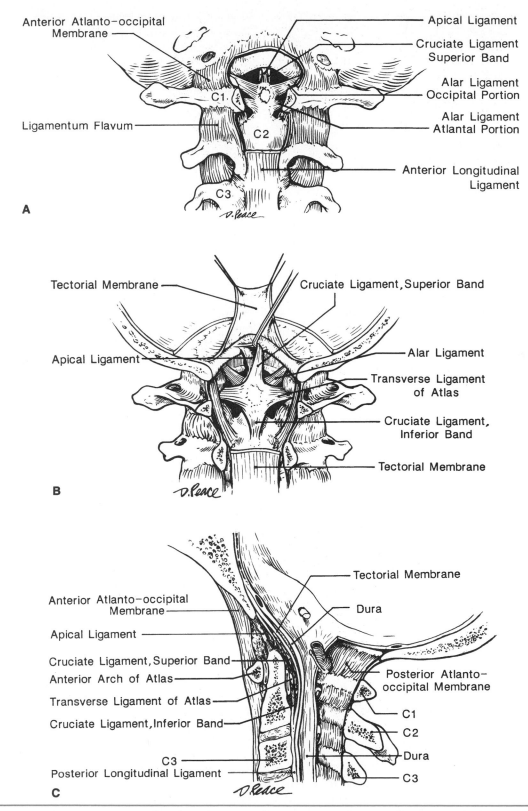

Figure 8–8 (A) Anterior, (B) posterior, and (C) lateral views of the upper cervical spine. Significant stability of this region is achieved through the transverse ligaments, the alar ligaments, and the facet joint capsules. *(Rockwood, C. A., et al. (1996). Rockwood & Green's Fractures in Adults. 4th ed. Philadelphia: Lippincott-Raven.)*

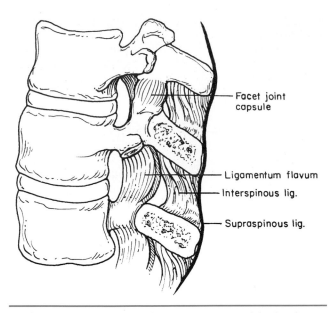

Facet joint
capsule

Ligamentum flavum

Interspinous lig.

Supraspinous lig.

Figure 8–9   Posterior ligamentous structures of the lumbar spine. *(Bridwell & DeWald (1997). The Textbook of Spinal Surgery. Philadelphia: Lippincott-Raven.)*

the external occipital crest to the spinous process of the seventh cervical vertebra. The nuchal ligament play an important role in holding the head erect.

MOVEMENTS OF THE VERTEBRAL COLUMN

The range of movement possible between any two adjoining vertebrae is restricted by the limited flexibility in the intervertebral disc between the vertebral bodies. Although movement between adjoining vertebrae is small, the sum of the movements gives a relatively wide range of motion to the vertebral column as a whole.

Flexion (forward bending), extension (backward bending), lateral flexion (bending to one side), circumduction (turning), and rotation (twisting) are all possible movements of the vertebral column. In flexion, the anterior longitudinal ligament is relaxed and the anterior parts of the intervertebral discs are compressed. At the limit of flexion, the posterior longitudinal ligament, the ligaments flava, and the intraspinous and supraspinous ligaments are stretched, and the posterior fibers of the intervertebral discs are decompressed. In extension, the opposite takes place. Extension is limited by the tension of the anterior longitudinal ligaments and by the approximation of the spinous processes. In lateral flexion, the sides of the intervertebral discs are compressed, with the extent of motion being limited only by the tension of antagonist muscles and surrounding ligaments. Circumduction is merely a succession of the preceding movements. Rotation is produced by the twisting of the vertebrae relative to each other with torsional deformation of the intervening intervertebral discs.

MUSCLES PRODUCING VERTEBRAL MOVEMENTS

The spinal column may be moved by muscles attached to it or by muscles attached to other bones that act on

it. Flexion involves the longus cervicis, the scaleni, the sternocleidomastoid, and the rectus abdominis of both sides. In extension, the erector spinae and the splenius and semispinalis capitis of both sides are involved. During lateral flexion, the longissimus and iliocostocervicalis components of the erector spinae and the oblique muscles of the side flexed are involved. In rotation, the rotatores, multifidus, and splenius cervicis are involved.

SPINAL NERVES

There are 31 pairs of spinal nerves; 8 pairs are cervical, 12 pairs are thoracic, 5 pairs are lumbar, 5 pairs are sacral, and one pair is coccygeal. The first pair of cervical nerves arises from the medulla oblongata and leaves the spinal canal between the occipital bone and the atlas. The other spinal nerves arise from the spinal cord, and each leaves the spinal canal through the intervertebral foramen behind the vertebra whose number it bears; for example, the sixth thoracic nerve emerges through the foramen between the sixth and seventh thoracic vertebrae. The coccygeal nerve passes from the lower extremity of the spinal canal.

Nerve plexuses are formed in the cervical, brachial, lumbar, and sacral segments. The cervical plexus is formed by the anterior branches of the first four cervical nerves. There is communication from the cervical plexus to the hypoglossal, vagus, and accessory nerves of the head and neck. The brachial plexus is formed by the union of the anterior branch of the last four cervical and the first thoracic nerves. Important nerves formed from the plexus are the median, ulnar, and radial nerves that supply the upper extremity. The lumbar plexus is formed by a few fibers from the twelfth thoracic and the anterior primary divisions of the first four lumbar nerves. The largest peripheral nerves formed are the femoral and obturator nerves. The sacral plexus is formed by a few fibers from the fourth lumbar nerve and the first three sacral nerves. The largest peripheral nerve is the sciatic, which supplies the muscles of the lower extremity. Other major nerves from the sacral plexus are the medial and posterior popliteal and tibial nerves, and the lateral popliteal and anterior tibial nerves.

CERVICAL SPINAL COLUMN

The cervical spine is completely encircled by intricate layers of muscles that function to control its movement and stabilize it. In the upright position, the cervical spine assumes a lordotic or convex inward curve known as the "relaxed" position. Any deviation from that position brings the muscles into play. Pain in and from the neck region can originate from many different tissue sites by many different mechanisms.

CERVICAL SPRAIN

Cervical sprain may be defined as a stretching disruption of the soft tissues that support the cervical spine.

The degree of injury may vary from a slight separation of a few fibers to an actual interruption of the gross ligament structure. Injuries that stretch the ligaments also involve other structures (e.g., disc, articular cartilage, and bone), damage to which must be assessed in every case. The most common ways of injuring the cervical vertebrae are by hyperflexion and hyperextension of the neck.

In a *hyperflexion* injury, the most superficial stabilizing ligamentous structure on the posterior aspect, the ligament nuchal, bears the brunt of the stretching force. It may be stretched or torn but usually heals rapidly. At times, however, it becomes elongated and permits excessive mobility of the cervical vertebrae at the affected level. An extreme forcible flexion injury, such as that sustained in a diving accident, usually tears the ligament nuchal at the lower cervical level (i.e., the C5–6, C6–7, or C7–T1) and can also involve the interspinous ligament. In such an extreme hyperflexion injury, the nuchal ligament may be torn or avulsed from the tips of the spinous processes.

In a *hyperextension* injury, when the head is thrust backward, the vertebrae are forced into an extremely lordotic position, the superior articulating processes displace inferiorly to an extreme degree, and the capsular ligaments are stretched. The anterior longitudinal ligament, which is very strong except when softened by disease, is rarely disrupted. The apex of the lordotic curve, from C3 to C6, receives the maximum amount of stress and is therefore the site of the patient's symptoms. A considerable amount of hyperextension force is usually necessary to produce posterior subluxation of one vertebra upon another. When it does happen, however, fractures of the posterior articulations or damage to laminae and discs often occur.

TYPES OF SPRAINS

A *mild sprain,* the most common type of cervical injury, involves mainly the muscles, and the symptoms usually last only a few days to a few weeks. The immediate discomfort is minimal but gradually intensifies in the hours after the injury. Motion in the neck becomes limited and painful, and the affected muscles are tender and painful when stretched. When these muscles are relaxed by heat and positioning, the discomfort is usually reduced.

A *moderate sprain* involves the ligaments as well as the muscles, with symptoms that persist well beyond the usual time required for recovery from a mild sprain. An initial short period of acute pain is usually followed by an interval of aching pain that is intensified by movements that exert tension on the affected ligaments. Over the hours following the injury, the pain usually becomes more severe, and protective muscle spasms become intense and persistent even while the patient is recumbent. The patient usually complains of generalized pain about the neck and referred pain to some distant point such as the occiput, the scapula, the upper extremity, or even the upper anterior chest area where it may be confused with pain of cardiopulmonary origin. Only

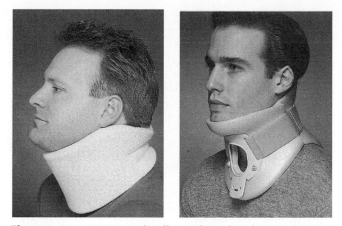

Figure 8–10 (A) Cervical collar with neck in hyperextension or reversed for flexion. (B) Philadelphia cervical collar. *(Courtesy of Zimmer, Inc.)*

absolute immobilization and strong sedation are usually effective in reducing the pain. During the initial acute phase, there are frequently vague complaints such as blurred vision, diplopia, vertigo, nausea, and headache. Those symptoms rapidly subside, although the headache may persist for a few weeks.

A *severe sprain* is one in which complete interruption of the ligaments takes place and is the result of a severe hyperflexion or hyperextension injury. The intensity of the trauma and the fragility of the tissues involved lead to a tearing of soft tissues and a displacement of the cervical vertebrae. Initially, the patient's symptoms are like those of a patient with a moderate sprain, but additional symptoms demonstrate the severity of the injury. Headache is typically occipital, although it may radiate forward. Vague symptoms such as vertigo, nausea, tinnitus, and blurred vision quickly subside, but the headache may continue indefinitely. Pain, paresthesia, and weakness in one or both upper extremities may develop at the time of injury or gradually over the first few hours. Those symptoms are often transitory and usually subside before medical attention can be obtained. Persistence of those symptoms is serious, as they may indicate associated neurologic damage.

TREATMENT

For moderate and severe sprains, a hot pack several times daily and analgesics usually help reduce pain from muscle spasms. Cervical traction is contraindicated in most instances, because traction stretches the damaged ligaments. However, light cervical traction (see Chapter 6) might be used, and sandbags may be placed beside the head to prevent unguarded motion. After a few days, a cervical collar (Fig. 8–10) may be applied, and the patient is then allowed to be ambulatory. If pain is provoked by bending the neck forward, the collar should be higher in front to hold the neck in a slight degree of extension. If extension is painful, the collar should be reversed. The collar is worn for several weeks or until all movement can be performed painlessly.

Physical therapy modalities such as infrared, diathermy, and ultrasound may also be used, but some physicians doubt their efficacy. Massage and manipulation are contraindicated, as they may tear the ligaments that are already softened by hemorrhage and edema. Restriction of cervical motion is continued until the ligaments are reconstituted and fixation is secured, which generally requires 4 to 6 weeks in cases of complete ligamentous separation.

CERVICAL DISLOCATIONS AND FRACTURES

Trauma to the cervical spine may produce a variety of injuries, varying from dislocations without fractures to massive fractures without dislocations. Frequently, both a fracture and a dislocation are sustained. Dislocations vary from mild spontaneously reduced subluxations to complete dislocations of the articular facets. Fractures associated with dislocations vary from small chip fractures of the distal border of a vertebra to complete separation of the pedicles, fractures of the articular processes, or marked compression fractures of the vertebral body. Milder injuries, such as crush or compression fractures of vertebral bodies or subluxations of the articular facets, usually respond satisfactorily to traction followed by immobilization in a cast or brace. More severe injuries may require surgery.

FRACTURE OF THE C1 VERTEBRA (JEFFERSON'S FRACTURE)

Ring fractures of the C1 vertebra (Jefferson's fracture) occur when a vertical compression force impacts downward on the articular facets of the skull, pushing the lateral masses outward and disrupting the ring of the atlas (Fig. 8–11). Normally, the articular processes of the atlas (C1 vertebra) face upward, inward, and slightly backward. The injury often results from a diving accident.

The patient's complaints may vary from minimal to severe pain, usually accompanied by gross limitation of movement. Tenderness is usually present posteriorly over the atlas. There is pain on extension of the neck, but rotation may be relatively pain free. There is a potential for injury to the suboccipital nerve, which crosses the posterior ring of the atlas to each lateral mass, and to the greater occipital nerve, which emerges just below the posterior ring of the atlas and supplies the skin over the occiput. If the fracture causes damage to the spinal cord, however, immediate death usually occurs.

Fractures of the C1 vertebra are normally treated conservatively, with cervical traction during the evaluation process, followed by a halo vest/cast (see Chapter 6) for 8 to 12 weeks. Rarely does the ring fracture heal completely (Meyers, 1997). When instability is identified, posterior arthrodesis between the occiput and the upper cervical segment is usually indicated. For a discussion of the halo vest/cast and nursing care, see Chapter 6. Fusion of the C1 to C2 may also be necessary to relieve painful arthrosis after Jefferson fractures (Main et al., 1998).

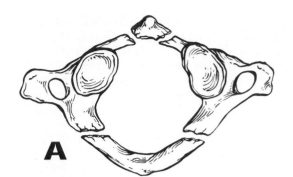

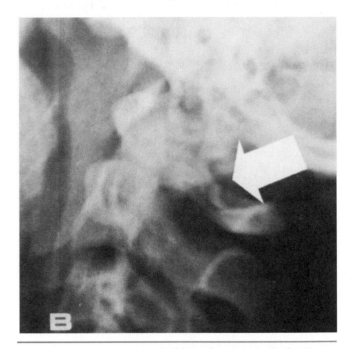

Figure 8–11   Diagram (A) and lateral x-ray (B) of a fracture of the ring of C1 (Jefferson's fracture).   *(Rockwood, C. A., et al. (1996). Rockwood & Green's Fractures in Adults. 4th ed. Philadelphia: Lippincott-Raven.)*

FRACTURE OF THE ODONTOID PROCESS

The C1 vertebra and the odontoid process of the C2 vertebra are a single functional unit. When the cruciate ligaments on the posterior aspect of the odontoid process remain intact following a flexion or extension injury to the upper neck, the result can be a fracture of the base of the odontoid process. The patient may have only minimal pain, but in most instances there is severe pain behind the ears and stiffness of the neck. Patients often complain of a feeling of instability at the base of the skull and hold or turn the head with their hands on top of the skull. There is usually no weakness or numbness of the extremities, but there is usually tenderness in the suboccipital region. The C1 vertebral fracture is the most common cervical fracture in individuals 70 years and older and probably presents more management problems than any other (Main et al., 1998).

Most often only type II fractures (Fig. 8–12) of the odontoid (i.e., fractures across the waist of the odon-

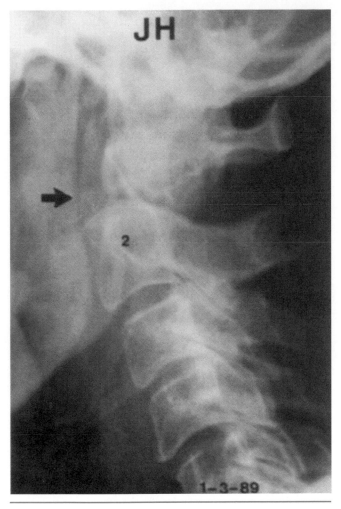

Figure 8–12   A type II odontoid fracture resulting from an extension-induced load. *(Bridwell & DeWald (1997). The Textbook of Spinal Surgery. Philadelphia: Lippincott-Raven.)*

toid) require surgical stabilization that is achieved by a C1–C2 posterior fusion. Type II fractures pass transversely across the base of the odontoid, leaving primarily cortical bone surfaces for healing. Some type II fractures through the waist of the odontoid are thought to result from a lateral force applied to the head with loading of the odontoid process against the lateral mass of C1. Others believe the fracture results from extension-induced loading.

In most instances, odontoid fractures are managed conservatively with a halo vest/cast (Meyers, 1997). Once reduction is accomplished, which is commonly done by placing the patient in cervical traction, the head and the neck are immobilized and held in position by a halo vest/cast. The cast is applied as soon as possible so that the patient can sit up and get out of bed. Immobilization is continued until the fracture is healed, usually about 3 months. Progressive mobilization of the neck is then initiated, and a soft collar is used until muscle strength has returned. If flexion and extension roentgenography do not demonstrate union 4 months after surgery, a posterior C1–C2 fusion is

usually done. In the elderly population, a posterior C1–C2 fusion is preferred over the halo. For discussion about the halo vest/cast and nursing care implications, see Chapter 6.

FRACTURE OF THE C2 VERTEBRA (HANGMAN'S FRACTURE)

Described first by Wood-Jones in 1913 and later named and described by R. C. Schneider in 1965, the hangman's fracture (Fig. 8–13) describes a group of fractures involving the C2 vertebra. The Levine classification of hangman's fractures is as follows: grade I is a bilateral pedicule, grade II is when both angulation and displacement of the body of the C2 vertebra are present, and grade III is when the fracture demonstrates gross instability (Meyer, 1997). The classic hangman's fracture injury is a bilateral fracture that passes through the posterior part of lateral masses and pedicles of the axis and into the intervertebral notch. The body of the axis is then subluxated or dislocated in relation to the body of the C3 vertebra. The skull and the C1 vertebra move as a unit with the body of the C2 vertebra, whereas the posterior elements of the C2 vertebra move with the posterior elements of C3.

Although hanging causes this injury by distraction and extension, other mechanisms that produce the same fracture occur in automobile accidents when persons catch their chin on the steering wheel or dashboard (causing flexion) or strike their forehead on the sun visor (causing extension). If the spinal cord is involved, most persons do not survive the initial trauma. Those who do may only complain of local pain, stiffness, and tenderness over the C2 spinous process. The injury is occasionally accompanied by other injuries in the lower part of the cervical spine.

Surgical management, should it be required, is a posterior fusion. Most of the cases are managed conservatively. Reduction of the fracture is usually accomplished with the neck in a neutral position and the application of traction (Fig. 8–14). Traction can produce distraction and subsequent nonunion or ligamentous instability if left on for too long. Patients may require intubation or a tracheotomy because of initial severe retropharyngeal swelling. Once reduction is achieved, the head and the neck are immobilized and held in position by a Philadelphia collar (see Fig. 8–10) or halo vest/cast, which is continued for 3 months. For discussion of the halo vest/cast and nursing care, see Chapter 6.

FRACTURES AND DISLOCATIONS OF THE C3 TO C7 VERTEBRAE

An *extension* injury to the neck can produce tearing of the anterior longitudinal ligament with or without an avulsion fracture of the anterior aspect of one of the vertebral bodies. Fractures of the pedicles (Fig. 8–15) and posterior subluxation may also occur. This injury is commonly associated with a rear-end automobile accident. Subsequent symptoms may last for a prolonged period of time without objective documentation of any

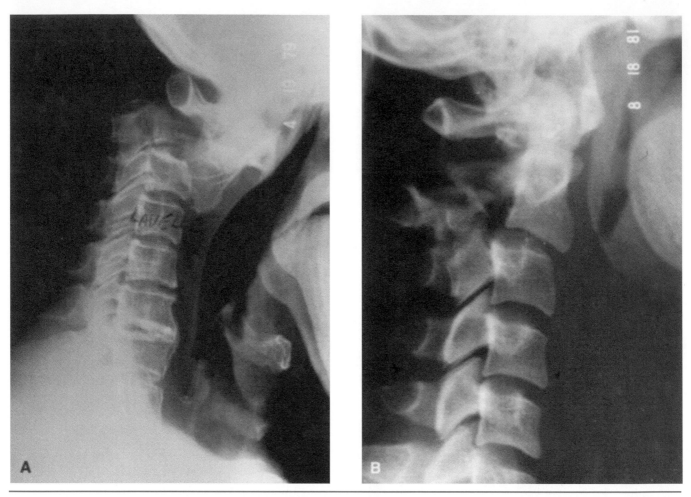

Figure 8–13   (A) Lateral radiograph of cervical spine demonstrating gross displacement grade III hangman's fracture with disruption of anterior and posterior longitudinal ligaments and bipedicle fractures. (B) Lateral radiograph of cervical spine demonstrating pedicle fracture of C2 (hangman's fracture) with resulting anterior displacement of C2 secondary to unilateral facet dislocation and disruption of the posterior longitudinal ligament. Both fractures were reduced by traction and managed conservatively with a halo vest.   *(Bridwell & DeWald (1997).* The Textbook of Spinal Surgery. *Philadelphia: Lippincott-Raven.)*

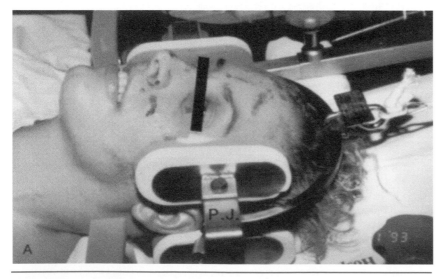

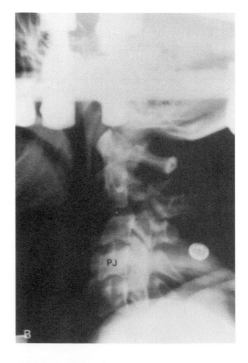

Figure 8–14   (A) P. J., a 29-year-old female unrestrained front seat victim of a motor vehicle accident. Patient's head struck windshield resulting in multiple facial lacerations. Neurologically, the patient remained intact. (B) Radiographs of the cervical spine revealed Type II C hangman's fracture. Fracture was managed in cervical fraction followed by a halo vest.   *(Bridwell & DeWald (1997).* The Textbook of Spinal Surgery. *Philadelphia: Lippincott-Raven.)*

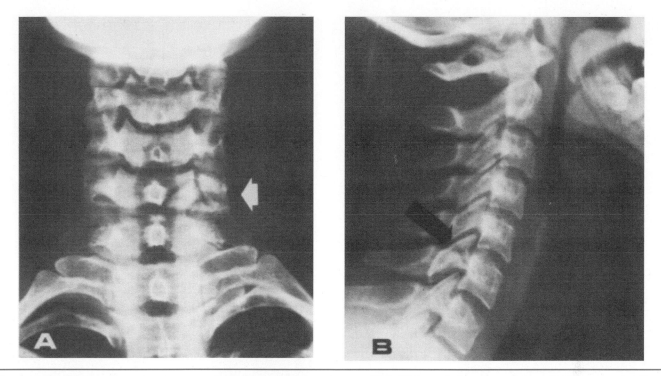

Figure 8–15   (A) An anteroposterior x-ray of a fracture of the lateral mass of C6. (B) Lateral view demonstrates the fracture extending through the pedicle and the facet.   *(Rockwood, C. A., et al. (1996). Rockwood & Green's* Fractures in Adults. *4th ed. Philadelphia: Lippincott-Raven.)*

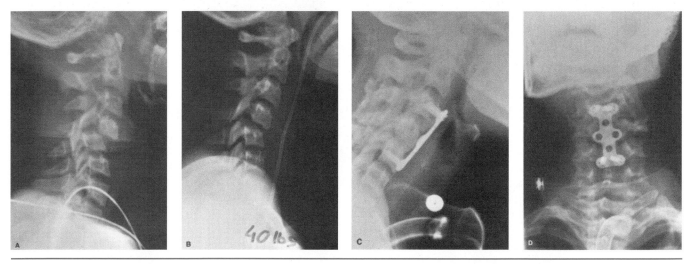

Figure 8–16   (A) After a diving accident, this patient presented with severe neck pain and a complete spinal cord injury. (B) Cervical fraction with 40 pounds results in reduction of the facets. (C) Surgical stabilization was performed with an anterior cervical plate and bone grafting. (D) Anteroposterior view of construct.   *(Rockwood, C. A., et al. (1996). Rockwood & Green's* Fractures in Adults. *4th ed. Philadelphia: Lippincott-Raven.)*

osseous or soft-tissue abnormalities. With *flexion* injuries, a unilateral dislocation or fracture-dislocation of the facets on one side of the neck can occur, whereas the interarticular facets on the other side usually remain intact. If a fracture is present, it is usually of the dislocated facet. Unilateral dislocation and interlocking of the cervical facets usually affect the lower cervical spine. The patient with a C3 to C7 fracture-dislocation usually complains of tenderness over one or more spinous processes and has limitation of movement and muscle

spasms. There may also be motor or sensory neurologic injuries including quadriplegia.

Whether or not neurologic damage is present, reduction of any displacement is essential. Reduction of dislocations and fracture-dislocations is accomplished with skull tongs. The patient is usually placed in skull tong traction with 15 pounds of weight, which may be increased by 5 pounds every hour until reduction is accomplished (Fig. 8–16; a discussion of skull tongs and the nursing care of a patient in a turning frame are pre-

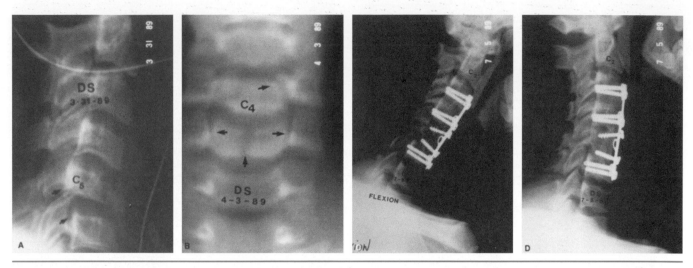

Figure 8–17   (A) Cervical radiograph revealing flexion axial loading injury at C5–C6. (B) Anterior tomogram reveals multiple associated posterior element fractures. (C, D) Fractures stabilized by A–O plate screw at C3–C6 because of fractures also identified at C4. Appropriate interbody fusions were accompanied at each intervening level.   *(Bridwell & DeWald (1997).* The Textbook of Spinal Surgery. *Philadelphia: Lippincott-Raven.)*

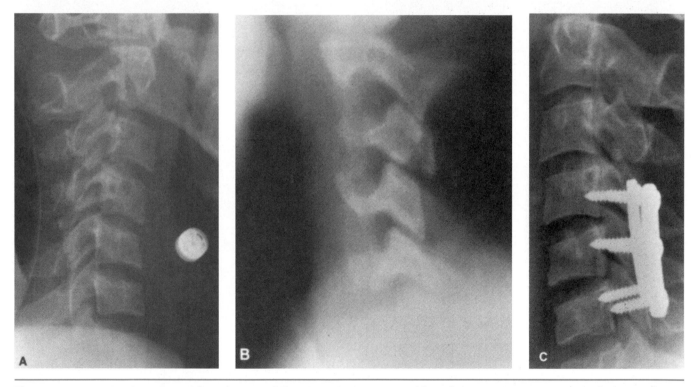

Figure 8–18   (A) C4–C5 unilateral facet fracture-dislocation. (B) Tomogram of facet fracture. (C) Posterior cervical plating of injury.   *(Rockwood, C. A., et al. (1996).* Rockwood & Green's *Fractures in Adults. 4th ed. Philadelphia: Lippincott-Raven.)*

sented in Chapter 6). After reduction is accomplished, immobilization using light skull traction may be continued for several days. In the absence of significant neurologic deficit, the patient may then be placed in a halo vest/cast. If the injuries are unstable, skull calipers with a halo vest/cast are used to immobilize the neck.

Stable fractures are treated nonoperatively with a brace, whereas unstable injuries with ligamentous tearing are usually considered for surgical treatment.

Unstable fractures are reduced by traction or surgical reduction of facet dislocations, followed by anterior (Fig. 8–17) or posterior instrumentation and fusion. Unilateral facet dislocations with nerve root impingement usually require early open reduction and fusion (Fig. 8–18 & Fig. 8–19).

Posterior Cervical Fusion with Instrumentation. A posterior cervical fusion is performed to relieve pain and

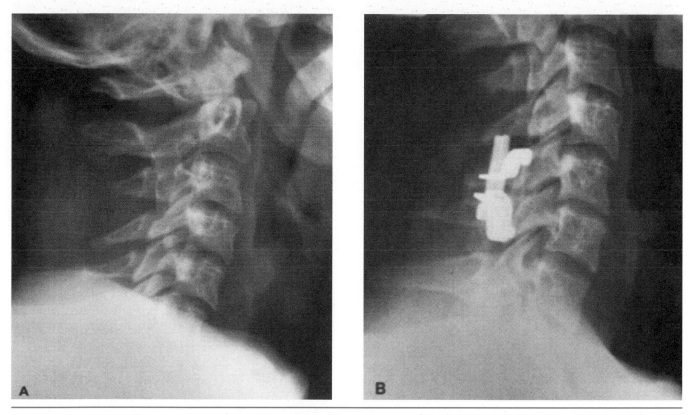

Figure 8–19 (A) C5–C6 unilateral facet fracture dislocation. (B) Reduction and fixation with laminar clamps. *(Rockwood, C. A., et al. (1996). Rockwood & Green's* Fractures in Adults. *4th ed. Philadelphia: Lippincott-Raven.)*

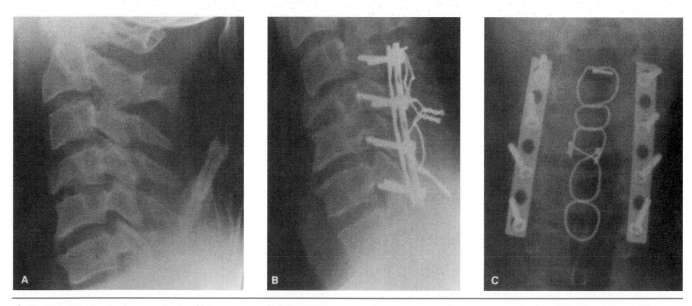

Figure 8–20 (A) Anterior column fracture with "hidden" posterior ligamentous failure. Note degenerative changes beneath fracture. (B) Posterior cervical plating to include degenerative segment. (C) Anterior view. *(Rockwood, C. A., et al. (1996). Rockwood & Green's* Fractures in Adults. *4th ed. Philadelphia: Lippincott-Raven.)*

provide stability in the cervical spine. This procedure may involve cervical fusion with bone grafting alone; cervical fusion with bone grafting and wiring; or cervical fusion with bone grafting and plates, screws, and wires (Fig. 8–20). When wires are used, holes are drilled through the cortices of the spinous process in each cervical vertebra being fused. A wire is then passed through each hole and twisted into place. One additional wire is placed around all of the vertebrae being fused. When screws and plates are used, the screws are placed through the middle portion of the vertebra into the body of the vertebra. Corticocancellous bone strips are taken from the iliac crest and laid along the vertebrae to aid in vertebral fusion. Postoperatively, a soft collar or brace is worn for 4 to 6 months until bony fusion occurs.

NURSING PROCESS (Patient with a Posterior Cervical Fusion with Instrumentation)

The following nursing process presents the care of a patient with a posterior cervical fusion with instrumentation (i.e., wiring) following a cervical fracture. The nursing process begins after the patient returns from surgery.

ASSESSMENT

The initial assessment of a typical patient following a posterior spinal fusion should emphasize the neurovascular status of the upper and lower extremities (see Chapter 2). Assess neurovascular status every 15 minutes for 2 hours, then every 30 minutes for 2 hours, every 2 hours for the next 24 hours, and then at the beginning of every shift, as spinal cord compression may produce rapid or delayed onset of paralysis. Assess the patient's blood pressure and pulse to determine cardiovascular status. Assess the patient's respiration for rate and depth and auscultate the lungs for clearness. Determine if the patient has any signs of nausea.

Determine that the suction and drains are working properly and note the amount of drainage. Inspect the dressing for serosanguineous drainage, which suggests a dural leak. Assess for signs of a headache. Check the dressing at the iliac crest if that area was used as a donor site for the bone fusion. Make sure that the patient is in correct body alignment and that the bed is either flat or with the head elevated but with no flexion at the neck. Assess for the severity, location, and duration of pain.

NURSING DIAGNOSIS

Based on all of the assessment data, the major nursing diagnoses for a typical patient following a posterior cervical fusion may include the following:

- Pain and discomfort related to trauma and immobility in the cervical area
- Impaired physical mobility related to instability of the cervical spine
- Anxiety related to knowledge deficit about the surgery and the rehabilitation process

COLLABORATIVE PROBLEMS

- Spinal nerve root injury or spinal cord injury
- Hematoma at the surgical site
- Infection

GOAL FORMULATION AND PLANNING

The goals are to have the patient experience (1) a decrease in pain through nursing measures and prescribed medications, (2) an increase in mobility with the use of a cervical collar, (3) a decrease in anxiety through patient education about the surgery and rehabilitation process, and (4) an absence of complications. Long-term goals are to have the patient free of pain and to have return of function and activities within 4 to 6 months.

INTERVENTIONS

ALLEVIATE PAIN

Following a posterior cervical fusion with wiring, the patient usually complains of pain at the surgical and donor sites. The donor site will usually cause the patient the most discomfort, and movement always produces pain in the beginning. Check the donor site for signs of a hematoma formation as this increases the amount of pain. Reposition the patient for comfort, reassure the patient that pain is normal but that it can be relieved with prescribed medications, and administer the analgesics.

INCREASE MOBILITY

Nursing interventions to increase mobility focus on position, exercises, and ambulation.

Position. Postoperatively the patient may wear a cervical collar or brace that contributes to limiting neck motion. The neck should be kept in a neutral (midline) position. During the immediate postoperative period, assist the patient in turning. As the patient changes position, make sure that the head, shoulders, and thorax are kept in alignment. Teach the patient to turn their body as a unit instead of turning the neck when looking from side to side.

Exercises. Exercises for the patient following a posterior cervical fusion include active range of motion to all joints except the spine and doing activities of daily living while keeping their shoulder, head, and neck working as one unit.

Ambulation. In the beginning, assist the patient in sitting up or getting out of bed by supporting the patient's neck and shoulders. Make sure the patient is wearing shoes, is not dizzy, and is steady on their feet before attempting to walk.

PATIENT TEACHING AND HOME CARE CONSIDERATIONS

The patient's hospital stay will probably be very short. The patient, the patient's family, and significant others need to understand the required home care for a smooth recovery. The patient needs to wear the cervical collar or brace for 4 to 6 months, until fusion is complete. The collar should be worn at all times until directed otherwise. A silk scarf can be placed under the collar/brace to increase comfort, but it must not be allowed to wrinkle or get bunched up under the collar. Caution the patient against flexing, extending, or rotating the neck to any extremes. Assist the patient in identifying strategies to cope with activities of daily living and to minimize risks to the surgical site. Instruct the patient to avoid sleeping in the prone position and to not prop themselves up in bed with pillows to minimize neck flexion.

To prevent infection, instruct the patient to wash the neck and incisional areas twice a day with a mild soap. With the patient sitting and supporting the front of the collar, an assistant removes one side tab and opens the posterior portion of the collar to wash the area. That tab is then closed, the other tab is opened, and the same procedure is done. The patient must keep their neck still while the collar is opened. The same procedure may be utilized for a man to shave. Men are also instructed to shave without moving or twisting their neck.

Staying as long as 30 minutes in one position (standing or sitting) can cause neck strain. Instruct the patient to alternate tasks in which greater body movement is required with nonmovement activities like reading or watching television. The patient is to avoid long automobile rides, as the vibration from the car on the highway is jolting to the spine.

MONITORING AND MANAGING POTENTIAL PROBLEMS

The major complications following a posterior cervical fusion include damage or contusion to the nerve root or to the spinal cord, hematoma, or infection. Damage to the nerve root or to the spinal cord can be due to retraction during surgery or from the initial injury if the fusion was done as the result of a cervical fracture. A contusion of the spinal cord or nerve root can also occur. Both result in weakness of muscles supplied by the nerve root or cord.

INFECTION

Check the donor and surgical sites for signs of redness or drainage, which may indicate infection. Determine that the patient's complaints of pain are not related to symptoms of infection. Verify that the patient's vital signs are within normal limits. Monitor the patient's cervical dressing for any signs of serosanguineous drainage. This could indicate a cut or tear in the dura and leakage of cerebrospinal fluid and could lead to meningitis.

HEMATOMA

Check the patient's initial drains to make sure they are working. Assess the patient for pain that may indicate the development of a hematoma. Inspect the incisional areas for any swollen or red areas. Blood can pool in the incisional or donor site areas if bleeding occurs and there is no exit for release.

EVALUATION/OUTCOMES

The patient should be free of pain or have reduced pain with cervical immobilization. The patient should be able to verbalize the restrictions in their mobility. The patient, the patient's family, and significant others should have acquired knowledge for self care and the detection of potential complications.

CLINICAL PATHWAY (Patient Having a Posterior Cervical Fusion and Instrumentation)

An example of a generic clinical pathway for a patient having a posterior cervical fusion with instrumentation is presented in Figure 8–21.

DEGENERATIVE DISEASES OF THE CERVICAL SPINE

Degenerative disease of the cervical spine is a fairly common problem and usually involves one of four major pathologic conditions. They are *cervical disc degeneration, degenerative arthritis* (see Chapter 3) *herniation of a cervical disc,* and *cervical nerve root compression.* Although the basic causes of these conditions are not yet known, the pathologic changes that occur in them are quite similar, differing only in degree. For example, cervical disc degeneration and degenerative arthritis of the cervical spine basically cause symptoms of pain and stiffness in the neck. Moreover, degenerative arthritis of the cervical spine and a herniated cervical disc may cause compression of the adjacent spinal nerve roots.

CERVICAL DISC DEGENERATION

Degeneration of a cervical intervertebral disc represents premature aging of the disc. The pathophysiology of disc degeneration involves the deterioration of the nucleus pulposus and annulus fibrosus and the lessening of the mechanical efficiency of the disc as a shock absorber or insulator between the adjacent vertebral bodies. The anterior margins of the involved vertebrae soon begin to show wear and osteophyte formation. With the decrease in the space between the vertebral bodies, the axis of motion shifts posteriorly to the apophyseal joints. Those joints cannot withstand the increased stress, and degenerative changes follow that alter the smooth contour of the apophyseal joints.

These patients are usually younger than those with degenerative arthritis of the cervical spine and more frequently are women. They complain of an acute onset of neck pain on one side that extends into the interscapular area. The symptoms may occur spontaneously or be the result of trauma. The patient typically complains of neck pain being worse upon rising in the morning, pain associated with occipital headaches, or pain radiating into the trapezium muscle and into the shoulder area.

Figure 8–21

Clinical Pathway: Posterior Cervical Fusion with Instrumentation

Admission Date: _____   **Discharge Plan:** _____ **Home** _____ **Skilled Nursing** _____ **Extended Care Facility**

Pathway	Preadmission Office/OP clinic	Admission Day Op day	Hosp Day 2 Post-op 1	Hosp Day 3 Post-op 2	Hosp Day 4 Post-op 3	Hosp Day 5 Post-op 4	Outcomes
Consultation	Primary Care/ Medical physician	Case Manager Anesthesia, PT					Cont. @ Home
Assessment	Nrsg database H & P Exam. by MD, NP or PA	Review & add Review H & P Postop routine				Resolved	
	Rehab/ECF/home Assessment of the Neurovasuclar status of extremities		Referral if nec. N/V status of ext.	Cont.	Cont.	Cont.	Cont.
Tests	ECG/UA/CXR/ chem 7 Coag. studies if app Cervical Spine X-rays, MRI, & CTM	H & H in PACU & repeat in pm					
Medications	D/C NSAIDs/ASA/ b/4 OR	Anticoagulant Routine meds	Cont. Anticoag.	Cont.	Cont.	Cont.	States meds, when to take and purpose
	Instruct on preop meds b/4 OR	✓ preadm meds IV Antibiotics		D/C antibiotics			
	Analgesics as nec	PCA/Epidural pump		D/C IV and begin Oral pain meds			Pain managed with Analgesics @ home
		Bowel protocol					Normal bowel function
Diet	Assessment wt. balanced diet	NPO @ MN b/4 OR Ice chips	Liquids	Advance as tol Roughage & liquids			Tolerating diet
Activity	Preop mobility	Ankle Pumps	Cont.				
		Turn upper body as a unit q 2 hrs	Turn q 2hrs				
		Quad & Glut q 2	Cont.				
		Bed rest with HOB elevated 45	OOB to BR with C. Collar	Walking with C. collar assistance			Walking @ home with cervical collar without assistance
Treatments		IV fluids/blood if necessary, I&O					
		TEDs or IPCD					Cont. TEDS § home
		Hemovac/output	Do not change	D/C			No complications
		Incisional dressing	Do not change	Change dressing		Change PRN	No infection
		Donor site dressing		Change dressing		Change PRN	
		IS/TCDB q hr w/a		PRN			Clear lungs
Education	Review pre & postoperative care procedures (moving upper ext. as a unit)	Reinforce	Cont.	Cont.			
	Rev. rehabilitation, body mechanics & exercises		Rev. hosp routine Review rehab			Reinforce	Continue with exc. regime and walking with C. collar on
	Attends gp ed class		Reinforce Ed.				
	Pain management	Rev. pain mgmt	Reinforce				
	Rev. basic back care						
	Review hosp LOS						

(continued)

Figure 8–21

Clinical Pathway: (continued)

Pathway	Preadmission Office/OP clinic	Admission Day Op day	Hosp Day 2 Post-op 1	Hosp Day 3 Post-op 2	Hosp Day 4 Post-op 3	Hosp Day 5 Post-op 4	Outcomes
D/C Plan	Identify discharge plan Caregivers & home situation (LOS 2–3 days)		Notify Social Worker Or Home Health if nec.				Discharged to home States reasons to contact physician

The majority of patients gain relief by heat applications or hot showers, salicylates and anti-inflammatory drugs, and resting the neck with the use of a soft cervical collar, especially during sleep.

CERVICAL NERVE ROOT COMPRESSION

Any condition of the neck that causes impingement or entrapment of a cervical nerve root or encroachment on its intervertebral foramen may cause cervical nerve root compression syndrome. The most frequent causes over the entire spine are degenerative arthritis and a herniated intervertebral disc, although in the cervical spine, degenerative changes with accompanying posterior spur formation are the most common. Less frequent causes include cervical subluxations and dislocations, cervical fractures with backward displacement of the fragments, congenital anomalies of the cervical spine, and tumors. The most common areas of involvement are C5–6 and C6–7, with entrapment of the sixth and seventh cervical nerve roots. Treatment depends on the cause, but most react to conservative treatment of immobilization, salicylates, and anti-inflammatory drugs. Cervical fusion is the surgical treatment.

Anterior Interbody Cervical Fusion. In an anterior interbody cervical fusion, the approach is commonly made through an anterolateral incision. The cervical disc is removed, the interbody space is curetted, and any osteophytes of the vertebral body are excised. A bone graft taken from the iliac crest is cut to fit into the space from which the disc was removed. The bone graft is put into place and the surgical incision closed. Following closure and the application of a dressing, the patient is placed in a soft cervical collar. At about the seventh to tenth day after surgery, the patient may be placed in a more rigid brace. Excessive extension of the neck is to be avoided to prevent unsatisfactory impaction or anterior displacement of the graft. Accurate and continuous observation is essential to prevent respiratory distress, neurologic deficits, and hematoma formation at the neck and at the donor site. Bony fusion is usually established in approximately 5 to 6 months. The wearing of the neck brace is gradually reduced as the fusion becomes complete.

NURSING PROCESS (Patient with an Anterior Interbody Cervical Fusion)

The following nursing process presents the care of a patient following an anterior interbody cervical fusion. The nursing process begins after the patient returns from surgery.

ASSESSMENT

The initial assessment of a typical patient following an anterior interbody cervical fusion should emphasize the neurovascular status of the upper and lower extremities (see Chapter 2). Assess neurovascular status every 15 minutes for 2 hours, then every 30 minutes for two hours, every 2 hours for the next 24 hours, and then at the beginning of every shift, as spinal cord compression may produce rapid or delayed onset of paralysis. Assess the patient's blood pressure and pulse to determine their cardiovascular status. Assess the patient's respiration for rate and depth, and auscultate the lungs for clearness. Determine if the patient has any signs of nausea.

Verify that the suction and drains are working properly and note the amount of drainage. Inspect the dressing for serosanguineous drainage, which suggests a dural leak. Note any complaint of a headache. Check the dressing at the iliac crest if that site was used as a donor site for the bone fusion. If the patient complains of excessive pressure in the neck or severe pain in the incisional area, check for bleeding.

Determine that the patient is in correct body alignment and that either the bed is flat or the head of the bed is elevated without any flexion at the neck. Assess the severity, location, and duration of pain. Observe the patient for the return of any radicular (spinal nerve root) pain, which may indicate that the spine is unstable. Throughout the postoperative course, monitor the patient to detect any signs of respiratory difficulty, neurologic deficits, or hematoma formation at the neck and donor site.

NURSING DIAGNOSIS

Based on all of the assessment data, the major nursing diagnoses for a typical patient following an anterior interbody cervical fusion may include the following:

- Pain and discomfort related to trauma and immobility in the cervical area
- Impaired physical mobility related to instabiliy of the cervical spine
- Anxiety related to knowledge deficit about the surgery and the rehabilitation process

COLLABORATIVE PROBLEMS

- Neurologic deficit
- Respiratory distress
- Hematoma
- Infection

GOAL FORMULATION AND PLANNING

The goals are to have the patient experience (1) a decrease in pain through nursing measures and prescribed medications, (2) an increase in mobility with the use of a cervical collar, (3) a decrease in anxiety through patient education about the surgery and the rehabilitation process, and (4) an absence of complications. Long-term goals are to have the patient free of pain and to have return of function and activities.

INTERVENTIONS

ALLEVIATE PAIN

Following an anterior interbody cervical fusion, the patient usually complains of pain at the surgical and donor sites. The donor site will usually cause the patient the most discomfort, and movement always produces pain in the beginning. Check the donor site for signs of hematoma formation, as this increases the amount of pain. Check for bleeding that is manifested by the complaint of excessive pressure in the neck or severe pain in the incisional area. Reposition the patient for comfort, reassure the patient that pain is normal but that it can be relieved with prescribed medications, and administer the analgesics. If the patient experiences a sudden reappearance of pain, report that to the physician immediately, as an extrusion of the graft may have occurred, requiring a return to surgery and a repositioning of the graft.

Usually the major complaint of the patient is a sore throat, hoarseness, and dysphagia due to temporary edema. These symptoms are usually relieved by throat lozenges, voice rest, and humidification. A blenderized or full liquid diet may be given if the patient has dysphagia.

INCREASE MOBILITY

Interventions to increase mobility are correct positioning, turning, exercises, and ambulation.

Position. Postoperatively, the patient is placed in a soft cervical collar, which contributes to limiting neck motion. The patient is kept flat for 12 to 24 hours with their neck in a neutral (midline) position. Instruct the patient to keep their shoulders flat on the bed and not to try raising up in bed.

Turning. Assist the patient in turning during the immediate postoperative period. As the patient changes position, make sure that the patient's head, shoulders, and thorax are kept in alignment. The patient should be taught to turn the body as a unit instead of turning the neck when looking from side to side.

Exercises. Exercises for the patient following a cervical fusion include active range of motion to all joints except the spine and doing activities of daily living while keeping their shoulder, head, and neck working as one unit.

Ambulation. In the beginning, assist the patient in sitting up or getting out of bed by supporting the patient's neck and shoulders. Make sure the patient is wearing shoes, is not dizzy, and is steady on their feet before attempting to walk. Walk with the patient until they are safe to walk by themselves.

PATIENT TEACHING AND HOME CARE CONSIDERATIONS

The patient's hospital stay will probably be very short. The patient, the patient's family, and significant others need to understand the home care required for a smooth recovery.

The patient needs to wear the soft cervical collar at all times until directed otherwise, usually for 7 to 10 days after surgery. At that time, the patient is placed in a more rigid brace that is worn until bony fusion, which is usually established in 5 to 6 months. The wearing of the brace is gradually reduced as the fusion becomes more complete. A silk scarf can be placed under the collar to increase comfort, but it must not be allowed to wrinkle or get bunched up under the collar. Caution the patient against flexing, extending, or rotating the neck to any extremes to prevent unsatisfactory impaction of the graft or anterior displacement. Assist the patient in identifying strategies to cope with the activities of daily living and to minimize risks to the surgical site. Instruct the patient to avoid sleeping in the prone position and to not prop themselves up in bed with pillows to minimize neck flexion.

To prevent infection, instruct the patient to wash the neck and incisional areas twice a day with a mild soap. With the patient sitting and supporting the back of the collar, an assistant removes one one side tab and opens the anterior portion of the collar to wash the area. That tab is then closed, the other tab is opened, and the same procedure is done. The patient must keep their neck still while the collar is opened. The same procedure may be utilized for a man to shave. Men are also instructed to shave without moving or twisting their neck.

Staying as long as 30 minutes in one position (standing or sitting) can cause neck strain. Instruct the patient to alternate tasks in which greater body movement is required with nonmovement activities like reading or watching television. The patient is to avoid long automobile rides as the vibration from the car on the highway is jolting to the spine even with the collar or brace in place.

MONITORING AND MANAGING POTENTIAL PROBLEMS

Uncommon complications following an anterior interbody cervical fusion include injury to the carotid or vertebral artery, recurrent laryngeal nerve dysfunction, esophageal perforation, and airway obstruction. The major complications are neurologic deficit, respiratory distress, hematoma, and infection.

NEUROLOGIC DEFICIT

Throughout the postoperative period, the patient must be monitored to detect any signs of neurologic deficit. Both the upper and lower extremities must be assessed. Weakness because of cord compression, due either to swelling, bleeding, or dislocation of the graft, may produce rapid or delayed onset of paralysis.

RESPIRATORY DISTRESS

Throughout the postoperative period, the patient must be monitored to detect respiratory problems. As a result of the trauma from surgery, swelling in the incisional area can apply pressure that impedes adequate respirations. Occasionally, during surgery, the recurrent laryngeal nerve may be injured by retractors, resulting in hoarseness and inability to cough effectively. Without an effective cough, the elimination of pulmonary secretions becomes a problem that requires more extensive chest physical therapy. If not resolved, the patient can develop pneumonia.

HEMATOMA

Check the patient's initial drains to make sure they are working. Assess the patient for pain that may indicate the development of a hematoma at the neck and at the donor site. Inspect the incisional area for any swollen or red areas. Blood can pool in the incisional and donor site areas if bleeding occurs and there is no exit for release.

INFECTION

As a norm, patients are usually placed on prophylactic antibiotics with one dose before surgery and continued doses for 24 to 72 hours after surgery. Check the donor and surgical sites for signs of redness or drainage, which may indicate infection. Determine that the patient's complaints of pain are not related to symptoms of infection. Verify that the patient's vital signs are within normal limits. Monitor the patient's cervical dressing for any signs of serosanguineous drainage. This could indicate a cut or tear in the dura

and a leakage of cerebrospinal fluid, which could lead to meningitis.

EVALUATION/OUTCOMES

The patient should be free of pain or have reduced pain with cervical immobilization. The patient should be able to verbalize restrictions in their mobility. The patient, the patient's family, and significant others should have acquired knowledge for self-care and the detection of potential complications.

CLINICAL PATHWAY (Patient with an Anterior Interbody Cervical Fusion)

An example of a generic clinical pathway for a patient having an anterior interbody cervical fusion is presented in Figure 8–22.

HERNIATION OF A CERVICAL DISC

Herniation of a cervical disc (Fig. 8–23) occurs laterally where the annulus fibrosus is weakest and the posterior longitudinal ligament is thinner. Thus, on the herniated side, there are symptoms of nerve root compression with radicular pain and paresthesia corresponding to the nerve root dermatome. Persistent pain in the neck and arm is usually caused by cervical nerve root compression at an intervertebral foramen. The processes that lead to herniation are (1) the formation of osteophytes that encroach on the intervertebral foramen and cause a narrowing of the intervertebral disc, and (2) an acute posterolateral rupture of a cervical disc with immediate compression of the nerve root in the foramen. They usually occur at the site of maximum mobility, that is, 95% herniate at the fifth and sixth cervical junction and the remainder at the fourth and seventh.

When there is a herniation of the fifth cervical disc, the symptoms usually are (1) paresthesia in the thumb and the radial side of the hand; (2) hypesthesia in the sixth cervical dermatome on the dorsal and lateral aspects of the thumb and the radial side of the hand; (3) weakness and atrophy in the biceps; and (4) reduction of the biceps reflex, which is indicative of sixth cervical nerve root involvement. With a herniation of the sixth cervical disc, the symptoms usually are (1) pain and paresthesia in the index and middle fingers and in the dorsum of the hand on compression testing; (2) hypesthesia in the seventh cervical dermatome, that is, the index and middle fingers and the dorsum of the hand; (3) weakness and atrophy in the triceps; and (4) reduction of the triceps reflex, which is indicative of seventh cervical nerve root involvement.

Most of the patients with a herniated cervical disc obtain satisfactory relief from conservative treatment. This includes the use of a cervical head halter (see

Figure 8–22

Clinical Pathway: Anterior Interbody Cervical Fusion

Admission Date: _____   **Discharge Plan:** _____ **Home** _____ **Skilled Nursing** _____ **Extended Care Facility**

Pathway	Preadmission Office/OP clinic	Admission Day Op day	Hosp Day 2 Post-op 1	Hosp Day 3 Post-op 2	Hosp Day 4 Post-op 3	Hosp Day 5 Post-op 4	Outcomes
Consultation	Primary Care/ Medical physician	Case Manager Anesthesia, PT					Cont. @ Home
Assessment	Nrsg database	Review & add					
	H & P Exam. by MD, NP or PA	Review H & P					
		Postop routine				Resolved	
	Rehab/ECF/home		Referral if nec.				
	Neurovascular status	Note hoarseness/ swelling in the cervical area	N/V status of ext.	Cont.	Cont.	Cont.	No N/V deficiet
			Cont. to assess	Cont. to assess			No complications
Tests	ECG/UA/CXR/ chem7	H & H in PACU & repeat in pm					
	Coag. studies if app						
	Cervical Spine X-rays, MRI, & CTM						
Medications	D/C NSAIDs/ASA/ b/4 OR	Anticoagulant	Cont. Anticoag.	Cont.	Cont.	Cont.	States meds, when to take and purpose
	Instruct on preop meds b/4 OR	Routine meds					
		✓ preadm meds					
		IV Antibiotics		D/C antibiotics			
	Analgesics as nec	PCA/Epidural pump		D/C IV and begin Oral pain meds			Pain managed with Analgesics @ home
		Bowel protocol					Normal bowel function
Diet	Assessment wt. balanced diet	NPO @ MN b/4 OR	Liquids	Advance as tol			Tolerating diet
		Ice chips		Roughage & liquids			
Activity	Preop mobility	Ankle Pumps	Cont				
		Turn upper body as a unit q 2 hrs	Turn q 2hrs				
		Quad & Glut q 2	Cont.				
		Bed rest with HOB elevated 45	OOB to BR with C. Collar	Walking with C. collar assistance			Walking @ home with cervical collar without assistance
Treatments		IV fluids/blood if necessary, I&O					Cont. TEDS § home
		TEDs or IPCD					No complications
		Hemovac/output		D/C			
		Dressing	Do Not Change	Change Dressing		Change PRN	No infection
		IS/TCDB q hr w/a		PRN			Clear lungs
Education	Review pre & postoperative care procedures (moving upper ext. as a unit)	Reinforce	Cont.	Cont.			
			Rev. hosp routine				Continue with exc. regime and walking with C. collar on
	Rev. rehabilitation, body mechanics & exercises		Review Rehab			Reinforce	
	Attends gp ed class		Reinforce Ed.				
	Pain management	Rev. pain mgmt	Reinforce				

(continued)

Figure 8–22

Clinical Pathway: *(continued)*

Pathway	Preadmission Office/OP clinic	Admission Day Op day	Hosp Day 2 Post-op 1	Hosp Day 3 Post-op 2	Hosp Day 4 Post-op 3	Hosp Day 5 Post-op 4	Outcomes
D/C Plan	Rev. basic back care Review hosp LOS Identify discharge plan Caregivers & home situation (LOS 2–3 days)		Notify Social Worker Or Home Health if nec.				Discharged to home States reasons to contact physician

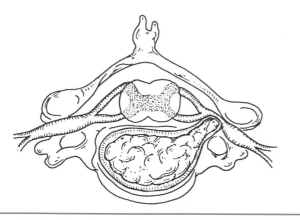

Figure 8–23 Typical posterolateral herniated nucleus pulposus in the cervical spine. *(Bridwell & DeWald (1997). The Textbook of Spinal Surgery. Philadelphia: Lippincott-Raven.)*

Chapter 6) at home, soft cervical collar or brace, bed rest, sedatives, hot packs applied to the neck at frequent intervals to reduce muscle spasms, and possibly the use of muscle relaxants. The patient needs to continue with the treatment for a long period of time and may even be advised to set up a cervical skin traction apparatus at home. Surgery is done only for persistent or frequently recurring pain and disability.

Cervical Laminectomy. A cervical laminectomy is a surgical procedure to remove a herniated nucleus pulposus. A midline incision is usually made from the spinous process of the fourth cervical vertebra to the first thoracic vertebra, and the posterior muscles are separated at the midline by blunt dissection. The laminae of the fifth, sixth, and seventh cervical vertebrae are then denuded, and the attachment of the ligamentum is separated from the anterior surface of the laminae above. The caudal third of the lamina above the lesion and the cephalic third of the lamina below the lesion are then removed laterally. If a herniated disc is present, the adjacent nerve root has probably been flat-

tened and displaced posteriorly. The nerve root is retracted upward, and the herniated disc is removed. The removal of the disc is usually easy unless there are bone spurs from osteoarthritis that displace the nerve root backward. The surgical wound is then closed, and in many instances a wound drain is put into place. The nursing care for a posterior or anterior laminectomy follows closely those of the posterior and anterior fusion procedures discussed earlier. However, there is less restriction on mobility, and with a laminectomy the patients only have a recovery period of about 6 weeks.

THORACIC SPINAL COLUMN

FRACTURES

The most common injury to the thoracic region of the back is a compression fracture of a vertebral body. This injury can arise in many ways, including a fall from a height, the effects of an explosion, or a hyperflexion of the spine. The most frequent is a wedge compression fracture of a vertebral body. In that injury, one or more vertebral bodies collapse anteriorly, become wedge-shaped, and create a prominence of the spinous process posteriorly. Neurologic deficits may occur, depending on the severity of the injury. The fracture is basically stable in that no further deformity is likely to occur. The usual treatment is a short period of bed rest followed by the redevelopment of the spinal muscles. Hyperextension jackets and posterior spinal supports are usually contraindicated, as they cause stiffness in the uninjured parts of the spine and thus may do more harm than good.

There are other types of compression fractures of the thoracolumbar spine. One is when a vertebral body is invaded by both of its adjacent discs and a biconcave prominence is produced; that *codfish* is seen in advanced cases of osteoporosis, and the bone deformity is caused by chronic compressive stress. A *burst* or

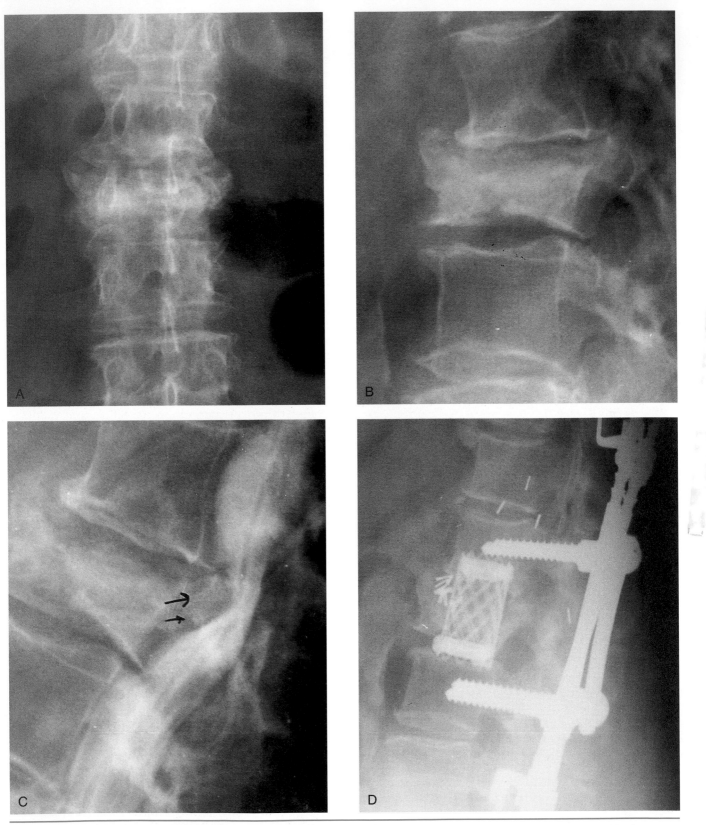

Figure 8–24   (A) AP view of osteoporotic burst fracture in a 63-year-old woman. (B) Lateral view reveals collapse of both anterior and middle columns. (C) Myelogram demonstrates compression of the column of dye by retropulsed bone fragment. (D) Postoperative plain film after posterior stabilization, anterior vertebrectomy, and vertebral body reconstruction with a titanium mesh cylinder.   *(Koval & Zuckerman (1998).* Fractures in the Elderly. *Philadelphia: Lippincott-Raven.)*

explosion (Fig. 8–24) fracture is caused by extreme compression on a vertebral body that produces a vertical fracture, which splits the body in two. The fracture is stable unless the posterior portion displaces posteriorly into the spinal canal, causing a neurologic deficit. There is normally little stress on ligamentous structures. If a large compressive force is applied to the spine with degenerated and extensively fibrosed intervertebral discs, the most likely result is a uniform flattening of a vertebral body.

Compression fractures of the thoracolumbar spine are usually treated with bed rest on a firm mattress followed by early mobilization. While on bed rest, sitting is not permitted. The head of the bed should not be elevated more than 20 to 30 degrees, and turning the patient from side to side must be done by logrolling. Analgesics are usually given for pain relief if there is no complication from head injuries. When the initial pain subsides, progressive muscle strengthening exercises for the spine are started. When the patient begins to ambulate, a reinforced thoracolumbar garment (corset) or orthosis is usually worn for 6 to 8 weeks for comfort. During that time, exercises to strengthen the spinal extensor muscles are encouraged so that use of the orthosis can be discontinued. Exercises that involve spinal flexion, such as sit-ups, are discouraged.

In fracture-dislocations of the thoracolumbar spine that do not involve paraplegia, open reduction and fusion by means of plating the spinous processes and bone grafting are indicated to prevent subsequent neurologic damage. With incomplete paraplegia of sudden traumatic onset, treatment may include bed rest on a turning frame. A spinal fusion is done later. Even with complete paraplegia, early open reduction, plating, and bone grafting are necessary to reduce the risk of subsequent injury to nerve roots that have been spared, to facilitate nursing care, and to get the individual up safely.

SCOLIOSIS

Scoliosis is a lateral curvature of the spine that can result from either a specific pathology or from unknown causes. It may develop in a localized area or involve the entire spinal column, and the degree of curvature may be mild, moderate, or severe. Scoliosis is classified by the nature of the lateral curvature produced, specifically, (1) functional curvature, where there are no structural alterations within the vertebral column; (2) structural curvature, where there are structural alterations within the vertebral column; (3) S-shaped curvature, a double curvature comprised of a major curve and a compensatory curve; (4) C-shaped curvature, where the lateral curvature involves all or most of the lumbar and thoracic areas; and (5) double major curvature, where there are two primary curves of equal or almost equal size. For a more in-depth discussion of pediatric scoliosis, see references at the end of the chapter.

After vertebral growth is completed (at approximately age 15 for women and age 17 for men), an existing scoliosis persists into adult life. The major impairments are the cosmetic deformity, pulmonary complications, and pain. The involved vertebrae may rotate, producing rib cage deformities and decreasing pulmonary capacity. In severe scoliosis, when the curvature exceeds 50 degrees in the thoracic region, cardiopulmonary complications are possible. Patients with a large curvature in the lumbar region may experience considerable pain. Confirmation of adult scoliosis is based on clinical examination and roentgenograms.

Treatment of adult scoliosis is different from that of the childhood disease. The adult spine is less flexible and thus less correctable by flexibility exercises, bracing, casting, or use of a scoliotron. The progress of adult scoliosis is not a result of vertebral epiphyseal deformation, but of asymmetrical intervertebral disc compression and degeneration on the concave side of the curves. In adult scoliosis, the increase in spinal curvature due to disc deterioration may be one degree per year. A scoliotic curve of 45 degrees in a patient aged 17 might be considered acceptable, but 20 years later, when the patient is 37, the curvature could approach 65 degrees. Advances in the past few decades have improved surgical methods of correcting the curvature in adult scoliosis and preventing the progression of the deformity. Even with surgical intervention, however, it is impossible to totally correct the curvature or eliminate the deformity.

POSTERIOR SURGICAL INTERVENTIONS

Surgical interventions for the management of spinal curvatures have changed greatly over the years. In 1914, Hibbs performed the first successful surgical treatment for curvatures of the spine, treating patients with tuberculosis and scoliosis. He fused the patient's spine without instrumentation and used a cast for immobilization. There were many failures due to the inability to determine when the fusion was solid and how long the back needed to be immobilized. In the 1930s, spinal fusions were done in conjunction with discectomies because it was thought that the spine was rendered unstable by the removal of a disc. Later, bone grafting was added to surgical fusion to increase the stability to the spine (Ficner, 1993).

The *Harrington rod instrumentation system* (Fig. 8–25), named for Paul Harrington, was the first instrumentation used to correct the deformed spine. In the 1950s, Harrington developed his system for the correction and stabilization of spine through the use of distraction. The use of such implants added to the stability of the spine, improved fusion healing, and allowed earlier mobility in a molded cast. Today, the Harrington rod instrumentation procedure is used to treat adolescent idiopathic scoliosis, juvenile idiopathic scoliosis if the curve is unresponsive to bracing, individuals with a large kyphosis unresponsive to bracing, and adult patients with a large kyphosis of the spinal column. The system is usually contraindicated for use in patients

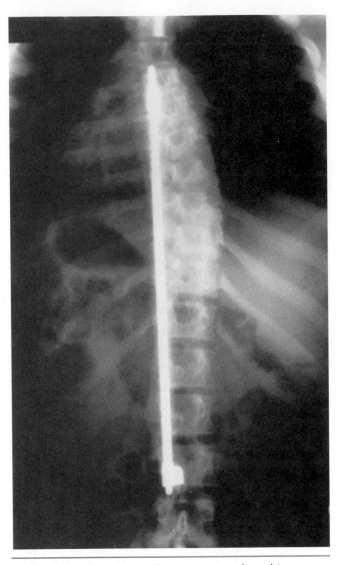

Figure 8–25   Spinal fusion for progressive idiopathic scoliosis using Harrington distraction instrumentation. *(Weinstein & Buckwalter (1994). Turek's Orthopaedics: Principles and Their Application. 5th ed. Philadelphia: J. B. Lippincott.)*

with congenital scoliosis and paralytic curvatures due to neuromuscular disease. A disadvantage of the Harrington technique is that two levels above and below the injured segment are also fused, and thus spinal mobility is significantly reduced.

The surgical procedure for Harrington rod instrumentation involves having the patient placed on the operating table in the prone position, and a midline incision is made down the center of the patient's back (even though the spinous processes deviate due to the curvature). All soft tissue and cortical bone are denuded from the spinous processes laterally to the transverse processes on both sides of the spine. Hooks are then placed in vertebrae at the upper and lower portions of the curve, and the Harrington rod is attached. Distrac-

tion forces are exerted as the rod is extended, reducing the spinal curvature. (The amount of correction of the curvature obtained varies according to the flexibility of the spine; on average, the curvature is reduced approximately 50%.) Large amounts of cortical and cancellous bone are then placed over the rods and the denuded area. Some bone for the graft may have been obtained from the iliac crest. The incision is closed with wound catheters in place.

Postoperatively, physicians would apply a body jacket cast immediately. However, the norm today is to place the patient in a regular bed for some 5 to 7 days and then apply a cast/brace. The cast/brace is used to immobilize the spine and promote the healing of the surgical fusion. If a cast is used, it can extend in front from the axilla or suprasternal notch of the upper chest down to the symphysis pubis, and in the back from the scapulae over the iliac crest to the tip of the coccyx so as to prevent the slightest degree of spinal flexion. Some body jacket casts may include the thighs and the pelvis or even the cervical spine. After the cast is applied, the nurse must repeat the assessment and nursing measures used immediately after the patient's return from surgery.

The *Luque rod instrumentation procedure* (Fig. 8–26), developed by Edward Luque, uses rods and sublaminar wires in a posterior fusion technique as an attempt to increase the points of fixation of the spine to increase stability. It is usually reserved for patients with neuromuscular conditions who cannot tolerate the reduced respiratory capacity associated with the application of a cast. However, some physicians utilize Luque rod instrumentation for all surgical conditions of the spine. The Luque rod procedure involves inserting a large amount of instrumentation (sublaminar wires) near the spinal cord, requires a longer period under general anesthesia, increases the risk of neurologic problems, and increases blood loss. Blood loss is especially great for patients with neuromuscular problems due to poor muscle tone.

A midline incision is made down the back, usually from the high thoracic area to the sacral area. The posterior elements in the thoracic area are exposed laterally to the facet joints, in the lumbar area to the transverse processes, and at the lumbosacral junction to the sacral alae. The facet joints are removed and packed with bone grafts from the iliac crest. The spinous processes are then removed, and the ligamentum flava is detached between each lamina to expose the neural canal. Loops of 16-gauge stainless steel wire are passed under and around each lamina. The L-shaped aspect of the Luque rod is then driven through the iliac wing along the superior border of the sacral alae. The first rod is placed on the convex side of the curve. The wires are then sequentially tightened by twisting distally to proximally. The second Luque rod is then placed on the concave side and wires tightened. Finally, the Luque rods are wired together transversely in two or three places with double

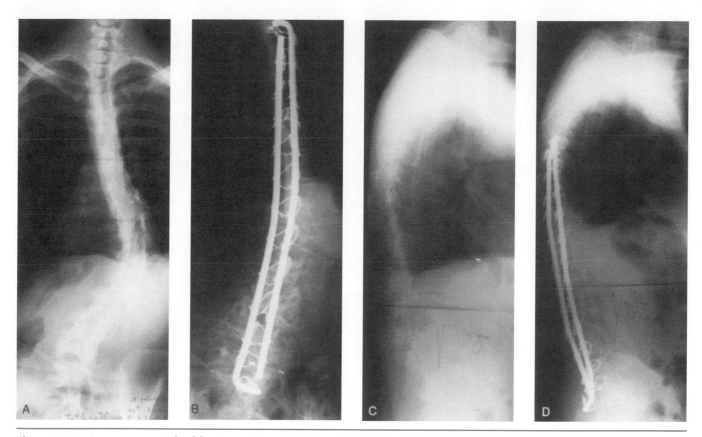

Figure 8–26 Luque segmental sublaminar wiring. (A, B) A painful progressive thoracolumbar curve reduced from 60 degrees to 46 degrees with pain alleviation. Fusion was to L5. (C, D) Lordosis was increased L–S1 from 8 degrees to 20 degrees. *(Bridwell & DeWald (1997).* The Textbook of Spinal Surgery. *Philadelphia: Lippincott-Raven.)*

wire loops. The posterior elements are decorticated, and the bone graft is placed along the entire area for fusion. The wound is then closed and a compression dressing applied.

Postoperatively, the patient with Luque instrumentation is cared for very much like a patient with Harrington rod instrumentation, but the patient with Luque rod instrumentation is active after surgery. The patient may be allowed to sit up in bed the evening of surgery, but most patients do not sit up until the second, third, or later postoperative day. Patients need to wear a brace or orthoplast jacket as a protective body splint. By the fifth to tenth postoperative day, most patients begin to return to their moderate preoperative activity levels. Potential postoperative complications are atelectasis, retention of secretions in the lung, decreased circulatory volume, and neurovascular deficit.

The *Wisconsin technique*, using Harrington rods and spinous process wiring, provides stability with decreased risk to neural elements. Harrington rod instrumentation with sublaminar wiring is indicated for the same type of patients as the Harrington procedure. The addition of sublaminar wires increases stability through segmental fixation and helps to decrease thoracic hypokyphosis (Green, 1997). Most patients with

this form of segmental instrumentation require no postoperative immobilization.

In 1963, Roy Camille used transpedicular screws to attach posterior spinal plates to the spine with excellent results. However, the technique did not become popular until the 1980s. Today, there are many systems (e.g., Cotrel-Dubousset, TSRH, Steffee, Danek, and others not listed here) that utilize plates or rods with screws to provide rigid fixation of the spine during fusion. For more information on pedicle screw instrumentation in the lumbar spine, see spinal fixation with pedicle screws later in this chapter.

The *Cotrel-Dubousset (CD) system* (Fig. 8–27), developed by Dr. Yves Cotrel and Dr. Jean Dubousset in the 1980s, is a system with many points of fixation and the capability to compress, distract, and derotate the spine. The Cotrel-Dubousset system uses a series of hooks that are vertically placed on both sides of the spine and connected by parallel rods. Because of its ability to derotate the vertebral bodies and reduce the patient's rib hump deformity, it is utilized to correct kyphosis and lordosis in scoliotic spines. Many surgeons believe the Cotrel-Dubousset system is secure enough to entirely eliminate a postoperative brace in adolescents. The *TSRH implant system* is a modification of the

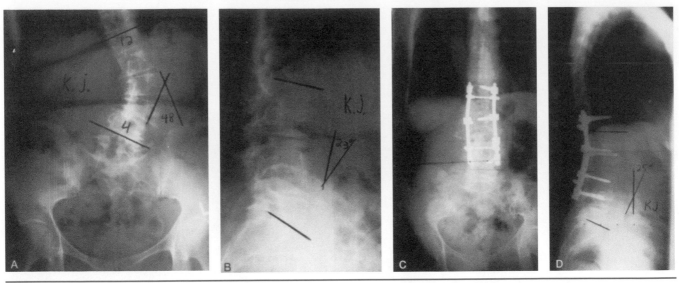

Figure 8–27   A 58-year-old female. (A) Progressive painful curve. Stage 1: Multiple anterior discotomies with morselized bone graft. Stage 2: Cotrel-Dubousset instrumentation and fusion. (B) Preoperative lateral view. Note significant loss of lordosis (–23 degrees L1–S1). (C) Postoperative anteroposterior view. (D) Postoperative lateral view. Note significant return of lumbar lordosis due to derotation and anterior release (increase of 48 degrees).   *(Bridwell & DeWald (1997). The Textbook of Spinal Surgery. Philadelphia: Lippincott-Raven.)*

Cotrel-Dubousset system that was developed by the physicians at Texas Scottish Rite Hospital for Crippled Children in Dallas.

NURSING PROCESS (Patient with Posterior Instrumentation for Scoliosis)

The following nursing process presents the care of a patient following a posterior instrumentation for scoliosis. The nursing process begins after the patient returns from surgery.

ASSESSMENT

The initial assessment of a typical patient following a posterior spinal fusion with instrumentation should emphasize the neurovascular status of both lower extremities (Chapter 2). Assess neurovascular status every 15 minutes for 2 hours, then every 30 minutes for 2 hours, every 2 hours for the next 72 hours, and then at the beginning of every shift. Check the patient's vital signs. Verify that the wound suction is working properly, and determine the amount of drainage. A cell saver may be used since these patients have significant blood loss during surgery. The patient's bed should be flat, and the patient should be in correct body alignment with no elevation of the shoulders. Assess the severity, location, and duration of pain. Determine if the patient has any signs of nausea.

Continuing assessment should include an evaluation of the patient's understanding of postoperative care. Monitor the patient's intake and output, and check the specific gravity of the patient's urine. Assess anal sphincter control by digital examination, and assess urinary sphincter control after the Foley catheter is discontinued. Continue to assess the amount of pain, and be especially alert for sudden onset of pain between the shoulders. Check bowel sounds. Assess the patient's anxiety level, and note any signs of depression.

NURSING DIAGNOSIS

Based on all of the assessment data, the major nursing diagnoses for a typical patient following a posterior instrumentation for scoliosis may include the following:

- Pain and discomfort related to surgery
- Impaired physical mobility related to the instability of the spine
- Anxiety related to knowledge deficit about the surgical procedure and the rehabilitation process

COLLABORATIVE PROBLEMS

- Neurologic injury
- Pulmonary complications
- Gastrointestinal complications
- Circulatory complications
- Infection
- Hematoma
- Fluid and electrolyte imbalance
- Instrumentation failure
- Nonunion of the fusion

GOAL FORMATION AND PLANNING

The goals are to have the patient experience (1) a decrease in the amount of pain through nursing measures and prescribed medications, (2) an increase in mobility through the use of a body cast/body brace and through controlled ambulation, (3) a decrease in anxiety through increased knowledge, and (4) an absence of complications from surgery and decreased activity. Long-term goals are to have the patient free of pain and to have return of function and activities.

INTERVENTIONS

ALLEVIATE PAIN

Following a posterior spinal fusion with instrumentation, the patient will usually have a fair amount of back pain from the surgery. Injections of narcotics such as morphine sulfate (subcutaneous) every 2 to 4 hours PRN or the use of a PCA are usually necessary for the first 48 to 72 hours after surgery. After 72 hours, oral narcotics such as hydrocodone or propoxyphene are usually sufficient. For anxious patients, hydroxyzine and, for muscle spasms, diazepam may be used in addition to the pain medications. Pain at the graft site on the iliac crest is also common. Movement always produces pain in the beginning, though medications for muscle spasms are not usually needed. Each patient has a different level of pain tolerance. The use of noninvasive measures such as conveying a sense of concern by talking softly to the patient, and using therapeutic touch, distraction, relaxation techniques, and visual imagery are also effective in reducing the degree of pain.

INCREASE MOBILITY

Early ambulation after posterior spinal instrumentation is optimal to prevent problems of immobility such as loss of muscle tone and decreased endurance. The major activities to increase mobility are correct positioning, turning, exercises, ambulation, and bracing.

Position. Following spinal surgery, the patient's bed should be kept flat and have a solid bottom or a board under the mattress. The patient is usually kept on their back for the first 8 hours to keep compression on the operative site and is tilted only briefly to assess the dressing. After the first 8 hours, the patient is usually turned every 2 to 3 hours as ordered. Some physicians restrict the patient's turn to only 20 to 30 degrees on either side. Patients should not lift their shoulders off the bed. If the patient should start to sneeze or vomit, assist the patient by holding their shoulders to keep stress off the spine. While the patient is supine, some physicians allow the knee gatch to be raised or pillows placed under the knees to reduce stress on the back. The patient is usually on bed rest for the first 24 hours and then advanced to sitting in bed.

Turning. The patient is turned by log-rolling and by using a turning sheet. The turning sheet should be about 78 inches long and 65 inches wide so that it will extend from the patient's shoulders to the knees. A draw sheet is not always adequate, but a folded top sheet generally

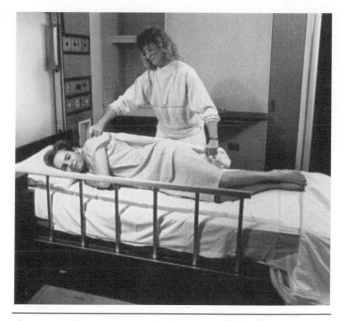

Figure 8–28 Draw sheet, placed from shoulders to pelvis, provides uniform support for the back as the patient is turned from side to side. *(Bridwell & DeWald (1997).* The Textbook of Spinal Surgery. *Philadelphia: Lippincott-Raven.)*

works. Ideally, one nurse should be able to turn the patient with a turning sheet (Fig. 8–28), but for the first couple of turns, immediate postsurgical for a large or obese patients may require two nurses to turn the patient safely and also to ensure safety for the nurses.

When two persons are needed to move and turn a patient lying on a turning sheet, they should stand on opposite sides of the bed. If the patient is very heavy or is unconscious, a third person is usually needed to support the head and neck or the legs. Before starting to move the patient, the patient's arms should be crossed over their chest, the pillow under the head removed, and one or two pillows placed between their legs. Take hold of the turning sheet at the level of the patient's buttocks and shoulders. Using an overhand grasp, both persons should roll or gather the sheet until their hands touch the patient's body, and then pull the draw sheet taut.

The person on the side of the patient that is to be raised calls the signals. The first step is to move the patient to the signal caller's side of the bed. Grasp the turning sheet and stand facing the patient with one foot closer to the bed than the other. The person who will move the patient toward them (the signal caller) has their weight on the forward foot. The other person has their weight on the back foot.

Both movers should flex their hips and knees. The signal caller gives the count, and the movers shift their weight from one foot to the other as they move the patient to the side of the bed. To turn the patient, the signal caller grasps the turning sheet at the level of the patient's shoulders and buttocks. The other person reaches across the patient and grasps the turning sheet at the level of the patient's knees and waist. That positioning makes it possible to turn the patient's trunk, hips,

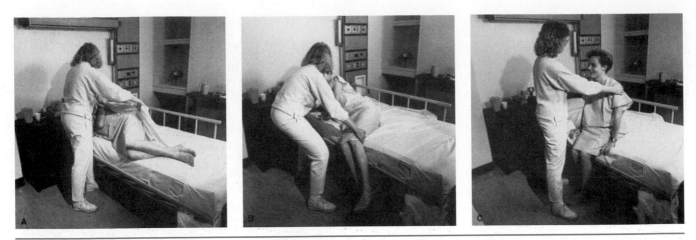

Figure 8–29 Mobilization activities include sitting. (A) Using an appropriately placed draw sheet, the patient is turned to the side-lying position. (B and C) The patient pushes up with the arms as the legs swing over the side of the bed in one motion. *(Bridwell & DeWald (1997). The Textbook of Spinal Surgery. Philadelphia: Lippincott-Raven.)*

and knees simultaneously, thus reducing the chances of twisting the patient's spine. The movers should flex their hips and knees and turn at the signal caller's count.

Once the turn is completed, the person on the side the patient is turned toward helps the patient maintain that position, while the signal caller places pillows for support. A pillow is placed under the patient's head, and two pillows may be used to support the patient's back and buttocks. Reposition the pillow or pillows between the patient's legs. A pillow can be placed in front of the patient's chest to support the patient's uppermost arm.

To turn a patient to their left side without a turning sheet, both persons should stand on the right side of the bed. Each person has the same foot forward and that leg is braced against the bed. The movers bend at the hips and knees and place their arms under the patient. One person places their hands and forearms all the way under the patient's upper trunk. The other person places their hands and forearms under the patient's buttocks, keeping the arms close together so the buttocks will not sag and make lifting the patient difficult. The person who is lifting the buttocks calls the signals. Turning the patient is done in approximately the same manner as with a turning sheet. Follow the procedure already described, moving the patient with your arms instead of the sheet.

Once the patient is able to help to some extent, log-rolling can be accomplished by one person with or without a turning sheet. Eventually, the patient may feel able to turn on his or her own, but patients with Harrington rod instrumentation should not do so. Other patients may be allowed to turn themselves but not until after proper instructions so that they will be able to keep their spine straight.

Exercises. Check with the patient's physician on the type of exercises allowed. Most patients do muscle-setting exercises (such as quadriceps- and gluteal-setting exercises) and some mild active exercises to the lower

extremities (such as plantar and dorsiflexion and active range-of-motion of the ankles). Some institutions utilize a footboard or flexion pillow at the foot of the bed to support the patient during the exercises. Exercises for the upper extremities involve muscle-setting exercises, activities of daily living (such as bathing the face and the arms), and other mild range-of-motion exercises to help maintain muscle strength.

Ambulation. By the third or fourth day after surgery, patients are usually allowed to stand by the side of the bed and to ambulate to the bathroom with assistance. Some patients may progress more rapidly. The rationale for ambulation is that loading the spine helps to lay down new bone and thus facilitates calcification. In the beginning, a tilt table may be used to get the patient up if there is concern about orthostatic hypotension. For some patients, it may take a day or two before they can stand upright without dizziness or other symptoms of hypotension. Patients need assistance in log-rolling to the side of the bed and getting to a sitting position before actually standing (Fig. 8–29). Patients will also need assistance in ambulating until they learn to maintain balance.

Bracing. Most patients will wear a thoracolumbosacral (TLSO) orthosis (Fig. 8–30) after surgery to support their back. Since the patient has to be able to stand for 10 minutes for the orthosis to be molded, it is usually molded approximately 5 or 6 days after surgery (Ficner, 1993). Once the brace is prepared, the patient will wear it for approximately 7 months and is then weaned off the brace over the next 2 to 3 weeks. For patients in a cast, see cast care in Chapter 5.

PATIENT TEACHING AND HOME CARE CONSIDERATIONS

Patient teaching for a patient having a posterior spinal fusion with instrumentation begins preoperatively. Review with the patient how to properly turn in bed, how to get out of bed, how to get in and out of a chair,

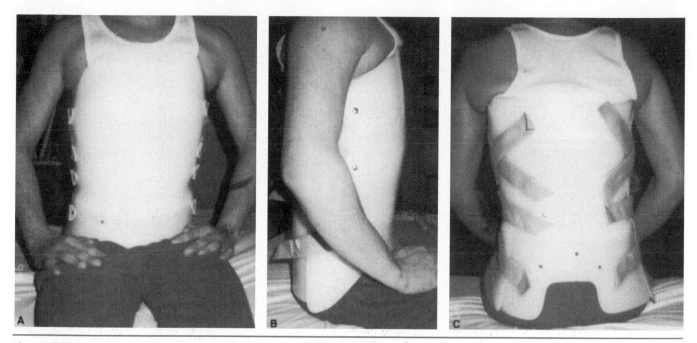

Figure 8–30   A patient lie with a custom thoracolumbosacral orthosis (TLSO) labricated from a body cast mold. Note the contouring over the iliac crests. (A) Anterior view (B) Lateral view. (C) Posterior view.   *(Rockwood, C. A., et al. (1996). Rockwood & Green's Fractures in Adults. 4th ed. Philadelphia: Lippincott-Raven.)*

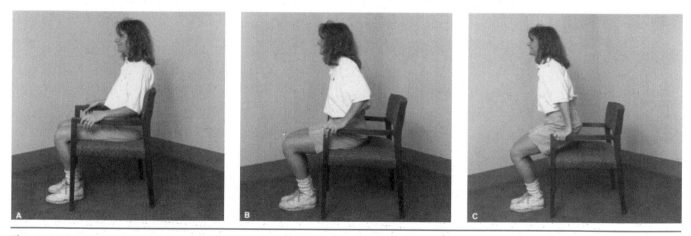

Figure 8–31   (A) Patient is sitting correctly in a suitable chair with armrests. (B) Preparing to arise, the patient moves the buttocks to the front edge of the chair. (C) Using the arms and legs, the patient arises, keeping the back straight.   *(Bridwell & DeWald (1997). The Textbook of Spinal Surgery. Philadelphia: Lippincott-Raven.)*

and how to do activities of daily living. Reinforce proper body mechanics, especially the use of the legs instead of the back in getting in out of a chair (Fig. 8–31) and how to get in and out of a car.

Instruct the patient, family, and significant others on cast/brace care. Discuss activity/rest levels, incisional care, and pain management. Since the cast/brace can cause some people to feel full after only a small amount of food, discuss utilizing small frequent feedings to maintain their weight. Focus on foods high in iron to help restore blood loss, foods high in calcium to help with fusion, and foods high in roughage and fluids to counteract the side effects of pain medications. It is

essential to have therapeutic communication to determine the patient's understanding of the rehabilitation process and to reinforce any weak points. Make sure the patient knows the signs and symptoms of potential problems, such as infection, or problems with the cast or brace that may develop after the patient returns home.

MONITORING AND MANAGING POTENTIAL PROBLEMS

Following a posterior spinal fusion with instrumentation, the patient is a potential candidate for all of the complications of immobility (especially respiratory, integumentary, and musculoskeletal problems), and nursing measures should be instituted to prevent those difficulties (see Chapter 4). There are also potential surgical complications, however, including neurologic impairment, altered gastrointestinal status, wound complications, urinary infection, fluid and electrolyte imbalance, instrumentation failure, and fusion failure.

NEUROLOGIC COMPLICATIONS

The most feared complication of spinal surgery is neurologic injury. To reduce this risk, the wake-up test was devised to be done after instrumentation and distraction but before closure. The patient is prepared before surgery so they can follow orders. The patient is awakened, and movement is assessed in both lower extremities. If one or both pyramidal tracts of the spinal cord have been injured, clonus is absent on the affected side. If neurologic function is abnormal, the instrumentation is removed and neurologic function is retested. If neurologic function does not return, the instrumentation is not replaced. However, if the neurologic function has returned, the spine may be reinstrumented but with slightly less distraction force. The patient is tested with the wake-up test again. If it is again abnormal, the instrumentation is removed and not replaced.

Other potential neurologic complications are muscle weakness, paresthesia, and dural lacerations. Neurovascular checks help in the early detection of potential problems. Subjective data presented by the patient may be complaints of "heaviness" in the legs indicating muscle weakness, or of "tingling" or "pins and needles" in the legs indicating sensory nerve impairment. A neurologic injury can also include loss of bowel and bladder control. Lacerations of the dura are usually detected and corrected in surgery. If the laceration was undetected, however, the patient may complain of a headache similar to that experienced after a spinal tap.

RESPIRATORY COMPLICATIONS

Patients are prone to pulmonary infections in the first 72 hours, especially without proper pulmonary hygiene. Teach the patient to cough and deep breathe and to use an incentive spirometer. Turning also assists in helping to excrete respiratory secretions. Note any rise in the patient's temperature as a potential sign of respiratory infection, and auscultate the patient's chest for clearness.

GASTROINTESTINAL COMPLICATIONS

The patient will probably have decreased to absent bowel activity for at least one day after surgery and then have hypoactive bowel activity on the following day. The patient should receive no oral fluids until bowel sounds are heard for several hours or until the patient expels flatus, usually on the second or third day postoperatively. Start fluids with a teaspoon of ice chips every hour. When no nausea or abdominal distention occurs, "sips" of clear liquids may be given with a syringe. This prevents the patient from swallowing air, which usually occurs when drinking through a straw.

Gradually increase the amount of liquids as bowel sounds and the feeling of hunger return. The slow increase in liquid intake is absolutely necessary because patients with midthoracic or lower spine surgery are predisposed to develop a paralytic ileus. The sudden correction of the spinal curve by internal fixation may narrow the angle at which the superior mesenteric artery leaves the aorta, thereby partially or completely obstructing the blood flow to the duodenum.

GENITOURINARY TRACT INFECTION

The patient with posterior spinal fusion and instrumentation will have an indwelling catheter for the first 3 or 4 days. Catheters are always a source of potential infection, but they provide comfort for the patient during the first few postoperative days and allow for an accurate assessment of the patient's kidney function. Once the catheter is removed, make sure the patient is voiding in adequate amounts, has no pain on voiding, and has a normal temperature. If an infection is suspected, get a urine culture. Patients with an infection are placed on a course of medications, and fluids are increased.

WOUND COMPLICATIONS

Two potential problems that can occur at the wound site are infection and the development of a hematoma. All surgical patients are at risk of wound infections because there has been a break in skin integrity. A body temperature of 102° F that persists for a couple of days after surgery is not uncommon due to the patient's reaction to surgery, stress, and dehydration, but it should be reported and recorded because it is also a sign of a potential infection. The initial dressings may be left in place for 36 to 48 hours at both the incision site and the donor site to allow initial healing to occur and to prevent bacteria from entering the wound. Each time the patient is turned, check the wound site for edema, redness, hardness, warmth, drainage, and the presence of an odor. Most patients have wound catheters inserted, but they may be obstructed, work ineffectively, or be removed too soon, and thus a hematoma may develop. Most patients are placed on prophylactic antibiotics at the time of surgery.

FLUID AND ELECTROLYTE DISTURBANCE

Because of the stress and the large amount of blood and fluid lost during surgery, fluid and electrolyte disturbances such as sodium and water retention, potassium excretion, and a negative nitrogen balance can occur. The amount and kind of fluid replacement the patient has received, the amount of urine output and its specific gravity, and other clinical conditions determine the fluid replacement therapy to be used.

Water intoxication can develop secondary to an inappropriate release of antidiuretic hormone (SIADH). The symptoms are usually headache, weight gain, weakness, mental confusion, lethargy, and progressive central nervous system deterioration. Urinary output diminishes, and urine concentrates to a specific gravity of 1.025 or more. Treatment is usually the restriction of fluid intake to establish a negative water balance; diuresis usually begins after 2 or 3 days.

INSTRUMENTATION FAILURE

Dislocation of the hooks, screws, cables, wires, and rods is not common. Physical predisposing factors are osteoporosis and degeneration in the adult spinal column. Other predisposing factors are twisting or stressing the spinal column when turning, ambulating, sneezing, coughing, or vomiting. The patient must understand that the back needs to be kept straight, especially once the immobilizing device is removed.

FUSION FAILURE

Fusion failure (or a non-fusion or partial fusion of the bone graft) can result from infection, inadequate diet, and as the result of instrumentation failure.

EVALUATION/OUTCOMES

Determine that the patient is obtaining adequate relief from pain. Use indicators such as irritability, restlessness, elevated systolic blood pressure, and increased heart rate to help determine the presence of pain. If nausea or vomiting occur after those signs are exhibited, pain is usually extreme. Evaluate how well the patient does muscle-setting and range-of-motion exercises. Check muscle tone and strength. The patient should not turn or be turned prone.

The patient should be free of complications from immobility or surgery. Check that the patient does not have more than 500 cc of drainage within 8 hours. Urinary output should not be less than 150 cc in 8 hours. In monitoring vital signs, the patient's blood pressure should not be below 90/50, pulse should not be above 120, and the oral temperature should not be above 102° F. The patient should be free of any signs of infection or neurologic impairment. If the patient has a cast, evaluate the patient's ability to ambulate with the cast on, to demonstrate proper body mechanics, and to verbalize cast care.

CLINICAL PATHWAY (Patient with Posterior Instrumentation for Scoliosis)

An example of a generic clinical pathway for a patient having posterior instrumentation for scoliosis is presented in Figure 8–32.

ANTERIOR SURGICAL INTERVENTIONS

The Dwyer and Zielke approaches are the two major anterior spine instrumentation systems. The *Dwyer* procedure is done for idiopathic thoracolumbar and lumbar scoliosis and lordosis, especially when there are spinal deficiencies. In surgery, the patient is placed on the table in a lateral decubitus position with the convex side of the curve in the upward position. An intercostal incision is made, and a rib is removed to provide exposure of the spinal column. The rib is saved for use as a bone graft. After the spinal column is exposed, the intervertebral discs along the curve are removed. A staple and a screw are then placed laterally into each vertebral body, and bone grafts are placed into each vertebral space. A heavy wire cable is passed through the heads of the vertebral screws and tightened. The screw heads are then crimped to the cable, and the incision is closed with chest tube drainage in place.

Because of the shortcomings of the Dwyer approach (i.e., kyphosis caused by ventral convex-side compression without derotation, pseudarthrosis as a

---

Figure 8–32

Clinical Pathway: Posterior Instrumentation for Scoliosis

Admission Date: _____ **Discharge Plan:** _____ Home _____ Skilled Nursing _____ Extended Care Facility

Pathway	Preadmission Office/OP clinic	Admission Day Op day	Hosp Day 2 Post-op 1	Hosp Day 3 Post-op 2	Hosp Day 4 Post-op 3	Hosp Day 5 Post-op 4	Outcomes
Consultation	Primary Care/ Medical physician	Case Manager Anesthesia, Dietitian Acute Pain Service	Social Work PT, OT if nec.				Cont. @ Home
Assessment	Nrsg database H & P Exam. by MD, NP or PA	Review & add Review H & P Postop routine			Resolved		
	Rehab/ECF/home		Referral if nec.				
	Home equipment		Referral if nec.		✓ if obtained		
	N/V status of legs	N/V status of legs	Cont.	Cont.	Cont.	Cont.	Will have nec. equipment @ home

(continued)

Figure 8–32

Clinical Pathway: Posterior Instrumentation for Scoliosis: *(continued)*

Pathway	Preadmission Office/OP clinic	Admission Day Op day	Hosp Day 2 Post-op 1	Hosp Day 3 Post-op 2	Hosp Day 4 Post-op 3	Hosp Day 5 Post-op 4	Outcomes
Tests	ECG/UA/CXR/1– 2 units autol. blood Coag. studies Spine X-rays & MRI	X-ray in OR H & H in PACU & repeat in pm	✓ CBC/Diff Transfuse per protocol	✓ CBC/Diff Transfuse per protocol			
Medications	D/C NSAIDs/ASA /b/4 OR Instruct on preop meds b/4 OR Prophylatic Antibiotics Analgesics as nec Start on Iron Med	Anticoagulant Routine meds ✓preadm meds IV Antibiotics PCA/Epidural pump Cont. Iron meds Bowel protocol	Cont. Anticoag	Cont. D/C antibiotics D/C IV and begin Oral pain meds	Cont.	Cont.	States meds, when to take, and purpose Pain managed with Analgesics @ home Normal bowel elim.
Diet	Assessment wt. balanced diet	NPO @ MN b/4 OR Ice chips/return bowel sounds	Liquids/as tolerated	Advance as tolerated Roughage & liquids			Tolerating diet
Activity	Preop mobility	Ankle Pumps Log roll turn q 2 hrs Quad & Glut q 2 Bed rest	Cont. Turn q 2hrs Cont Tilt Table	 Cont OOB to BR with and assistance		Walking with assit.	Walking @ home with Brace on without asst.
Treatments	Set blood donation dates, 1 wk between units & 14 days between last unit and OR day	IV fluids/blood if necessary, I&O TEDs, IPCD or foot pumps Hemovac/output Dressing IS/TCDB q hr w/a Foley to drain	Cont. Cont. Do Not Change	DC if liq tolerated Cont. D/C Dressing change PRN D/C		Cont. Change PRN	Cont. TEDS @ home No complications No infection Clear lungs Normal bladder elim.
Education	Review pre & postop. care procedures (Log-rolling & getting OOB) & Brace Rev. rehabilitation, body mechanics & exercises Attends gp ed class Pain management Review hosp LOS	Reinforce Rev. pain mgmt	Cont. Rev. hosp routine Review Rehab Reinforce Ed. Reinforce	Cont.		Reinforce	Knows care of & how to live with the Brace
D/C Plan	Identify discharge plan Caregivers & home situation (LOS 5–7 days) Discuss wearing & care of TLSO		Notify Social Worker Or Home Health if nec. Care as appropriate Rev. back care and Brace				Discharged to home States reasons to contact physician Wears Brace as app.

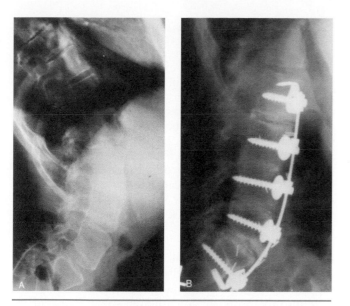

Figure 8–33 (A) Marked paralytic hyperlordosis. (B) Lordosis has been reduced to 60 degrees L1–S1 by anterior Zielke instrumentation. Note the anteroposterior orientation of the screws. *(Bridwell & DeWald (1997). The Textbook of Spinal Surgery. Philadelphia: Lippincott-Raven.)*

consequence of cable fractures, and insufficient fixation of the cable in the screw heads), Zielke and Stukat developed (Fig. 8–33) the VDS. It includes the basic principle of compression on the convex side as in the Dwyer operation but also offers the possibility of derotation. The VDS *(Zielke)* implants (Giehl & Zielke, 1997) are extremely simple and inexpensive in comparison to modern dorsal systems, and the VDS compression rod has a higher degree of mechanical stability than the Dwyer cable.

Postoperatively, the care of a patient with anterior instrumentation focuses on immobilizing the spinal column and preventing complications (as discussed under posterior fusion with instrumentation), with additional efforts to promote the return of lung function. The patient will have a chest tube for several days after surgery. Care must be taken to encourage pulmonary hygiene, as the patient's chest tube often makes it uncomfortable for the patient to cough and deep breathe. Splinting the chest during coughing and deep breathing, as well as proper positioning, will help facilitate adequate pulmonary hygiene. Careful assessment of the lungs to detect any abnormal or diminished breath sounds is essential to prevent atelectasis or pneumonia in patients with an anterior fusion with instrumentation.

LUMBAR SPINAL COLUMN

The lumbar spine connects the upper portion of the skeleton with the lower, furnishes support for the torso, and transmits weight from the torso to the pelvis. As there are no ribs attached to the lumbar spine, it has a relatively wide range of motion.

LOW BACK PAIN

Low back pain has always been a human problem. Today, possibly because of obesity and a sedentary lifestyle, backache is second only to headache as the most common complaint of pain. Data from the National Center for Health Statistics indicate that, in the United States, chronic impairments of the back and the spine are the most common cause of activity limitations for persons under age 45. Back and spine impairment ranks third, after heart conditions and arthritis, as a cause of activity limitation for persons 45 to 64. Although numerous theories, techniques, and treatments have been advocated, low back pain remains a great dilemma for the health professions.

ACUTE BACK PAIN

There are normally three types of injuries to the back. They are (1) injury to the disc or endplate of a vertebra from hyperflexion; (2) disruption or sprain of the ligaments of the posterior elements, particularly the posterior facets, following twisting; and (3) a herniated intervertebral disc. A flexion injury is more likely to cause a disruption or a fracture of the endplate than an injury to the ligaments. The healing of a flexion injury is generally rapid, and the patient responds well initially to bed rest and then to gradual activity. However, a later sequela may be an invasion of the disc by fibroblasts that can lead to disc degeneration and subsequent subluxation of the posterior facet joints.

The second type of injury is caused by torsion or twisting and accounts for approximately 70% of all causes of acute low back pain. Twisting injuries usually occur at the L4–5 level. Frequently, there is a ligamentous injury to the posterior facets with a sprain of the posterior facet capsule. Patients usually have pain on hyperextension and rotation of the spine and are initially treated with bed rest and then placed in a back brace. A plastic, molded spinal orthosis usually works well (Fig. 8–34). If a brace is not worn continuously during healing, posterior facet syndrome, that is, instability of the facets and chronic low back pain, may develop. Patients with twisting injuries generally heal more slowly than patients with flexion injuries.

An acute herniated disc may be the result of natural degeneration with age or repeated torsional stress to the annulus. For that reason, a patient may sustain a herniated disc without any definite acute injury, although the nucleus pulposus may rupture and cause an acute injury to the disc. Initially, the major complaint may be back pain, but severe leg pain develops when the nerve root becomes inflamed. Not all patients with an acute herniated disc need surgery, as most will respond to bed rest. Surgery is considered if the patient has a marked neurologic deficit, such as bowel or bladder symptoms, or a marked motor weakness, such as dropped foot, or severe, unrelenting leg pain.

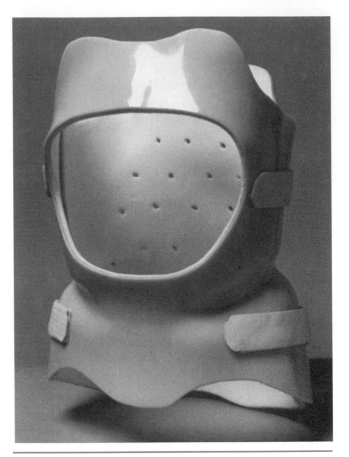

Figure 8–34   Thoracolumbosacral orthosis (TLSO).   *(Bridwell & DeWald (1997). The Textbook of Spinal Surgery. Philadelphia: Lippincott-Raven.)*

CHRONIC BACK PAIN

Chronic back pain refers to pain lasting more than 3 months or repeated episodes of incapacitating back pain. Its most common cause is a chronic instability of the posterior facets together with a degeneration of the intervertebral disc. Those changes in the facet joint and disc may result from aging and the effects of normal daily activities. The instability and degeneration may be accentuated by weakness in the extrinsic stabilizing systems, that is, the abdominal and back muscles. Weak abdominal and back muscles also increase the chance for injury to discs and facet joints. Chronic back pain may also come about through nerve root compression due to either a long-standing herniated disc or a bony impingement. The reason certain persons experience back pain and others with similar body structures and lifestyles do not still remains an unanswered question.

To enhance the patient's understanding, reduce the pain associated with daily activities, and increase compliance with the rehabilitation program, some physicians advocate a "back school." The school program usually consists of a series of lectures by physicians, physical therapists, and psychologists who discuss the influence of stress on daily life and its effect on pain, how to do activities with reduced pain, and how to develop and maintain an exercise program. Some patients need more than an explanation and an exercise program to reduce their pain. Other methods for possible pain relief are (1) transcutaneous electrical nerve stimulation, which works by blocking pain sensations; (2) injections of cortisone into a facet joint, which provides temporary relief; and, occasionally, (3) a percutaneous rhizotomy, which is a neurectomy of the posterior dorsal rami. Surgery for chronic back pain is usually a last resort but may be indicated for patients with long-standing leg pain secondary to nerve root compression from either a herniated disc or stenosis of the spinal canal.

HERNIATED INTERVERTEBRAL DISC

A herniated intervertebral disc is one with a rupture or herniation of the nucleus pulposus (the center of the disc) into the posterior longitudinal spinal ligament or spinal canal, causing pressure on the adjacent spinal nerve root. Ninety-five percent of herniations in the lumbar region occur at the vertebral interspaces L4–5 and L5–S1.

The nucleus pulposus is enclosed by a thick fibrous band called the annulus fibrosus. Stresses that suddenly or continually increase intervertebral pressure can eventually cause the posterior fibers of the annulus to give way. Examples of stressful activities include lifting, a fall on the buttocks, direct trauma to the back, twisting movements, or repeated flexion and lifting motions. Ruptures are particularly likely when the annulus has been weakened or has gone through degenerative changes. The annulus is notably softened and liable to rupture during pregnancy and labor and after prolonged confinement to bed. Disc rupture can also occur without apparent cause, indicating that the degenerative process alone is sufficient to cause the annulus to yield to mere weight bearing. An acute episode of pain from a herniated intervertebral disc usually subsides within a few days; typically, the patient will have many such episodes lasting longer and coming on after a shorter period of time.

Clinical manifestations of a herniated intervertebral disc are (1) sciatic pain that usually appears gradually over subsequent episodes; (2) paresthesia and numbness referred to the involved dermatome of the spinal nerve (L5–S1 lesion causes pain and paresthesia in the sole and outer border of the foot; an L4–5 lesion causes referred sensations to the dorsum of the foot and big toe; and an L2–3 or L3–4 lesion causes referred sensations to the anterior thigh, radiating to the antereomedial aspect of the leg); (3) tilting or listing of the trunk away from the affected side as in an attempt to relieve pressure on the nerve; (4) decreased mobility; (5) tenderness in the lower back; (6) abnormal results in straight-leg raising or La Segue tests; and (7) decreased motor and sensory function in the legs. The pain first appears as an ache in the buttocks, and later the pain tends to radiate to the posterior thigh area, the popliteal area, the calf or anterolateral aspect of the leg, and even into the heel, the ankle, and the foot. The sciatic pain is generally unilateral and is aggravated by coughing, sneezing, and straining while having a stool. A common complaint by the patient with a herniated intervertebral disc is the sensation of muscle cramping in the posterior thigh or calf. As the sciatic pain increases in intensity and extent, the low back pain diminishes and occasionally may even disappear entirely.

Other diagnostic measures are roentgenograms of the spine, myelograms, epidural venograms, MRIs, and CT scans (see Chapter 2). Anteroposterior, lateral, and oblique roentgenographic views are usually taken. A newly herniated disc does not show any narrowing of the disc space, but degenerative changes in the posterior articulations, a predisposing factor, are visible. On a myelogram, a defect, with rare exceptions, indicates a disc protrusion. A small disc protrusion, particularly in the spacious lower lumbar canal, however, may fail to indent the dura and thus may go undetected. In addition, the dura may not extend sufficiently caudally to allow the column of fluid to reach the level of the disc. An epidural venogram uses the veins of the epidural to allow the contrast medium to extend beyond the spinal canal and caudally to the L5–S1 level. The venogram demonstrates impingement upon an epidural plexus, a neural foramen, or a radicular vein. The MRI is more accurate than the CT and myelography for many spinal disease processes.

Conservative Treatment. Ninety percent of the episodes subside with conservative treatment. Removal of pressure on the nerve root relieves the symptoms, allowing protruded disc tissue to be reabsorbed by the body and the defect in the annulus repaired by fibrous tissue. The healed area of the posterior annulus is thinner, more fragile, and less resistant to pressure; and fibrosis may engulf the dura and the nerve root and cause persistent low-grade symptoms. In most instances, the patient becomes less responsive to conservative treatment with each subsequent episode. Repeated dissolutions of a small portion of the disc may lead, however, to complete loss of the disc and a permanent cure.

Conservative treatment may vary, but usually involves some combination of the following: (1) bed rest to relieve stress on the inflamed tissue (note that recent research indicates that two days of bed rest are as beneficial as seven days); (2) traction to reduce the pressure on the protruding disc and nerve root and to apply countertension against back muscle spasms; (3) muscle relaxant medications; (4) analgesics; (5) local heat application to improve circulation in the skin and superficial muscles and help reduce local muscle spasm or tension; (6) local cold applications to

---

Box 8–1
Low Back Exercises

1. *Pelvic tilt.* Lying supine, the patient tightens the stomach muscles and then rocks the pelvis, flattening the low back. The patient holds that position for a count of 5.
2. *Sit-up.* Lying supine with the abdominal muscles tightened, the patient raises their head and shoulders and reaches toward the knees, holding the position for a count of 5. As the patient's muscles become stronger, they may fold their arms across the chest and even advance to putting their hands behind their head.
3. *Knee-chest.* Lying supine with the abdominal muscles tightened, the patient raises their head and shoulders and brings one knee up toward the nose, holding the position for a count of 5.
4. *Double knee.* The same as (3), except that the patient brings both knees up at the same time.
5. *Straight leg raises.* The patient lies supine with one knee bent and held to the chest with the hands. The patient then lifts the other leg, keeping the knee straight and the ankle flexed.

---

provide an analgesic or to counter irritating effects; (7) radiant energy applied in the form of ultrasound or diathermy to penetrate deeper into the body than topical heat or cold applications; (8) massage to provide a rolling, rubbing, pressing, kneading, and gently pounding effect on tender areas, which helps to relax tight muscles and improve local circulation; (9) back supports in the form of corsets, braces, and belts, which afford another means to reduce mobility for back pain relief; (10) topical medications; and (11) low back exercises designed to increase abdominal strength and endurance, stretch the low back, and develop and maintain the correct pelvic tilt. Back exercises should be done twice a day for the first 3 months and once a day thereafter. Each exercise should be done every day, as it builds on the day before to increase strength and endurance. The number of repetitions of each exercise depends on the patient's condition (Box 8-1). It is also very important to teach the patient how to flex, stand, get in and out of a car, and to support their lumbar back area while they are driving (Fig. 8–35).

Surgical Treatment/Lumbar Laminectomy. When symptoms are persistent and intolerable, the disc is removed by a laminectomy. A surgical incision is made down the midline of the back over the affected disc. The lamina over the involved nerve root and the underlying ligamentum flavum are excised. The nerve root is gently retracted, and the herniated nucleus pulposus is removed. The incision is then closed with wound catheters in place.

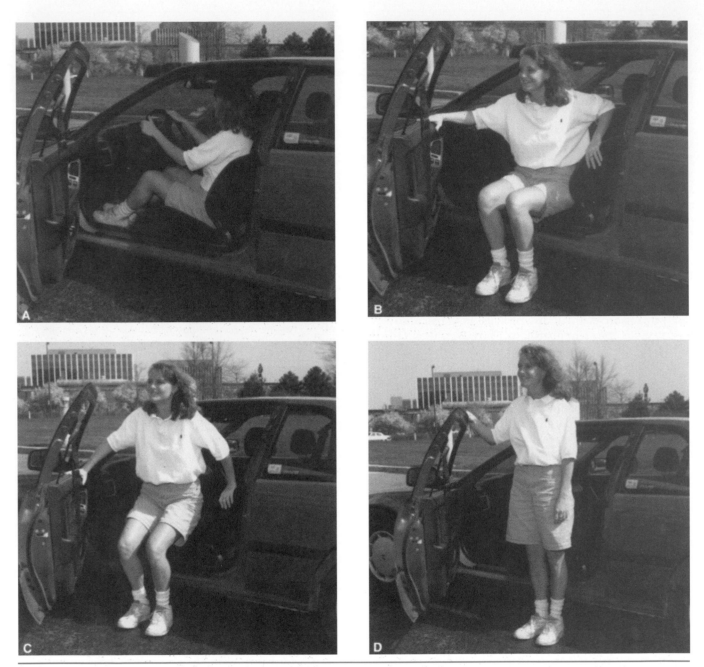

Figure 8–35 (A) The patient should have proper lumbar support while driving. (B) Turning the entire body to place both feet firmly on the ground. (C) Identifying stable points on the car, the patient uses the upper and lower extremities to stand, limiting the amount of forward flexion, as possible. (D) Standing is accomplished without flexing the lumbar spine. *(Bridwell & DeWald (1997). The Textbook of Spinal Surgery. Philadelphia: Lippincott-Raven.)*

NURSING PROCESS (Patient with a Lumbar Laminectomy)

The following nursing process presents the care of a patient following a lumbar laminectomy. The nursing process begins after the patient returns from surgery.

ASSESSMENT

The initial nursing assessment of a typical patient following a posterior lumbar laminectomy should include a general assessment of the patient and emphasize the neurovascular status of both lower extremities (see Chapter 2). Assess the neurovascular status every 15 minutes for the first 2 hours after surgery, then every 30 minutes for 2 hours, every 2 hours for the next 18 hours, and subsequently at the beginning of every shift. Check that the hemovac is working properly, and determine the amount of drainage in the hemovac. The patient's bed should be flat, and the patient should be in correct body alignment. Assess the severity, location, and duration of pain. Determine if the patient has any signs of nausea.

Continuing assessment should include exploring the patient's understanding of postoperative care. Check for bowel sounds, and monitor the patient's intake and output of fluids. Continue to assess for pain, the patient's anxiety level, and signs of depression.

NURSING DIAGNOSIS

Based on all of the assessment data, the major nursing diagnoses for a typical patient following a lumbar laminectomy may include the following:

- Pain and discomfort related to trauma and surgery
- Impaired physical mobility related to instability of the lumbar spine
- Anxiety related to knowledge deficit about the surgery and rehabilitation process

COLLABORATIVE PROBLEMS

- Infection
- Neurologic deficit
- Gastrointestinal complications
- Spinal instability
- Residual leg and back pain

GOAL FORMULATION AND PLANNING

The goals are to have the patient experience (1) a decrease in the amount of pain through nursing measures and prescribed medications, (2) an increase in mobility through controlled ambulation and correct body mechanics, (3) a decrease in anxiety through increased knowledge, and (4) an absence of complications from surgery and decreased activity. Long-term goals are to have the patient free of pain with full return of function.

INTERVENTIONS

ALLEVIATE PAIN

The amount of pain following a laminectomy varies with each patient. Intramuscular or PCA intervenous narcotic medications are usually needed to relieve pain during the first 48 to 72 hours. After that period, oral medications are usually sufficient to relieve discomfort. For some patients, however, additional medication for pain and the relaxation of muscle spasms is needed, as they experience those difficulties throughout their postoperative period in the hospital. Noninvasive measures such as conveying a sense of concern by talking softly to the patient and using therapeutic touch, distraction, relaxation techniques, and visual imagery are also effective in reducing the degree of pain.

INCREASE MOBILITY

The focus of nursing efforts to increase mobility is on correct positioning, turning, exercise, and ambulation.

Position. Following a laminectomy, the patient needs to be kept in correct body alignment to maintain a straight spinal column. The patient's bed needs to have a firm mattress or a bedboard under the mattress. Immediately after surgery, the patient may be kept supine for a number of hours before being allowed to turn. Many physicians require that the patient's bed remain flat at all times. However, some will allow the head of the bed to be elevated a few degrees if the patient's hips are positioned at the flex of the bed, so that when the head of the bed is elevated the patient's spinal column remains straight and in good alignment. Other physicians allow only the knee gatch to be raised or pillows to be placed under the patient's knees to reduce stress on the back. The nurse should remind the patient not to keep the pillows under the knees at all times as that promotes venous stasis in the lower extremities.

Turning. Once the patient is allowed to turn, he or she is turned on a regular schedule. The patient should be turned by log-rolling (see nursing care for a patient with posterior spinal fusion earlier in this chapter) to prevent twisting the body. The patient may be log-rolled with or without the use of a turning sheet, but whatever method is used, perfect alignment of the body should be maintained at all times. Gradually, patients become able to move and turn themselves.

Exercises. Check with the patient's physician regarding the type of exercises allowed. Most patients do muscle-setting exercises (such as quadriceps- and gluteal-setting exercises) and some mild active exercises of the lower extremities (such as plantar and dorsiflexion and active range of motion of the ankles). Some institutions utilize a footboard or flexion pillow at the foot of the bed to support the patient during the exercises. Exercises for the upper extremities involve muscle-setting exercises, activities of daily living (such as bathing the face and arms), and other mild range-of-motion exercises to help maintain muscle strength.

Ambulation. Some physicians allow the patient to dangle their legs on the side of the bed as early as the evening after a morning surgery. To dangle the patient's legs for the first time, explain the procedure to the patient, administer pain medication, and let enough time elapse for the medication to take effect. Then log-roll the patient onto one side as close to the edge of the bed as safety permits. Have the patient flex their hips and knees, and make sure the pillow is still between the patient's legs. Raising the patient requires coordinated movement. The patient pushes up with one hand as one nurse supports the patient's shoulders and another nurse brings the patient's legs over the edge of the bed. In this way, the patient is brought to a sitting position on the side of the bed without twisting their body. If the patient's bed has upper and lower side rails, the upper rail can be left up so the patient can use it to help push up. Once the patient is sitting on the side of the bed, support the patient's back and shoulders to prevent slumping. Have the patient take deep breaths and move their feet up and down to exercise the ankles and increase circulation. To put the patient back to bed, reverse the procedure.

Within 24 hours (or even less), the patient is allowed out of bed and encouraged to walk. Get the patient up by using the foregoing technique. Once the patient is sitting on the side of the bed, wait a few moments before helping the patient stand. It is usually better to have two persons assist the patient in ambulating for the first time. The patient will have discomfort when standing and will need to be encouraged to move. Walking helps to relieve the pain by making it intermittent rather than continuous and promotes venous return from the lower extremities.

Once the patient is out of bed, he or she may be allowed to sit for a short period of time in a firm chair with good back support and armrests. To ease the process of getting into and out of the chair, the patient should use their arm and leg muscles and keep their back straight.

PATIENT TEACHING AND HOME CARE CONSIDERATIONS

Patient teaching for a patient with a posterior lumbar laminectomy should begin preoperatively. An important aspect of care is psychological support, including an explanation of the procedure and the expected results. Demonstrate the proper way to turn, get in and out of bed, get in and out of a chair, and do activities of daily living. Have a male patient practice voiding while lying supine or on one side. After surgery, reinforce proper body mechanics, especially the use of the legs instead of the back. Discuss positions for sleeping such as (1) sleeping in a side-lying position with knees bent, (2) not sleeping on the back unless the knees are supported by a pillow, (3) using flat pillows under the head and neck to avoid straining the neck and shoulders, and (4) never sleeping on the abdomen, as that leads to lordosis and puts stress on the shoulders. The patient should be advised to rest the back when he or she feels tired, avoid riding in a car unless absolutely necessary, and make sure the knees are higher than the hips when in a sitting position.

The patient should not undertake any exercise or activity that has not been permitted by the physician. Ask the patient to write down questions or concerns at the time they occur so the patient will remember to ask about them. In particular, patients are often concerned about when they can resume sexual activities but may be reluctant to ask the physician. The nurse may need to remind the patient to do so or ask the physician to discuss the matter with the patient.

MONITORING AND MANAGING POTENTIAL PROBLEMS

Potential complications following a laminectomy are infection, neurologic deficit, and gastrointestinal complications as discussed under posterior spinal fusion. Other potential complications include spinal instability requiring spinal fusion and residual leg and back pain.

EVALUATION/OUTCOMES

Determine that the patient is obtaining adequate relief from pain. After 48 to 72 hours, most patients require only oral pain medications. The patient should be able to walk for increasingly longer periods of time without fatigue and should remain free of any complications from immobility or surgery. Through therapeutic discussions, evaluate how well the patient understands the rehabilitation process and his or her capacities and limitations. Have the patient discuss the activities of a typical day at home.

CLINICAL PATHWAY (Patient with a Lumbar Laminectomy)

An example of a generic clinical pathway for a patient having a lumbar laminectomy is presented in Figure 8–36.

Surgical Treatment/Spinal Fusion. Loss of a disc through a laminectomy may cause increased stresses on the posterior articulations leading to degenerative changes. These changes may produce disabling symptoms and instability requiring a spinal fusion. A spinal fusion may also be done in conjunction with a laminectomy to provide spinal stability for patients who will engage in heavy lifting. In a lumbar spinal fusion, the transverse process of the sacrum, and the fifth, fourth, and a portion of the third lumbar vertebrae are decorticated. The lateral portion of the pedicle and the lateral portion of the superior articular facets are also decorticated. Large amounts of cortical and cancellous bone are taken from the iliac crest and placed over the decorticated areas. The procedure may be carried out on both sides of the lumbar spine. The incision is closed with wound catheters in place.

COMMON CONDITIONS

INTRASPINAL TUMORS

Intraspinal tumors may give rise to back and leg pain similar to that from radiculitis or a herniated lumbar disc. Approximately 1% of the patients operated on for a herniated lumbar disc are found to have an intraspinal tumor. In general, two types of intraspinal tumors may occur: extradural and intradural. *Extradural tumors* are usually secondary and represent metastatic carcinoma from lymphatic system tumors such as Hodgkin's disease, lymphosarcoma, and reticulum cell sarcoma. *Intradural tumors* are most often primary and include meningioma, neurofibroma, glioma, medulloblastoma, and ependymoma. For further information on these tumors, see Chapter 3.

The existence of an intraspinal tumor rather than a herniated lumbar disc is suspected when (1) there is a failure to respond to conservative treatment and the pain remains intractable, or there is an unusual progression of the neurologic signs; (2) a neurogenic type of bladder or bowel dysfunction exists; (3) nocturnal

Figure 8–36

Clinical Pathway: Lumbar Laminectomy

Admission Date: _____   **Discharge Plan:** _____ **Home** _____ **Skilled Nursing** _____ **Extended Care Facility**

Pathway	Preadmission Office/OP clinic	Admission Day Op day	Hosp Day 2 Post-op 1	Hosp Day 3 Post-op 2	Hosp Day 4 Post-op 3	Hosp Day 5 Post-op 4	Outcomes
Consultation	Primary Care/ Medical physician	Case Manager Anesthesia, PT					Cont. @ Home
Assessment	Nrsg database	Review & add					
	H & P Exam. by MD, NP, or PA	Review H & P	Referral if nec.				
		Postop routine	N/V status legs			Resolved	
	Rehab/ECF/home						
		Assessment of the Neurovascular status of lower extremities		Cont.	Cont.		Cont.
Tests	ECG/AU/CXR/ Spine X-rays & MRI Coag. studies if app.	H & H in PACU & repeat in pm	Cont. Anticoag.			Cont.	
Medications	D/C NSAIDs/ASA /b/4 OR	Anticoagulant		Cont.	Cont.	Cont.	States meds, when to take and purpose
	Instruct on preop meds b/4 OR	Routine meds ✓ preadm meds					
	Prophylatic Antibiotics	IV Antibiotics		D/C antibiotics			
	Analgesics as nec	PCA/Epidural pump		D/C IV and begin Oral pain meds			Pain managed with Analgesics @ home
		Bowel protocol	Liquids				Normal bowel function
Diet	Assessment wt. balanced diet	NPO @ MN b/4 OR		Advance as tol Roughage & liquids			Tolerating diet
		Ice chips/return bowel sounds	Cont. Turn q 2hrs				
Activity	Preop mobility	Ankle Pumps	Cont.				
		Log-roll turn q 2 hrs					
		Quard & Glut q 2	OOB to BR with assistance				
		Bed rest with HOB elevated 45 if app.		Walking with assistance			Walking @ home without assistance
Treatments		IV fluids/blood if necessary, I&O TEDs, IPCD or foot pumps	Do not Change				Cont. TEDS @ home No complications
		Hemovac/output		D/C			
		Dressing		Change Dressing		Change PRN	No infection
		IS/TCDB q hr w/a		PRN			Clear lungs
				D/C			Normal clim. using elevated toilet seat
		Foley to drain if app.	Cont.				
Education	Review pre & post operative care procedures (Log rolling & getting OOB)	Reinforce	Rev. hosp routine	Cont.			
			Review Rehab				Continue with exc. regime and walking
	Rev. rehabilitation, body mechanics & exercises					Reinforce	
			Reinforce Ed.				
	Attends gp ed class						

(continued)

Figure 8–36

Clinical Pathway: Lumbar Laminectomy: *(continued)*

Pathway	Preadmission Office/OP clinic	Admission Day Op day	Hosp Day 2 Post-op 1	Hosp Day 3 Post-op 2	Hosp Day 4 Post-op 3	Hosp Day 5 Post-op 4	Outcomes
D/C Plan	Pain management Rev. basic back care Review hosp LOS Identify discharge plan Caregivers & home situation (LOS 4 days)	Rev. pain mgmt	Reinforce Notify Social Worker Or Home Health if nec.				Discharged to home States reason to contact physician

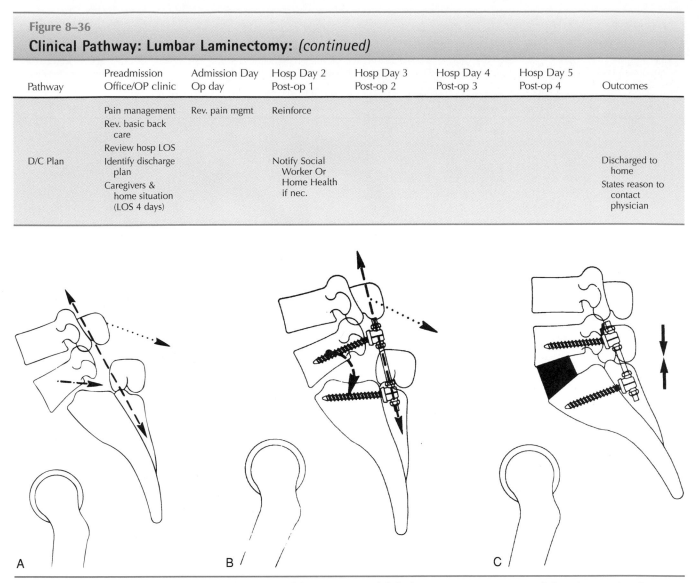

Figure 8–37   Schematic illustration of reduction and fusion in spondylolisthesis. (A) Distraction and dorsal extension forces. (B) Reduction is maintained by pedicle-screw-rod system. Screws are loaded in distraction, and L5–S1 interspace is still kyphotic. (C) After anterior support, posterior compression is applied.   *(Bridwell & DeWald (1997).* The Textbook of Spinal Surgery. *Philadelphia: Lippincott-Raven.)*

pain awakens the patient and such pain is essentially unrelated to movement, position, or activity; (4) patient's complaints cannot be localized to a single nerve root; or (5) there is upper motor neuron dysfunction. For example, the presence of spasticity, hyperactive reflexes, clonus, and positive Babinski signs all indicate a tumor in the central nervous system and not the lower neuron type of involvement found in herniated disc disease. The presence of a spinal cord tumor can be confirmed by lumbar puncture, cystometric test of bladder function, myelogram, MRI, or CAT scan. In some instances, however, surgical exploration is necessary. Others may require posterior surgical intervention for the removal of the tumor and spinal fusion with or without pedicle screws to stabilize the spine. If the tumor has caused significant anterior destruction, an anterior decompression and stabilization may be necessary. For more information on spinal tumors, see Chapter 3.

SPONDYLOLISTHESIS

In spondylolisthesis, there is a forward subluxation of the body of one vertebra on the vertebra below it. The term is derived from "spondylo" meaning vertebra and "listhesis" meaning slipping, sliding, or falling (Fig. 8–37). The body and pedicles of the affected vertebra tend to slip forward, whereas the laminae and spinous process remain in approximately the correct position. Normally, sliding is prevented by the mechanical relationship of the articular facets and the ligaments.

Spondylolisthesis occurs because of the development of a defect or break in the pars interarticularis,

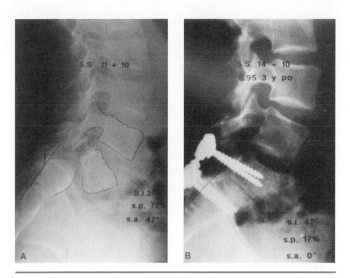

Figure 8–38 Reduction and fusion of congenital spondylolisthesis with improvement of all objective parameters. *(Bridwell & DeWald (1997). The Textbook of Spinal Surgery. Philadelphia: Lippincott-Raven.)*

giving rise to a bony discontinuity between the anterior and posterior halves of the neural arch. Most causes of spondylolisthesis are undetected fatigue fractures occurring in an elongated and mechanically weak portion of the pars interarticularis of the fifth lumbar vertebra. Another type seen frequently in the lumbosacral joint is due to a congenital anomaly. A third type, which is degenerative, occurs at the fourth lumbar vertebra, usually in women over 50. Degenerative spondylolisthesis is not associated with a neural arch defect, but frequently produces spinal stenosis at the level of the vertebral slipping.

Patients with spondylolisthesis usually have chronic low back pain. If there is lumbosacral nerve root involvement, the patient may have pain that radiates into the hips, the thighs, and even the feet, but usually there is only numbness or "tingling" noted in the legs. The patient typically complains of back stiffness, limited forward flexion of the lumbar spine, muscle spasms, and discomfort when lifting or bending.

The vast majority of patients are treated conservatively. The back pain can best be controlled by the use of a back support such as a corset, brace, or cast combined with back strengthening exercises and the avoidance of bending and lifting. Spinal fusion of the involved vertebrae is indicated in patients who fail to respond to conservative methods or who are likely to experience further slippage. The fusion usually involves L4 to S1 or L5 to S1 and in severe cases total hip replacements (Fig. 8–38). It is most commonly done using a posterior approach (with or without pedicle screws); however, it may also be accomplished by an anterior interbody fusion.

SPINAL STENOSIS

Spinal stenosis is the narrowing of any region of the spinal canal or nerve root foramina and usually involves

pressure on spinal nerves or the vessels supplying those nerves. Spinal stenosis may be caused by a congenital anomaly such as achondroplasia, or it may develop following severe degenerative spinal changes, spondylolisthesis, spinal surgeries such as laminectomy or spinal fusion, trauma to the spine, or Paget's disease.

Pain may be caused by ischemia and compression from a blockage or restriction to the flow of cerebrospinal fluid due to the stenosis. The onset of the discomfort may be tingling, weakness, or clumsiness; and the "pain" may be only minimal. As the condition progresses, pain develops in the back and buttocks, and there is often intermittent claudication, that is, severe pain in the calf muscles during walking that subsides with rest. The leg pain is not relieved by standing. In many instances, the patient can obtain pain relief by sitting down and assuming a flexed back posture.

The first step is conservative treatment (see herniated disc earlier in this chapter) to decrease the lumbar lordosis and relieve pain. Emphasis should be placed on the importance of good body mechanics and the need to reduce stress on the spinal column. Surgical intervention is considered when the patient has (1) daily activities unacceptably restricted or intolerable pain in spite of conservative treatment; for example, the patient has difficulty walking 50 yards or sitting for 30 minutes or has recurrent leg cramps that interfere with sleep; (2) a progressive neurologic deficit such as a motor weakness of the quadriceps that causes one knee to "buckle" or an ankle dorsiflexion paresis; or (3) a bladder dysfunction from a neurogenic cause. Prevention of further disabilities, lessening of pain, and improvement in daily function are the major objectives of the surgery. Complete relief from pain is not assured, nor is marked improvement in functional activities predictable following surgical decompression. Surgical decompression may involve spinal fusion at multiple levels and the use of pedicle screws to help stabilize the spine.

Spinal Fixation with Pedicle Screws. A spinal fusion and the insertion of a pedicle screw fixation system uses stainless steel rods, cables, and/or plates that are attached to the spine with screws anchored to the pedicles of the vertebrae. The surgeon makes a posterior approach through a midline incision. Muscles and ligaments are separated and removed from the vertebrae. If the patient has spinal stenosis or nerve root compression, decompression is accomplished by doing a laminectomy, a hemilaminectomy, or a laminotomy and then decorticating the transverse processes. A fluoroscopy (C-Arm) is used to help visualize the exact placement of the pedicle screws and the rods or slotted plates, depending on the system utilized. The plates or rods are placed along the processes from the upper to the lower vertebrae, and screws are inserted into the pedicles. The procedure is carried out on both sides of the lumbar spine. Once the screws and plates are in place, autogenous or allograft bone grafts are laid down. Pedicle screw fixation provides stability and alignment to the lumbar spine until bone fusion is complete. This approach is utilized in the treatment of multiple problems, including fractures, tumors, spinal stenosis, spondylolisthesis, and failed low back surgery.

NURSING PROCESS (Patient with a Spinal Fixation with Pedicle Screws)

The following nursing process presents the care of a patient with a spinal fixation with pedicle screws. The nursing process begins after the patient returns from surgery.

ASSESSMENT

The initial assessment of a typical patient following spinal fixation with pedicle screws should emphasize the neurovascular assessment of the lower extremities. The first 48 to 72 hours are the most critical in the patient's postoperative recovery phase. Accurate and frequent neurologic assessment is essential to prevent neurologic deficit. Assess neurovascular status (see Chapter 2) every 15 minutes for 2 hours, then every 30 minutes for 2 hours, and every 2 to 4 hours for the next 72 hours. Log-roll the patient and check the patient's posterior lumbar dressing (and donor site if an allograft was utilized) for drainage. Check the suction(s) drain and note the amount and color of drainage. The patient's bed should be flat and the patient in correct body alignment. Assess the severity, location, and duration of pain. Determine if the patient has any signs of nausea. Auscultate the patient's lungs, and check for clearness. Check the nasogastric tube and Foley catheter if they are present. Check the patient's IV. Continuing assessment should include checking neurovascular status in the lower extremities and evaluating the patient's understanding of their postoperative care and anxiety level.

NURSING DIAGNOSIS

Based on all of the assessment data, the major nursing diagnoses for a typical patient following a spinal fixation with pedicle screws may include the following:

- Pain and discomfort related to surgical trauma
- Impaired physical mobility related to instability of the spine
- Potential infection related to surgical site (and donor site if an allograft was used)
- Anxiety related to knowledge deficit about the surgical procedure and rehabilitation process

COLLABORATIVE PROBLEMS

- Pulmonary complications
- Circulatory impairment
- Neurologic deficit

- Screw breakage or loosening
- Delayed or nonunion of fusion

GOAL FORMULATION AND PLANNING

The goals are to have the patient experience (1) a decrease in pain through correct positioning, nursing interventions, and medications; (2) an increase in physical mobility through the use of positioning, exercises, and ambulation; (3) no signs of infection at the incision site(s); (4) a decrease in anxiety through patient education about the surgery and rehabilitation process; and (5) an absence of complications. Long-term goals are to have the patient free of pain and to have a return of mobility.

INTERVENTIONS

ALLEVIATE PAIN

Patients with pedicle screw fixation appear to have less pain following surgery than patients having spinal fusions. However, pain must be evaluated on an individual basis. Determine the amount, location, and severity of the patient's pain. Some patients will receive intramuscular injections, while others will be using a patient controlled analgesia (PCA) machine to administer a narcotic analgesic (usually morphine or meperidine). Most patients will also need a muscle relaxant to reduce muscle spasms. All need to be evaluated regarding the effectiveness of pain relief, with dosages adjusted accordingly. Administer or have the patient administer pain medications before doing activities that will increase the patient's pain.

INCREASE MOBILITY

Early and less painful mobility is one of the advantages of lumbar spinal fixation with pedicle screws. Measures to increase mobility are log-rolling, positioning, sitting, exercising, ambulating, and using a thoracolumbosacral orthosis.

Position. Patients who have received a dura tear during surgery will need to be on bed rest for the first 48 to 72 hours after surgery. Verify that the patient is in correct body alignment, and make sure that there are pillows between their legs when they turn. Log-roll the patient (see care of the patient following posterior fusion with instrumentation earlier in this chapter.)

Sitting. If there were no complications in surgery, most patients are allowed to sit up the first day after surgery (exact time depends on the time of surgery the previous day). Log-roll the patient to the side of the bed, and then assist the patient to a sitting position as discussed in the care of the patient with a spinal fusion earlier in this chapter. At first, the patient may only be allowed to sit for 10 to 20 minutes at a time. Sitting time is limited to prevent further swelling and trauma to the lower lumbar spine during initial healing, as sitting at 90 degrees increases pressure to the lumbar area.

Exercises. Exercises include doing plantar and dorsiflexion (ankle pump) exercises and quadriceps- and gluteal-setting exercises. Patients can do these exercises while they are in bed or while they are sitting.

Ambulation. By the second postoperative day, the patient is usually allowed to stand and even take a few steps. Ambulation slowly progresses over the next few days, and the patient may be allowed to walk to the bathroom and to go for short walks out of the room. Physical therapy also works with the patient to increase their strength and to assist their progress with ambulation, stair climbing, and gait training (Brosnan & Berda, 1990)

Thoracolumbosacral orthosis. Patients will wear a thoracolumbosacral orthosis (TLSO) when they are out of bed (except for showering). The brace is molded and made specifically for each patient. The purpose of the TLSO (Fig. 8–39) is to give added support and immobility to the lumbar spine. In the beginning, most patients do not want to wear the brace, but they then begin to grow dependent on it. A number of patients will wear it part-time for months.

WOUND INFECTION

Precautions should be taken to prevent wound infections. The patient's temperature is monitored at least every 4 hours. Antibiotic therapy is usually administered as a prophylactic measure. The initial dressing is not changed for 48 hours after the surgery to allow time for the epithelial layers of the incision to begin to heal. Once the dressing has been changed, check the area at least every shift for any signs of redness, swelling, drainage, or any increase in complaints of pain in the area. Check the patient's laboratory tests for any increase in white cell count. In the event that an infection should occur, long-term antibiotic therapy is required, and in some instances the instrumentation must be removed until the infection is resolved.

PATIENT TEACHING AND HOME CARE CONSIDERATIONS

Each patient reacts differently to pain. Management of pain at home includes oral medications and a discussion with patients on ways to reduce the need for prescribed pain medications to approximately 6 to 8 weeks after surgery.

Personal care includes showering, the use of mild soap and water over the incision area (covered with steri strips), and the avoidance of powders, lotions, and oils. Instruction includes knowing the signs and symptoms of infection and when to notify their physician.

The patient is instructed to refrain from sexual activity for a few weeks until surgical pain and discomfort have subsided. The main concern is to prevent flexion-extension motion of the lumbosacral spine and to maintain support for the spine. The patient is instructed to keep the brace on and to maintain a position of full back support (by staying supine or in a side-lying position). Women in their childbearing years need to refrain

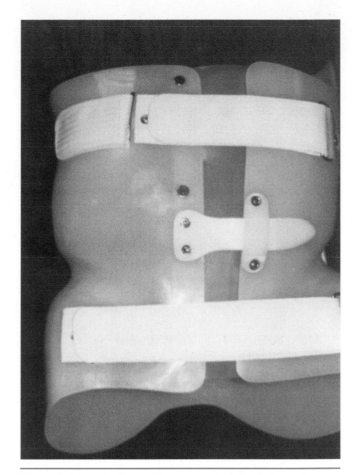

Figure 8–39.   Underarm brace (TLSO): frontal view of one model.   *(Weinstein & Buckwalter (1994). Turek's Othopaedic: Principles and Their Applications: Philadelphia: J.B. Lippincott Company.)*

Box 8–2
Guidelines for Orthotic Care

Wear a T-shirt or other light cotton garment under the brace at all times.
Change the T-shirt or other garment several times a day to maintain comfort.
Remove the brace to take a shower.
Avoid putting powders, lotions, or oils under the brace.
Wash the brace with a mild soap and water; do not soak.
Keep the Velcro closures clean.

Source: Brosnan, H., & Berda, P. (1990). Pedicle screw fixation in the lumbar spine. *Orthopaedic Nursing, 9*(6), 29.

from getting pregnant for 18 to 24 months following surgery to prevent additional stress on the back.

Patients go home wearing a thoracolumbosacral orthosis (Box 8–2, Guidelines for Orthotic Care). They are encouraged to maintain a nutritionally balanced diet and not to gain or lose weight as it affects the fit of the orthosis and may affect healing. Eating 3 times a day is encouraged, but some individuals find the orthosis causes a fullness during meals and limits oral intake. These individuals will need more frequent but smaller feedings. Emphasis is on foods that are high in iron to counteract the effects of blood loss, calcium for bone healing, and fluids and roughage to help with constipation due to their pain medications.

Home activity levels include rest periods during the first few weeks to help the patient regain their strength and stamina. Patients need to set a schedule of daily activities that includes personal hygiene, meals, and exercise. They are placed on a progressive ambulation program to increase the length of their walks, but not to over do physical activity. Between 8 and 12 weeks, upper and lower extremity muscle strengthening exercises, progressive ambulation, treadmill, and stationary bicycling are started. The average adult is able to return to work 3 months after surgery. Patients employed in heavy manual labor occupations are encouraged to change their vocation.

MONITORING AND MANAGING POTENTIAL PROBLEMS

The immediate potential complications following a spinal fixation with pedicle screws are the same as those associated with any surgical procedure. They are pulmonary complications, circulatory impairment, neurological deficit, and a urinary tract infection if a Foley catheter was utilized. (If used, the catheter is usually removed by the 3rd or 4th day.)

Long term complications that may occur are breakage or the pulling-out of instrumentation from the spine, delayed or nonunion, and pseudarthrosis, all of which may require additional surgery.

PULMONARY COMPLICATIONS
The two major pulmonary complications are pulmonary infection and pulmonary emboli.

Pulmonary Infection. Pneumonia is a concern for any surgical patient who has received general anesthesia, especially if the patient is obese, a smoker, or has a history of respiratory problems. Encourage the patient to cough and deep breathe. Some patients receive blow bottles or other additional pulmonary hygiene measures to assist them in excreting the residue from the anesthesia. Log-rolling the immobilized patient also helps with the drainage and expulsion of these secretions.

Pulmonary Emboli. The term *pulmonary emboli* refers to the obstruction of one or more pulmonary arteries by a thrombus (or thrombi), which originates somewhere in the venous system or the right side of the heart, becomes dislodged, and is carried to the lung. An infarction of lung tissue occurs due to the interruption of the lung's blood supply. The best treatment is prevention. Keep the patient well hydrated, doing active and passive exercises, and ambulating as tolerated. Pharmacologic prophylaxis measures may include aspirin, low-dose

heparin or coumadin, and utilizing compression or elastic stockings. See Chapter 4 for further discussion.

CIRCULATORY IMPAIRMENT
There is always the potential for excessive bleeding. An unforeseen coagulopathy may lead to a cauda equina syndrome and partial or complete paralysis. The major circulatory impairment that occurs following a spinal fixation with pedicle screws is phlebitis. Patients who are obese, who smoke, or who have been immobilized preoperatively are at a higher risk, and the rule is to prevent the complication. Patients are placed on anticoagulation therapy (see Chapter 4) and thigh-high antiembolic stockings, leg pumps, and other products to alternate pressure in the patient's legs. Patients are also taught to do ankle pumps, and quadriceps- and gluteal-setting exercises. Log-rolling the patient while they are in bed and getting the patient out of bed as soon as allowed by the physician also help.

NEUROLOGIC DEFICIT
The two potential neurologic deficits that occur following a spinal fixation with pedicle screws are dura tears and paralysis.

Dura tears. A tear in the dura mater, the cover for the spinal cord, is a risk during any spinal surgery. If a tear is detected during surgery, the physician can repair it at that time. If there has been a tear and it was repaired, the patient is usually kept flat for 48 to 72 hours after surgery to allow the dura to heal and to prevent spinal headaches.

Paralysis. To prevent paralysis, the neurologic deficit that concerns most patients, the patient is constantly monitored by somatosensory evoked potential (SSEP) monitoring, which monitors the integrity of the nerve conduction pathways throughout surgery. Once the instrumentation is in place, the Stagnara wake-up test is performed. Although asleep, the patient can respond to commands to move their lower extremities in plantar dorsi flexion, inversion, and eversion to reaffirm that motor function is intact. If not, the instrumentation is removed, the patient evaluated, the instrumentation replaced, and the patient reevaluated once more to ensure that the patient's motor function is intact. There is significant reduction in risk of paralysis for these patients because the lumbar spine is below the conus (Brosnan & Berda, 1990). Continue to check the neurovascular status of both extremities every 2 to 4 hours for the first 72 hours after surgery.

BREAKAGE OR LOOSENING
The purpose of the pedicle screw instrumentation system is to hold the spine in corrected and stable position until fusion occurs. Delayed bone healing, injury, or an accident could lead to screw breakage or pseudarthrosis. If the screw loosens or breaks, it is usually due to delayed healing of the bone fusion. If the fusion does not occur within 6 to 7 months,

increased stresses are placed on the device, and eventually the metal will fatigue and fail. Another operation is required to repair the devices and supplement the bone graft.

DELAYED UNION OR NONUNION

Delayed union or nonunion can occur as the result of an infection or of manipulation of the site. The process of calcification is usually monitored by periodic roentgenograms. Initial healing is expected to occur within 6 to 7 months. It is also believed that the bone fusion will continue to calcify for up to 2 years.

EVALUATION/OUTCOMES

Determine that the patient is obtaining adequate relief from pain. The patient should be free of complications of surgery or bed rest. The patient should understand their limitations and how to progress with ambulation, know how to do self-care activities in a safe manner, and understand the signs of complications and when to notify their physician.

CLINICAL PATHWAY (Patient with a Spinal Fixation with Pedicle Screws)

An example of a generic clinical pathway for a patient having a spinal fixation with pedicle screws is presented in Figure 8–40.

ANKYLOSING SPONDYLITIS

Ankylosing spondylitis (or Marie-Strümpell disease or Bechterew's disease) is a disease of the spinal column that occurs predominantly in men in late adolescence or early adulthood. It is characterized by a slow, progressive inflammation of the spine, the sacroiliac, and the larger joints of the extremities (particularly the hips, knees, and shoulders), leading to a fibrous or bony ankylosis and deformity (Fig. 8–41). The cause is unknown, and it is not clear whether it is a variant of rheumatoid arthritis or a totally different entity. The pathologic joint changes are indistinguishable in the two diseases, but the majority of patients with ankylosing spondylitis have a negative rheumatoid factor.

The condition usually starts insidiously with the first symptoms being most often vague and poorly localized. The patient complains of aching and stiffness about both sacroiliac joints, which usually occur as a morning backache. The pain subsides with activity but returns after sitting in one position for a long period of time. The patient commonly has a sciatic radiating pain, either unilateral or bilateral. Initially, the patient rarely has discomfort in the lumbothoracic or the cervicothoracic area. After 6 months to a year, the pain and the stiffness become progressively worse and slowly spread to the rest of the spine. There are severe spasms in the paraspinal muscles with the flexors predominating and pulling the entire spine into forward flexion, so that the cervical and lumbar curves are obliterated. The thoracic curve is exaggerated, and the end result is a single kyphotic rounding of the entire back. Although the deformity is occurring in the spine, the hips, the knees,

---

Figure 8–40
Clinical Pathway: Spinal Fusion with Pedicle Screws

Admission Date: _____   **Discharge Plan:** _____ **Home** _____ **Skilled Nursing** _____ **Extended Care Facility**

Pathway	Preadmission Office/OP Clinic	Admission Day Op day	Hosp Day 2 Post-op 1	Hosp Day 3 Post-op 2	Hosp Day 4 Post-op 3	Hosp Day 5 Post-op 4	Outcomes
Consultation	Primary Care/ Medical physician	Case Manager Anesthesia, Dietitian	Social Work				
			PT, OT if nec.				Cont. @ Home
		Acute Pain Service					
Assessment	Nrsg database	Review & add					
	H & P Exam. by MD, NP or PA	Review H & P					
		Postop routine				Resolved	
	Rehab/ECF/home		Referral if nec.				
	Home equipment		Referral if nec.		✓ if obtained		Will have nec. equipment @ home
		N/V status legs	Cont.	Cont.	Cont.	Cont.	
Tests	ECG/UA/CXR/1– 2 units autol. blood	X-ray in OR	✓ CBC/Diff				
		H & H in PACU & repeat in pm	Transfuse per protocol				
	Coag. studies						
	Spine X-rays & MRI						

(continued)

Figure 8–40

Clinical Pathway: Spinal Fusion with Pedicle Screws: *(continued)*

Pathway	Preadmission Office/OP Clinic	Admission Day Op day	Hosp Day 2 Post-op 1	Hosp Day 3 Post-op 2	Hosp Day 4 Post-op 3	Hosp Day 5 Post-op 4	Outcomes
Medications	D/C NSAIDs/ ASA/b/4 OR	Anticoagulant Routine meds ✓ preadm meds	Cont. Anticoag.	Cont.	Cont.	Cont.	States meds, when to take, and purpose
	Instruct on preop meds b/4 OR						
	Prophylatic Antibiotics	IV Antibiotics		D/C antibiotics			
	Analgesics as nec	PCA/Epidural pump		D/C IV and begin Oral pain meds			Pain managed with Analgesics @ home
	Start on Iron Med	Cont. Iron meds					
		Bowel protocol					Normal bowel elim.
Diet	Assessment wt. balanced diet	NPO @MN b/4 OR	Liquids/as tolerated	Advance as tolerated			Tolerating diet
		Ice chips/return bowel sounds		Roughage & liquids			
Activity	Preop mobility	Ankle Pumps	Cont				
		Log-roll turn q 2 hrs	Turn q 2hrs				
		Quad & Glut q 2	Cont.				
		Bed rest	OOB to BR with TLSO Brace	Walking with brace on and assistance			Walking @ home with Brace on without asst.
Treatments	Set blood donation dates, 1 wk between units & 14 days between last unit and OR day	IV fluids/blood if necessary, I&O					
		TEDs, IPCD or foot pumps					Cont. TEDS @ home
		Hemovac/output		D/C			No complications
		Dressing	Do Not Change			Change PRN	No infection
		IS/TCDB q hr w/a		PRN			Clear lungs
		Foley to drain		D/C			Normal bladder elim.
Education	Review pre & postop. care procedures (Log-rolling & getting OOB) & Brace	Reinforce	Cont. Rev. hosp routine	Cont.			
	Rev. rehabilitation, body mechanics & exercises		Review Rehab			Reinforce	Knows care of & how to live with the Brace
	Attends gp ed class		Reinforce Ed.				
	Pain management	Rev. pain mng	Reinforce				
	Review hosp LOS						
D/C Plan	Identify discharge plan		Notify Social Worker Or Home Health if nec.				Discharged to home
	Caregivers & home situation (LOS 5–7 days		Care as appropriate				States reason to contact physician
	Discuss wearing & care of TLSO						

and the shoulders become painfully distended with increased synovial fluid. The muscles around the joints develop painful spasms that produce flexion adduction deformities of the hips, flexion of the knees, and adduction and internal rotation of the shoulders. At that stage, the typical "stooped-over" position is usually evident. The patient faces downward, as the entire back is rounded, the hips and the knees are semiflexed, and the arms cannot be raised more than a limited amount. Complaints include radicular pain in the upper extremities, in the intercostal and anterior abdominal areas, in the groin, and in the lower extremities.

At present, no treatment effectively cures or arrests the progression of ankylosing spondylitis. Conservative treatment is directed toward relieving the pain and keeping the spine erect. Treatment usually consists of drugs, positioning, exercises, and physical therapy. A common back surgery is an osteotomy of the spine where a wedge of bone is removed from the posterior portion of the spinal column, usually at the lumbar level (L2–3 or L3–4). That area is usually selected because the thoracic spine is fixed by rib attachments, the lumbar canal is wider, and that level is below the level of the cord.

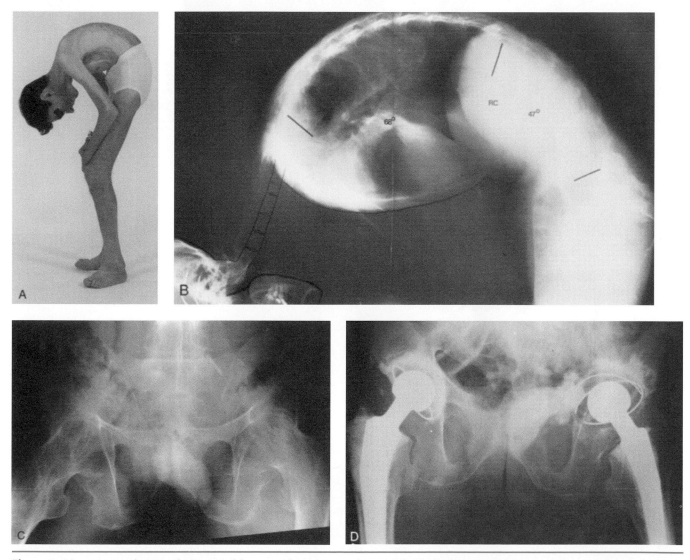

Figure 8–41 (A) Lateral view of 36-year-old man with an 18-year history of ankylosing spondylitis presenting combined kyphotic deformities. The patient was able to see only backward and had to walk backward. The lateral view shows a chin-brow to vertical angle of 134 degrees. Cervical kyphosis is present but not the area of main deformity. (B) Lateral standing radiograph showing cervical kyphosis, thoracic kyphosis of 68 degrees with complete loss of lumbar lordosis, and additional 47 degrees of lumbar kyphosis with hip flexion deformities. (C) Anteroposterior radiograph of pelvis showing fused hip joints in flexion. Bilateral total hip replacement arthroplasties were done at one sitting, under regional anesthesia. (D) Anteroposterior view of total replacement arthroplasties. *(continued)*

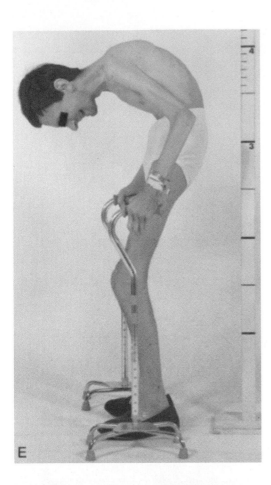

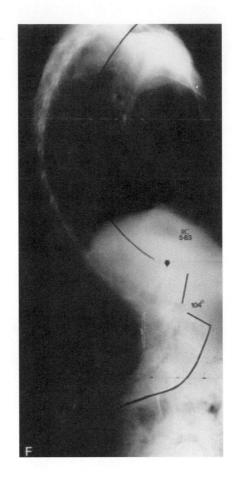

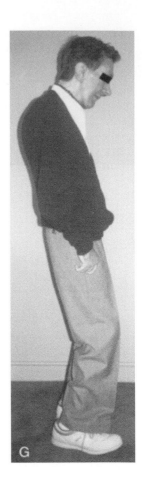

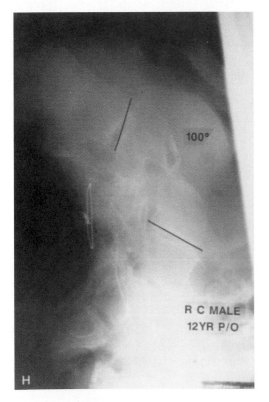

Figure 8–41   (E) Lateral view of the patient showing improvement following hip arthroplasties, but the patient is now not able to see backward nor forward for walking. (F) Lateral standing 3-ft radiograph of spine following resection-extension osteotomy at L3-4 of 104 degree done under local anesthesia. Note shift of weight-bearing line well posterior to osteotomy site. (G) Standing lateral view of patient 12 years postoperatively showing correction of major deformities. He still has some kyphosis of neck and knee flexion but is able to stand and look ahead. He is able to enjoy normal daily activities and walks in a normal fashion. His major areas of deformity have been corrected. (H) Lateral standing radiograph of lumbar spine showing remodeling and maintenance of correction in the area of main deformity.
(Bridwell & DeWald (1997). The Textbook of Spinal Surgery. *Philadelphia: Lippincott-Raven.)*

PELVIS

SACROILIAC STRAIN

Sacroiliac strain is a painful stretching of the ligaments about one or both sacroiliac joints. The condition is uncommon because the sacroiliac ligaments are very strong, and the movements of bending, lifting, or hyper-extending the back, which are likely to produce a torsion strain on the sacroiliac joints, will probably first cause a strain on the smaller lumbosacral ligaments. Individuals are most prone to sacroiliac strain when the ligaments are softened and elongated by pregnancy, prolonged periods of bending and lifting, or degenerative arthritis. The injury usually occurs in the act of straightening up from a stooped position. The hip flexors may hold the ilium forward while the sacrum is rotated backward, or the hamstrings and the gluteus maximus may extend the hip, rotating the ilium backward, while the sacrum is held forward by the weight of the trunk.

SACROILIAC SUBLUXATION

Sacroiliac subluxation implies that ligamentous stretching has been sufficient to permit the ilium to slip on the sacrum. Typically, an irregular prominence on one articulating surface becomes wedged on another prominence of the opposite articulating surface. The ligaments become taut, reflex muscle spasms are intense, and pain is severe and continuous until reduction is effected. The displacement may be so slight that it cannot be recognized in roentgenograms. The condition is differentiated from sacroiliac strain in that pain is more intense and is not relieved by sitting, recumbency, or a tight encircling bandage. The pain is often relieved dramatically and suddenly by manipulation.

PELVIC FRACTURES

Pelvic (Fig. 8–42), sacral, and coccygeal fractures are often associated with multiple life-threatening injuries that occur in vehicular accidents, crush injuries, or falls that cause trauma to the pelvis (directly or indirectly through the femur). After head injuries, pelvic fractures are the most common cause of traumatic death. The life-threatening nature of pelvic injuries arises from the multiple fractures, soft-tissue injuries, hemorrhages, and shock that typically accompany them. Pelvic hemorrhages are especially serious because of the rich blood supply to the pelvis, the possibility of massive and hidden bleeding in the cancellous surfaces of the fracture fragments, and the laceration of veins and arteries (including the iliac artery) by bone spicules (fragments). The assessment in the ER or trauma unit focuses on the standard trauma triage protocols and will not be discussed here.

TREATMENT

Most fractures of the pelvis heal rapidly because the innominate bones are mostly cancellous bone, which have a rich blood supply. Surgery is usually required

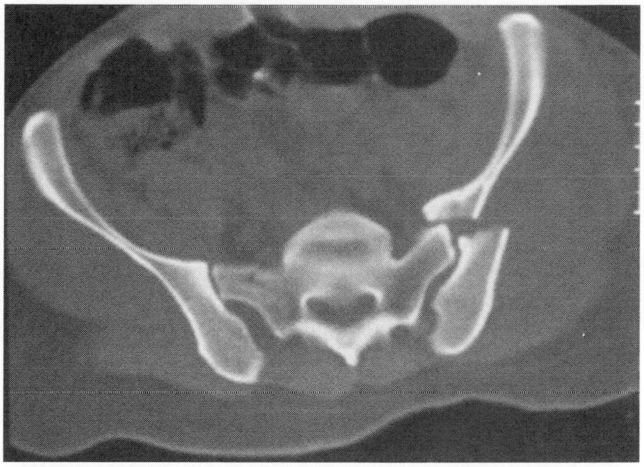

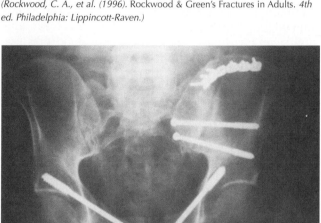

Figure 8–42   CT scan showing pelvic ring disruption. *(Rockwood, C. A., et al. (1996).* Rockwood & Green's Fractures in Adults. *4th ed. Philadelphia: Lippincott-Raven.)*

Figure 8–43   AP view of the pelvis after ORIF of bilateral anterior ring fractures.   *(Rockwood, C. A., et al. (1996).* Rockwood & Green's Fractures in Adults. *4th ed. Philadelphia: Lippincott-Raven.)*

for ruptured abdominal or pelvic viscera and occasionally for hemorrhage. In the past, pelvic slings, skeletal traction, and spica casts were used to manage these fractures. Today it is more common for the initial stabilization of fractures to be accomplished with external fixation devices, either used alone or in conjunction with open reduction and internal fixation (ORIF; Fig. 8–43). For a discussion of the use of external fixation devices and the nursing care for such patients, see Chapter 7. The type of immobilization depends on the nature and location of the fractures.

Earlier and more aggressive use of the ORIF method of treating pelvic fractures has increased in recent years due to new surgical procedures and instrumentations that provide for immobilization immediately after surgery. Using plates that conform to the anatomy of the pelvis in pelvic fracture stabilization leads to improved survival and decreases the incidence of adult respiratory distress syndrome from immobilization. Early ambulation not only reduces complications from bed rest but also shortens the length of hospital stay (in some cases from 68 to 25 days or less).

NURSING PROCESS (Patient with Closed Pelvic Fracture and ORIF)

The following nursing process demonstrates the nursing care of a patient with a pelvic fracture following an ORIF. The nursing process begins after the patient returns from the postanesthesia room or intensive care unit.

ASSESSMENT

The immediate postoperative assessment (which may take place in the intensive care unit) for a typical patient following an ORIF for a pelvic fracture involves taking vital signs (i.e., pulse, respiration, and blood pressure) and observing the patient's general color and warmth. A neurovascular assessment (pulse, temperature, color, capillary filling, edema, and sensory and motor nerve function) of the lower extremities should be made (see Chapter 2) and the position of the patient's legs in relation to the patient's trunk noted. Check that the incisional dressing is dry and intact and that drains or wound catheters (if utilized) are functioning. Check the patient's level of consciousness and orientation. Assess the type, severity, and location of pain, and determine whether the patient received pain medications in the operating room. Have the patient cough and deep breathe, and auscultate their lungs. Note the type of intravenous solutions, the rate of flow, and the amount left in the bag. Determine blood loss in surgery and replacement of fluids. Check the patient's urinary catheter for amount of output.

Frequent assessments of the patient should be made during the postoperative period. These include the auscultation of the patient's chest, assessment of the neurovascular status of the lower extremities, determining the amount of intake and output of fluids and noting the presence of bowel sounds. Note any signs or symptoms of shock, pulmonary emboli, deep vein thrombosis, or infection.

NURSING DIAGNOSIS

Based on all of the assessment data, the major nursing diagnoses for a typical patient with pelvic fractures and an ORIF may include the following:

- Pain and discomfort related to bone and soft-tissue trauma
- Impaired physical mobility related to instability of the pelvis
- Risk of impaired skin integrity related to immobility
- Constipation related to decreased activity and pain medications

- Ineffective individual coping related to the trauma and rehabilitation process
- Increased anxiety related to knowledge deficit about the procedure and the rehabilitation process

COLLABORATIVE PROBLEMS

- Deep vein thrombosis
- Pulmonary emboli
- Hypovolemic shock
- Infection

GOAL FORMULATION AND PLANNING

The goals are to have the patient experience (1) a decrease in pain through nursing measures and medications; (2) an increase in mobility with the use of crutches or a walker; (3) no break in skin integrity; (4) normal bowel elimination; (5) effective coping; (6) a decrease in anxiety through increased knowledge of the surgical procedure, rehabilitation process, and prognosis; and (7) an absence of complications.

INTERVENTIONS

ALLEVIATE PAIN

Pain management is essential for a patient following a pelvic fracture and an ORIF. Pain must be controlled to allow the patient to actively participate in the rehabilitation process. Patient-controlled analgesia with morphine is usually used for the first 24 to 48 hours. The patient will then be placed on oral narcotics.

Assess the patient's pain for amount, severity, and cause. Verify that the patient is correctly positioned while in bed or in a chair and that the correct amount of weight or nonweight was applied to the extremities during transfer. Teach the patient relaxation techniques and utilize activities as a means of distraction to help relieve the patient's feelings of pain. For further discussion of pain management, see Chapter 2.

INCREASE MOBILITY

Methods to increase the patient's mobility focus on correct positioning, exercises, and ambulation.

Position. While the patient is in bed, they should be turned and repositioned every 2 hours. If their fracture site is only on one side, turn the patient to the unfractured or nonoperative side. If the patient has bilateral fracture involvement, the patient can be turned from their back to either side. However, when on their side, the patient should be tilted at a 45-degree angle. Use log-rolling to turn the patient (see care of a patient following a posterior fusion with instrumentation earlier in this chapter).

Exercises. The patient should start muscle-setting exercises immediately after surgery. These exercises should include quadriceps- and gluteal-setting, ankle pumps, and range of motion to the ankle. In patients with associated acetabular fractures, continuous passive motion (CPM) machines may be used to prevent loss of range of motion in the hip (see total knee replacement in Chapter 10). The patient should also work on exercises for the upper extremities to assist with crutch walking (see Chapter 4).

Ambulation. On the first postoperative day, if not contraindicated by other injuries, the patient may be gotten out of bed and into a chair. Be alert to the fact that the patient may feel weak or dizzy because of the blood lost (and replaced) since the trauma and during surgery. Patients who have associated bilateral acetabular fractures are nonweight bearing and must transfer to a chair using a sliding board. Patients with unilateral posterior injuries are permitted early weight bearing on the noninjured side and non-weight bearing or toe touch on the injured side 8 to 12 weeks postoperatively. After 12 weeks postoperatively, patients with bilateral injuries are allowed limited weight bearing (e.g., standing for transfers) on the less disrupted side only.

MAINTAIN SKIN INTEGRITY

In administering care, make sure that there are no signs of redness or pressure on bony prominences. Reposition the patient every 2 hours as discussed under positioning. Turning every 2 hours not only prevents pressure areas but also aids in preventing pooling of blood and tissue fluid in the dependent areas. Keep the prominent bony areas soft and well lubricated. Massage to those areas should be done gently with a circular motion. Keep linen dry and free of wrinkles. A number of institutions place these patients on a low-air-loss bed (e.g., Kinair® Mediscus®, and Flexicare®). Keep the patient well hydrated and maintain a well-balanced diet with adequate protein.

CONSTIPATION

Following a pelvic fracture with an ORIF, patients have limited activity and are taking pain medications, which put them at risk for constipation. Most will be on stool softener medication, but also make sure the patient takes in plenty of fluids to keep their stool soft, eats a high fiber diet that includes fresh fruits and vegetables, and does as much activity as allowed. At the same time, maintain a diet that does not cause the patient to gain weight as that would adversely affect their mobility.

COPING MECHANISMS

Depression can occur in patients following surgery and during the rehabilitation process. Patients feel "helpless" and are unwilling to try to do anything for themselves. Look for decreased concentration, fatigue, increased restlessness, increased complaints, or withdrawal from staff and others. Encourage the patient and family to verbalize questions. Keep the patient actively involved in their care and involved in any decisions that need to be made. To help prevent or reduce boredom and self-centeredness, find activities that can occupy the patient's time and that they like to do. Try to make the activities mentally stimulating as a change from the passive role of television viewer. The occupational therapy department can be of assistance in the hospital as well as in planning activities for home care.

PATIENT TEACHING AND HOME CARE CONSIDERATIONS

Patient teaching focuses on the exercise and rehabilitation regime. The accident was both a physical and emotional shock to the patient, so be aware that they may be suffering from anxiety and stress related to the trauma. Most of the activities up to this time have focused on physical well-being; it is now time to let the patient talk about the accident and what occurred. The patient may also have symptoms related to posttraumatic stress syndrome (see Chapter 4). See Chapter 1 for a discussion of how patients adjust to a possible debilitating injury or long rehabilitation process.

Know what the physician has told the patient and what the plan of treatment will be. Reinforce these objectives and help the patient plan a realistic home rehabilitation program. Make sure the patient understands the purpose of the exercises, how they are to be done, how often they are to be done, and what to do should pain or swelling develop after exercising. Make sure the patient is safe doing crutch walking and knows how to go up and down stairs and how to get in and out of a car before going home (see Chapter 4). Discuss with the patient home care issues such as activities of daily living and food preparation.

MONITORING AND MANAGING POTENTIAL PROBLEMS

The major complications that may arise following a pelvic fracture with an ORIF are (1) deep vein thrombosis, (2) pulmonary emboli, (3) hypovolemic shock, and (4) infection.

DEEP VEIN THROMBOSIS

Unless precluded by the patient's general physical condition, some institutions use a combination of pneumatic sequential compression stockings, elastic stockings, and low-dose heparin or coumadin as a prophylaxis against thromboembolism. Some physicians perform pre- or postoperative duplex ultrasound screening (which combine real time imaging and pulsed Doppler) capabilities to identify deep venous thrombosis.

PULMONARY EMBOLI

The term *pulmonary emboli* refers to the obstruction of one or more pulmonary arteries by a thrombus (or thrombi), which originates somewhere in the venous system or the right side of the heart, becomes dislodged, and is carried to the lung. An infarction of lung tissue occurs due to the interruption of the lung's blood supply. The best treatment is prevention. Keep the patient well hydrated, doing active and passive exercises, and ambulating as tolerated. Pharmacologic prophylaxis measures may include aspirin, low-dose heparin or coumadin, and utilizing compression or elastic stockings. Inferior vena caval filters may be used to minimize the risk of pulmonary embolism. See Chapter 4 for further discussion.

HYPOVOLEMIC SHOCK

Hypovolemic shock is the result of hemorrhage and loss of extracellular fluid into damaged tissues. The patient has had a relatively large blood loss before, during, and immediately following surgery. Make sure adequate intake and output records are maintained. Assess the balance between them, as the patient could still develop shock. The greatest risk for the patient was before surgery, but risks persist after surgery. The prevention and/or treatment of shock consists of replacing depleted blood volume.

INFECTION

Check to see if the entire dressing is dry and intact. Reinforce the dressing and notify the physician if there is excess bleeding. The initial postoperative dressing is usually left in place until the drains, if used, are removed 48 hours postoperatively, and then standard wound management care is implemented. Because these patients are at risk for infection, most are placed on prophylactic antibiotic therapy before, during, and after surgery. Note any signs and symptoms of infection not only near the incision but also involving the pulmonary and urinary tracts.

EVALUATION/OUTCOMES

For a typical patient recovering from a pelvic fracture with an ORIF, pain will be controlled by nursing interventions and medications. With a unilateral fracture, the patient is able to ambulate safely using a three-point gait with non-weight bearing (or toe touch) on the injured side. Before going home, the patient is able to demonstrate compliance in doing exercises and going up and down stairs safely with crutches. If the patient received a bilateral injury, they are able to transfer safely to a chair using a sliding board. The patient will verbalize an understanding of the goals and objectives of rehabilitation and their role in achieving them. The patient will be free of complications.

CLINICAL PATHWAY (Patient with Closed Pelvic Fracture and ORIF)

An example of a generic clinical pathway for a patient with closed pelvic fracture and ORIF is presented in Figure 8–44.

Figure 8–44

Clinical Pathway: Closed Pelvic Fracture with ORIF

Admission Date: _____   Discharge Plan: _____ Home _____ Skilled Nursing _____ Extended Care Facility

Pathway	Preadmission Office/OP clinic	Admission Day Op day	Hosp Day 2 Post-op 1	Hosp Day 3 Post-op 2	Hosp Day 4 Post-op 3	Hosp Day 5 Post-op 4	Outcomes
Consultation	Primary Care/ Medical physician	Case Manager Anesthesia, Dietitian Acute Pain Service	Social Work PT, OT if nec.				Cont. @ Home
Assessment	Nrsg database H & P Exam. by MD, NP, or PA	Review & add Review H & P Postop routine				Resolved	
	Rehab/ECF/home		Referral if nec.				
	Home equipment		Referral if nec.		✓ if obtained		Will have nec. equipment @ home
	N/V status of legs	N/V status legs	Cont.	Cont.	Cont.	Cont.	
Tests	ECG/UA/CXR/Chem7	X-ray in OR	✓ CBC/Diff Transfuse per protocol	✓CBC/Diff Transfuse per protocol			
	X & Type units of blood	H & H in PACU & repeat in pm					
	Coag. studies						
	Pelvic x-rays & MRI						
Medications	Trauma patient ✓ Routine meds	Anticoagulant Restart routine meds.	Cont. Anticoag.	Cont.	Cont.	Cont.	States meds, when to take, and purpose
	Instruct on preop meds b/4 OR	✓ preadm meds					
	Prophylatic Antibiotics	IV Antibiotics		D/C antibiotics			
	Pain meds as approp.	PCA/Epidural pump		D/C IV and begin Oral pain meds			Pain managed with Analgesics @ home

(continued)

Figure 8–44

Clinical Pathway: *(continued)*

Pathway	Preadmission Office/OP clinic	Admission Day Op day	Hosp Day 2 Post-op 2	Hosp Day 3 Post-op 3	Hosp Day 4 Post-op 4	Hosp Day 5 Post-op 4	Outcomes
	Start on Iron Med	Cont. Iron meds Bowel protocol					Normal bowel elim.
Diet	Assessment pre. admission diet	NPO @MN b/4 OR	Liquids/as tolerated	Advance as tolerated			Tolerating diet
		Ice chips/return bowel sounds		Roughage & liquids			
Activity	Preop mobility	Ankle Pumps	Cont.	Cont.	Cont.		
		Unlt fr. turn (log) to Nonop. side q 2 hrs	Turn q 2hrs	Cont.	Cont.		
		Quad & Glut q 2	Cont.	Cont.	Cont.		
		CPM affected side	Cont.	Cont.	Cont.		
		Bed rest	Unil-OOB to Chair NWB - 3-pt gait	OOB to BR with CW -3 pt			CW -3pt. Gait. @ home for 8–12 wks.
Treatments		IV fluids/blood if necessary, I&O TEDs, IPCD or foot pumps	Cont.	DC if liq tolerated			Cont. TEDS @ home
			Cont.	Cont.	Change PRN		No complications
		Hemovac/output	Cont.	D/C			
		Dressing	Do Not Change	Dressing change			No infection
		IS/TCDB q hr w/a		PRN			Clear lungs
		Foley to drain		D/C if approp.			Normal bladder elim.
Education	Review postop. care procedures	Reinforce	Cont.	Cont.			
			Rev. hosp routine			Reinforce	
			Review Rehab				
	Pain management Review hosp LOS	Rev. pain mgmt	Reinforce				
D/C Plan	Identify discharge plan		Notify Social Worker Or Home Health if nec.				Discharged to home or ECF Knows when to contact physician
	Caregivers & home situation (LOS up to 25 days)		Care as appropriate				

References

Alonso, J. E. (1994). Pelvic and acetabulum fractures. In V. R. Masear (Ed.), *Primary care orthopaedics* (pp. 63–71). Philadelphia: W. B. Saunders.

Baldus, C., & Blanke, K. (1997). Preoperative nursing care. In K. H. Bridwell & R. L. DeWald (Eds.), *The textbook of spinal surgery* (2nd ed., pp. 3–10). Philadelphia: Lippincott-Raven.

Bates, B. (1995). *A guide to physical examination and history taking.* Philadelphia: J. B. Lippincott.

Belinsky, J. D. (1993). Acetabular fracture: ORIF. *Orthopaedic Nursing, 12*(1), 42–50.

Berg, E. E. (1998). Radiology review: Open book (AP compression) pelvis fracture. *Orthopaedic Nursing, 17*(2), 59–62.

Bigoas, S., Bowyer, O., Braen, G., et al. (1994, December). *Acute low back problems in adults: Assessment and treatment* (AHCPR Publication No. 95-0643). Rockville, MD: U.S. Department of Health and Human Services.

Bolesta, M. J., Viere, R. G., Montesano, P. X., & Benson, D. R. (1996). Fractures and dislocation of the thoracolumbar spine. In C. A. Rockwood, D. P. Green, R. W. Bucholz, & J. D. Heckman (Eds.), *Rockwood and Green's fractures in adults* (4th ed., pp. 1529–1574). Philadelphia: Lippincott-Raven.

Borrelli, J., Koval, K. J., & Helfet, D. L. (1998). Pelvis and acetabulum. In K. J. Koval & J. D. Zuckerman (Eds.), *Fractures in the elderly* (pp. 159–174). Philadelphia: Lippincott-Raven.

Brosnan, H., & Berda, P. (1990). Pedicle screw fixation in the lumbar spine. *Orthopaedic Nursing, 9*(6), 22–30, 32.

Brown, J. C. (1997). Cotrel-Dubousset instrumentation in the treatment of adolescent idiopathic scoliosis. In K. H. Bridwell & R. L. DeWald (Eds.), *The textbook of spinal surgery* (2nd ed., pp. 489–534). Philadelphia: Lippincott-Raven.

Brown, K. L. (1998). Cauda equina syndrome: Implications for the orthopaedic nurse in a clinical setting. *Orthopaedic Nursing, 17*(5), 31–35.

Burgess, A. R., & Jones, A. L. (1996). Fractures of the pelvic ring. In C. A. Rockwood, D. P. Green, R. W. Bucholz, & J. D. Heckman (Eds.), *Rockwood and Green's fractures in adults.* (4th ed., 1575–1616). Philadelphia: Lippincott-Raven.

Chase, J. A. (1992). Outpatient management of low back pain. *Orthopaedic Nursing, 11*(1), 11–20.

DeWald, R. L. (1997). Spondylolisthesis. In K. H. Bridwell & R. L. DeWald (Eds.), *The textbook of spinal surgery* (2nd ed., pp. 1199–1210). Philadelphia: Lippincott-Raven.

Doheny, M., Linden, P., & Sedlak, C. (1995). Reducing orthopaedic hazards of the computer work environment. *Orthopaedic Nursing, 14*(1), 7–15.

Enke, P., & Steffee, A. D. (1997). Total disc replacement. In K. H. Bridwell & R. L. DeWald (Eds.), *The textbook of spinal surgery.* 2nd ed., pp. 2275–2288). Philadelphia: Lippincott-Raven.

Feingold, D. J., Peck, S. A., Reinsma, E. J., & Ruda, S. C. (1991). Complications of lumbar spine surgery. *Orthopaedic Nursing, 10*(4), 39–58.

Ficner, H. B. (1993). Revision surgery in adult scoliosis patients. *Orthopaedic Nursing, 12*(2), 23–32.

Gates, S., (1995). Development of the practice guidelines for acute low back pain in adults. *Orthopaedic Nursing, 14*(5), 35–36.

Giehl, J. P., & Zielke, K. (1997). Anterior Zielke instrumentation in thoracolumbar and lumbar curves. In K. H. Bridwell & R. L. DeWald (Eds.), *The textbook of spinal surgery* (2nd ed., pp. 627–649). Philadelphia: Lippincott-Raven.

Green, N. E. (1997). The role of Harrington rods and Wisconsin wires. In K. H. Bridwell & R. L. DeWald (Eds.), *The textbook of spinal surgery* (2nd ed., pp. 627–640). Philadelphia: Lippincott-Raven.

Gruen, G. S, & Engle, C. (1993). Vertical shear fractures of the pelvis. *Orthopaedic Nursing, 12*(5), 55–59.

Halverson, P. B. (1997). The spondyloarthropathies. *Orthopaedic Nursing, 16*(4), 21–25.

Jackson, R. P. (1997). Lumbar burst fractures: Fixation with pedicle instrumentation and reduction by adjustable contoured translating axes. In K. H. Bridwell & R. L. DeWald (Eds.), *The textbook of spinal surgery* (2nd ed., pp. 1881–1898). Philadelphia: Lippincott-Raven.

Jerva, M. J. (1993). Automated percutaneous lumbar discectomy: A review. *Orthopaedic Nursing, 12*(3), 27–31.

Johnson, J., Anderson, C., Barrett, A., Duke, K., & Sharp, D. (1995). Roller traction: Mobilizing patients with acetabular fractures. *Orthopaedic Nursing, 14*(1), 21–24.

Johnston, C. E., Ashman, R. B., Richards, B. S., & Herring, J. A. (1997). TSRH universal spine instrumentation. In K. H. Bridwell & R. L. DeWald (Eds.), *The textbook of spinal surgery* (2nd ed., pp. 535–568). Philadelphia: Lippincott-Raven.

Kirkpatrick, J. S., & Ghavan, C. (1996). Injuries to the spinal column. In V. R. Masear (Ed.), *Primary care orthopaedics* (pp. 50–62). Philadelphia: W. B. Saunders.

Kopp, M. (1997). Caring for the adult patient undergoing anterior/posterior spinal fusion. *Orthopaedic Nursing, 16*(2), 55–59.

Kostuik, K. P. (1997). Intervertebral disc replacement. In K. H. Bridwell & R. L. DeWald (Eds.), *The textbook of spinal surgery* (2nd ed., pp. 2257–2266). Philadelphia: Lippincott-Raven.

Kuslich, S. D. (1997). Anterior interbody fusion of the lumbar spine using a bone graft containing hollow, rigid interbody device—The Bagby and Kuslich method of spinal fusion. In K. H. Bridwell & R. L. DeWald (Eds.), *The textbook of spinal surgery* (2nd ed., pp. 2243–2257). Philadelphia: Lippincott-Raven.

Leininger, S. M. (1997). *Building clinical pathways.* Pitman, NJ: National Association of Orthopaedic Nursing.

Lisanti, P., & Verdisco, L. A. (1994). Perceived body space and self-esteem in adult females with chronic low back pain. *Orthopaedic Nursing, 13*(2), 55–63.

Main, W. K., Cammisa, F. P., O'Leary, P. F., Bryan, B. M., Hoffman, B. D., & Klein, J. D. (1998). The spine. In K. J. Koval & J. D. Zuckerman (Eds.), *Fractures in the elderly* (pp. 143–158). Philadelphia: Lippincott-Raven.

Meyers, P. R. (1997). Cervical spinal fractures: Changing management concepts. In K. H. Bridwell & R. L. DeWald (Eds.), *The textbook of spinal surgery* (2nd ed., pp. 1679–1742). Philadelphia: Lippincott-Raven.

Motte, K. M. (1991). Making a thoraco-lumbo-sacral orthosis. *Orthopaedic Nursing, 10*(4), 59–62.

Neuwirth, M., & Marsicano, J. (1996). Cervical spondylosis: Diagnosis, symptomatology, and treatment. *Orthopaedic Nursing, 15*(1), 31–42.

Olson, B., & Ustanko, L. (1990). Self-care needs of patients in the halo brace. *Orthopaedic Nursing, 9*(1), 27–33, 52.

Olson, B., Ustanko, L., & Warner, S. (1991). The patient in a halo brace: Striving for normalcy in body image and self-concept. *Orthopaedic Nursing, 10*(1), 44–50.

Patel, P. R., & Lauerman, W. C. (1997). Radiology review: The use of magnetic resonance imaging in the diagnosis of lumbar disc disease. *Orthopaedic Nursing, 16*(1), 59–65.

Popkess-Vawter, S., & Patzel, B. (1992). Compounded problem: Chronic low back pain and overweight in adult females. *Orthopaedic Nursing, 11*(6), 31–35, 43.

Rodts, M. F. (1997). Perioperative and postoperative nursing care for the spinal surgery patient. In K. H. Bridwell & R. L. DeWald (Eds.), *The textbook of spinal surgery* (2nd ed., pp. 11–30). Philadelphia: Lippincott-Raven.

Rodts, M. F. (1998). Disorders of the spine. In A. B. Maher, S. W. Salmond, & T. A. Pellino (Eds.), *Orthopaedic nursing* (2nd ed., pp. 545–585). Philadelphia: W. B. Saunders.

Stauffer, E., & MacMillan, M. (1996). Fractures and dislocations of the cervical spine. In C. A. Rockwood, D. P. Green, R. W. Bucholz, & J. D. Heckman (Eds.), *Rockwood and Green's fractures in adults.* (4th ed., pp. 1473–1528). Philadelphia: Lippincott-Raven.

U.S. Department of Health and Human Services. (1995). Acute low back problems in adults: Assessment and treatment (AHCPR Publication No. 95-0643, December 1994). *Orthopaedic Nursing, 14*(5), 37–52.

Weinstein, S. L. (1994). The thoracolumbar spine. In S. L. Weinstein & J. A. Buckwalter (Eds.), *Turek's orthopaedics: Principles and their application* (pp. 447–488). Philadelphia: J. B. Lippincott Company.

Chapter

9

Care of a Patient with Hip and Femoral Surgery

Chapter 9 focuses on the care of patients with traumatic and pathologic conditions of the hip and femur, including the proximal femur. Surgical procedures that correct hip and femoral deformities and their associated nursing are discussed, from minor hip dislocations through total hip arthroplasties to traumatic injuries of the femoral shaft. The chapter begins with a review of the anatomy of the hip.

ANATOMY

The hip joint is a ball and socket joint with movements of flexion-extension, adduction-abduction, and a combination of circumduction and medial and lateral rotation. The head of the femur articulates with the cup-shaped fossa of the acetabulum. The head of the femur is completely covered with articular cartilage except over the small, roughened pit to which the ligament of the head of the femur is attached. The articular surface of the acetabulum forms an incomplete ring, termed the lunate surface, broadest at its upper part where the pressure of the body weight falls in the erect position, and narrowest where it covers the pubic constituent. The ligamentous structures of the joint are the fibrous capsule; the acetabular labrum; the ligament of the head of the femur; and the iliofemoral, ischiofemoral, pubofemoral, and transverse acetabular ligaments. The pubofemoral ligament forms the inferior and medial part of the anterior capsule. The ischiofemoral ligament reinforces the posterior surface of the capsule. Its fibers spiral laterally and upward, arching across the femoral neck to blend with the fibers of the zona orbicularis (Fig. 9–1).

The capsule is surrounded by muscles on all sides. Different muscles produce different movements. Flexion is accomplished by the psoas major and the iliacus, assisted by the pectineus, the rectus femoris, and the sartorius with the adductor longus assisting in the early stages. Extension is accomplished by the gluteus maximus and the hamstring muscles. Abduction is achieved by the glutei medius and minimus, assisted by the ten-

sor fasciae latae and the sartorius. Adduction is achieved by the adductors longus, brevis, and magnus, assisted by the pectineus and the gracilis. Medial rotation is accomplished by the tensor fasciae latae and the anterior fibers of the glutei minimus and medius. Lateral rotation is accomplished by the obturator muscles, the gemellus, and the quadratus femoris, assisted by the piriformis, the gluteus maximus, and the sartorius.

The arteries that supply the joint are derived from the obturator, the medial circumflex femoral, and the superior and inferior gluteal arteries. The nerves are derived from the femoral nerve, directly or through its muscular branches, the obturator, the accessory obturator, the nerve to the quadratus femoris, and the superior gluteal (Buckwalter, 1994; Wasielewski, 1998).

DISLOCATIONS OF THE HIP JOINT

A dislocation occurs when the bones that make up a joint are out of anatomical alignment. Adult hip dislocations are most commonly traumatic, following such events as difficult deliveries, athletic injuries, and vehicular accidents, or are postoperative complications of a hip arthroplasty.

POSTERIOR DISLOCATIONS

Posterior dislocations of the hip are becoming more common and account for the majority of all hip dislocations (Jaffe, Killian, & Morris 1996). The injury usually occurs when a forceful blow applied to a flexed knee drives the femoral head posteriorly out of its socket, frequently fracturing the rim of the acetabulum. If the hip is in a neutral position or in adduction at the time of impact, there is usually a simple dislocation without a fracture. However, if the hip is slightly abducted, an associated fracture of the posterosuperior rim of the acetabulum usually occurs (DeLee, 1996, p. 1771). The involved limb is clinically shortened, internally rotated, and adducted (Fig. 9–2).

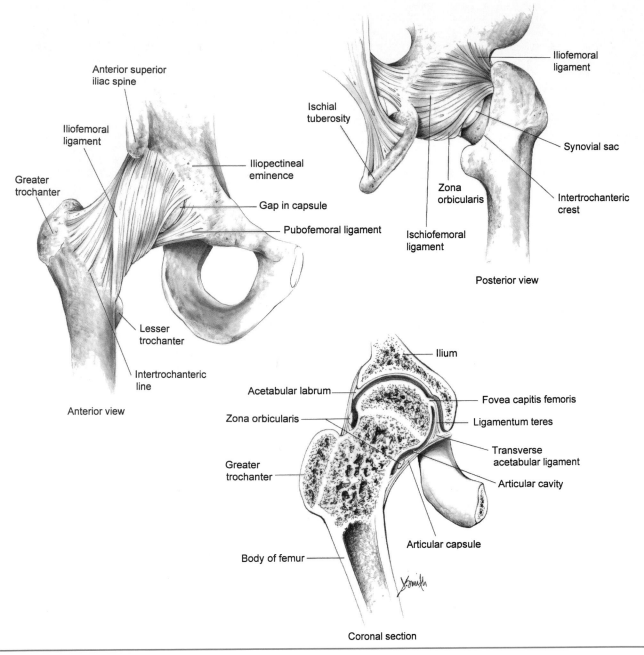

Figure 9–1   Ligaments of the hip joint.   *(Callahagen, et al. (1998). The Adult Hip. Philadelphia: Lippincott-Raven.)*

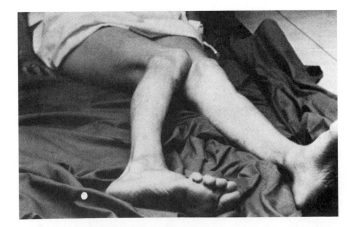

Figure 9–2   The clinical appearance of a posterior dislocation of the right hip.   *(Rockwood, et al. (1996).* Rockwood & Green's Fractures in Adults. *Philadelphia: Lippincott-Raven.)*

If high-energy trauma has occurred, assess for associated musculoskeletal injuries. In other instances, the dislocation may be due to abduction, where the head of the femur dislocates inferiorly and then assumes the posterior position. When that occurs, the hip internally rotates and is locked in a position of adduction and flexion, and the leg is shortened up to 5 cm (2 inches). Only the foot can be actively moved. The greater trochanter is abnormally prominent, whereas palpation beneath the inguinal ligament for the femoral head yields only an indentation. Passive rotation of the femur is absent. The pain is severe and constant in the inguinal region and thigh.

METHODS OF REPAIR

The most common treatment of a posterior dislocation is immediate closed reduction within 24 hours following injury. Reduction is usually accomplished in the emergency department with the patient under intravenous analgesic and muscle relaxants; others may require a general or spinal anesthesia in the OR. Although there are several different methods of reduction, the Allis maneuver is presented here (Fig. 9–3). The patient is positioned supine, and the patient's pelvis is stabilized by pressure on both anterior spines by an assistant. The physician then applies traction in the direct line of the deformity followed by gentle flexion of the hip to 90 degrees. The hip is then gently rotated internally and externally with continued longitudinal traction until reduction is accomplished (DeLee, 1996, p. 1774). Most reductions can be accomplished without open surgery, but occasionally the iliopsoas, the capsule, or both may prevent a nonsurgical reduction. An unstable reduction usually requires an open reduction to stabilize the hip.

ANTERIOR DISLOCATIONS

Anterior dislocations of the hip are rare, accounting for only 10% to 15% of hip dislocations (Jaffe, Killian, and Morris, 1996). Anterior dislocations occur when, in a vehicular accident, the knee strikes the dashboard with the thigh abducted; when a person lands on their feet after a fall from a height; or secondary to a blow to the back while in a squatting position. The femur is forcefully externally rotated and abducted, causing the femoral head to dislocate through a ruptured anterior capsule of the hip, which usually results in an associated femoral head fracture. The lower extremity is held in a position of abduction and external rotation with slight flexion. Often the femoral head can be palpated beneath the inguinal ligament in the anterior part of the thigh. There is no shortening of the limb, because the head is impaled anteriorly in the iliofemoral ligament (Fig. 9–4). The femoral artery and nerve, which run in that area, can be compromised at that point (DeLee, 1996).

METHODS OF REPAIR

Early diagnosis and prompt closed reduction under general or spinal anesthesia (or even under intravenous

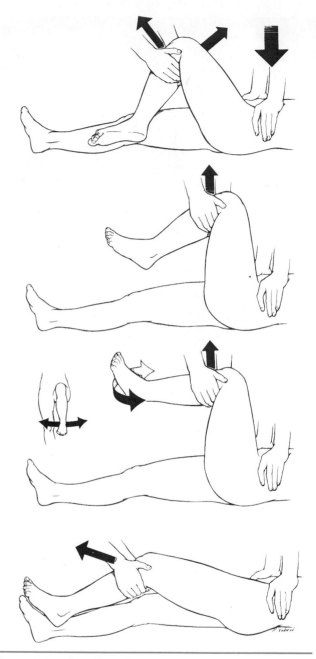

Figure 9–3   The Allis reduction maneuver for a posterior dislocation of the hip (see text for description).   *(Rockwood, et al. (1996). Rockwood & Green's Fractures in Adults. Philadelphia: Lippincott-Raven.)*

analgesia in some situations) are the treatment of choice. There are three common methods of closed reduction: Stimson's gravity method, the reverse Bigelow maneuver, and the Allis maneuver. In the Allis maneuver (Fig. 9–5), the patient is placed in the supine position. The patient's knee is flexed to relax the hamstrings. An assistant stabilizes the patient's pelvis and applies a lateral traction force to the inside of the thigh (DeLee, 1996; Jaffe, Killian, & Morris, 1996).

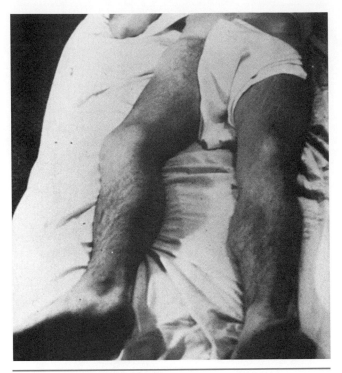

Figure 9–4 Clinical appearance of a superior-type anterior dislocation of the hip. (*Courtesy of Herman Epstein, M.D.*) *(Rockwood, et al. (1996). Rockwood & Green's Fractures in Adults. Philadelphia: Lippincott-Raven.)*

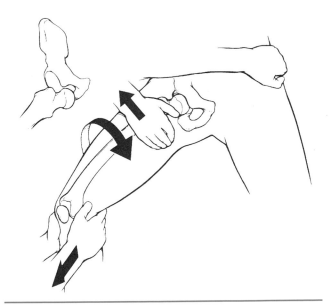

Figure 9–5 The Allis reduction maneuver for an anterior dislocation of the hip (see text for description). *(Rockwood, et al. (1996). Rockwood & Green's Fractures in Adults. Philadelphia: Lippincott-Raven.)*

CENTRAL DISLOCATIONS

A central dislocation of the hip can occur with a central fracture of the acetabulum, the mechanism of the injury being a direct blow to the trochanteric area.

NURSING PROCESS (Patient with a Dislocated Hip)

ASSESSMENT

The initial assessment of a typical patient admitted with a dislocated hip includes an evaluation of the patient's physical and emotional status. Emphasis should be placed on a complete description of what happened to cause the injury and a thorough physical assessment of the hip. The physical position of the involved leg is important. For a posterior hip dislocation, the leg is in adduction and flexion and may be shortened by up to 5 cm (2 inches). The greater trochanter is abnormally prominent, and only the foot can actually be moved. Pain is usually severe and constant in the inguinal region and the thigh. For anterior dislocations, the leg is in abduction and external rotation, slight flexion, and sometimes the femoral head is palpable beneath the inguinal ligament in the anterior part of the thigh. There is no shortening of the leg, but because of the position of the dislocated femoral head, the femoral artery and nerve can be compromised. Their function should be assessed quickly.

Postoperatively, the assessment is the same as for a patient recovering from general anesthesia and in skin or skeletal traction. Special considerations include neurovascular checks (Chapter 2) of the affected leg and of the traction apparatus (Chapter 5).

NURSING DIAGNOSIS

Based on all of the assessment data, nursing diagnoses for a typical patient with a reduced dislocated hip include the following:

- Pain and discomfort related to soft-tissue trauma
- Impaired physical mobility related to instability of the hip joint
- Anxiety related to knowledge deficit about rehabilitation and prognosis

COLLABORATIVE PROBLEMS

- Pin site infection (if the patient has skeletal traction)
- Myositis ossificans
- Aseptic necrosis of the femoral head
- Posttraumatic arthritis

GOAL FORMULATION AND PLANNING

The goals are to have the patient experience (1) a decrease in pain through nursing measures, traction, and prescribed medications; (2) an increase in mobility through positioning and controlled exercises; (3) a decrease in anxiety through patient education; and (4) an absence of complications from surgery and decreased activity.

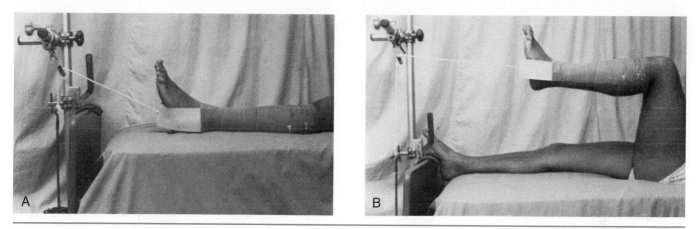

Figure 9–6 A modified Apley traction. This type of traction can be applied as skin of skeletal traction depending on hip stability. (*Top*) The thigh rests flat on the bed. (*Bottom*) Distal traction allows active hip and knee flexion. *(Rockwood, et al. (1996). Rockwood & Green's Fractures in Adults. Philadelphia: Lippincott-Raven.)*

INTERVENTIONS

ALLEVIATE PAIN

A large amount of the pain following a hip dislocation is from muscle spasms and soft-tissue trauma. Traction, by applying a continuous pull, helps to reduce pain by reducing muscle spasms. Consequently, when patients are first removed from traction, the pain may temporarily increase somewhat. Maintain the traction with a continuous pull, and avoid hitting or jarring the traction when providing care. Utilize nursing comfort measures, and provide pain and muscle relaxant medications as needed. Also teach the patient relaxation techniques they can utilize as well as providing other activities to take their mind off their injury. (For further information on treatment of pain, see Chapter 4.)

INCREASE MOBILITY

To increase hip joint stability and thus increase the patient's mobility, the nursing focus is on correct positioning, maintaining traction, doing exercises, and controlled-weight-bearing ambulation.

Position. The patient is maintained in traction with correct body alignment. Utilizing a spica cast after reduction is usually contraindicated because it prevents early range of motion (DeLee, 1996). The patient utilizes the trapeze and the unaffected leg to change position in bed and uses a fracture bedpan for elimination and linen changes while maintaining their traction in correct alignment. To do so, the patient should grip the trapeze with both hands and pull their body up while pushing down with their unaffected leg (with knee flexed and foot flat on the bed).

Traction. Because of the instability of the hip joint immediately after reduction, the involved leg is placed in 5 to 8 pounds of traction (Fig. 9–6) until the joint capsule and soft tissue heals, usually 5 days to 2 weeks for posterior and 5 to 7 days for anterior dislocations.

For a posterior dislocation, the traction is used to prevent the hip from flexing, internally rotating, and adducting. For a patient with an anterior dislocation, the traction maintains the leg in slight flexion and internal rotation. Skeletal traction with a pin through the tibia is utilized when the patient will be in traction for a long period of time or the patient's traction requires a large amount of weight to immobilize the leg, keep the hip in anatomical alignment, and reduce muscle spasms. Traction is maintained until the hip has painless range of motion. More specific details on the care of patients in traction are given in Chapter 6.

Exercises. Muscle rehabilitation is essential following a hip dislocation. The objective of exercise is to help restore muscle tone, develop muscle strength, and prevent the hip from dislocating again. The patient must do quadriceps- and gluteal-setting exercises, ankle pumps (plantar and dorsiflexion of the foot), flexion and extension of the leg, and active range of motion of the unaffected hip. Protected range of motion of the affected hip is begun while the leg is in traction to aid nutrition to the articular cartilage. Care must be taken to avoid extremes of abduction and external rotation for the patient following an anterior dislocation. A skateboard exercise is utilized twice a day to obtain full hip motion, especially abduction (Fig. 9–7). While the patient is utilizing the skateboard for adduction and abduction exercises, make sure the affected leg does not cross the midline (place the unaffected leg on a pillow at the midline). The patient must do exercises to prepare their arms and shoulders for weight bearing during crutch walking (see Chapter 4).

Ambulation. Once the patient has obtained painless range of motion in the affected hip, weight bearing is resumed. Ambulation usually begins with crutches and weight bearing as tolerated for patients following an anterior dislocation. There is a difference of opinion among physicians on when is the best time to resume

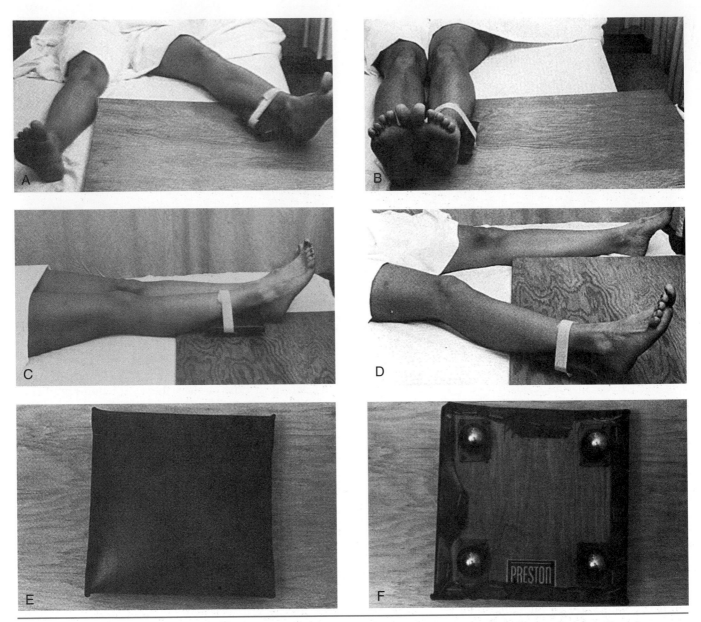

Figure 9–7   A pad with rollers (skateboard) is applied to the patient's heel and then placed on a piece of plyboard on the patient's bed. This allows active abduction and adduction exercises of the hip. (*Top*) Abduction and adduction viewed from the front. (*Center*) Abduction and adduction viewed from the side. (*Bottom*) Superior and inferior views of the padded roller.   *(Rockwood, et al. (1996). Rockwood & Green's Fractures in Adults. Philadelphia: Lippincott-Raven.)*

ambulation for individuals following a posterior dislocation, since some 25% to 30% of the patients develop avascular necrosis of the head of the femur due to interference with the blood supply. Most surgeons, however, believe that no treatment can alter the incidence of that condition (DeLee, 1996). Therefore, some physicians recommend weight bearing 2 to 4 weeks after reduction. Others restrict weight bearing for up to 12 weeks, and still others avoid weight bearing for 6 to 12 months.

PATIENT TEACHING AND HOME CARE CONSIDERATIONS
Most patients are healthy individuals with no other major medical problem. Once the hip is back in anatomical posi-

tion, the patient, family, and significant others need to understand the necessity for immobilization, exercise, and controlled ambulation (see increase mobility). Some may find it harder to understand immobilization and restriction for a dislocation as opposed to a fracture. Stress the importance of muscle rehabilitation following a dislocation to restore joint function and prevent recurrence.

MONITORING AND MANAGING POTENTIAL PROBLEMS

The major potential complications are infection related to the skeletal pin site (if skeletal traction is utilized) and the effects of bed rest (see Chapter 4). More long-term complications may be myositis ossificans, aseptic necrosis of the femoral head, and posttraumatic arthritis. See the references at the end of the chapter for further information related to collaborative problems.

EVALUATION/OUTCOMES

The patient is maintained in a level of comfort with traction, which is applied to the reduced hip joint until there is painless range of motion (usually for a relatively short period of time). There will be a return to full range of motion and weight-bearing without complications verified by an MRI done 2 to 6 months postdislocation.

CLINICAL PATHWAY

An example of a generic clinical pathway for a patient with a reduced posterior hip dislocation is presented in Figure 9–8.

Figure 9–8
Clinical Pathway: Dislocated Hip with Traction

Admission Date: _____   **Discharge Plan:** _____   **Home** _____   **Skilled Nursing** _____   **Extended Care Facility**

Pathway	ER/Trauma Unit	Admission Day Op day	Hosp Day 2 Post-op 2	Hosp Day 3 Post-op 3	Hosp Day 4 Post-op 4	Hosp Day 5	Outcomes
Consultation	Orthopaedic MD, Medical MD	Case Manager, Anesthesia	Social Work, PT	Dietitian			Cont. PT @ home, Assistance @ home If needed
Assessment	Nrsg database, H & P Exam. by MD, NP, or PA, CMST of involved Ext. q 15 x 4 then q hr, Other injuries	Review & add, Review H & P, Postop routine, CMST q 15 x 4 q 30 x 2, q 1 hr x 2, q 4 hrs.	Home environment			Resolved	Home safe for C/W
Tests	ECG/UA/CBC, SMA, AP & Lateral of Pelvis & hips	X-ray in OR Hip/Pelvic- H & H in PACU	✓ CBC				
Medications	✓ Home Meds, Demerol/ Morphine IM or IV for pain, Antibiotics, PCA, Preop meds b/4	preadm meds, Routine meds, Anticoagulant, Antibiotics, PCA/Epidural, Bowel protocol	D/C antibiotics, D/C begin oral pain meds				States meds, when to take and purpose, States purpose, Pain managed with oral medications, Normal bowel function
Diet	NPO.	NPO @ MN b/4 OR	Liquids, diet as tol.	Advance as tol, Encourage fluids			Tolerating diet
Activity	Bed rest	Bed rest with TX, Correct alignment, HOB elevated, No hip flexion, No internal rotation, No adduction	BRR with TX, Correct alignment, HOB elevate	Cont			Ambulate with a Walker or crutches, Using NWB or Toe-touch gait
Treatments	Start IV, Foley Catheter	IV fluids/, Intake & Output, Foley to drain, Antiembolic hose on unaffected leg	D/C if taking fluids, Continue, Continue	D/C, D/C, Continue			Normal bladder function

(continued)

Figure 9–8

Clinical Pathway: (continued)

Pathway	ER/Trauma Unit	Admission Day Op day	Hosp Day 2 Post-op 2	Hosp Day 3 Post-op 3	Hosp Day 4 Post-op 4	Hosp Day 5	Outcomes
Treatments (Continued)		Apley's Traction ____ lbs ____ leg	Continue	Continue	Continue	Continue	Able to ambulate safely on crutches
		Trapeze	Utilizes to reposition				
		Quadriceps-setting	Continue				
		Gluteal-setting q. 2 h	Continue				
		Ankle Pumps q. 2 h.	Continue				
		Skateboard x 2	Continue				
		Exercise Upper ext.	Continue				
		Hemovac/ output		D/C			No signs of infection
		IS/CDB q hr w/a		PRN			Clear lungs
		Dressing	Do Not Change	Change PRN (Wound care protocol)			No infection, States When to Call MD>
Education		Preoperative ed.	Operative routine				Verbalizes knowledge of the rehab. process
		Review hosp LOS	Rehab. Process				
D/C Plan		Identify discharge plan					Discharged to home
		Assistance at home					
		LOS 6 days to 2 weeks					

FRACTURES OF THE HIP

Hip fractures remain one of the most potentially devastating injuries of the elderly. The incidence of hip fracture increases with age, doubling for each decade beyond age 50, and occurs twice as often in women as in men (Koval & Zuckerman, 1998, p. 175; Kannus, Parkkasi, Hievanen, Heinonen, Uuori & Jarvinen., 1996). There is also a 2 to 3 times higher incidence of hip fractures in white females than in black and Hispanic women.

Approximately half of the individuals who break a hip will never walk independently again (Lindsay & Cosman, 1992), and a third will require placement in a long-term care institution (Cosman, Nieves, Horton, Shen, & Lindsay, 1994). Hip fracture results in a 12% to 20% excess mortality within the first year (Magaziner, Simonsick, Kashner, Hebel, & Kenzora, 1989), and the highest mortality rate occurs in the institutionalized elderly and those 85 years and older (Koval & Zuckerman, 1998, p. 175).

A fracture of the hip refers to a fracture of the proximal third of the femur, which extends up to 5 cm (2 inches) below the lesser trochanter. It occurs most commonly through the neck or the intertrochanteric region of the femur. Fractures of the hip are classified as either intracapsular of extracapsular. Intracapsular fractures are those occurring within the hip joint capsule, that is, within the fibrous tissues that enclose the hip joint. The intracapsular fractures are (1) capital (fractures of the head of the femur), (2) subcapital (fractures just below the head of the femur), and (3) transcervical (fractures of the neck of the femur). Extracapsular fractures are those outside of the joint capsule, through the femur's greater or lesser trochanter, in the intertrochanteric area, or in the subtrochanteric area.

NURSING PROCESS (Patient with an Unreduced Hip Fracture)

PREOPERATIVE ASSESSMENT

The patient admitted with a chief complaint of hip injury generally arrives on a stretcher. The first step in assessment is usually a visual inspection of the affected extremity. The classic features of the patient with a fractured hip are that the patient is usually elderly, has fallen, and has pain in the hip with shortening, adduction, external rotation, and slight flexion of the affected leg. However, different types of hip fractures may cause a slightly different positioning of the affected extremity. With extracapsular fractures, the leg rests in external rotation of 90 degrees and there is shortening and a lot of bruising. With intracapsular fractures, the joint capsule restrains rotation to about 45 degrees, and there is considerable swelling of the upper thigh. In patients having displaced intracapsular fractures, the extremity usually assumes a position of shortening and external rotation due to displacement at the fracture site and muscle spasms, which shorten and externally rotate the involved leg. When the femur separates at the time of the fracture, the strong gluteus medius muscle pulls the distal portion upward. The iliopsoas tends to rotate the leg outward, as does the gluteus maximus.

The major exception to the foregoing description is that patients with impacted intracapsular fractures are usually relatively pain free at first. The patient may have walked into the hospital after having walked on the fractured hip for a week or more before the discomfort increased enough to require medical attention. Upon observation of the affected leg, the nurse may notice that there is no shortening and the leg is in good alignment. The patient will limp only minimally. There is usually no deformity to the leg, but there may be marked valgus, that is, the patient will display a knocked knee. Pain can be elicited by slightly forcing the hip into internal rotation. A way to distinguish an impacted fracture from a displaced fracture is that the patient with an impacted fracture can lift the foot off the bed.

Subtrochanteric fractures usually involve younger patients, with the fracture produced by severe trauma. The fracture may be open or closed, and typically there is extensive hemorrhage into the soft tissue. The affected leg appears shortened, and there may be an anterior and lateral rotation. The line of pull and the great strength of the muscles of the hip and the thigh tend to produce marked displacement of bone fragments. Many powerful short muscles pull on the neck fragment, especially the iliopsoas, and tend to flex and rotate the proximal fragment.

An assessment of the injured hip must include a neurovascular check of the area distal to the injury. The neurovascular check must include capillary filling, color, temperature, edema, pulse, sensory nerve function, and motor nerve function. An adequate assessment of the entire extremity is imperative to guard against permanent neurovascular damage.

The complete assessment of the patient must include not only the assessment of the obvious injury but also an assessment of the patient's general status. That must be accomplished quickly, but thoroughly, before proceeding with nursing actions concerning the obvious injury. An open subtrochanteric fracture of the femur may appear to be the most serious injury but in many instances may in fact not be the most urgent. Pertinent observations of the patient can be made while personal clothing is being exchanged for a hospital gown and the patient is helped into a position of comfort. The injury may have just occurred, or the patient may have fallen at home and was unable to get help for several hours. Some patients who live alone may have abrasions or other skin lesions from dragging themselves trying to get help.

The major points in the general assessment are to assess for (1) chest pain or difficulty breathing; (2) possible internal bleeding at the fracture site, shock, or dehydration (e.g., vital signs, swelling at the site of the fracture, ecchymosis if the fracture occurred some hours before, skin turgor, and condition of the mucous membranes); (3) level of consciousness; orientation to time, place, and person; and ability to communicate; (4) the condition of other extremities (e.g., perhaps the patient has previously had a stroke or just suffered one that caused the fall); (5) pain; (6) the presence of other health problems; and (7) anxiety level. Find out who the patient's significant others are, if they are there, or whether they have been notified. If those persons cannot come to the hospital before surgery, it may be possible to have them talk directly to the patient by phone. If the family or significant others of the patient are available, this may be a good time to give them information about the patient's condition and also gain knowledge about the patient from them. Information needed may be on the mental alertness of the patient, the patient's ability to do activities of daily living, ambulatory status before injury, and other health problems, as well as the patient's likes and dislikes on food, fluids, allergies, and daily routines. Depending on the patient's condition and the time of the surgery, the nurse can do a more complete assessment and nursing history before surgery.

PREOPERATIVE NURSING DIAGNOSIS

Some patients with a fractured hip will go from the ER or trauma unit to OR, some will be admitted to the nursing unit until they can be taken to the OR (usually within 24 hours), while still others may be admitted to the nursing unit for a day or two until their general physical condition is stabilized for surgery. If the patient is to be maintained on the nursing unit, they will be placed in skin traction (except in cases of an impacted fracture). For a typical patient, preoperative hip fracture, the major nursing diagnoses related to the fracture include the following:

- Pain and discomfort related to bone and soft-tissue trauma
- Impaired physical mobility related to femur instability and pain
- Urinary incontinence related to age and reaction to trauma
- Impaired tissue integrity related to immobilization and immobilization device
- Altered peripheral tissue perfusion related to traction or other immobilization device
- Anxiety related to knowledge deficit about the trauma and rehabilitation

PREOPERATIVE COLLABORATIVE PROBLEMS

- Dehydration
- Additional damage to soft tissue and blood supply to the hip
- Lack of immobilization of the fracture site
- Other health problems

PREOPERATIVE GOAL FORMULATION AND PLANNING

The goals are to have the patient experience (1) a decrease in pain through nursing measures, traction, and prescribed pain medications; (2) an increase in mobility through the stabilization of the unreduced fracture with traction; (3) no urinary incontinence; (4) no break in skin integrity; (5) no neurovascular deficit from the traction or other immobilization device; and (6) a decrease in anxiety through increased knowledge.

PREOPERATIVE INTERVENTIONS

ALLEVIATE PAIN

The primary nursing interventions to relieve pain in a patient with an unreduced hip fracture are the administering of pain medications per order (after assessment of pain) and keeping the affected extremity in correct anatomical alignment. Repositioning the body and even the affected extremity can also relieve pain and discomfort. Speak in a quiet calm voice and explain to the patient what you are going to do and how they are involved. The patient needs to trust that the nurse will not cause them more pain. Work with the patient slowly and gently so the patient will relax, let the medications work, and thus ease the muscle tension and spasms in the affected hip to reduce the pain.

INCREASE MOBILITY

For the patient in the preoperative stage with a fractured hip, immobilization is key.

Position. Immobilization of the affected hip can be achieved through traction or pillows, sandbags, and trochanter rolls. Keep the affected leg from moving or externally rotating by placing a trochanter roll along the lateral aspect of the hip and/or a sandbag along the lateral aspect of the lower leg. Make sure there is no pressure applied against the proximal portion of the fibula (near the location of the peroneal nerve) or the external malleolus.

Turning. To turn a patient with an unreduced hip fracture, the nurse (with the assistance of another person if necessary) places a pillow between the patient's legs and then *turns the patient onto the side of the fracture.* The bed provides support to the fracture site to maintain hip stability. Usually a Foley catheter is inserted, but for the patient to have an elimination, turn the patient to the side of the fracture and use a fracture bedpan.

Traction. Depending on the size of the patient, skin traction is usually 3 to 5 pounds, but no more than 8 pounds are applied to the affected extremity (Fig. 9–9). The purpose of Buck's traction is to help reduce muscle spasms and keep the affected hip in position through immobilization (see Chapter 6 on traction). If the patient is in traction, maintain the traction at all times.

URINARY INCONTINENCY

Urinary incontinency afftects some 15% of the elderly population. However, because of disorientation from trauma and medications, the prevalence increases to approximately 40% in the hospitalized elderly population. Age-related physiologic changes result in decreased bladder capacity, incomplete emptying, and increased residual urine. With age, the sensation to void is delayed. Medications also decrease the sensation to void and thus shorten the time period from when they feel the urge and the actual time of voiding. Some elderly patients may require Foley catheters presurgery and for a short time postsurgery.

MAINTAIN SKIN INTEGRITY

Nursing measures need to be implemented preoperatively to prevent a break in skin integrity from bed rest and immobilization devices. Subcutaneous fat tends to decrease with age, reducing the cushioning of bony prominences and putting elderly patients at risk for pressure ulcers. Change the patient's position every 2 hours, within the constraints of the immobilizing device. Check the immobilizing device (e.g., traction, sandbags) to make sure there are no pressure areas.

PERIPHERAL TISSUE PERFUSION

On the injured leg, check the neurovascular status every hour for the first 8 hours, and then every 2 to 4 hours. The neurovascular check must include capillary filling, color, temperature, edema, pulse, sensory nerve function, and motor nerve function. Check the circulation and neurovascular status after any readjustment of the traction straps or splint/boot. Check the traction straps and splint/boot to make sure they are not too tight. Report any change in status.

PREOPERATIVE PATIENT TEACHING AND HOME CARE CONSIDERATIONS

The elderly patient is typically quite anxious about having a fractured hip. They may be frightened about what will happen to them in the short term and in the long term. Questions that may be going through their mind are: (1) Does my family know where I am and what has happened to me?; (2) Will I be able to walk and take care of myself?; and (3) Will "they" put me in a nursing home? There is still a fear, which is to some extent realistic, that they may never leave the hospital alive.

The nurse needs to give them correct information regarding their care and treatment by explaining the nature of the injury, the procedures to be done, and the follow-up care that will be provided. Contact their family or significant other if they have not been notified.

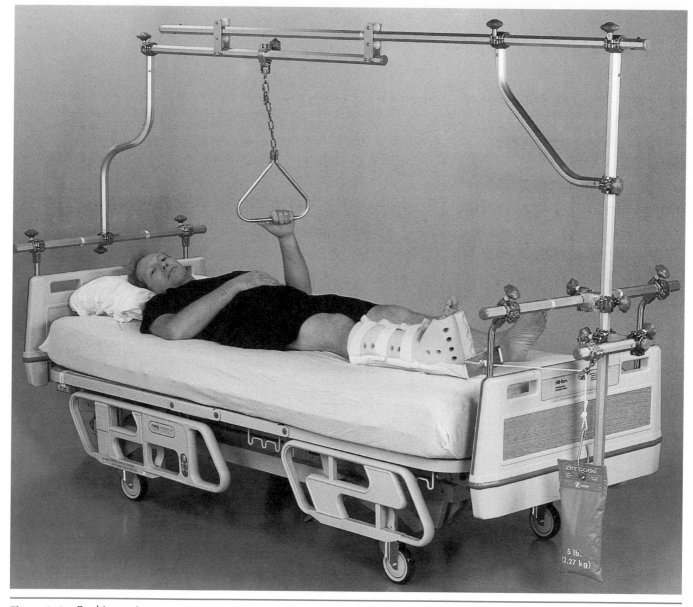

Figure 9–9   Buck's traction.   *(Provided Courtesy of Zimmer, Inc.)*

PREOPERATIVE MONITORING AND MANAGING POTENTIAL PROBLEMS

Immediate reoperative complications include possible dehydration, further damage to soft tissue and blood supply to the hip because of lack of immobilization, and neurovascular deficit due to traction or other immobilizing devices.

PREOPERATIVE EVALUATION/OUTCOMES

Immobilization of the affected hip is achieved without complications. The patient is comfortable and relatively free of pain. The patient is physically and emotionally prepared for surgery without complications of immobility.

METHODS OF SURGICAL REPAIR

The choice of procedure in the treatment of a hip fracture depends primarily upon the type of fracture and secondarily upon the patient's general physical and emotional condition, the length of time since the fracture was sustained, and the surgeon's preference and judgment. Most patients with hip fractures, being elderly, have chronic health problems. The hip fracture is complicated by, or perhaps has complicated, an existing cardiac condition, diabetic problem, or other health deficit that frequently accompanies the aging process. In view of modern surgical techniques, many surgeons feel that the sooner operative fixation is done the better, but in some instances, reduction and fixation of the fracture must be delayed one or two days or even longer to permit a complete medical evaluation and treatment of an existing health problem. The primary consideration in delaying surgery is the patient's general condition. If surgery is delayed for intracapsular or extracapsular fractures, the application of skin traction (Buck's extension, Russell's traction, or a similar apparatus; see Chapter 6) will help to immobilize the fracture and lessen muscle spasms, thus making the patient more comfortable. Patients with impacted intracapsular fractures will probably not need to be placed in traction because the fracture site is stabilized by the impaction itself. In the case of a subtrochanteric fracture, the flexion pull of the iliopsoas muscle make 90-90 traction effective in aligning the distal fragment with the proximal fragment.

The treatment of hip fractures usually consists of realigning the fragments by either closed or open methods, followed by operative insertion of some metallic internal fixation device (such as a compression screw or multiple threaded pins) to fasten the broken fragments together until healing occurs. In selected frail or aged patients, in those few patients for whom the head fragment cannot be reduced, or in some fractures of the proximal neck of the femur, the femoral head may be removed and a metallic femoral head prosthesis inserted. All things considered, however, it is usually better for the patient to obtain healing of the fracture by means of internal fixation than to have prosthetic replacement of the femoral head.

INTRACAPSULAR FRACTURES

An intracapsular fracture is a serious orthopaedic problem because the fracture may severely restrict the blood supply to the femoral head. The restriction or destruction of the blood supply may occur at the time of the fracture or any time prior to internal fixation. The proximal fragment of the femur, being inside the joint, is almost devoid of soft-tissue attachments. Its major blood supply (the retinacular or epiphyseal arteries) runs along the femoral neck in a distal to proximal direction to enter the base of the head of the femur. All interosseous vessels are interrupted by the fracture, leaving the femoral head dependent on the ligament of the head of the femur, which carries little or no circulation. For that reason, a *femoral neck fracture* (Fig. 9–10) is a vascular emergency that demands immediate attention. The blood supply is disturbed in some 25% to 40% of the patients, and at the present time there are no known methods whereby avascular necrosis can be avoided. It is believed that the more efficient the internal fixation, the less the chance of avascular necrosis. In contrast, for fractures of the intertrochanteric area or below, the blood supply to both portions of the femur is almost always satisfactory.

An *impacted intracapsular fracture* (Fig. 9–11a) of the femur usually is in a position that allows for fairly good function, as even in the acute injury phase the patient may be able to walk on the affected leg with only minimal pain. That type of fracture is stabilized without manipulation and can be treated with success conservatively (i.e., prolonged period of toe-touch weight-bearing ambulation), but there has to be absolute cooperation from the patient. When that is not possible, and because the fracture usually occurs in persons for whom prolonged bed rest would be unsuitable, such patients are usually treated by internal fixation in the form of pins (i.e., Knowles, Hagie, or Moore pins) or screws (i.e., cannulated cancellous lag screws, see Fig. 9–11b) to prevent further displacement of the femoral head. Large implants, such as compression hip screws or other nail plate devices, may increase the risk of disimpaction at surgery and therefore are not used (DeLee, 1996, p. 1673; Koval & Zuckerman, 1998, p. 178).

On the other hand, the treatment of *displaced intracapsular fractures* is either reduction and internal fixa-

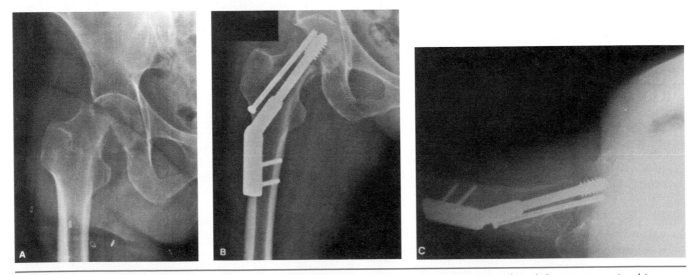

Figure 9–10   A femoral neck fracture (A) treated by anatomic closed reduction and fixation with a sliding compression hip screw and a superiorly placed cannulated screw to prevent rotation (B and C). A two-hole side plate gives adequate fixation to the shaft of the femur.   *(Rockwood, et al. (1996).* Rockwood & Green's Fractures in Adults. *Philadelphia: Lippincott-Raven.)*

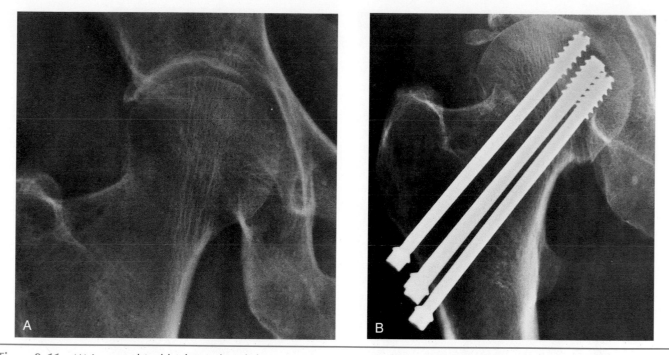

Figure 9–11   (A) Impacted (stable) femoral neck fracture. (B) An impacted femoral neck fracture stabilized with three parallel cancellous lag screws.   *(Koval & Zuckerman (1998).* Fractures in the Elderly. *Philadelphia: Lippincott-Raven.)*

tion of the femoral head or replacement by a prosthesis. The procedure is to utilize a sliding hip screw with a single Knowles pin above the sliding screw to prevent rotation (Fig. 9–12). Because these fractures frequently occur in elderly patients with other serious health problems and high mortality within a year of the accident, some surgeons believe an immediate replacement endoprosthesis is the correct treatment. Problems with reduction and fixation are particularly severe for the displaced subcapital intracapsular fracture, which has been named "the unsolved fracture."

EXTRACAPSULAR FRACTURES

Intertrochanteric fractures of the femur (Fig. 9–13) occur most commonly in women. As a general rule, these patients are older than those fracturing the neck of the femur, but healing at the intertrochanteric location is more favorable because of the blood-rich cancellous bone. Treatment of the fracture usually consists of an open reduction and internal fixation by means of a metallic, nail-plate device with or without a compression element. Typical devices are the intramedullary nail and sliding compression hip screw (e.g., Gamma nail or intramedullary hip screw, see Fig. 9–14). Koval and Zuckerman (1998) suggest that the sliding hip screw (Fig. 9–15) is the implant of choice for the elderly. The sliding hip screw implant allows weight-bearing ambulation as tolerated. The others allow only partial-weight or non-weight-bearing ambulation until calcification. Partial- and non-weight-bearing ambulation are difficult for the elderly.

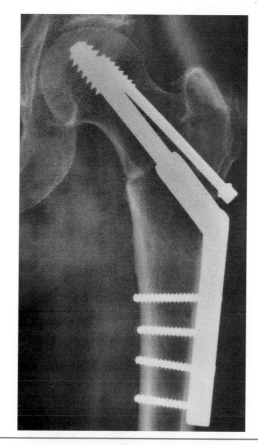

Figure 9–12   A basicervical hip fracture stabilized with a sliding hip screw and a supplemental antirotation cancellous screw.   *(Koval & Zuckerman (1998).* Fractures in the Elderly. *Philadelphia: Lippincott-Raven.)*

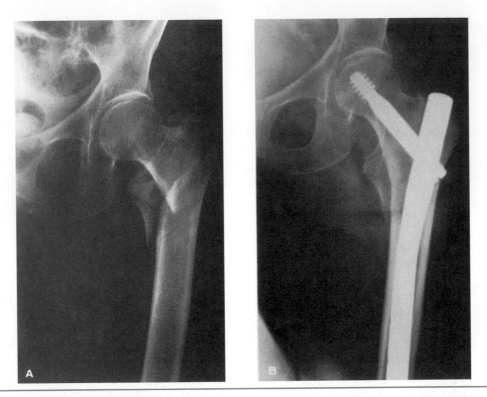

Figure 9–13   Displaced intertrochanteric hip fracture.   *(Rockwood, et al. (1996). Rockwood & Green's Fractures in Adults. Philadelphia: Lippincott-Raven.)*

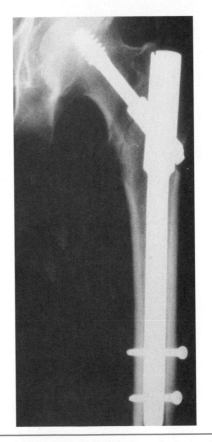

Figure 9–14   Stabilization of an intertrochanteric fracture with an intramedullary hip screw.   *(Koval & Zuckerman (1998). Fractures in the Elderly. Philadelphia: Lippincott-Raven.)*

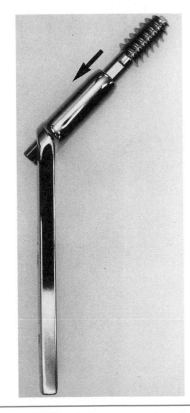

Figure 9–15   The sliding hip screw consists of a large-diameter screw that provides fixation in the femoral head and neck and a side plate and barrel that allow the screw to telescope within the barrel.   *(Koval & Zuckerman (1998). Fractures in the Elderly. Philadelphia: Lippincott-Raven.)*

A *subtrochanteric fracture* of the femur, one below the lesser trochanteric region, has been viewed by physicians as being difficult to manage either surgically or conservatively. In the elderly, this fracture is usually the result of a simple fall. It is also the site for pathologic fractures caused by neoplastic disease (Koval & Zuckerman, 1998, p. 189). In younger adults, these fractures may occur with other body trauma and may be either open or closed fractures. The muscle forces in that area cause problems with the maintenance of reduction by either closed or open methods. Treatment is by immediate surgery, if possible, with either a locking intramedullary nail (Fig. 9–16), a Russell-Taylor reconstruction nail, or a sliding compression hip screw. Bone grafting is sometimes necessary, depending on the type of fracture.

After surgery, only toe-touch weight bearing is allowed for 6 to 8 weeks when the compression screw is used. DeLee (1996, p. 1752) states that he uses a modified cast brace with pelvic band knee hinges after

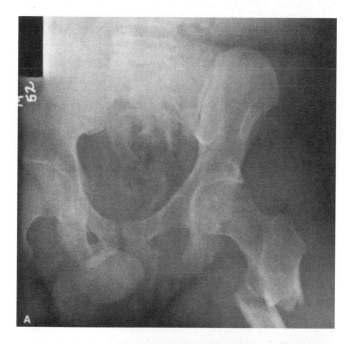

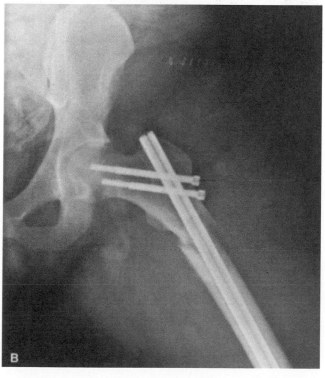

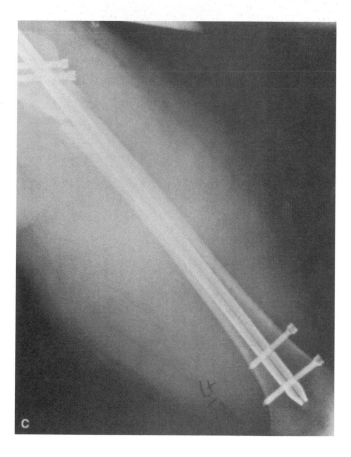

Figure 9–16 (A) Anteroposterior radiograph of a subtrochanteric fracture. (B) Anteroposterior view of the proximal femur stabilized with a cephalomedullary nail. (C) Anteroposterior view of the distal femur stabilized with a cephalomedullary nail. *(Rockwood, et al. (1996). Rockwood & Green's Fractures in Adults. Philadelphia: Lippincott-Raven.)*

surgery to allow early knee motion in patients who are not likely to comply with the postoperative regime. For patients treated with intramedullary nailing, partial weight bearing is allowed when muscular control of the limb is present, and progression to full weight bearing is based on the amount of pain.

Although rare, conservative treatment is sometimes utilized. It is usually with skeletal or Russell's traction modified for skeletal application. During traction, it is necessary to keep the patient's leg in slight adduction and moderate flexion because the proximal fragment is pulled in the upward direction (toward the body) by the iliopsoas muscle.

Isolated avulsion fractures of the *lesser trochanter,* usually occurring in young athletes, can usually be treated symptomatically with excellent return of function. Open reduction is usually not necessary. However, recently this fracture has been recognized as pathognomonic for pathologic lesions of the femur. Thus, these fractures should be further investigated (Koval & Zuckerman, 1998, p. 186). Fractures of the greater trochanter, also avulsion injuries, are generally essentially undisplaced. They can usually be treated symptomatically with bed rest for a few days with the leg held slightly abducted. Healing is usually complete in about 6 weeks.

SURGICAL COMPLICATIONS

The most serious complication of intracapsular fractures of the femoral neck is avascular necrosis. The second is nonunion. It has been estimated that one out of four patients sustaining a fracture through the neck of the femur fails to obtain a successful union. Because of those two problems, some physicians prefer endoprosthesis surgery to internal fixation. Loss of reduction of the fracture usually occurs only if the fixation is not good because of too few pins, poor pin placement, or inadequate impaction of the fractured fragments. Infection occurs in older patients because of poor subcutaneous tissues, but even in those patients the infection rate can be reduced to as low as 2% with prophylactic antibiotics.

Avascular necrosis and nonunion are rarely encountered following intertrochanteric fractures of the hip because of the relative abundance of the blood supply in the cancellous segment of the femur. An intertrochanteric fracture is a more severe injury than an intracapsular fracture, however, because of the high incidence of complications involving blood loss, shock, fat embolisms, pulmonary embolisms, and pneumonia. Shortening of the affected leg is common. Some patients will have a shortening of one-half to three-fourths of an inch because of the collapse of the fragments at the fracture site, which frequently occurs during the healing phase. Those fractures commonly unite with considerable varus because the lesser trochanter has usually been avulsed from the femur. For that reason, there is no effective action of the psoas muscle, and the uncompensated action of the gluteal muscles produces a coxa vara deformity. Attempts have been made by physicians to

overcome that by weakening the abductor muscles at the time of surgery by dividing them at their point of insertion into the greater trochanter.

Other complications that can occur in patients with hip fractures are nail or pin penetration into the acetabulum, breakage of the fixation device, deep infection around the implant, thrombophlebitis, and pulmonary embolism. Deep infection around the implant often develops slowly. The patient usually complains of increased pain in the hip. Roentgenograms in the early stage of the infection are generally negative, but the sedimentation rate is usually elevated. With deep infections, the physician usually tries to keep the implant in place at least until the fracture has healed. If that is not possible, the implant is removed and irrigation with large amounts of antibiotics is usually done by means of closed-tube drainage or antibiotic beads. Patients with fractures of the hip repaired by internal fixation are usually elderly, and the implant can easily remain in place without difficulty. Younger patients, whose life span can be expected to be many years, should have the device removed about one year after healing has occurred. That will avoid a weakening of the bone from any reaction to the implant.

A high incidence of thrombophlebitis and pulmonary embolism occurs in injured patients. Patients with fractured hips are in particular jeopardy, as about 30% develop thrombophlebitis and about 2% die of pulmonary embolism. Several drugs have been used to try to prevent these problems, including heparin, warfarin, low-molecular-weight dextran, Lovenox, and aspirin. With heparin and warfarin, some patients, especially the elderly, develop sensitivities to the drug. Dextran has the complications of congestive heart failure, allergic reaction, renal failure, and anemia. Aspirin, also a drug with anticoagulant properties, has been used with various dosages. It has been the drug of choice for a large number of physicians to treat and prevent the problems of thrombophlebitis and pulmonary embolism. A major side effect is gastrointestinal distress, which can be prevented by taking aspirin with food. Some physicians use enteric coated aspirin to decrease gastrointestinal symptoms, but the absorption rate is not always consistent and some patients have been known to excrete the enteric coated aspirin without its being dissolved. A major reason is the inconsistent amount of coating each aspirin receives in the coating process.

NURSING PROCESS (Postoperative Patient with a Fractured Hip)

POSTOPERATIVE ASSESSMENT

The immediate postoperative assessment for a typical patient following the repair of a fractured hip involves taking vital signs (e.g., pulse, respiration, and blood pressure) and observing the patient's general color and warmth. A neurovascular assessment of the affected leg and comparison with the nonaffected leg (pulse, temperature, color, capillary filling, edema, and sensory and motor nerve function) should be made (Chapter 2) and the position of the leg checked for proper alignment. The patient's level of consciousness and orientation should be determined. The incisional dressing and the area posterior to the dressing should be checked for drainage. If the patient has wound catheters in place, note the color and amount of drainage and whether the suction is working. Assess the type, severity, and location of pain and the patient's verbal and nonverbal expressions of pain, and note whether the patient received medication in surgery or in the postanesthesia room. Have the patient cough and deep breathe, and auscultate the chest for clearness of the lungs and any cardiac abnormalities. Note the type of intravenous solution, the rate of flow, and the amount left in the bottle or bag. Obtain from anesthesia and postanesthesia records or personnel the amount of blood loss in surgery and the amount of fluid replacement. Check the patient for bladder distention, urgency, or the need to void.

Frequent assessment of the patient should be made during the postoperative period. Auscultation of the patient's chest should be done at least once a shift. For the first few postoperative days, the nurse will also need to assess for bowel sounds. Neurovascular assessments of the affected extremity are usually done every 15 minutes for 2 hours, then every 30 minutes for 2 hours, then every hour for 2 hours, then every 2 hours for 18 hours, and then every 4 hours.

POSTOPERATIVE NURSING DIAGNOSIS

Based on all of the assessment data, the major nursing diagnoses for a typical patient following a surgical repair of a hip fracture include the following:

- Pain and discomfort related to the soft-tissue and bone trauma
- Impaired physical mobility related to bone instability and soft-tissue trauma
- High risk for injury related to decreased orientation and decreased mobility
- Impaired skin integrity related to aging skin and decreased mobility
- Alteration in elimination related to aging and surgery
- Anxiety related to knowledge deficit about the rehabilitation process

POSTOPERATIVE COLLABORATIVE PROBLEMS

- Wound infection
- Venous stasis
- Pulmonary emboli
- Fat emboli
- Paralytic ileus
- Flexion contractures

POSTOPERATIVE GOAL FORMULATION AND PLANNING

The goals are to have the patient experience (1) a decrease in pain through positioning, nursing interventions, and prescribed medications; (2) an increase in mobility through positioning, turning, exercises, and ambulation; (3) no falls as a result of orientation or mobility; (4) no break in skin integrity through nursing measure; (5) normal bowel and bladder elimination patterns; (6) a decrease in anxiety through patient education; and (7) an absence of complications.

POSTOPERATIVE INTERVENTIONS

ALLEVIATE PAIN

The first step is to assess for the location, severity, and degree of physical and emotional pain. Remember that sympathoadrenal signs indicating pain include changes in pulse rate, blood pressure, and respiration and the occurrence of diaphoresis, depression, or mood swings. Today, many patients are on PCAs for pain control and may need reinstructions on how to use the PCA or encouragement to initiate the medication. If the nurse is administering pain medications, do not hesitate to medicate during the first 24 hours following surgery should the patient's condition warrant, even if the patient does not request medication. However, reassure the patient while trying physical nursing measures for pain relief. Sometimes the patient becomes anxious and tense and tightens their muscles to prevent any movement. This increases the discomfort and leads the patient to tighten their muscles even more. After reassuring the patient and getting the patient to relax the affected leg in your hands, use both hands and gently lift the leg and move it through its range of motion several times before repositioning it. Frequently, the pain will go away or at least be greatly reduced. In general, muscle-setting exercises, which increase circulation, help to relieve pain.

With the pain due to muscle tension eased by exercise, it is much easier to determine the amount of pain medication needed for the patient's underlying condition. Caution should be exercised to prevent oversedation or excessive doses of pain medication. Especially among the elderly, there is great variability in the absorption, distribution, metabolism, and excretion of drugs, and these factors may affect the patient's immediate and long-term responses to medications. Be alert for physical, behavioral, and mental changes that may be drug induced. Elderly patients on the whole do not tolerate sedatives well, particularly barbiturates, because they tend to produce drowsiness and a "hangover" the next day.

Do give medications for pain relief, but assess pain, try nursing measures for pain relief, note the dosage of all medications given, and definitely observe for physical and mental reactions to the drugs.

INCREASE MOBILITY

Following hip surgery, efforts to increase the patient's mobility involve correct positioning, turning, exercise, and ambulation.

Position. Immediately after surgery, when the patient is supine, the affected leg should be in correct alignment (which for some patients may mean being in sight abduction), but often the leg will have a tendency to move toward slight external rotation. To prevent external rotation, the affected leg is placed in a sling. Other methods are to place a trochanter roll beside the lateral aspect of the thigh or, if need be, place a sandbag or trochanter roll along the lateral aspect of the lower leg. Make sure that it is not placed in a position that will apply pressure against the proximal portion of the fibula (near the location of the peroneal nerve) or the external malleolus. Teach the patient where the support should be positioned and why it is necessary. Another way to prevent external rotation is to teach the patient to keep the toes straight up toward the ceiling when lying supine.

Check to see if there are any specific restrictions on positions or activities for the patient. In general, the patient can have the head of the bed elevated for meals and activities of daily living. Most patients will not want the head elevated more than 30 to 40 degrees because of the stress that is placed on the muscles of the hip and the fracture site. The patient should not have the head of the bed elevated at all times (unless medically warranted) because of the possibility of developing hip flexion contractures and the shearing effect on the skin at the coccyx.

Turning. When the patient returns to the unit from the postanesthesia room and the initial assessment is satisfactory, one of the first things to do is to turn the patient to the unaffected side. The patient may have been lying supine for several hours on a variety of firm surfaces and hence have some stiffness and discomfort. Turning immediately also lets the patient know that he or she is able to move. Movement helps the patient in expelling respiratory secretions and in improving circulation, and turning is usually done every 2 or 3 hours.

When helping a patient with a hip fracture turn following insertion of an internal fixation, avoid extremes of motion, prevent strain on the hip, maintain alignment of the affected leg and hip, and handle the operated leg gently. At first, the patient may be somewhat uncooperative because of pain and apprehension, but that usually passes after a few turns. Nurses usually assume that they should not turn a patient to the affected side unless there are specific orders to do so. Most patients with internal fixations, however, are allowed to turn to either side because the bed acts as a splint for the injured hip. In the beginning, some patients cannot tolerate being turned completely onto their side, especially the affected side. In those instances, turn the patient at least 45 degrees. If the patient is not allowed to turn for some reason, he or she may be able to lift straight up periodically for back care and linen changes with the use of the trapeze.

When turning the patient onto the unoperated side, place one pillow between the patient's thighs and another one or possibly two pillows, depending on the amount of abduction and the size of the patient, between the lower legs and the feet. The pillows help keep the operated leg aligned with the trunk, or in slight abduction when warranted, and prevent a twisting movement of the leg. A slight abduction reduces the stress to the incisional area and fracture site. In the beginning, at least two persons are needed to turn the patient. In turning a patient with a fractured right hip onto the unaffected left side, one person gently places their hands under the patient's right side with one hand under the patient's right shoulder and the other near the buttocks under the upper right thigh. The second person, on the left side of the bed, reaches across the patient, places one hand in the patient's lumbar area and the other under the right upper thigh distal to the first person's hand. The person on the left side of the bed is in a position to support the affected leg during the turn. The patient is then rolled toward the left side of the bed onto the unaffected side. The side rails should be up on the left side of the bed before the turn is started, and the patient should be encouraged to breathe out or at least breathe normally during the turning. Once the patient is turned to the side, the patient can use the side rails for support until complete positioning is done. The pillows prevent the operated leg from dropping down into adduction. While the patient is turned to the side, the knee of the affected leg may be flexed, and a slight flexion of the hip is also allowed. To foster mobility, make sure that the position of the hip changes in the turn. Before leaving the patient, ensure that the upper leg is securely positioned on the pillows.

If a patient takes a deep breath and holds it during the turn, it evokes the Valsalva maneuver. The Valsalva maneuver (filling the lungs, closing the glottis, and forcibly attempting to exhale) raises intrathoracic pressure and resists venous blood from entering the large veins. When the glottis is released and the lungs are allowed to exhale, the intrathoracic pressure falls, causing a large volume of blood to enter the heart. This may pose a serous problem for patients with cardiac conditions and for the elderly because of the stress it places on the heart. Prevent the problem by having the patient breathe with their mouth open during the turn.

Exercises. Exercises should be started as soon as possible to restore normal joint function and muscle tone. If time and conditions allow, the patient may be taught some of the exercises before surgery, such as doing leg exercises with the unaffected leg. Exercises for the patient having hip surgery include breathing exercises; abdominal exercises; gluteal- and quadriceps-setting exercises; plantar and dorsiflexion exercises (also known as ankle pumps), which exercise the muscles of the calf and foreleg; active range of motion of the ankle on the affected side; exercises for the upper extremities (see Chapter 4, exercises for crutch walking); and active range of motion for all unaffected joints. Most exercises are started on the first postoperative day.

At first, the patient should not be left alone to do the exercises. In assessing the degree of supervision required, consider the age of the patient, motivation, and understanding of what is being asked. Most patients need some assistance and probably need to have the instructions for the exercises gone over several times, possibly even every exercise time. Some of the exercises can be incorporated into self-care activities, which makes the patient more independent. Observe the patient for signs of fatigue, weakness, or stiffness. Encourage quadriceps- and gluteal-setting exercises hourly for the first 2 to 3 days and then every 2 to 4 hours.

To begin quadriceps-setting exercises (see Box 6–2, Exercise for the Lower Extremity), the patient should sit or lie in a comfortable position and have the exercise demonstrated on the unaffected leg. Place a hand behind the knee and instruct the patient to press the knee down against the hand or have the patient pretend he or she is pushing the knee into the bed. A strong contraction of the quadriceps should occur when the patient presses. This tightening should be followed by complete relaxation. The patient should be taught to press for a slow count of 3 and then to relax for a slow count of 3. The alternating contractions and relaxations of the muscle should be built up so that they can be performed 20 times an hour. The quadriceps femoris muscle extends the leg and is one of the major muscles necessary for ambulation.

The abdominal exercises (discussed under gastrointestinal complications in Chapter 4), the breathing exercises (discussed under respiratory complications in Chapter 4), and the gluteal-setting exercises are isometric exercises that strengthen the muscles but do not move any joint. Gluteal-setting exercises, which simply tighten and relax the gluteal muscles on a slow count of 3, help to increase circulation to the gluteal area and preserve muscle tone.

Ankle pumps involve doing plantar and dorsiflexion exercises of the foot and ankle. The exercise maintains the range of motion of the ankle needed for walking and increases the circulation in the calf muscles.

Performing arm exercises (flexion and extension of the arms) strengthens the muscles in the shoulder girdle and upper extremities, which must be strong enough to bear the patient's weight so that the patient can use an assistive device for walking. The use of the trapeze, which strengthens the biceps of the arm, helps, but the major muscle in the arm that needs strengthening is the triceps. Strengthening of the triceps can be accomplished by the following exercises. The patient, in a sitting position, takes a weight in each hand and flexes both arms while extending both hands above the head toward the ceiling. Another exercise uses sawed off crutches or books placed in the bed on each side of the patient. The patient pushes down on the books or crutches and lifts the buttocks off the bed.

Trapeze. Teach patients how to use the trapeze correctly. It will greatly help patients reposition themselves while supine, help them get out of bed, and enable them to assist when nurses have to reposition them in bed, give them the bedpan, administer skin care, and change the linen. Use of the trapeze helps maintain muscle tone and builds up strength in the arms and shoulders as well as helping to improve the functioning of the respiratory and circulatory systems. In using the trapeze, the patient should grasp it with both hands and, flexing the unaffected knee and hip, bring the unaffected foot up and place it flat on the bed at least to the level of the knee of the affected leg. Next, the patient should pull on the trapeze and push down on the unaffected foot, lifting the buttocks off the bed. If the patient needs to move up in bed after lifting the buttocks, the patient should push with the unaffected foot to move the body toward the head of the bed. In the beginning, the nurse may have to assist because the patient lacks arm strength.

Ambulation. In most instances, patients who have had an internal fixation for a hip fracture may be allowed to dangle their legs on the side of the bed the day of surgery and sit in a chair on the first postoperative day. Before attempting to get the patient up to move to a chair, explain every step of the procedure. Tell the patient how he or she can be of help, and make sure the patient is informed about weight bearing on the affected leg. Commonly, patients with internal fixation devices are not allowed weight bearing on the affected leg in the early postoperative period. However, Koval and Zuckerman (1998, p. 177) state that if a sliding compression hip screw is utilized for the repair, weight bearing can be allowed as tolerated. They feel this method of repair and weight bearing is less physically stressful on the patient and should be utilized when possible. However, depending on the size and age of the individual, weight bearing before bone union may exert too much stress to the fracture site and thus cause bending, breaking, or displacement of the implant, crushing of bone at the fracture site, or loss of fixation due to the device's cutting through the bone.

Do not rush or try to hurry the patient through the transfer. First, move the patient so that the unaffected hip is at the side of the bed, and bring the patient to a sitting position on the edge of the bed. Let the patient sit there for a few minutes to prevent orthostatic hypotension. (It has been noted that some institutions have the nurse keep an ammonia capsule with them to use if needed.) Next, pivot the patient into a chair, ensuring that there is no weight bearing on the affected leg (or weight bearing as tolerated when that is permitted). The first time, the assistance of another person may be advisable. Talk to and reassure the patient during the activity. The patient can assume a normal sitting position. Encourage the patient to do exercises such as deep breathing, abdominal, gluteal- and quadriceps-setting, and ankle exercises while in the chair. If a chair that allows a rocking motion is available, it will help the patient to flex and extend the knees and ankles. After the patient gains confidence and if the chair has armrests, encourage the patient to periodically push down on the chair arms and raise their buttocks off the chair. The raising allows circulation to the buttocks and also helps build up muscles in the upper extremity for crutch walking.

Most patients start ambulation by first transferring to a chair as just described. The time up in the chair may be gradually increased but not so much that the patient becomes fatigued. Next, the patient will be able to use a walker. After developing a safe, steady gait, the patient can progress to crutches using a three-point gait (either non-weight bearing or toe-touch). Crutches allow for more and easier mobility, and the patient should be encouraged to use them even if he or she feels less sure at first. However, a number of the elderly patients feel safer with a walker and will not progress to crutches. Patients should be taught how to get in and out of a chair and on and off the toilet, how to go up and down stairs with or without arm rails, and how to get in and out of a car. How to do these movements is discussed in Chapter 4.

FALLS PREVENTION

Nurses should recognize that most patients are not only weak from the trauma and shock of the injury and surgery but are elderly. Nurses need to implement their institutional protocol for falls prevention.

SKIN INTEGRITY

Elderly persons typically have a thinning of their skin, rendering it susceptible to abrasions and contusions. Avoid using tape (or use paper tape) when applying dressings or securing intravenous needles to the patient. When ordinary tape is removed, damage to their skin is likely to occur, as some of their skin may be removed with the tape. The use of adhesive removers is advised to reduce the risk of a break in skin integrity.

An older person's skin is also more sensitive to pressure and will tend to break down much quicker than that of a younger adult. Make sure there is adherence to the turning schedule, and observe and intervene if red areas occur (see Chapter 4 on the effects of immobility and the geriatric patient).

NORMAL ELIMINATION

Postoperative care of elderly patients includes a focus on bladder and bowel elimination because of the aging process, decreased mobility, and the effect of medications. If an elderly female is left in bed for urination, she may not be able to empty her bladder completely, leaving a large amount of residual urine. That can lead to incontinency, or some of the urine can flow into her vagina because of positioning during urination. Older men may have problems with bladder elimination because of an enlarged prostate. Get the patient to as normal a position of urination as possible to prevent the use of a catheter with its added potential for infection. For both men and women, it is better to get them up as soon as possible. Females may use a bedside commode and men may stand at the side of the bed, but it is better to utilize an assistive device and get them to the bathroom.

Postoperative care also needs to focus on bowel elimination. Make sure the patient has plenty of fluids,

roughage in their diet, and as much activity as tolerated. Stool softeners are standard orders for most surgical patients. However, we need to be aware that some elderly individuals may have been overusing laxatives. Patient education may be needed to help them gain a return to normal (for their age) bowel elimination.

POSTOPERATIVE PATIENT TEACHING AND HOME CARE CONSIDERATIONS

Patients have rights whether they are coherent or confused, and one of those rights is the right to considerate and respectful care. For confused patients, the first step is orientation to self, place, and time. Call them by name instead of using terms such as "grandma" unless the patient requests otherwise. Once the person is oriented, explain what has happened and what is being done. Patients have a right to receive information concerning diagnosis, treatment, and prognosis in terms they can reasonably be expected to understand. Most of that information is usually provided by the physician, but the nurse may need to go over it several times before the patient is able to comprehend what it means. Remember, having a fractured hip is very traumatic psychologically as well as physiologically. Most patients are elderly and have a fear of death, because many remember when an elderly person taken to the hospital with a fractured hip died. Most fear a fractured hip because it means not being able to walk and care for themselves. This fear is realistic if you consider that half of the patients following a fractured hip will not walk independently again and up to one third may need the use of a long-term care facility.

The nurse must gain the confidence and trust of the patient. Spend time with the patient talking with the realistic assurance of someone who cares and wants to help. Use a lot of touch and direct eye contact. When possible, let the patient have a say in decisions being made about care. Encourage as much self-care as possible within medical limits.

A knowledgeable patient is a much more cooperative patient. Education begins when the patient is first seen on admission, in the emergency room, or on the unit. When the patient understands the rationale for specific exercises and positioning, he or she is much more willing to cooperate. Older individuals can and do learn. They just do it a little more slowly. It should be remembered that if one can simplify the demands of the task and make it meaningful, older people will do relatively well (though caution seems to increase with age).

Teaching the patient should be as well planned as the other aspects of care. Teaching sessions should be scheduled for when the nurse is unhurried and the time is right for the patient to learn. Patients under stress tend not to hear or comprehend all that is being said, and adults want to know how the information is relevant to them. Teaching materials can be collected from numerous sources. Many orthopaedic supply companies have educational materials available on request, either from their representative in the area or from the home office. Materials are also available at a cost from companies that develop patient education materials (i.e., Pritchett and Hull, Krames, NAON, and the American Association of Orthopaedic Surgeons [AAOS]). You may create your own, individualized to the patient. Once you, the plan, the materials, and the patient are all ready, go over the material in simple steps, allowing time for the patient to comprehend and ask questions. If necessary have the patient demonstrate understanding by, for example, actually putting on those elastic stockings with an assistive device. Evaluate how well the patient understands the procedure.

Discharge planning should begin when the patient is admitted and include all members of the health team (i.e., physician, nurse, physical therapist, social worker, and the patient's family and significant others). Spend time with the patient discussing the realistic options for care once he or she leaves the hospital. The anticipated date of discharge to an extended care facility or a nursing home is usually about 5 days; for discharge to home it may be 7 days, depending on the patient's medical condition. The patient, family, and significant others need to be aware of the approximate length of stay. Utilize the assistance of a social worker, home health nurse, or individuals from the extended care facility when warranted.

If the patient is to return to his or her own home or to the home of a family member or significant other, the home must be made safe. The patient will be using a walker or crutches and should be able to safely go up and down stairs. Pets such as cats and dogs can cause an unsteady person to fall. Loose rugs should be removed, and a comfortable chair should be available. Those who will be living with the patient should be aware of the extent to which the patient will not be self-sufficient and should know how to provide the necessary nursing care without making an invalid out of the patient.

POSTOPERATIVE MONITORING AND MANAGING POTENTIAL PROBLEMS

Most postoperative complications are related to the trauma, surgery, and imposed immobility and are discussed in Chapter 4.

Patients having internal fixations for fractured hips are particularly susceptible to *pulmonary emboli,* one of the leading causes of death following hip surgery. *Fat emboli* are especially likely in patients with fractures of the intratrochanteric or subtrochanteric regions. A *paralytic ileus* can occur because of the patient's age, surgical procedure, and immobility; make sure bowel sounds are present before administering food. However, most common musculoskeletal complications are *flexion contractures* of the *hip* and the *knee* and *equinus contractures* of the *foot* ("footdrop").

In preventing complications, therefore, it is frequently necessary to consider both orthopaedic and gerontologic nursing concepts. Elderly patients are more likely to be affected by circulatory overload, skin breakdown, and constipation. Lower tract urinary infections are of special concern. Elderly men usually have an enlarged prostate and an atonic decompensated bladder. Elderly women may have interstitial cystitis, a contracted bladder, stress incontinency due to a prolapsed uterus, and urine collecting in the vagina because of their unaccustomed position during voiding.

WOUND INFECTION

To enhance wound healing and avoid or control infection, physicians may place wound catheters (usually two) into the wound before closing the incision line. The wound catheters are generally inserted through the skin a few inches from the incision line. They may be connected to a device (i.e., Hemovac, J Vac, or Gomco) for continuous suction. The placement of the catheters and the continuous suction are to prevent pooling of blood within muscle layers, which can be a source of infection. The catheters are usually in place 24 to 36 hours.

The initial dressing is usually removed the same day that the wound catheters are removed. Utilizing strict asepsis, the best procedure is to remove the wound catheters first and leave a pressure dressing on for an hour or so before changing the surgical dressing. Reinforce a dressing if it becomes soiled or loosened. Once the initial dressing is removed, a variety of methods to care for the incision may be employed. One is to leave the incision open to the air. A second is to use alcohol swabs and do a daily cleansing of the incision, which toughens the skin. A third is to do a daily betadine scrub of the incision. The nurse needs to follow the protocols developed by the institution for wound care and utilize strict asepsis.

POSTOPERATIVE EVALUATION/OUTCOMES

For a typical patient recovering from surgery for a fractured hip with an internal fixation device, the patient should be free of pain. The patient should have a safe gait utilizing an assistive device and be able to go up and down stairs, get in and out of a chair, and get on and off the toilet without the assistance of another person. They should be free of complications and be able to articulate the goals and objectives of their rehabilitation.

CLINICAL PATHWAY (Patient with a Fractured Hip and Internal Fixation)

An example of a generic clinical pathway for a patient with a fractured hip and an internal fixation device is presented in Figure 9–17.

Figure 9–17

Clinical Pathway: Fractured Hip with Internal Fixation

Admission Date: _____ Discharge Plan: _____ Home _____ Skilled Nursing _____ Extended Care Facility

Pathway	ER/Trauma Unit	Admission Day Op day	Hosp Day 2 Post-op 2	Hosp Day 3 Post-op 3	Hosp Day 4 Post-op 4	Hosp Day 5	Outcomes
Consultation	Orthopaedic MD Medical MD	Case Manager Anesthesia, Acute Pain Service	Social Work PT Home Health Svs	Dietitian			Cont. PT @ home ECF
Assessment	Nsrg database H & P Exam. by MD, NP, or PA CMST of involved Ext. q 15 x 4 then q hr	Review & add Review H & P Postop routine CMST q 15 x 4 q 30 x 2, q 1 hr x 2, q 4 hrs. Rehab/ECF/ home Home equipment	Home environment	Referral if nec. Referral if nec.		Resolved ✓ if obtained	Home Care Nurse ECF\ Will have nec. equipment at home
Tests	ECG/UA/CXR/ T & C Blood PT, PTT, SMA AP & Lateral of Pelvis & hips	X-ray in OR Hip/Pelvic x ray in PACU H & H in PACU & repeat @ pm	✓ CBC Transfuse per protocol	✓ CBC Transfuse per protocol			
Medications	✓ Home Meds Demerol/ Morphine IM or IV for pain Antibiotics PCA Instruct on preop meds b/4 OR	✓ preadm meds Routine meds Anticoagulant Antibiotics PCA/Epidural Bowel protocol	Cont. D/C antibiotics	Cont. D/C begin oral pain meds	Cont.		States meds, when to take and purpose States purpose Pain managed with oral medications Normal bowel function
Diet	NPO.	NPO @ MN b/4 OR	Liquids	Advance as tol Encourage fluids			Tolerating diet
Activity		Bed rest Turn q 2 hr Dangle	BRP with assist Turn q 2 hrs during day & q 4 hrs @ noc. with 1–2 pilllows between legs. Up in Chair 30 x 2	Amb with walker			Ambulates with a Walker or crutches Using NWB or Toe-touch gait
Treatment	Start IV Foley Catheter	IV fluids/blood if necessary, Intake & Output Foley to drain Antiembolic hose on unaffected leg Buck's Traction ——— lbs ——— leg	D/C not nec. Cont. Cont. D/C traction post Surgery	D/C Cont. hose on affected leg	Cont.	Cont.	Normal bladder function Cont. @ home Cont. @ home

(continued)

Figure 9–17

Clinical Pathway: (continued)

Pathway	ER/Trauma Unit	Admission Day Op day	Hosp Day 2 Post-op 2	Hosp Day 3 Post-op 3	Hosp Day 4 Post-op 4	Hosp Day 5	Outcomes
		Trapeze	Utilizes to position				
		Fall precautions	Cont. precautions				
		Bed alarm if nec.	Cont.				
		Hemovac/output		D/C			No signs of infection
		IS/TCDB q hr w/a		PRN			Clear lungs
		Dressing	Do Not Change	Change PRN Wound care protocol			No infection, States When to call MD
Education		Preoperative ed.	Operative routine				
		Review hosp LOS	Rehab. Process				Verbalizes knowledge
D/C Plan		Identify discharge plan					Discharged to home with home health Services
		Caregivers & home, LOS 5 days to ECF (7 days to home)					

OTHER HIP PROCEDURES

OSTEOTOMY

A femoral osteotomy involves surgery on the femur, which changes its alignment, altering weight bearing in the hip joint and transferring a greater part of the body's weight to healthier parts of the joint. The procedure, which has a number of variations, may also be used to correct angulation or deformities (Fig. 9–18a,b). Postoperatively, the femur is immobilized in some manner, and the care of the patient is the same as that of a patient who has had a hip fracture. The time when weight bearing may begin and the amount of weight bearing that will be allowed depend on the specific type of surgical procedure used.

HANGING HIP

The "hanging hip" operation, developed by Voss, releases the fasciae latae and the adductor muscles in an attempt to decrease pressure on the articular cartilage of the hip. Many versions of this procedure have been developed. Some physicians release different muscles, others do the muscle release in combination with another procedure, such as the osteotomy, and still other physicians do a closed adductor tenotomy. The effects of the muscle release operation are muscular decompression, correction of contractures, and improvement of weight-bearing surfaces. The main

goals of the muscle-release operation are the relief of pain and the correction of harmful soft-tissue contractures. The degree of joint motion does not usually increase postoperatively, but the correction of contractures places it into a more useful range. The main complications are thrombophlebitis and pulmonary embolism. Other complications, such as anterior subluxation of the femoral head and marked and prolonged abductor limp, can be prevented with proper surgical technique and adequate postoperative muscle reeducation.

GIRDLESTONE PROCEDURE

G. R. Girdlestone developed a procedure to cut away the lip of the acetabulum and trim the femoral neck to create gliding surfaces between the bones. By leaving the lip of the acetabulum alone and keeping much of the inferior neck of the femur, a cleft is created between the greater trochanter and the inferior neck. A new articulation can then develop between the inferior neck of the femur and the acetabular lip. Different versions of the procedure have been developed. Girdlestone recommended the procedure for any infection of the hip that failed to respond to conservative treatment. The Girdlestone operation is so extensive that it produces a marked shortening of the leg (2 or more inches) and can result in an ankylosis or in a nearly useless pseudarthrosis (i.e., false joint) on which weight bearing may be virtually impossible. For those reasons, most physicians

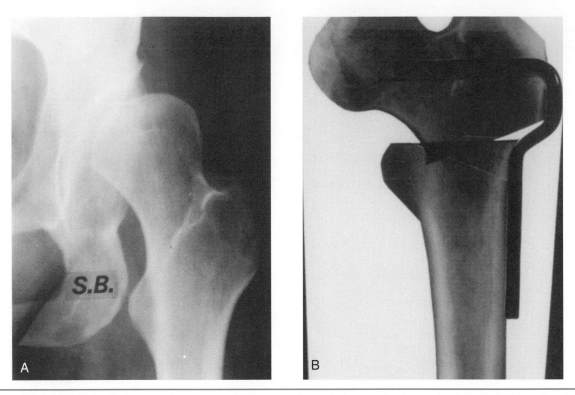

Figure 9–18 (A) Radiograph of a patient whose proximal femur and acetabulum are both grossly abnormal. This patient is a candidate for combined intertrochanteric varus derotation osteotomy and periacetabular redirection osteotomy. (B) Intertrochanteric osteotomy is indicated when the major deformity or incongruity can be attributed to the proximal femur. The osteotomy is always performed at the proximal border of the lesser trochanter. The blade plate is always inserted about 1.5 to 2.4 cm proximal to the osteotomy. *(Weinstein & Buckwalter (1994). Turek's Orthopaedics: Principles and Their Application. 5th ed. Philadelphia: J. B. Lippincott.)*

consider the procedure a last resort. It is mainly used for patients with pyogenic infection after hip surgery (i.e., salvage a failed total hip arthroplasty (THA), or with a chronic infection secondary to infectious arthritis or tuberculosis, or in instances involving osteomyelitis of the hip joint with surrounding muscle infection.

ARTHRODESIS

A hip arthrodesis is the surgical fusion of a hip joint (Fig. 9–19). Its purpose is to halt the disease process, provide stability, and relieve pain. Some physicians feel that it is the best type of surgery for young men with chronic hip joint infection, for with a good spinal column and no problems with the other hip, fusing the infected hip gives it stability and allows the patient to do heavy manual labor. With the present extensive use of the total hip replacement procedure, however, there is a decreased use of hip arthrodesis. It is most strongly indicated for tuberculosis of the hip, a pyogenic hip joint, and osteoarthritis (especially of a traumatic nature in a young patient). There are major complications with the hip arthrodesis. Specifically, (1) there is a high rate of nonunion, especially in infected hips; (2) in hip fusions where internal fixation is used, fatigue fractures may develop at the level where the metallic implants end; (3) because 4 or more months of bed rest typically follow surgery, there is a danger from the disabilities that develop during immobility; and (4) the

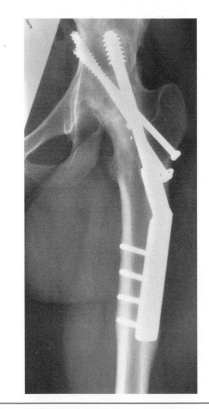

Figure 9–19 Hip arthrodesis using a two-incision technique and a compression screw for fixation. *(Callahagen, et al. (1998). The Adult Hip. Philadelphia: Lippincott-Raven.)*

femur may be malpositioned in surgery. The most obvious disadvantage for the patient is that there is no motion in the joint, and, for that reason, many patients avoid the procedure.

TOTAL HIP ARTHROPLASTY

An arthroplasty is the surgical formulation or reformation of a joint. The goals of a hip arthroplasty are to relieve pain and deformity and to restore hip joint mobility. Three common types of hip arthroplasty are the cup or mold arthroplasty, the total hip arthroplasty, and the total hip surface replacement arthroplasty. With the cup arthroplasty, the acetabulum and the head of the femur are reamed down to an untraumatized surface, and an appropriate size metal cup is fitted over the head of the femur. Presently, that kind of arthroplastic surgery is largely being replaced by the other two. The procedure for a total hip arthroplasty is to remove the femoral head and neck, ream the femoral canal, and insert a metal femoral component (which includes a head, neck, and stem) into the femoral shaft. The acetabulum is reamed to accept a polyethylene acetabular cup. The third procedure, the total hip surface replacement arthroplasty, consists of reaming out the acetabulum and implanting an acetabular cup, while the femoral head is only reamed down to accept a metal femoral cup (Fig. 9–20).

Cemented and noncemented total arthroplasties are both utilized, but for different populations. A plastic cement (polymethyl methacrylate) is used for fixation of the femoral and acetabular components of patients who are elderly or have compromised bone strength due to osteoporosis or other conditions. Cemented prostheses loosen as a result of cement failure at a rate of 1% per year (Altizer, 1998). Younger, active, and heavier patients may experience a higher rate of loosening. Thus, in younger patients, prostheses with a porous surface that allows fixation of the prostheses by growth of the patient's bone into the porous surface are utilized. In other areas of concern (e.g., dislocation rate, infection rate, and so on), the experience with cementless prostheses has been equal to that of cemented hip arthroplasties.

Another procedure, the insertion of an endoprosthesis (i.e., Austin-Moore, Bateman, Thompson, or Cathcart) is sometimes referred to as a hemiarthroplasty (Fig. 9–21). It is used in the treatment of some intracapsular fractures of the femur and involves replacing

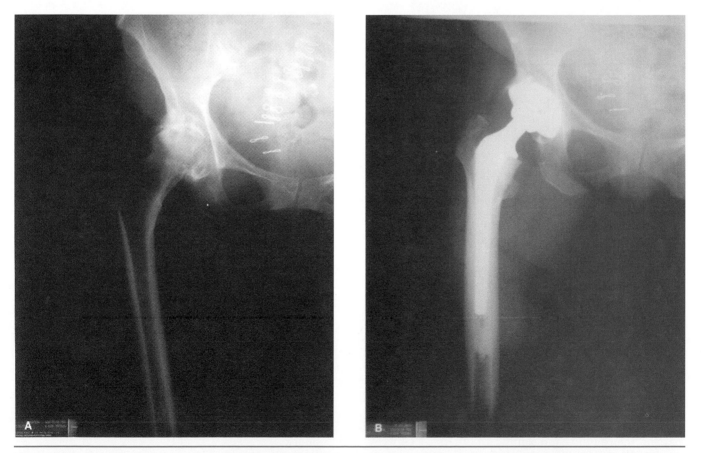

Figure 9–20   Preoperative (A) and postoperative (B) radiographs in a 67-year-old woman with osteoarthritis of the right hip joint. The patient underwent a hybrid total hip arthroplasty with uncemented acetabular component and cemented femoral component. The femoral side illustrates cement technique that can be achieved with plugging of the femoral canal, vacuum mixing of methylmethacrylate, and pressurization injection techniques into the proximal femur. *(Weinstein & Buckwalter (1994). Turek's Orthopaedics: Principles and Their Application. 5th ed. Philadelphia: J. B. Lippincott.)*

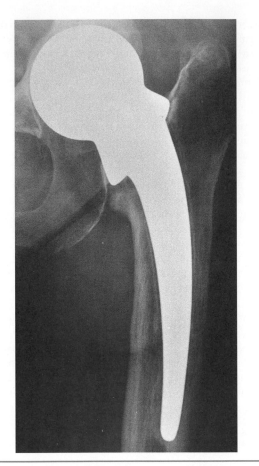

Figure 9–21   Hemiarthroplasty of the left hip with evidence of progressive acetabular erosion.   *(Koval & Zuckerman (1998). Fractures in the Elderly. Philadelphia: Lippincott-Raven.)*

the patient's femoral head and neck with a metal component the same size as the patient's original femoral head. Because the principles of care for a hemiarthroplasty are very similar to those for a hip arthroplasty, the nursing care of both kinds of patients are discussed together. Care specific to one or the other procedure is indicated. It should be understood that the postoperative care required depends on the operative procedure and the condition of the patient.

Patients scheduled for a total hip arthroplasty usually arrive at the hospital the morning of their surgery, and most are discharged within 5 days. Their preoperative blood testing and blood donations, x-rays, history, physical examination, and patient teaching has been completed before admission. With the emphasis on shorter hospital stays, many outpatient clinics and physician's offices have developed some form of preoperative education classes. They vary greatly in scope and content, from giving a printed pamphlet to providing formal classes. Most have an organized class for the patient, their family, and significant others 2 to 4 weeks prior to the surgical date, when the patient comes in for tests. At that time, the nurse usually performs a nursing assessment and provides perioperative teaching that includes perioperative routines, hygiene care, pain man-

agement, anticoagulant therapy, antibiotics, wound care, exercises, use of equipment, and a preview of home care needs. Formal class presentations may also include physical therapy.

NURSING PROCESS (Patient with a Total Hip Arthroplasty)

ASSESSMENT

Immediately after surgery (as discussed for a patient with an ORIF), the patient with a total hip arthroplasty should be observed closely for any evidence of shock or cardiopulmonary abnormality. The chief cause of hypotension in postoperative shock is a failure to maintain blood volume, but it could also result from cardiac abnormalities. Some hip arthroplasties can be performed without giving blood in surgery, but blood may be necessary postoperatively. (Most patients donate at least two units of blood before surgery to have available should they need blood during or postsurgery.) Monitor central venous pressure, especially to avoid overhydration in the elderly, and record urinary output. Patients who were on steroids preoperatively may need them intravenously after surgery. Assess the neurovascular status in the involved leg, which should be in abduction and neutral rotation (or as specified under the section on position). The leg may be held in position by splints, pillows, traction, or casts. The age of the patient undergoing a hip arthroplasty ranges from the late teens to over 80. Assess physical and emotional needs specific for age. (For a more detailed assessment, see the care of a patient having an internal fixation of the hip, Chapter 2 on assessment, and Chapter 3 on arthritis).

NURSING DIAGNOSIS

Based on all of the assessment data, the major nursing diagnoses for a typical patient with a hip arthroplasty include the following:

- Pain and discomfort related to surgery and immobility
- Impaired physical mobility related to instability in the hip joint
- Anxiety related to knowledge deficit of the rehabilitation process

COLLABORATIVE PROBLEMS

- Neurovascular impairment
- Wound infection
- Hip dislocation
- Shock
- Urinary retention
- Deep venous thrombus (DVT)
- Pulmonary emboli
- Fat emboli

GOAL FORMULATION AND PLANNING

The goals are to have the patient experience (1) a decrease in pain from medications and nursing measures, (2) an increase in mobility through positioning and exercises, (3) decreased anxiety with patient education, and (4) an absence of complications.

INTERVENTIONS

ALLEVIATE PAIN

Some patients will not complain of pain after a hip arthroplasty, saying that the postoperative pain is so much less than what they were suffering that they do not want anything for pain. Those patients need to be encouraged to take (or self-administer) pain medications for the first 24 to 48 postoperative hours so that they will receive adequate rest and comfort. Most will have an epidural catheter or PCA in place to give them control over the pain medications, while others will need nurse administered medications. Do not wait for the patients to ask, and make sure that they understand that if they are in pain they should ask for medication or assistance. Giving pain medication before physical therapy also helps the patient perform the required exercise regime.

INCREASE MOBILITY

The most important interventions to increase mobility are correct positioning, turning, exercises, and controlled ambulation.

Position. Correct positioning of the hip joint is essential at all times, because dislocation of the new joint can occur easily. (A dislocation is of even greater concern for a patient with a hemiarthroplasty, because the head of the prosthesis is larger and it must fit within the patient's acetabulum.) Postoperative positioning to prevent a dislocation is based to a large extent on the surgical approach. Postoperative positioning for a patient who has a posterolateral surgical approach (the one more commonly used, see Fig. 9–22) consists of keeping the leg externally rotated and in abduction with the hip in extension. If the surgical approach was anterior (used less frequently, see Fig. 9–23), the patient should be maintained in internal rotation, adduction, and hyperflexion. (See Box 9–1.)

There are a variety of methods utilized by different physicians and institutions to help keep the involved leg in the correct position. These are (1) a Thomas splint with a Pearson attachment, with or without traction; (2) a Hodgen splint, with or without traction; (3) a Kirschner wire inserted through the proximal tibia for traction and control of rotation (Fig. 9–24); (4) Hamilton-Russell traction; (5) Buck's traction; (6) an Amsterdam sling; (7) abductor pillows (Fig. 9–25) or an abductor splint; (8) a short leg cast with attached spreader bar; and (9) regular pillows between the legs. A modified above-knee spica cast may be used for approximately 3 weeks if the hip was unstable at the completion of the operation.

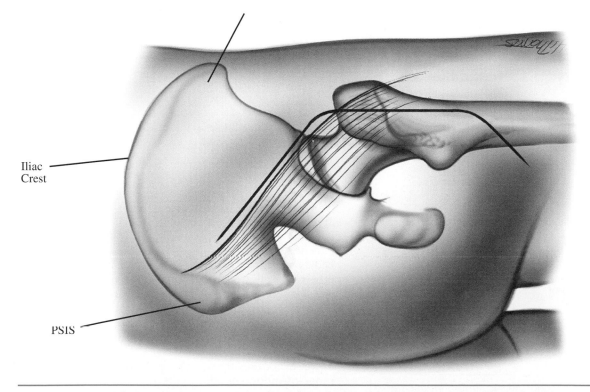

Iliac Crest

PSIS

Figure 9–22   Modified posterolateral incision. The proximal of the three limbs extends proximal to the superior border of the gluteus maximus. The middle limb is placed slightly anterior to the middle of the greater trochanter but posterior to the tensor muscle. The distal limb is made at a 45-degree angle to assist the mobility of the posterior flap.   *(Callahagen, et al. (1998). The Adult Hip. Philadelphia: Lippincott-Raven.)*

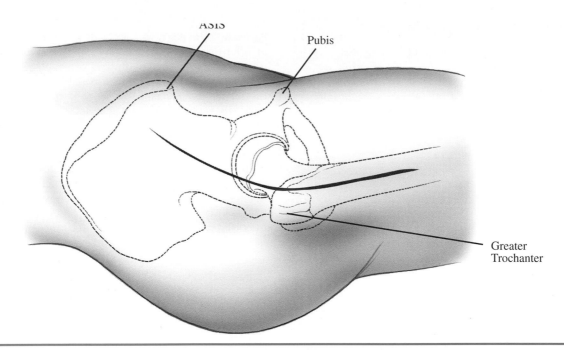

Figure 9–23   Anterolateral approach. The typical curvilinear incision for the anterolateral approach. For hip arthroplasty where greater exposure is needed, the apex of the incision may be placed more posterior to the level of the posterior edge of the greater trochanter.   *(Callahagen, et al. (1998). The Adult Hip. Philadelphia: Lippincott-Raven.)*

Box 9–1
Positioning Don'ts

POSTEROLATERAL APPROACH
   Don't cross legs.
   Don't bend at the hip >90 degrees.
   Don't turn toes inward.

ANTERIOR APPROACH
   Don't use Bedpans.
   Don't turn toes outward.

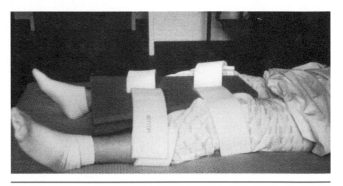

Figure 9–25   Abduction pillow.   *(Callahagen, et al. (1998). The Adult Hip. Philadelphia: Lippincott-Raven.)*

Turning. Turning is based on the type of surgical approach and the physician's preference. Some only allow the patient to turn onto the unaffected side and use pillows or an abductor pillow between the patient's legs to keep the involved leg in abduction. Others will only allow the patient to be turned onto the affected side, utilizing the bed as a splint to keep the affected leg in alignment. Still others will allow the patient to be turned to either side. Check the institutional or physician protocols. If Buck's traction is used, disconnect the traction, turn the patient using pillows between their legs, reposition the traction on the other side of the bed, and reconnect the traction.

Exercises. Mild active and passive exercises (active range-of-motion ankle, ankle pumps, quadriceps- and gluteal-setting exercises) are started the day of surgery and are carried out every 2 hours while the patient is awake. Other exercises to be included are hip rotation, hip abduction, and hip flexion exercises (Fig. 9–26) On the second or third postoperative day, a patient with a

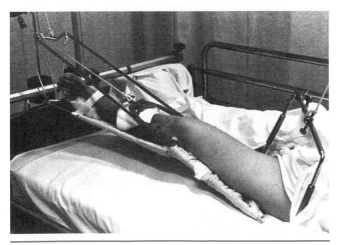

Figure 9–24   Skeletal traction and suspension for fracture of the distal femur demonstrating external rotation of the distal fragment and leg. This suspension device is the Harris-Aufranc design with Pearson attachment. Skeletal traction is by a Kirschner wire in the tibial tubercle.   *(Rockwood, et al. (1996). Rockwood & Green's Fractures in Adults. Philadelphia: Lippincott-Raven.)*

EXERCISES

You should have 2 to 3 exercise workouts every day. Do each exercise a minimum of 10 times, gradually increasing as you work with your therapist. These exercises will help you gain strength and mobility.

1.   Ankle pumps: Bend your ankles up and down.

2.   Quad sets: Tighten your thigh muscle and push the back of your knee into the bed. Hold for 6 seconds.

3.   Gluteal sets: Squeeze your buttocks together. Hold for 6 seconds.

4.   Hip rotation: Keep leg straight and roll out so kneecaps point to side. Return to starting position; kneecaps point to ceiling.

5.   Hip abduction: Keep leg straight and kneecap pointed toward ceiling; slide your leg out to side, then back to center.

6.   Hip flexion: Slide your heel toward buttock, bending your knee. DO NOT bend more than 70 degrees.

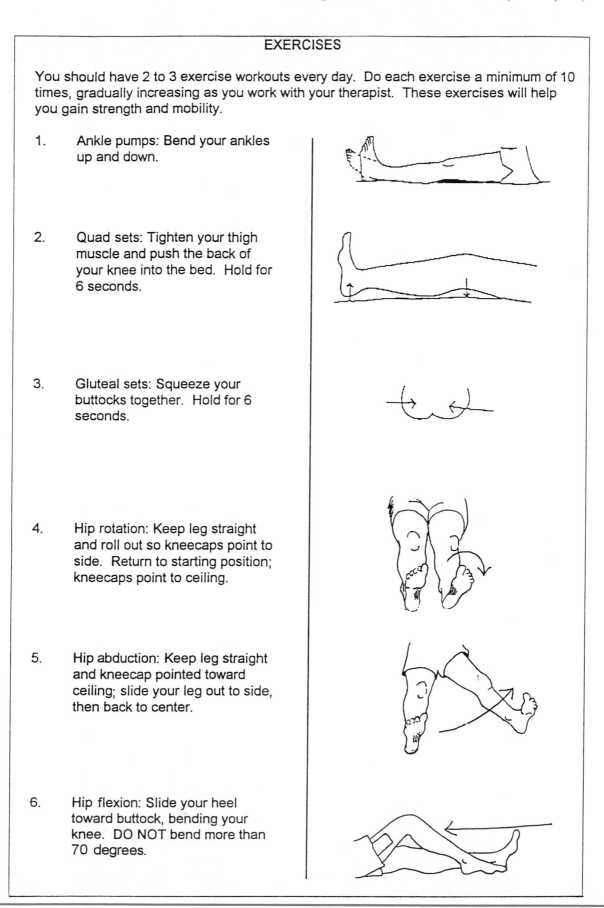

Figure 9–26   Exercises are started the day of surgery.   *(Callahagen, et al. (1998). The Adult Hip. Philadelphia: Lippincott-Raven.)*

posterolateral approach may begin using a skateboard (for abduction and adduction exercises, see Fig. 9–7), working up to a total of 30 minutes twice a day. To prevent the involved leg from going past the midline and into adduction, the uninvolved leg can be placed on a pillow that comes to the midline. Another exercise that patients may do later is riding a stationary bicycle. For the patient with an anterior approach, flexor and adductor strengthening exercises are initiated.

Sitting. Sitting in a chair may be started as early as the first or second postoperative day. The patient (with a posterolateral approach) should be in a semierect or slouched backward position, rather than a normal sitting position. The hip should not be flexed more than 90 degrees, and bending forward, such as when getting out of a chair, should be avoided. Such a semierect position can be achieved by placing pillows in the seat and the back of an armchair, which prevents the patient from sitting with their hip at a right angle. The hips should be kept higher than the knees. Another way is to utilize the total hip chair or EZ-up chair, but no recliner chairs. Bathroom privileges, which allow the use of the toilet stool, require the use of an elevated seat or "hi-john" to prevent too much hip flexion. Patients with the anterior approach are allowed to sit erect with 90 degrees of flexion at the hip postoperatively.

Ambulation. The patient usually comes to a standing position for the first time on the first or second postoperative day. The patient may get out of bed with the assistance of the nurse or physical therapist or with the use of a tilt table. With the posterior approach, getting out of bed without having the involved leg cross the midline or without flexing the affected hip more than 45 degrees is generally easier if it is done on the side of the uninvolved hip. For most patients, it is easier to keep the involved leg in abduction by returning to bed on the side of the affected hip. The patient usually begins walking using a walker with a four-point gait (see Chapter 4) and then progresses to crutches and even canes by 6 weeks after surgery. Only partial weight bearing is allowed at first, followed by weight bearing as tolerated, and then full weight bearing.

PATIENT TEACHING AND HOME CARE CONSIDERATIONS

Spend time with the patient, family, and significant others answering questions about the surgery, exercises, and planning for discharge. The usual hospital stay for a patient having a hip arthroplasty is 5 days; therefore, teaching and planning for discharge should start before admission. For patients with a posterolateral approach, points that are specific for recovery from hip arthroplasty and the prevention of dislocations (Fig. 9–27), especially during the first 6 weeks, are (1) continuing with exercises (see Fig. 9–26 and Fig. 9–28) so that hip flexion increases to 90 degrees, thus allowing the patient to sit erect in a straight chair with the hip at 90 degrees of flexion by 6 weeks postsurgery; (2) continuing to use the elevated toilet until 90 degrees of hip flexion is allowed; (3) avoiding crossing legs or ankles by keeping the feet about 3 to 6 inches apart and the knees 8 inches or more apart; (4) using pillows or an abductor pillow between the legs at night to prevent the involved leg from crossing the midline and rotating inward; (5) taking showers, not tub baths; (6) continuing with crutches and weight bearing as prescribed; (7) refraining from prolonged sitting or driving a car; (8) not bending at the waist or flexing the hip to pick anything up off the floor, tie a shoelace, or pull up linens in bed; (9) refraining from sexual intercourse until the 6-week checkup (some physicians do not impose that restriction, especially for women and, for certain positions, for men; discuss that point with the patient's physician); and (10) immediately reporting any signs of subluxation or dislocation of the hip; chest pain; excessive swelling in the leg; redness, tenderness, or swelling of the hip; bloody or purulent discharge from the incision; or urinary tract infection. (For further discussion, see the section on anxiety related to insufficient knowledge for the care of the patient with an internal fixation following a hip fracture.)

MONITORING AND MANAGING POTENTIAL PROBLEMS

Potential complications following a total hip replacement are neurovascular impairment, infection, hip dislocation, shock, urinary retention, deep venous thrombus (DVT), pulmonary embolism, and fat embolism.

NEUROVASCULAR IMPAIRMENT

A patient with a hip arthroplasty is at risk of peripheral neurovascular impairment or injury related to the surgical procedure, the abductor pillow, or other immobilizing devices utilized for positioning. It is imperative that nurses check the circulation, motor and sensory function, and temperature (CMST) of the affected hip and compare them with the unaffected hip (see Chapter 2). Any change in status needs to be reported immediately.

WOUND INFECTION

The initial postoperative dressing is usually left in place until the first postoperative day. Check to see if the entire dressing is dry and intact. The nurse may need to turn the patient to check beneath the patient, especially for patients who have had a posterolateral incision. Reinforce the dressing and notify the physician if there is excess bleeding. Once the initial dressing has been changed, change the dressing PRN and follow the institution's protocol for wound care. Because these patients are at increased risk for infection, they usually receive prophylactic antibiotics before, during, and immediately after surgery. Note any signs and symptoms of infection, not only near the incision but also involving the pulmonary and urinary tracts and other skin lesions.

HIP DISLOCATION

Positioning with correct alignment, exercising to gain control over the affected extremity, and sitting are all vital to preventing a hip dislocation. (See previous discussion of impaired physical mobility.)

Going Home

Precautions:

1.   NO hip bending beyond 70 degrees

2.   NO crossing of legs

3.   NO rolling kneecap in

4.   Limit riding in a car for 6 weeks, except for necessary appointments.

5.   DENTAL WORK:

After total joint surgery, you need to take antibiotics any time you have dental work done. This is to prevent infection of your new total joint. You will be given two dental cards telling you what to take and when. Please give one of the cards to your dentist, who can prescribe these antibiotics for you.

6.   SITTING:

- Choose a firm chair with arms. Avoid low or overstuffed chairs.
- Keep your knees apart.
- DO NOT bend forward (DO slouch so hips kept forward).
- DO NOT sit for longer than 45 minutes at a time.
- Use elevated toilet seat until told otherwise.

7.   SLEEPING:

- Use either your abductor pillow or two bed pillows between your legs.
- DO NOT sleep on your operated side.
- If you sleep on nonoperated side, keep your pillows between your legs.

8.   WALKING:

- Continue to use your walker/crutches for balance while standing or walking.
- Check the tips of your walker or crutches. Tighten the screws on your crutches daily.
- Remember to remove scatter rugs.

9.   STAIRS:

- Going up, lead with nonoperated leg.
- Going down, lead with operated leg and crutches/walker.

Figure 9–27   Going home precautions.   *(Callahagen, et al. (1998). The Adult Hip. Philadelphia: Lippincott-Raven.)*

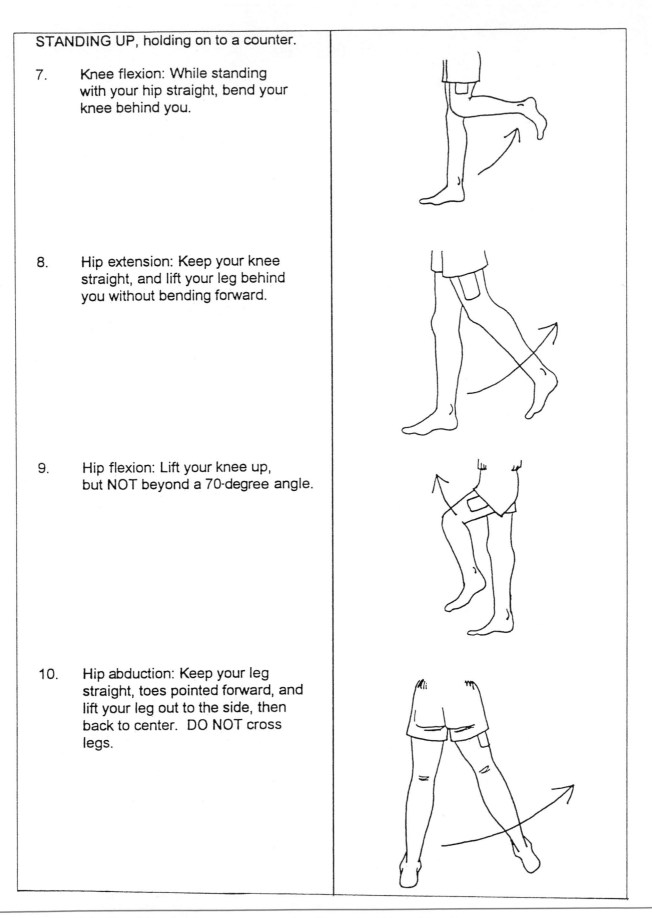

STANDING UP, holding on to a counter.

7.   Knee flexion: While standing with your hip straight, bend your knee behind you.

8.   Hip extension: Keep your knee straight, and lift your leg behind you without bending forward.

9.   Hip flexion: Lift your knee up, but NOT beyond a 70-degree angle.

10.   Hip abduction: Keep your leg straight, toes pointed forward, and lift your leg out to the side, then back to center. DO NOT cross legs.

Figure 9–28   Additional exercises.   *(Callahagen, et al. (1998). The Adult Hip. Philadelphia: Lippincott-Raven.)*

SHOCK

The patient has had a relatively large blood loss both in the operating room and in the immediate postoperative period. Make sure adequate intake and output records are maintained. Assess the balance between the intake and output, as the patient could develop shock. Hypovolemic shock is the result of hemorrhage and loss of extracellular fluid into damaged tissues. The prevention and/or treatment of shock consist of replacing depleted blood volume. Following a hip arthroplasty, the patient returns to the unit with postoperative wound drains to collect drainage from the surgical site and to prevent postoperative hematoma formation. However, in the immediate postoperative period, the physician may use an autotranfusion device (Fig. 9–29) or cell saver. This device collects the postoperative blood from the surgical site (usually 500–1,000 cc) for reinfusion back to the patient. The collection begins when the drains are placed in the patient in the operating room and can continue for 6 hours. The drain tubing is then reattached to a standard wound drainage (i.e., Hemovac, JVac). From insertion until the drains are removed (usually on the first postsurgical day), it is within normal limits for the patient to have a total output of 1,000–1,500 cc of drainage. The amount of drainage should be recorded each shift.

URINARY RETENTION

A Foley catheter is in place for the first 24 hours and is then removed. Once the catheter is removed, make sure the patient can void spontaneously. Keep the patient well hydrated. The first 24 hours the patient will have an IV and be allowed ice chips; the patient will then progress to liquids and to a normal diet as tolerated. Urinary retention is a common complication following a hip arthroplasty. Patients requiring prolonged catheterization are at higher risk of developing a urinary tract infection, which may pose a risk to the new prosthesis.

DEEP VENOUS THROMBUS

When a patient is immobile, venous return is slowed, partly because of the decreased muscular activity in the lower extremities, which would normally assist the return of blood from the legs back to the heart. When the walls of the vessels lose their tone, there may be stasis of some of the heavier components in the blood, leading to inflammation of the veins and the formation of clots (thrombi). Thrombophlebitis, intravascular clotting in an inflamed vein, can easily occur in patients postoperatively. Thrombophlebitis and the formation of thrombi can lead to pulmonary emboli.

PULMONARY EMBOLISM

The term *pulmonary embolism* refers to the obstruction of one or more pulmonary arteries by a thrombus (or thrombi), which originates somewhere in the venous system or the right side of the heart, becomes dislodged, and is carried to the lung. An infarction of lung tissue occurs due to the interruption of the lung's blood supply. The best treatment is prevention. Every effort should be made to keep the patient well hydrated, doing active and passive exercises (especially ankle pumps and quadriceps- and gluteal-setting exercises), and beginning ambulation as early as possible. Pharmacologic prophylaxis measures may include aspirin, warfarin, or heparin. Patients may wear elastic stockings or utilize an intermittent pneumatic compression device (Fig. 9–30) or arteriovenous foot pumps to increase blood flow to the deep veins and prevent deep venous thrombosis. See Chapter 4 for further discussion.

FAT EMBOLISM

A fat embolism occurs when fat in the blood becomes entrapped in the lung capillaries. There may also be occlusions of small vessels that supply the brain, kidneys, and other organs. The fat may originate at the surgical (or fracture) site or may be formed by an alteration of lipid stability in the blood caused by the stress (or trauma) of the surgery. The fat gains access to the venous circulation through ruptured narrow veins. Occlusion of a large number of small vessels in the lungs causes pulmonary pressure to rise, possibly even resulting in acute

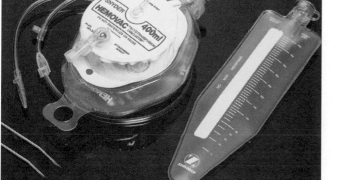

Figure 9–29 A postoperative orthopedic autotransfusion device. *(Courtesy of Zimmer, Inc.)*

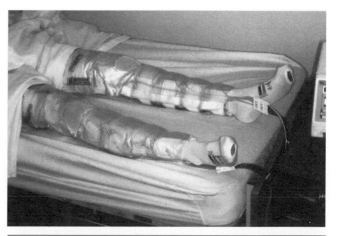

Figure 9–30 Thromboembolic stockings and an intermittent pneumatic compression device used for the prevention of deep venous thrombosis. *(Callahagen, et al. (1998). The Adult Hip. Philadelphia: Lippincott-Raven.)*

right-sided heart failure. Edema and hemorrhage in the alveoli impair oxygen transport, leading to hypoxia. See Chapter 4 for further discussion and treatment methods.

EVALUATION/OUTCOMES

The patient will have no complications, will be free of pain, and able to ambulate safely with a walker, crutches, or cane. The patient will be able to return to his or her normal activities of daily living.

CLINICAL PATHWAY (Patient with a Total Hip Arthroplasty)

An example of a generic clinical pathway for a patient with a total hip arthroplasty is presented in Figure 9–31.

FEMORAL FRACTURES

A fracture of the femoral shaft is a relatively common injury in adults. The fracture is usually produced by major trauma (e.g., car and motorcycle accidents, auto-pedestrian accidents, gunshot wounds, and falls from heights) and may be associated with multiple system injuries. Auto-pedestrian accidents tend to have a high prevalence of head, chest, pelvis, arm, and leg injuries. Motorcyclists tend to sustain associated pelvis and ipsi-lateral leg injuries.

Because the femur is the largest bone in the body and the principal weight-bearing bone of the leg, fractures may result in prolonged restrictions in mobility. With a fracture of the femoral shaft, the great strength of the muscles of the hip and thigh usually shortens the leg, and the thigh may present anterior and lateral angulation, with the lower portion of the leg lying in an abnor-

---

Figure 9–31

Clinical Pathway: Total Hip Arthroplasty (Replacement)

Admission Date: _____   **Discharge Plan:** _____ **Home** _____ **Skilled Nursing** _____ **Extended Care Facility**

Pathway	Preadmission Office/OP clinic	Admission Day Op day	Hosp Day 2 Post-op 2	Hosp Day 3 Post-op 3	Hosp Day 4 Post-op 4	Hosp Day 5	Outcomes
Consultation	Primary Care/ Rheumatologist or Medical	Case Manager Anesthesia, Dietitian AcutePain Service	Social Work PT, OT if nec.				Cont. @ Home or ECF
Assessment	Nrsg database H & P Exam. by MD, NP, or PA Rehab/ECF/home Home equipment Home environment	Review & add Review H & P Postop routine	Referral if nec Referral if nec		✓ if obtained Resolved		Home Care Nurse ECF Will have nec. equipment @ home
Tests	ECG/UA/CXR/ 1–2 units autol. blood Coag. studies AP & Lateral of pelvis/hips	X-ray in OR Hip/Pelvic X-ray in PACU H & H in PACU & repeat @ pm	✓ CBC Transfuse per protocol	✓ CBC Transfuse per protocol			
Medications	D/C NS AIDS 3d. b/4 OR D/C ASA 10 d. b/4 OR D/C anti coag. meds - c̄ MD Instruct on preop meds b/4 OR Analgesics as nec.	✓ preadm meds Routine meds Anticoagulant Antibiotics PCA/Epidural Bowel protocol	Cont. Anticoag. D/C antibiotics	D/C begin oral pain meds Analgesics			States meds, when to take and purpose Pain managed with oral medications Normal bowel function Analgesics @ home
Diet	Assessment wt. Overweight—lose weight slowly & sensibly Underweight—eat balanced diet	NPO @ MN b/4 OR	Liquids	Advance as tol		\	Tolerating diet

(continued)

Figure 9–31

Clinical Pathway: *(continued)*

Pathway	Preadmission Office/OP clinic	Admission Day Op day	Hosp Day 2 Post-op 2	Hosp Day 3 Post-op 3	Hosp Day 4 Post-op 4	Hosp Day 5	Outcomes
Activity	Preop mobility	Ankle pumps	Cont				Use cane/ walker safely
		Turn Protocol q 2	Turn q 2hrs				
	Fatigue level	If allowed HOB 45	NWB/WB as tol				
	ADLs & upper arm strength	Quad & Glut q 2 Bedrest	Cont OOB to Chair	Walking			Continue with exc
		OTC in bathroom	BRP with assist	BRP OTC			
		Obs. THA Precautions	Cont.				Observe THA Precautions
Treatment	Set blood donation dates 1 wk between units & 14 days between last unit and OR day	IV fluids/blood if necessary, I&O					
		TEDs, IPCD or foot pumps					Cont. TEDS @ home
		Hemovac/ouput		D/C			
		IS/TCDB q hr w/a		PRN			
		Foley to drain		D/C			Normal bladder function
		Dressing	Do Not Change	Change PRN			No infection
							States reason to contact MD
Education	Review Total hip precautions (THP)	Reinforce	Reviews Rehab Process			Reinforce	
						View Post-op THA video	Understands purpose of THA Precautions
	View THA video	Rev. hosp routine					
	Rev. THA booklet						
	Attends gp ed class						
	Pain management						
	Review hosp LOS						
D/C Plan	Identify discharge plan		Notify Social Worker Or Home Health Care as appropriate				Discharged to home
	Caregivers & home situation (LOS 5 days)						

mal rotation. The patient is unable to move the leg, and attempts to do so cause severe pain. The fracture is typically accompanied by extensive hemorrhage into the soft tissue of the thigh (2 to 4 units of blood are usually lost even in the simplest femoral fractures), which is sometimes severe enough to precipitate shock (Stephenson, 1996, p. 81). Additionally, these fractures can be life threatening from infection, fat embolism, respiratory syndrome, or multiple organ failure (Bucholz & Brumback, 1996, p. 1827). Generally, the fracture is closed rather than open, and damage to the sciatic nerve may occur.

METHODS OF REPAIR

Several methods are available for treatment of femoral shaft fractures. The type and the location of the fracture, the degree of comminution, the age of the patient,

and the patient's occupation are factors in determining the method of care. A femoral shaft fracture in an adult can rarely be reduced and held in immobilization by a cast, because a cast cannot prevent bone displacement and angulation from the large, powerful muscles of the thigh. In the past, femoral fractures were often treated in skeletal traction initially, followed by the use of a hip spica (worn for 3 to 6 months) or an ambulatory cast brace. Today, only distal third femoral fractures are treated with a cast brace (without other forms of traction), which is usually in place for 13 to 14 weeks.

Skeletal traction, the most common method of treatment for femoral shaft fractures before the 1970s, remains the method of choice for early fracture care (Bucholz & Brumback, 1996). Sufficient force can be applied by traction to the leg to achieve fracture reduction. The goal of the traction is to restore the fractured femur to proper length within the first 24 hours after

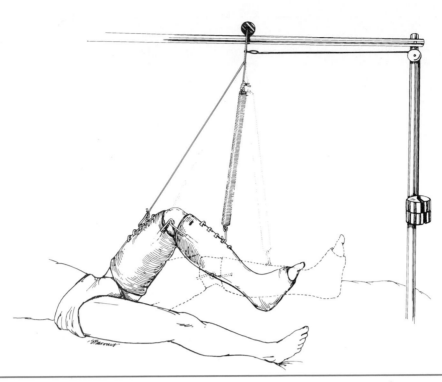

Figure 9–32 Diagram of a patient in a roller traction/suspension system. There are two separate lines—one for traction, and the other for suspension. Note the use of variable tension created by changing hook placement. *(Rockwood, et al. (1996).* Rockwood & Green's Fractures in Adults. *Philadelphia: Lippincott-Raven.)*

injury. Many variations of leg suspension for applying traction to a fractured femur have been devised; most are modifications of the Thomas splint with Pearson attachment. The half ring of the splint fits loosely around the upper thigh. Slings support the thigh while traction is applied in the general line of the femur, and the foot is supported in the Pearson attachment (See Chapter 6 nursing process for a patient in balanced suspension skeletal traction with a fractured femur). The traction is applied by utilizing a Kirschner wire or Steinmann pin through the proximal tibia. Another variation, Neufeld traction, incorporates the leg and Steinmann pin in plaster casts and applies traction through a roller system (Fig. 9–32) that permits greater early knee motion. Finally, 90–90 traction (Fig. 9–33), so called because the hip and knee are each positioned in 90 degrees of flexion, is also utilized. This traction is for the treatment of femoral shaft fractures that extend into the subtrochanteric region. External fixation (Fig. 9–34), using percutaneous pins inserted proximal and distal to the fracture, has yielded mixed results and is used most often in high-energy injuries in which rapid, rigid fracture stabilization is required because of the patient's associated injuries.

The treatment of femoral shaft injuries has shifted to an operative approach. When the fracture is treated surgically, one option is open reduction with a compression plate fixation. Although the open reduction with plating method overcomes the difficulties with respect to restoration of femoral length and rotational alignment that were associated with skeletal traction, it also has limitations and has decreased in popularity. In the 1980s, intramedullary techniques improved, and the

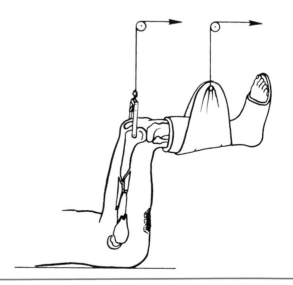

Figure 9–33 90-90 traction is especially applicable to fractures of the subtrochanteric area with associated wounds of the groin and buttocks. Traction of the femoral condyles is most effective. Suspension of the leg in a plaster cast usually is necessary. *(Rockwood, et al. (1996).* Rockwood & Green's Fractures in Adults. *Philadelphia: Lippincott-Raven.)*

use of the interlocking nail came into practice. The interlocking nail controls femoral length and rotation without the risks of tissue devitalization, quadriceps scarring, blood loss, and infection that were associated with plating. However, fractures that involve the distal metaphyseal-diaphyseal junction of the femur may still require open reduction and plating.

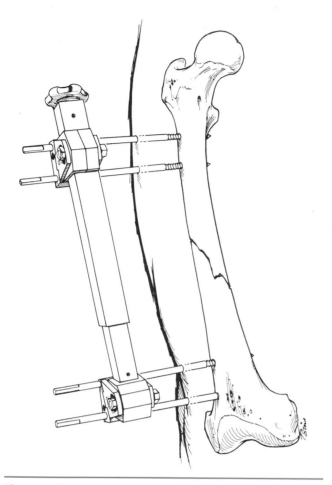

Figure 9–34   The Wagner leg-lengthening apparatus for lateral stabilization of femoral fractures.   *(Rockwood, et al. (1996). Rockwood & Green's Fractures in Adults. Philadelphia: Lippincott-Raven.)*

INTRAMEDULLARY FIXATION

In adults with closed uncomminuted fractures of the narrow portion of the medullary canal, intramedullary fixation (Fig. 9–35) is the treatment of choice. A variety of intramedullary fixation devices exist, including the Hansen-Street diamond-shaped nail with a tapered end, the flanged Schneider nail, the cloverleaf Küntscher nail, and the double I-Beam nail. For fixation to be secure, the nail must be of sufficient length and strength and be of a size that completely fills the medullary canal. The two most serious complications are nonunion and infection.

Open Method.   Open intramedullary nailing of the femur involves inserting a nail after surgical exposure of the fracture. After reaming the proximal and distal canals, a guidewire is driven up the proximal segment until it exits from the superior neck at the base of the trochanter or through its medial margin. Reduction is accomplished as the intramedullary nail is introduced over the guidewire and driven down the medullary canal, across the fracture site, and into the distal fragment, usually to the level of the proximal pole of the patella.

Closed Method   Closed intramedullary nailing is a method to nail shaft fractures of long bones without exposing the fracture site. It was first advocated by Küntscher in 1940, but has become more widely used with the development of image intensifier television fluoroscopy. With the closed method, an incision is made proximal to the greater trochanter, and a hole is made in the trochanter just medial to its tip. The nail is then driven down the medullary canal, across the fracture

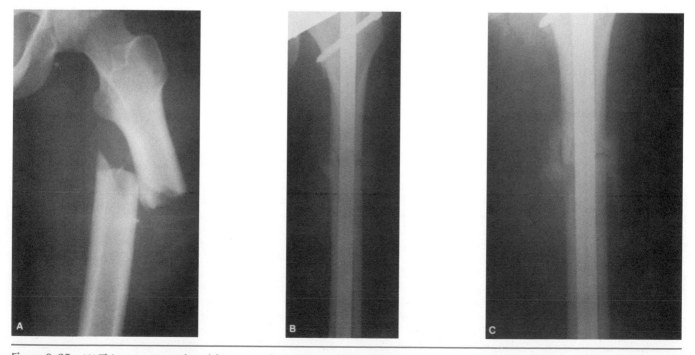

Figure 9–35   (A) This transverse, closed fracture at the junction of the proximal and middle thirds of the femur was managed by closed insertion of a dynamically locked intramedullary nail. (B) Abundant callus was formed within 3 weeks of the nailing. (C) By 5 weeks, bridging trabeculae of new bone were evident.   *(Rockwood, et al. (1996). Rockwood & Green's Fractures in Adults. Philadelphia: Lippincott-Raven.)*

site, toward the condyles. The fracture site may be manipulated to get the nail across the fracture, but the fracture site is never opened.

NURSING PROCESS (Patient with an Intramedullary Nail for a Fractured Femur)

ASSESSMENT

The patient with an intramedullary nail for a fractured femur is usually a young adult who has sustained a high-energy trauma. Thus, there may additional injuries beyond the affected leg. The patient may be placed in balanced suspension skeletal traction for a few days before surgery, or the patient may have gone directly to surgery after the accident. Assess for signs and symptoms of shock since a patient with a femoral fracture always has a large amount of blood loss. Assess other areas of the body for skin abrasions, which may lead to infection. Determine if there was a head injury or injuries to internal organs.

Upon return from the postanesthesia room, the immediate postoperative assessment involves taking vital signs (e.g., pulse, respiration, and blood pressure) and observing the patient's general color and warmth. A neurovascular assessment of the affected leg (pulse, temperature, color, capillary filling, edema, and sensory and motor nerve function) should be made (see Chapter 2) and the position of the leg checked for proper alignment in the support sling. The patient's level of consciousness and orientation should be determined. The incisional dressing and the area posterior to the dressing should be checked for drainage. If the patient has wound catheters in place, note the color and amount of drainage and whether the suction is working. Assess the type, severity, and location of pain and the patient's verbal and nonverbal expressions of pain; and note whether the patient received medication in surgery or in the postanesthesia room. Have the patient cough and deep breathe, and auscultate the chest for clearness of the lungs. Note the type of intravenous solution, the rate of flow, and the amount left in the bottle or bag. Obtain from anesthesia and postanesthesia records or personnel the amount of blood loss in surgery and the amount of fluid replacement. Check the patient for bladder distention or the need to void. Assess the status of any other injuries the patient may have received during the accident.

Frequent assessment of the patient should be made during the postoperative period. Auscultation of the patient's chest should be done at least once a shift. For the first few postoperative days, the nurse will also need to assess for bowel sounds. Neurovascular assessments of the affected extremity are usually done every 15 minutes for 2 hours, then every 30 minutes for 2 hours, then every hour for 2 hours, then every 2 hours for 18 hours, and then at the beginning of every shift.

NURSING DIAGNOSIS

Based on all of the assessment data, the major nursing diagnoses for a typical patient following an intramedullary nailing for a femoral fracture include the following (other potential injuries [e.g., head injury, a fractured arm, or internal injuries the patient may have received in the accident] are not addressed here):

- Pain and discomfort related to soft-tissue and bone trauma
- Impaired physical mobility related to instability of the femur
- Impaired skin integrity related to the trauma and surgery
- Posttrauma response related to the accident, as evidenced by recurring nightmares and expressions of survival guilt
- Anxiety related to knowledge deficit about the surgery and rehabilitation process

COLLABORATIVE PROBLEMS

- Shock
- Wound infection
- Venous stasis
- Pulmonary emboli
- Fat emboli
- Paralytic ileus
- Nonunion of the femur

GOAL FORMULATION AND PLANNING

The goals are to have the patient experience (1) a decrease in pain through positioning, nursing interventions, and prescribed medications; (2) an increase in mobility through positioning, turning, exercises, and ambulation; (3) skin integrity through nursing care measures; (4) no nightmares or feeling of guilt survival; (5) a decrease in anxiety through patient education; and (6) an absence of complications.

INTERVENTIONS

ALLEVIATE PAIN

The first step is to assess for the location, severity, and degree of physical and emotional pain. Remember that sympathoadrenal signs indicating pain include changes in pulse rate, blood pressure, and respiration and the occurrence of diaphoresis, depression, or mood swings. Today, many patients are on PCAs for pain control and may need instructions on how to use the PCA or encouragement to initiate the medication. If the nurse is administering pain medications, do not hesitate to medicate during the first 24 hours following surgery should the patient's condition warrant, even if the patient does not request medication. Reassure the patient while trying physical nursing measures for pain relief. Sometimes the patient becomes anxious and tense and tightens their muscles to prevent any movement. This increases the discomfort and leads the patient to tighten their muscles even more. After reassuring the patient and getting the patient to relax the affected leg in your hands, use both hands and gently lift the leg and move it through its range of motion several times before repositioning it. Frequently, the pain will go away or at least be greatly reduced. In general, muscle-setting exercises, which increase circulation, help to relieve pain.

With the pain due to muscle tension eased by exercise, it is much easier to determine the amount of pain medication needed for the patient's underlying condition. Do give medications for pain relief, but assess pain, try nursing measures for pain relief, note the dosage of all medications given, and note the patient's reaction. Determine the effectiveness of the pain relief measures taken.

INCREASE MOBILITY

The major interventions to increase mobility are correct positioning, exercises, and controlled ambulation.

Position. Whether the patient was in balanced suspension skeletal traction before surgery or not, most patients will be placed in a Thomas, Brady, or similar splint to support the affected leg for the first 3 to 5 days after surgery. The splint is for support only, not to immobilize the leg. No traction will be applied after surgery. The patient can have the head of the bed elevated for comfort but must stay supine. The patient can utilize the trapeze to lift themselves to change position, use a bedpan, and facilitate linen changes.

Turning. Postoperatively, while the patient's affected leg is in a sling, the patient will need to remain supine and not turn. Once the support splint is removed, the patient can turn to either side, since the intramedullary nail gives the necessary support to the fracture site. Some patients will not want to turn onto the affected side for fear of increasing pain or "hurting" the surgical site. In the beginning, when the patient turns to the unaffected side, the patient may find that placing a pillow between their legs helps to increase comfort in the affected leg. Encourage the patient to move freely in bed, since that movement is not restricted, and to turn to both sides.

Exercises. Exercises are very important for the rehabilitation of a patient with an intramedullary nail following a femoral fracture. Exercises maintain muscle tone and strength, which act to compress the fracture and probably to stimulate local vascularity. Quadriceps-setting and plantar and dorsiflexion exercises (see care of the patient with a fractured hip) on the affected side are started as the patient recovers from anesthesia. Make sure the patient does active exercises to the unaffected leg, and teach the patient exercises to prepare for crutch walking (as discussed in Chapter 4).

Ambulation. As soon as the patient gains muscle control of the affected leg, ambulation on crutches is permitted with no weight bearing. This may be within the first 24 hours after surgery. Progressively increasing weight bearing is permitted as roentgenograms indicate progress and complete union. Often union is rapid, and unrestricted weight bearing may be permitted by 10 to 12 weeks. When the stability of the fixation is not optimal because of comminution or other problems, alterations in the rehabilitation program and delays in weight bearing may be required. Other physical injuries from the accident may also impede or restrict this activity.

POSTTRAUMA RESPONSE

Be alert to the patient not sleeping or having disturbed sleep. Some patients will not want to go to sleep and state, "I just don't feel like sleeping." In fact, the patient may not want to go to sleep because they experience nightmares about the accident. Does the patient have a preoccupation with the accident or express guilt about surviving while others lost their lives? Does the family mention behavioral or personality changes since the accident?

The experience of traumatic situations differs from ordinary experiences in that it involves realistic danger of physiologic or psychologic destruction that could mobilize fear of death. The patient's initial response is to survive. A coping method of "numbing" is used to help reduce or suppress psychological and emotional impacts. However, in trying to suppress the traumatic experience, intrusive recollections or reenactments of the trauma erupt into conscious awareness. This oscillation between intrusive reenactment and "numbing" continues until the individual works through the trauma and assimilates the trauma into a meaningful and congruent whole.

Do not ask the patient to talk about the accident with others in the room, not even the patient in the other bed; that request may cause significant discomfort to the patient. Provide time for one-to-one interactions in a quiet, safe environment. Acknowledge that talking about the traumatic event may intensify the symptoms (e.g., nightmares, flashbacks, feeling of numbness), and proceed at the patient's pace. Listen with empathy in an unhurried manner. Reassure the patient that these feelings often occur in individuals who experience such traumatic events. Assist the patient in differentiating reality from fantasy. Help to identify the patient's strengths and resources. For the orthopaedic nurse, having a psychiatric clinical nurse specialist help with these activities may be advantageous (Carpenito, 1993).

PATIENT TEACHING AND HOME CARE CONSIDERATIONS

Spend time with the patient, family, and significant others answering questions about the surgery, exercises, and planning for discharge. Points that are specific for recovery from intramedullary nailing focus on exercises and prevention of infection. Make sure the patient understands their exercises, how to do them, how often they are to be done, and when they are to progress to more stressful exercises. Reinforce teaching on progressive weight-bearing ambulation. Have the patient demonstrate the exercises and tell how they will incorporate these exercises into their daily activity when they get home. Stress the need to progress but not to overdo the exercises or apply too much weight too soon when ambulating. Have the patient demonstrate going up and down stairrs. Go over the safety precautions for a patient going home on crutches (e.g., no loose rugs, no pets that jump on them). Make sure the patient knows how to get into and out of the car.

Review the signs and symptoms of infection (and wound care if necessary) and when to notify the physician. Also review with the patient the potential complications of immobility and why it is important that the patient remain as active as possible.

MONITORING AND MANAGING POTENTIAL COMPLICATIONS

The potential complications that can occur following a high-energy trauma and the intramedullary nailing of a femoral fracture involve (1) shock, (2) wound infection, (3) venous stasis (deep vein thrombosis), (4) pulmonary emboli, (5) fat emboli, (6) paralytic ileus, and (7) nonunion. If the patient was in traction for a few days before surgery, the potential for shock is reduced, but the patient must still be monitored for signs and symptoms of shock. Items 3 through 6 are discussed in the care of a patient with a fractured hip in this chapter and in Chapter 4. The patient was at risk for fat emboli immediately after the accident. However, the surgery again places the patient at risk for fat emboli.

WOUND INFECTION
The development of infection after intramedullary fixation is serious, as it greatly increases the likelihood of nonunion. Even if union does occur, it may take years. Amputation may be the ultimate result of an infection. Assess for signs and symptoms of infection, provide wound care per your facility's protocol, and administer antibiotics as prescribed.

NONUNION
Nonunion is usually the result of a failure to accomplish fixation. The nail may be too small to completely fill the medullary canal or too short to extend proximally and distally through the fracture site, thus being unable to adequately control rotation (Bucholz and Brumback, 1996). Fixation is also poor in fractures that are too comminuted.

EVALUATION/OUTCOMES

The patient should remain relatively free of pain, and, if pain occurs, it is controlled by medication. There should be an absence of complications from surgery and immobility. The patient should have a positive attitude toward recovery and returning to their normal life. Keep in mind that the patient will probably need to return to the hospital in 12 to 18 months (possibly as soon as 6 months) to have the intramedullary nail removed.

Figure 9–36

Clinical Pathway: Femoral Fracture with Intermedullary Nail

Admission Date: _____   Discharge Plan: _____ Home   _____ Skilled Nursing   _____ Extended Care Facility

Pathway	Preadmission Office/OP clinic	Admission Day Op day	Hosp Day 2 Post-op 2	Hosp Day 3 Post-op 3	Hosp Day 4 Post-op 4	Hosp Day 5	Outcomes
Consultation	Orthopaedic MD Medical MD	Case Manager Anesthesia, AcutePain Service	Social Work PT Home Health Svs	Dietitian			Cont. PT @ home/ECF
Assessment	Nrsg database H & P Exam. by MD, NP, or PA CMST of involved Ext. q 15 x 4 then q hr Other injuries	Review & add Review H & P Postop routine CMST q 15 x 4 q 30 x 2, q 1 hr x 2, q 4 hrs. Rehab/ECF/ home		Referral if nec.		Resolved	Home Care Nurse
Tests	ECG/UA/CXR/ T & C Blood PT, PTT, SMA AP & Lateral of Pelvis & hips	X-ray in OR Hip/Pelvic x ray in PACU H & H in PACU & repeat in pm	✓ CBC Transfuse per protocol	✓ CBC Transfuse per protocol			
Medications	✓ Home Meds Demerol/ Morphine IM or IV for pain	✓ preadm meds Routine meds Anticoagulant					States meds, when to take and purpose States purpose *(continued)*

Figure 9–36

Clinical Pathway: *(continued)*

Pathway	Preadmission Office/OP clinic	Admission Day Op day	Hosp Day 2 Post-op 2	Hosp Day 3 Post-op 3	Hosp Day 4 Post-op 4	Hosp Day 5	Outcomes
	Antibiotics PCA Instruct on preop meds b/4 OR	Antibiotics PCA/Epidural	D/C antibiotics	D/C begin oral pain meds			Pain managed with oral medications Normal bowel function
		Bowel protocol					
Diet	NPO.	NPO @ MN b/4 OR	Liquids to Diet as tol.	Advance as tol Encourage fluids			Tolerating diet
Activity	Bed rest	Bed rest with Splint	BR with Splint	BR with Splint	BR with Splint		
		Control over leg Muscles— CW/NWB	Continue	Continue	Continue	Continue	Ambulate safely for gait
		Quadricep- setting q. 2	Continue	Continue	Continue	Continue	Exercise at Home
		Gluteal-setting q. 2 h.	Continue	Continue	Continue	Continue	
		Ankle Pumps q. 2 h.	Continue	Continue	Continue	Continue	
		Exc. Upper Ext.	Continue	Continue	Continue	Continue	
		Trapeze to move Self in bed	Continue	Continue	Continue	Continue	
Treatments	Start IV	IV fluids/blood if necessary,	D/C not nec.				
		Intake & Output	Continue	D/C			
	Foley Catheter	Foley to drain		D/C			Normal bladder elim.
		Antiembolic hose	Continue.				Cont. AE stockings
		Thomas Splint to support the affected leg	Thomas Splint	Thomas Splint	Thomas Splint	??D/C	D/C t raaction post
		Trapeze	Utilizes to re- position				
		Hemovac/ output		D/C			No signs of infection
		IS/CDB q hr w/a		PRN			Clear lungs
		Dressing	Do Not Change	Change PRN (Wound protocol)			No infection, S & S of Infection and when to Call MD>
Education		Preoperative ed.	Operative routine				Verbalizes knowledge
		Review hosp LOS	Rehab. Process				
D/C Plan		Identify discharge plan					Discharged to home
		Assistance at home LOS 4 to 6 days					Assistance @ home
		Depending on other injuries that occurred.					

CLINICAL PATHWAY (Patient with a Femoral Fracture and Intramedulallary Nail)

An example of a generic clinical pathway for a patient with a femoral fracture and an intramedullary nail is presented in Figure 9–36.

FRACTURES OF THE DISTAL THIRD OF THE FEMUR

Fractures of the distal third of the femur can be classified into supracondylar fractures without joint involvement and condylar fractures with joint involvement. Supracondylar fractures not involving the joint, which are undisplaced impacted fractures, can usually be treated with a few days of traction followed by application of a cast brace. For severely displaced and comminuted fractures, the usual treatment is skeletal traction with a Kirschner wire near the tibial tuberosity (see Chapter 6 for nursing care of a patient in balanced suspension skeletal traction). After reduction has been obtained and maintained for 2 to 3 weeks, the leg can usually be placed in a femoral cast brace and ambulation permitted.

A *cast brace* (Fig. 9–37) is a combination cast and brace made up of three components. First, there is a patellar weight-bearing cast on the lower leg, either as a short leg cast or as a cylinder cast. Second, there is an ischial weight-bearing cast on the thigh, molded well around Scarpa's triangle, the ischial seat, and the greater trochanter. The thigh component is applied snugly to increase the hydrodynamic compressive effect of the thigh muslces and to provide for immobilization of the fracture fragments. Third, there is an external polycentric knee hinge that connects the below-the-knee portion to the thigh portion, which allows 90 degrees of knee flexion. The cast brace allows for mobility of both hip and knee joints and thus permits a fairly normal gait when ambulating.

Cast bracing is based on the concept that weight bearing is always a physiologic activity that will promote the formation of bone. It allows early ambulation and partial weight bearing, which promotes healing by adding pressure to the fracture site, by improving circulation, by mobilizing muscles, and by lessening edema in the capsules and joint structures of the knee.

For supracondylar fractures not involving the joint, open reduction and internal fixation is usually only done for fractures secondary to a pathologic process, or when the condition of the patient will not permit bed confinement for traction. Such internal fixations are usually repaired using Blount or Elliott blade plates, straight plates, Zickel nails, Rush pins, or other devices. Complications that can occur are infection, nonunion, and restriction of motion.

Condylar fractures involving the joint may be unicondylar or bicondylar. A common method of treatment is skeletal traction with a pin through the tibia near the

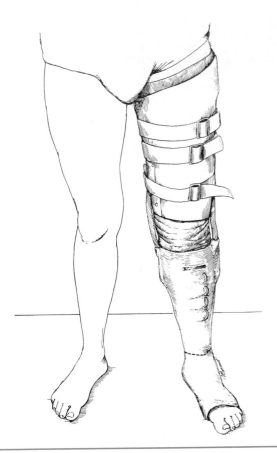

Figure 9–37   The femoral fracture brace with adjustable plastic (or plaster substitute) thigh section. Hooks incorporated in shank plaster are for roller traction suspension. The dotted line at the ankle demonstrates where the foot section can be removed, which is possible as long as suspension of the thigh section is still available. (Note the skeletal pin incorporated in the plaster.)   *(Rockwood, et al. (1996). Rockwood & Green's Fractures in Adults. Philadelphia: Lippincott-Raven.)*

tuberosity and, if necessary, an additional pin through the distal fragment of the femur, with light traction used to help with positioning. Open reduction may be necessary following a period of traction. Unicondylar displaced fractures may be treated with an open reduction and internal fixation using Knowles pins and cancellous screws. When the posterior part of the medial femoral condyle is sheared off, an open reduction and internal fixation with a lag screw may be used. For T condylar fractures, a common method of fixing the fracture is a plate, Knowles pins, and four screws.

NURSING PROCESS (Patient with a Cast Brace for a Supracondylar Fracture)

ASSESSMENT

Because the patient typically has been in skeletal traction, his or her overall condition has generally stabilized before the cast brace is applied. Assess the involved leg after the cast brace is applied. Determine the amount, kind, and location of pain. Check the neurovascular status of the affected extremity (see Chapter 2). Check the skin around the edges of both casts, and note any complaints or discomfort at the proximal or distal ends. Ensure that the hinges of the cast brace are functioning.

The assessment of the cast depends on the type of material used for casting. Here the emphasis is on the assessment of a patient with a cast brace made of plaster of Paris. (For more information on other types of casts, e.g., fabric tapes impregnated with resins and the general assessment of each cast, see Chapter 5.) Do a general assessment of each cast as discussed in Chapter 5. Always compare the affected leg with the unaffected leg.

Listen to the patient's complaints, and check for unrelieved pain, increased pain, or swelling. Ask the patient to specify the exact site of the pain. Check for any tightness or skin abrasions from the cast.

NURSING DIAGNOSIS

Based on all of the assessment data, the major nursing diagnoses for a patient in a cast brace following a distal femoral fracture typically include the following:

- Pain and discomfort related to soft-tissue and bone trauma
- Impaired physical mobility related to instability of the femur
- Anxiety related to knowledge deficit regarding the cast brace and rehabilitation

COLLABORATIVE PROBLEMS

- Neurovascular impairment
- Swelling above the knee
- Pressure areas from the cast brace

GOAL FORMULATION AND PLANNING

The goals are to have the patient experience (1) a decrease in pain with fracture immobilization and prescribed medications, (2) an increase in mobility with a weight-bearing cast brace, (3) a decrease in anxiety through patient education, and (4) an absence of complications.

INTERVENTIONS

ALLEVIATE PAIN

The cast brace helps to keep the fractured femur in alignment. Muscle-setting exercises increase circulation to the area and help reduce muscle spasms and pain. Elevating the affected leg helps to reduce the edema and pain; however, make sure that the patient is able to relax the leg in that position. Discuss with the patient their complaints of pain. There may be an increase in pain after removal from skeletal traction and the application of a cast brace. Offer prescribed analgesics as needed.

INCREASE MOBILITY

The major nursing interventions to increase mobility include correct positioning, turning, exercises, and ambulation. Exercises and turning procedures are the same as those for a patient with a long leg cast (discussed in Chapter 5).

Position. The patient with a femoral cast brace needs to be in bed with the casted leg elevated until the cast is dry, usually 24 hours but sometimes longer, depending on the cast (see Chapter 5). Make sure that there is no pressure on the soft tissue at the proximal end of the cast or on the patient's low back.

Exercises. The patient will continue to do the exercises started while he or she was in balanced suspension traction (see Chapter 6). The patient can now do flexion and extension exercises while sitting, which is probably a more comfortable position than standing or lying supine.

Ambulation. Even though the patient may start ambulating as soon as the cast is dry, care should be taken the first time the patient gets up because he or she has been on bed rest for some time. The patient will be using crutches with partial weight bearing on the affected log. The hinges at the knee are unlocked before the patient starts to get out of bed and are locked before the patient begins to walk. When the patient gets onto a commode or into a chair, the hinges are unlocked again. A priority for the nurse assisting with ambulation is to check the status of the hinges.

PATIENT TEACHING AND HOME CARE CONSIDERATIONS

First and foremost, the patient should understand the purpose of the femoral cast brace and how it works and why he or she should not try to adjust or alter it. Teach the patient, the family, and significant others about the general care of the cast brace and the involved leg, and discuss home care and safety precautions for a patient going home with a cast and crutches (see Chapter 4 and Chapter 5). Suggest to the patient ways to modify clothing for the affected extremity. One example is to open a seam in a pair of slacks and attach Velcro straps for closure. Discuss sponge bathing as a replacement for a tub bath or shower. Once in a while, a plastic cover can be placed over the leg for a shower, but the brace is too high to allow the patient to get into a tub even if only a small amount of water is present.

MONITORING AND MANAGING POTENTIAL PROBLEMS

The potential complications that occur following a supracondylar fracture and the application of a cast brace are swelling above the knee and the development of pressure areas from the cast.

SWELLING

Nursing care for a patient with a femoral cast brace is similar to that of a patient in a long leg cast. The major difference is that patients with a cast brace frequently have swelling above the knee. After traction is removed and the cast brace applied, the patient frequently has swelling about the knee and to some degree in the toes, especially after ambulation. The knee may swell up to twice the normal size and cause the cast to feel tight. Even though that is an expected outcome and will gradually subside over time, there are a number of measures that may reduce the swelling. Explain to the patient why swelling occurs and that it is not a cause for alarm. Encourage quadriceps-setting exercises, exercising the knee with flexion and extension, and elevating the complete leg when not weight bearing. Teach the patient to report any changes in neurovascularity, for example, tingling, numbness, or coldness in the involved leg (see Chapter 2) and how to elevate the leg (see Chapter 5).

IMPAIRED SKIN INTEGRITY

Pressure areas are a potential problem with any cast, but this is especially true with the femoral cast brace. The thigh component has a particular tendency to develop pressure areas, because the proximal edge extends well into the groin and gluteal areas and the distal edge presses against the swelling at the knee. An activity that seems to present added skin problems is getting on and off the toilet, because doing so may pinch the skin along the proximal edge of the cast. One measure to help relieve the discomfort is to reposition the casted extremity to ease pressure on specific areas. Also, make sure there are no rough edges on the cast. Petal the cast edges as indicated. Sometimes a small amount of cornstarch will help to smooth the skin and reduce irritation. Follow up on all complaints of pain or discomfort.

EVALUATION/OUTCOMES

Special emphasis should be given to evaluating the patient's response to the cast brace and their understanding of home care instructions and safety precautions. The patient should be able to explain cast care and demonstrate how the cast brace functions without assistance from others. The patient should be able to go up and down stairs.

References

Altizer, L. L. (1995). Total hip arthroplasty. *Orthopaedic Nursing, 14*(4), 7–18.

Altizer, L. L. (1998). Degeneration disorders. In A. B. Maher, S. W. Salmend T. A. Pellino (Eds). *Orthopaedic Nursing.* 2nd. ed. p. 480–544. Philadelphia: W. B. Saunders.

Anders, R. L., & Ornellas, E. M. (1997). Acute management of patients with hip fracture: A research literature review. *Orthopaedic Nursing, 16*(2), 31–46.

Anderson, L. P., & Dale, K. G. (1998). Infections in total joint replacements. *Orthopaedic Nursing, 17*(1), 7–10.

Berg, E. E. (1993). Editorial comment: Postoperative bold salvage systems. *Orthopaedic Nursing, 12*(3), 8.

Blaylock, B., Murray, M., O'Connell, K., & Rex, J. (1995). Tape injury in the patient with total hip replacement. *Orthopaedic Nursing, 14*(3), 25–28.

Bucholz, R. W., & Brumback, R. J. (1996). Fractures of the shaft of the femur. In C. A. Rockwood, D. P. Green, R. W. Bucholz, & J. D. Heckman (Eds.), *Rockwood and Green's fractures in adults.* (Vol. 2, pp. 1627–1918). Philadelphia: Lippincott-Raven.

Buckwalter, J. A. (1994). Musculoskeletal tissues and the musculoskeletal system. In S. I. Weinstein and J. A. Buckwalter (Eds.), *Turek's orthopaedics: Principles and their application* (5th ed., pp. 13–67). Philadelphia: J. B. Lippincott Company.

Callaghan, J. J., Rosenberg, A. G., & Rubash, H. E. (Eds.). (1998). *The adult hip.* Philadelphia: Lippincott-Raven.

Carpinto, L. J. (1993), Nursing diagnosis: Application to clinical practice (5th ed.) Philadelphia: J. B. Lippincott Company.

Christensen, C. (1997). Total hip arthroplasty: Positioned, prepped, and draped. *Orthopaedic Nursing, 16*(1), 43–48.

Conner, M. L. (1998). Hip fractures in older persons. In V. C. Williamson (Ed.), *Management of lower extremity fractures* (pp. 95–108). Pitman, NJ: National Association of Orthopaedic Nurses.

Cosman, F., Nieves, J., Horton, J., Shen, V., & Lindsey, R. (1994). Effects of estrogen on response to edetic acid infusion in postmenopausal osteoporotic women. *Journal of Clinical Endocrinology and Metabolism, 78*, 939–943.

Cummings, S., Black, D., & Rubin, S. (1989). Lifetime risks of hip, Colles', or vertebral fracture and coronary heart disease among white women. *Archives of Internal Medicine, 149*, 2445–2448.

DeLee, J. C. (1996). Fractures and dislocations of the hip. In C. A. Rockwood, D. P. Green, R. W. Buckholz, & J. D. Heckman (Eds.), *Rockwood and Green's fractures in adults* (Vol. 2, pp. 1756–1803). Philadelphia: Lippincott-Raven.

Evans, R. L. (1998). Nursing care of the surgical patient. In J. J. Callaghan, A. G. Rosenberg, & H. E. Rubash (Eds.), *The adult hip* (pp. 647–662). Philadelphia: Lippincott-Raven.

Evans, R. L., Rubash, H. E., & Albrecht, S. A. (1993). The efficacy of postoperative autotransfusion on total joint arthroplasty. *Orthopaedic Nursing, 12*(3), 11–18.

Howe, J. G., & Lambert, B. (1998). Critical pathways in total hip arthroplasty. In J. J. Callaghan, A. G. Rosenberg, & H. E. Rubash (Eds.), *The adult hip* (pp. 865–892). Philadelphia: Lippincott-Raven.

Jaffe, K. A., Killian, J. T., & Morris, S. (1996). Hip fractures and dislocations. In V. R. Masear (Ed.), *Primary care orthopaedics.* (pp. 72–80). Philadelphia: W. B. Saunders.

Kannus, P., Parkkari, J., Hievanen, H., Heinonen, A., Vuori, I., & Jarvinen, M. (1996). Epidemiology of hip fracture. *Bone, 18*, 57s–63s.

Koval, K. J., & Zuckerman, J. D. (1998). Hip. In K. J. Koval & J. D. Zuckerman (Eds.), *Fractures in the Elderly* (pp. 175–192). Philadelphia: Lippincott-Raven.

Lappe, J. M. (1998). Prevention of hip fractures: A nursing imperative. *Orthopaedic Nursing, 17*(3), 15–25.

Leininger, S. M. (1997). *Building clinical pathways.* Pitman, NJ: National Association of Orthopaedic Nursing.

Lichtenstein, R., Semaan, S., & Marmar, E. C. (1993). Development and impact of a hospital-based perioperative patient education program in a joint replacement center. *Orthopaedic Nursing, 12*(6), 17–25.

Lindsey, R., & Cosman, F. (1992). Primary osteoporosis. In F. Coe & M. Favus (Eds.), *Disorders of bone and mineral metabolism* (pp. 831–888). New York: Raven Press.

Mae, H. L., Reynolds, M. A., Treston-Aurand, J., & Henke, J. A. (1993). Comparison of autoreinfusion and standard drainage systems in total joint arthroplasty patients. *Orthopaedic Nursing, 12*(3), 9–25.

Magaziner, J., Simonsick, E., Kashner, T., Hebel, J., & Kenzora, J. (1989). Survival experience of aged hip fracture patients. *American Journal of Public Health, 53,* 274–278.

Mehlhoff, M. A. (1994). The adult hip. In S. E. Weinstein and J. A. Buckwalter (Eds.), *Turek's orthopaedics: Principles and application* (5th ed., pp. 521–572). Philadelphia: J. B. Lippincott Company.

Messer, B. (1998a). Reducing lengths of stays in the total joint replacement population. *Orthopaedic Nursing, Supplement,* 23–25.

Messer, B. (1998b). Total joint replacement preadmission programs. *Orthopaedic Nursing, Supplement,* 31–33.

Mourad, L. (1997). Fracture forum: Epstein types of fracture/dislocations of the hip. *Orthopaedic Nursing, 16*(1), 70.

Nelson, L., Taylor, F., Adams, M., & Parker, D. E. (1990). Improving pain management for hip-fractured elderly. *Orthopaedic Nursing, 9*(3), 79–83.

O'Brien, S., Engela, D. W., Trainor, P., & Beverland, D. E. (1996). Assessing the accuracy of femoral component placement in custom cemented hip replacement. *Orthopaedic Nursing, 15*(4), 47–53.

Sauenwhite, C. A., & Simpson, P. (1998). Patient and family perspective regarding early discharge and care of the older adult undergoing fractured hip rehabilitation. *Orthopaedic Nursing, 17*(1), 30–36.

Spica, M. M., & Schwab, M. D. (1996). Sexual expression after total joint replacement. *Orthopaedic Nursing, 15*(5), 41–44.

Stephenson, S. (1996). Fractures of the femur. In V. R. Masear (Ed.), *Primary care orthopaedics* (pp. 81–83, 106–109). Philadelphia: W. B. Saunders.

Thorngren, K. (1994). Fractures in older persons. *Disability Rehabilitation, 16,* 119–126.

Wasielewski, R. C. (1998). The hip. In J. J. Callaghan, A. G. Rosenbert, & H. E. Rubash (Eds.), *The adult hip* (pp. 57–74). Philadelphia: Lippincott-Raven.

Williams, M. A., Oberst, M. T., & Bjorklund, B. C. (1994). Posthospital convalescence in older women with hip fracture. *Orthopaedic Nursing, 13*(4), 55–64.

Yandrich, T. J. (1995). Preventing infection in total joint replacement surgery. *Orthopaedic Nursing, 14*(2), 15–19.

Chapter 10 focuses on the care of patients with traumatic and pathologic conditions affecting the knee and the lower leg. The chapter starts with a brief review of anatomy to help the nurse understand the rationale underlying nursing care. Next, discussions center on conditions affecting the knee from a minor sprain to a total knee replacement, with emphasis on the clinical assessment and the nursing care associated with surgical procedures. The final major sections of the chapter focus on traumatic and pathologic conditions that affect the lower leg.

ANATOMY

BONES

The bones of the knee and the lower leg are the femur (see Chapter 9), the tibia, the fibula, and the patella.

TIBIA AND FIBULA

The tibia and the fibula are the medial and lateral bones of the lower leg. The tibia is the stronger of the two and, except for the femur, is the longest bone of the skeleton. Its lower end is smaller than the upper end, and on its medial side a stout process, the medial malleolus, projects downward beyond the rest of the bone. The upper end is expanded, providing a weight-bearing surface for the weight transmitted through the lower end of the femur. The proximal end of the tibia is comprised of two prominent masses, the medial and lateral condyles, and a smaller projection, the tibial tuberosity. The fibula is much more slender than the tibia and is not a weight-bearing bone. The lower end, or lateral malleolus, projects downward to a lower level than the tibia and lies on a more posterior plane.

PATELLA

The patella is the largest sesamoid bone, that is, the largest bone that is embedded within a tendon. The anterior surface is convex, perforated by nutrient ves-

sels, and marked by numerous rough, longitudinal striae. The patella is anterior to the knee joint and embedded within the substance of the quadriceps tendon. A thin layer of quadriceps tendon passes over the anterior surface of the patella to join the patellar tendon, which inserts distally into the tibial tubercle. When a person is standing, the lower limit of the patella lies more than one cm above the line of the knee joint. The patella is separated from the skin over the joint by a bursa as well as by the tendon of the quadriceps femoris.

The function of the patella, in addition to protecting the femoral condyles from injury, is to increase the mechanical advantage of the quadriceps tendon. Active knee extension is achieved by the quadriceps muscles. The muscle forces are transmitted to the patella through the quadriceps tendon, then to the patellar tendon, and finally to the tibia at the tibial tubercle. When the knee is extended, the force the quadriceps muscles must exert is influenced by the patella, because the patella causes an increase in the length of the movement arm through which the quadriceps muscles work. If the patella is removed, the moment arm is shortened and the muscular force required to extend the knee increases. The quadriceps muscles cannot provide this additional force, and hence the knee cannot be fully extended if the patella is absent.

MUSCLES

The knee is a modified hinge (or ginglymus) joint between the femur and the tibia. It is surrounded by a thick synovial membrane that secretes the synovial fluid that lubricates the joint. Because flexion and extension are its principal movements, with only a small amount of rotation of the tibia possible, two main groups of muscles are involved in movements of the knee. The flexor (hamstring and gastrocnemius) muscles bend the knee, and the extensor (quadriceps femoris) muscles cause the knee to straighten (Fig. 10–1). A major function of both groups is to hold the knee in any desired position so that it is a stable and reliable supporting structure.

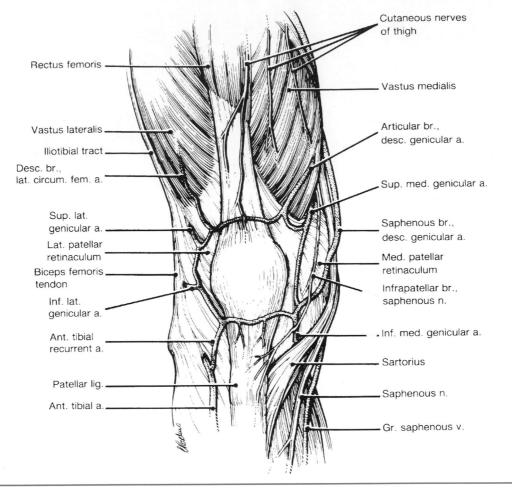

Figure 10–1   The anterior aspect of the knee joint.   *(Weinstein & Buckwalter (1994). Turek's Othropaedics: Principles and Their Application. 5th ed. Philadelphia: J.B. Lippincott-Raven.)*

NERVES

The muscles of the knee joint are enervated by the femoral nerve (see Fig.10–1) on the anterior position of the thigh (supplying the quadriceps) and the sciatic nerve on the posterior surface of the knee (supplying the hamstring and the gastrocnemius). Division of either or both of these nerves seriously impairs the action of the knee. The knee joint may also be deprived of its sensory nerve supply as a result of disease and is then vulnerable to repeated trauma because no pain is felt.

BURSAE

The knee is supplied extensively with protective bursae (Fig. 10–2). These are sacs composed of a synovial membrane that contains synovial fluid, and they are situated between two surfaces of the knee to minimize the friction between them. For example, one bursa extends up from about one third of the length of the thigh behind the quadriceps, and another is on the anterior surface of the tibia. As a result of infection, surgery, or trauma, these bursae can become distended with the products of the lesion, such as blood, pus, or increased synovial secretions.

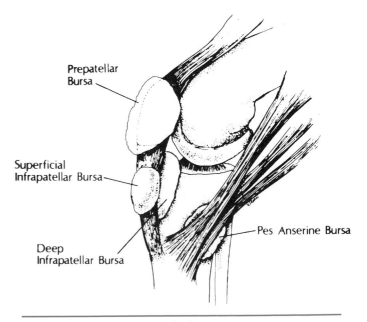

Figure 10–2   The bursae of the knee.   *(Weinstein & Buckwalter (1994). Turek's Othropaedics: Principles and Their Application. 5th ed. Philadelphia: J.B. Lippincott-Raven.)*

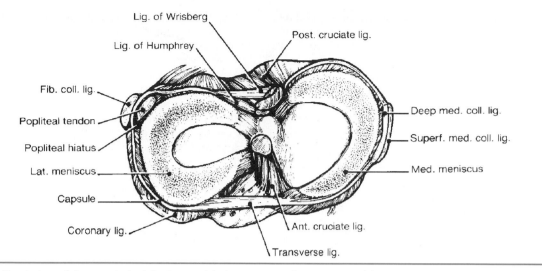

Figure 10–3   Depiction of the menisci of the knee with the associated intermeniscal ligaments.   *(Weinstein & Buckwalter (1994).* Turek's Othropaedics: Principles and Their Application. *5th ed. Philadelphia: J.B. Lippincott-Raven.)*

THE KNEE JOINT

The knee is the largest joint in the body and plays a key role in human locomotion. At the same time, it is one of the joints most frequently affected by trauma because of its anatomical structure, its exposure to external forces, and the functional demands placed upon it.

The bones of the knee joint are the femur, the patella, and the tibia. The joint surface of the distal femur has two condyles. Between the condyles anteriorly is the saddle-shaped femoral patellar surface, upon which the patella glides. Between the condyles inferiorly is the femoral tibial surface, which has a deep U-shaped notch, the intercondylar fossa. The joint surface of the proximal tibia, called the tibial plateau, has two articular indentations separated by the raised intercondylar eminence. All of the articular surfaces of the femoral condyles, the tibial condyles, and the dorsal aspect of the patella are covered by 3 to 4 mm of cartilage.

MENISCUS

The hinge effect of the knee joint is produced by the rounded femoral condyles and the shallow depressions of the tibial plateaus. The tibial spine (or intercondylar fossa) is a twin-peaked projection that lies between and separates the tibial plateaus. Lying on top of the tibia are two incomplete rings of semilunar-shaped pieces (or C-shaped wedges) of fibrocartilage known as the medial and lateral menisci (Fig. 10–3). The menisci cover one half to two thirds of the articular surfaces of each tibial plateau. The menisci move forward and backward with the tibia and promote a snug fit between the femur and the tibia when the joint is in extension.

One function of the menisci is weight bearing. At least 50% of the compressive load of the knee joint is transmitted through the menisci in extension, and about 85% of the load is transmitted through them when the knee is in 90 degrees of flexion. The menisci provide joint stability, increase the congruence between the condyles of the femur and tibia, and contribute significantly toward overall joint conformity. The menisci also have been shown to serve a proprioceptive role in the knee (Windsor, 1994).

THE FIBROUS CAPSULE

The ligaments of the joint comprise the fibrous capsule, which surrounds and supports the joint. Those ligaments are the patellar, the tibial (medial) and fibular (lateral) collateral, the oblique and arcuate popliteal, the anterior and posterior cruciate, and the transverse ligaments. The fibrous capsule is augmented by the tendons of the muscles that surround the joint. It is blended above on each side with the origin of the corresponding head of the gastrocnemius, and centrally it is strengthened by the oblique popliteal ligament. On the medial side, the fibers are attached to the medial surfaces of the femoral and tibial condyles beyond the articular surfaces. Thus, the fibrous capsule blends with the posterior part of the tibial collateral ligament of the joint. On the lateral side, the fibers are attached to the femur above the origin of the popliteus and descend over the tendon to the lateral condyle of the tibia and the head of the fibula. Anteriorly, the fibrous capsule is entirely absent above the patella and the patellar area.

Within the joint are two strong ligaments known as the anterior and posterior cruciate ligaments, named because they run in a crisscross fashion from the femur to the tibia. The anterior cruciate ligament goes from the anterior surface of the tibia to the posterior aspect of the femur and acts to prevent forward displacement of the tibia on the femur. The posterior cruciate ligament goes from the posterior surface of the tibia to the anterior aspect of the femur and acts to prevent backward displacement of the tibia on the femur.

The extracapsular ligaments are strong bands that pass from the femur to the tibia on the lateral and medial aspects of the knee and are known as the collateral ligaments. The medial stability of the knee joint is increased by the medial collateral ligament, which runs from the medial femoral condyle to the medial tibial condyle. The deeper layer of the ligament is attached to the outer border of the medial meniscus. The lateral stability of the knee joint is increased by the lateral collateral ligament, which runs from the lateral femoral condyle to the fibular head but has no attachment to the lateral meniscus.

BLOOD SUPPLY

The popliteal artery, a continuation of the femoral artery, has five branches in the area of the knee joint: the superior medial and superior lateral geniculars, the middle genicular, and the inferior medial and inferior lateral geniculars (see Fig. 10–1).

INTERNAL DERANGEMENT OF THE KNEE JOINT

The term *internal derangement* is loosely applied to a variety of intra-articular and extra-articular disturbances of the knee joint, usually of traumatic origin, which interfere with the function and mechanics of the joint. The pathologic changes that take place in the knee immediately after trauma depend on the nature and the severity of the injury.

LESIONS OF THE MENISCUS

Injuries to a meniscus are common and result from twisting strains applied to the knee when it is slightly flexed or when it is in full flexion. A twisting force applied to the knee joint may trap a meniscus between the femur and the tibia to produce the familiar "torn cartilage" lesion. To produce a tear, the knee joint must be first rotated in a flexed position to trap the meniscus and then extended to produce the tearing force on the tissue. This combination of motions is frequently encountered in athletics. The torn or detached portion of the meniscus may become displaced toward the joint and jammed between the articular surfaces of the femur and the tibia, arresting all movement and producing a "locked" knee.

MEDIAL MENISCUS
Medial meniscus tears are 9 times more common than tears of the lateral meniscus. This is believed to occur because the medial meniscus has less mobility, being more securely attached to such neighboring structures as the deep layer of the medial collateral ligament, and is therefore less able to adapt to sudden changes of position. Furthermore, during rotation of the flexed or partially flexed joint, the medial meniscus moves through a greater interval than the lateral meniscus and is there-

fore subject to more stress. At the same time, the medial fibers of the popliteus may prevent the lateral meniscus from being trapped between the articular surfaces.

Two types of medial meniscus tears occur most frequently. One, the "punch press" effect of the femoral condyle on the trapped meniscus, causes a splitting of the meniscus along its longitudinal axis, producing the so-called "bucket handle" tear. Here, the inner portion of the torn cartilage may get displaced into the joint and cause locking. The bucket handle tear is the lesion usually present in an athlete with a "trick knee." The joint may be unlocked by manipulation, but healing of the tear does not occur because the largely avascular meniscus has a limited capacity for regeneration, and a tear cannot be expected to heal unless it has occurred close to the capsule. Treatment is usually by the surgical removal of the torn meniscus.

In the second type of medial meniscus tear, the meniscus is torn along the transverse axis. The tear usually does not cause locking of the joint. Pain is produced by momentary impingement of the irregular meniscus between the femur and the tibia when the knee is in motion. Symptoms of a transverse tear of the meniscus can frequently be relieved by the use of anti-inflammatory drugs, combined with putting the joint at rest for a period of time. If symptoms persist, operative excision of the meniscus is indicated.

LATERAL MENISCUS
Lateral meniscus lesions include tears and cystic degeneration. Tears similar to those of the medial meniscus may occur, though they are much less common. On the other hand, cystic degeneration is more common in the lateral meniscus than in the medial. In this condition, thought to be caused by repeated trauma, multiple cysts containing gelatinous material appear within the peripheral border of the meniscus. The cysts may cause pain and often can be seen and palpated along the lateral border of the knee joint. Treatment is by surgical removal of the cysts.

POSTTRAUMA ASSESSMENT FOR INTERNAL KNEE DERANGEMENT

The differential diagnosis of internal derangement of the knee is somewhat difficult, but it can be made by taking a careful history and doing a thorough examination of the knee. It is often necessary for the examination to be supplemented by roentgenograms, arthrography, MRI, or arthroscopy (see Chapter 2). Accuracy rates of the MRI are 93% to 98% for medial meniscal tears, and 90% to 96% for lateral meniscal tears (Garth & Fagan, 1996). When a meniscus has been injured, the capsular and ligamentous structures and even the articular surfaces may also have been injured.

A history of the injury is important to establish that the lesion is of traumatic origin and that the meniscus was previously sound. In tears of abnormal or degenerative menisci, a history of specific injury may not be

---

Box 10–1
Symptoms of Meniscal Injuries

1. Locking
2. Giving Way
3. Effusion
4. Atrophy
5. Pain

---

obtained, for example, in middle-aged persons who sustain a weight-bearing twist of the knee or have pain after squatting. These patients may recall symptoms of mild catching, snapping, or clicking, and occasional pain and mild swelling in the joint, but may not seek medical care until the tear increases and causes locking or lack of stability in the knee.

The symptoms (Box 10–1) of the more typical traumatic tears of a normal meniscus follow: (1) Locking. Even though locking is a classic symptom of a meniscal tear, it must be emphasized that an intra-articular tumor, an osteocartilaginous loose body, and other conditions may also cause locking. A locked knee may not be recognized unless the extension of the affected knee is compared with that of the other knee. In "true" locking, there is something within the joint that prevents full extension. "False" locking is also possible, especially after an injury that causes hemorrhaging into the posterior part of the capsule or a spasm of the hamstring muscle. (2) "Giving way." A sensation of "giving way" may be felt by the patient during a rotary movement of the knee. The sensation may result from a tear in the posterior part of the meniscus but may also be produced by other conditions, especially loose bodies, chondromalacia of the patella, and instability of the joint resulting from injury to ligaments or weakness of the supporting musculature, especially of the quadriceps. (3) Effusion. Effusion indicates an irritation to the synovium. Alone, effusion has limited diagnostic value, especially as tears that occur within the body of the meniscus or in a degenerative area may not produce an effusion. To help determine if there is a large amount of fluid in the knee, a test for ballottable (i.e., rebounding) patella can be done. To do the test, instruct the patient to relax the quadriceps muscles and then gently extend the knee until the leg is straight. Next, push the patella backward into the trochlear groove, quickly releasing it (see Chapter 2). When the patella is forced into the trochlear groove, the fluid under the patella is forced to the sides of the joint. When the patella is quickly released, the fluid flows back to its former position, forcing the patella to rebound. If only a minimal amount of effusion is in the knee joint, the ballottable patella test is not diagnostic. To test for minimal effusion (see Chapter 2), have the patient's knee in extension, and then "milk" the fluid down from the suprapatellar pouch and over from the lateral side into the medial side of the knee. After the fluid is collected on the medial side of the knee joint, gently tap the medial side and observe how much fluid flows to the lateral side. (4) Atrophy of the musculature. Atrophy of the musculature about the knee, especially of the vastus medialis component of the quadriceps muscle, suggests a recurring disability of the knee but does not indicate its cause. (5) Pain. Probably the most important physical finding is localized tenderness over the medial and lateral joint line or over the periphery of the meniscus. Menisci are without nerve fibers, except at the periphery, but the pain may result from synovitis and traumatized capsular tissue. The pain is frequently aggravated by forced rotation of the foot and leg, and pain or a click may be produced by the McMurray test.

To do the McMurray test for the medial meniscus, stand to the patient's affected side and have the patient lie supine. Take hold of the patient's heel and flex the leg fully. Then place your other hand on the affected knee with your fingers touching the medial joint line. While keeping the knee completely flexed, externally rotate the knee as far as possible; then slowly extend the knee. As the knee passes over a tear in the meniscus, a click may be heard or felt. To examine the lateral meniscus, palpate the posterolateral margin of the joint while internally rotating the leg as far as possible. Then slowly extend the knee, listening and feeling for a click. A click produced by the McMurray test usually occurs between complete flexion of the knee and 90 degrees and indicates a posterior peripheral tear of the meniscus. Popping, which occurs at a greater degree of extension, suggests a tear of the middle and anterior positions of the meniscus. Thus, the position of the knee when the click occurs helps to identify the location of the lesion. A negative McMurray test, however, does not rule out a tear (Windsor, 1994).

Another test to aid in the diagnosis of a torn meniscus is Apley's grinding test. Begin with the patient lying prone on the examining table and flex the affected knee to 90 degrees. The affected leg is then pulled upward to distract the joint and then rotated to place rotational strain on the ligaments. If that part of the test is painful, it usually indicates a lesion or tear of the tibial collateral ligament. Next, with the knee in the same initial position, the foot and leg are pressed downward into the knee and rotated as the joint is slowly flexed and extended. When the medial meniscus is torn, popping and pain localized to the joint line may be noted.

TREATMENT

The initial treatment for a torn meniscus includes rest, ice, compression, and elevation (RICE). Once the initial swelling and pain subside, a conservative method of treatment usually follows. This nonoperative treatment method consists of anti-inflammatory medications and careful exercise (e.g., quadriceps-strengthening exercises) to allow the menisci to heal. In some cases, the patient's injured leg may also be immobilized in a

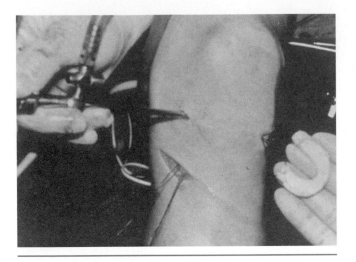

Figure 10–4   Arthroscopic insertion of a lateral meniscus.
(Aichroth, Cannon & Patel. Eds. (1992). Knee Surgery: Current Practice. *New York: Raven Press.)*

long leg cast with a walking heel for 3 to 6 weeks. The conservative method usually lasts 6 to 8 weeks to allow for the possibility that meniscal healing will occur.

Unfortunately, most meniscal tears occur in areas where healing cannot be expected, and consequently it is rare that the symptoms are permanently relieved without surgery. A tear of the meniscus along the inner two thirds generally will not heal due to the lack of blood supply to the area. If the pain and swelling are persistent and/or the patient continues to complain of symptoms after 6 to 8 weeks, surgery can be performed arthroscopically. One of two types of surgery are usually undertaken (Scuderi Scott, & Insall 1996). Patients with meniscal tears of the inner two thirds require an arthroscopic partial meniscectomy procedure. On the other hand, patients with a tear of the meniscus along its outer periphery, which is generally well vascularized, are treated with an arthroscopic meniscus repair procedure.

ARTHROSCOPY

One method of removing a torn meniscus is through the use of an arthroscope (Fig. 10–4). This method is less invasive than a meniscectomy because the scope is inserted into the joint through small puncture wounds that permit visual inspection, irrigation with a saline solution, and the introduction of instruments to either repair or remove portions of the meniscus. If a portion of the torn meniscus is removed, it is removed in very small pieces.

Because the knee joint is not opened with a conventional incision, arthroscopic surgery for the repair or removal of a meniscus is usually done on an outpatient basis and requires no hospitalization. The patient does not have an immobilizing device, only a small dressing,

and typically has few complaints of discomfort. Rehabilitation consists of quadriceps-strengthening and range-of-motion exercises, and the return to previous activities is allowed as soon as the patient has regained normal strength in the affected extremity. If the meniscus has been repaired, the patient is kept non-weight bearing, and range of motion of the knee is limited to protect the integrity of the repair. During this time, isometric, active, and resistive exercises are performed to maintain the strength of the quadriceps and hamstrings. Progression to full weight bearing and full range of motion is determined by the extent and location of the meniscal tear. Most patients with a partial removal of the meniscus are able to ambulate with weight bearing as tolerated soon after recovering from the anesthesia. Some may require crutches for a few days, and all will require exercises to regain full function in the knee.

CLINICAL PATHWAY (Patient with a Knee Arthroscopy)

An example of a generic clinical pathway for a patient having a arthroscopy is presented in Figure 10–5.

MENISCECTOMY

An alternative to arthroscopic surgery, now done relatively infrequently, is an open or conventional method of opening the knee joint called a meniscectomy. A meniscectomy or removal of a meniscus may be indicated for a knee that locks or for a patient who experiences recurrent pain and limitation of motion from a torn cartilage. In some instances, however, a torn meniscus can be repaired rather than being removed. A full meniscectomy begins with the knee in a flexed position. The meniscus is separated from its anterior tibial attachment, then from its middle and posterior peripheral attachments, and removed. After an examination of other structures in the knee for possible pathology, the incision is closed and a compression dressing with a knee immobilizer, posterior splint, or cylinder cast applied. In a partial meniscectomy, only the damaged portion of the meniscus is removed.

A partial meniscectomy requires little protection following the surgical procedure, and patients are generally back to full activity as early as 2 to 3 weeks after the operation. Meniscus repairs, however, must be protected for 3 weeks while waiting for the meniscus to heal. Rehabilitation otherwise does not differ from that of a total knee replacement. Generally, after a meniscus repair, the patient can return to full activity by 12 weeks.

Figure 10–5
Clinical Pathway: Knee Arthroscopy

Admission Date: _____   **Discharge Plan:** _____ **Home**   _____ **Skilled Nursing**   _____ **Extended Care Facility**

Pathway	Preadmission Office/OP clinic	Admission Day Op day	Discharge Postop 1	Postop 2	Postop 3	Postop 4	Outcomes Rehabilitation
Consultation	Primary Care/ Medical physician	Case Manager					Postoperative Appt with physician
		Anesthesia, PT	Cont.				Cont. with PT
Assessment	Nrsg database	Review & add					
	H & P Exam. by MD, NP, or PA	Review H & P					
	Including normal Activity, History of Injury	Postop routine					
	Results of Lachman, Anterior drawer, Pivot shift maneuver, or arthrometer						
Tests	ECG/blood/UA X-ray knee— Anterior/posterior, lateral, intercondylar notch, & a patellar view, MRI						
Medications	D/C NSAIDS 3d. b/4 OR	✓ preadm meds					
	D/C ASA 10 d. b/4 OR	Routine meds					
	D/C anti coag. meds - MD	Oral narcotic meds or analgesics as needed	Cont.				Minimal amount of pain and relieved with analgesics
	Instruct on preop meds b/4 OR	Ice along incision	Cont. If nec.				States the purpose of the ice
		Antibiotics	D/C antibiotics				
Diet	Assessment wt.	NPO b/4 OR (Min. 8 hours)	Advance as tol				Tolerating diet
	Balanced diet						
Activity	Preop mobility	CW with PWB to WB as tol	Cont.				Cont. with CW and Prog. to WB as tol.
	Crutch walking	Quad & Glut	Cont.				
		Ankle Pumps	Cont.				
		ROM exercises	Cont.				Cont at home
Treatments	Physical therapy	Exercises with PT	Cont.				Cont with excs.
Education	Teach pre & postoperative	Reinforce					
	Teaching regarding surgical preparation Rev. hosp routine						
	Exercises, assistive device cane/crutches and WB						Upon discharge, pt states purpose and demonstrated exercises

(continued)

Figure 10–5
Clinical Pathway: *(continued)*

Pathway	Preadmission Office/OP clinic	Admission Day Op day	Discharge Postop 1	Postop 2	Postop 3	Postop 4	Outcomes Rehabilitation
	Pain management						Pain controlled with meds.
D/C Plan	Review hosp LOS						Knows activity level and when to contact physician
	Include exercise & activity level, signs of infection, & when to notify their physician						
	DC when recovered from anesthesia, usually the same day as surgery						

LIGAMENTOUS INJURIES OF THE KNEE

The knee joint owes its stability to a strong and extensive capsule, formed by the collateral ligaments, cruciate ligaments, surrounding muscles, and tendons. Injury to any one of the ligaments affects locomotion and the stability of the knee. Knee ligaments are often injured in athletic activities and motor vehicle accidents. They may also occur in falls or when sudden severe stress or tension is placed on the ligament.

A *sprain* is defined as an injury limited to ligaments (which attach bone to bone) and a *strain* as a stretching injury of a muscle or its tendinous attachment to bone. Sprains of the knee are classified into categories depending on the degree of severity. A *mild sprain* of a ligament is a tear of a minimum number of fibers of the ligament with localized tenderness but no instability of the knee. A *moderate sprain* disrupts more ligamentous fibers with more loss of function and more joint reaction but no instability of the knee. A *severe sprain* is a complete disruption of the ligament with resultant instability. Severe sprains may be further classified as to the degree of instability demonstrated under stress testing of the joint. A 1+ instability indicates that the joint surfaces separate 5 mm or less; a 2+ instability indicates that they separate between 5 and 10 mm; and a 3+ instability indicates that they separate 10 mm or more.

Treatment of a mild sprain may be entirely symptomatic with the patient returning to normal activities within a few days. Usually rest, ice, and a compression bandage are all that is required. A moderate sprain usually requires some protection, because while the remaining untorn portion is able to stabilize the knee, the strength of the ligament has been significantly impaired. These patients are usually placed in a long leg cast with the knee flexed 30 to 45 degrees for 4 to 6 weeks. Recovery can usually be expected with no residual effects if a program of rehabilitative exercises is followed. Severe sprains often require surgical treatment and immobilization. Optimally, repair restores the anatomical integrity of, and tension in, the torn ligament. After most surgeries, the leg is immobilized in a long leg cast with the knee flexed 45 to 60 degrees. The patient, the family, and significant others as well as the nurse should understand that ligament healing and return to normal function require 9 to 12 months. Repair is distinct from reconstruction, which refers to the surgical treatment of ligamentous laxity that is present 3, 4, or more months following injury.

COLLATERAL LIGAMENT INJURIES

Stability to the knee joint is provided by several ligaments that attach bone to bone. The most important of these ligaments are the medial and lateral collateral ligaments that provide stability to the sides of the knee.

MEDIAL COLLATERAL LIGAMENT

Medial stability of the knee is accomplished by the joint capsule and the medial (tibial) collateral ligament, which runs from the medial femoral condyle to the medial tibial condyle. Injuries of the medial collateral ligament usually occur from forceful valgus bending of the knee joint. In such instances, the femoral attachment is usually torn, though less frequently the tibial attachment is detached. The midportion of the medial collateral ligament is attached to the medial meniscus, so its injuries are properly associated with ruptures of the meniscus.

With an incomplete rupture of the medial collateral ligament, pain is usually severe but function is not completely lost. The region around the ligament is tender and swollen. Lateral mobility of the joint is lacking. Individuals with a complete rupture of the ligament have pain and swelling at the site, and palpation may disclose a movable fragment of the bone where the ligament attaches to the bone. A slight lateral mobility indicates an accompanying rupture of the anterior cruciate ligament.

LATERAL COLLATERAL LIGAMENT

Rupture of the lateral (fibular) collateral ligament is produced by a severe varus bending of the knee and is rather uncommon. Usually the fibular attachment is torn, and the head of the fibula may be abused. Tenderness occurs on the lateral aspect of the bone between the lateral femoral epicondyle and the fibular head. If there is a complete severance of the lateral collateral ligament, the ends may be palpated. Crepitus may be elicited to indicate avulsion of the fibular head. A slight lateral mobility of the knee may be present. A frequent complication of a ruptured lateral collateral ligament is damage to the common peroneal nerve; thus the patient's ability to move the anterior and lateral muscles of the leg and the short extensors of the toes should be noted.

POSTTRAUMA ASSESSMENT FOR COLLATERAL LIGAMENT STABILITY

Besides the assessment already noted, a more extensive assessment of the lateral and medial collateral ligaments can be done through the posterior pivot shift test (Fig. 10–6) and the reverse pivot shift test (Fig. 10–7). To test the medial collateral ligament, secure the patient's ankle with one hand and place the other hand around the patient's knee, so that the thumb is against the fibular head. Push medially against the knee and laterally against the ankle in an attempt to open the knee joint medially (valgus stress). Palpate the medial joint line for any gapping. If a gap is present, the medial collateral ligament is not supporting the knee properly. When the stress on the knee is released, you can feel the tibia and femur "clunk" together. To test the lateral collateral ligament, reverse the procedure (e.g., reverse pivot shift test). Most liga-

ment injuries around the knee occur on the medial side. To summarize, an abnormal opening of the medial aspect of the knee joint noted when the medial collateral ligament is stretched with the knee partially flexed indicates damage to the medial collateral ligament. When an opening is noted on the lateral aspect of the knee joint, the lateral collateral ligament has been damaged.

TREATMENT

Immediate treatment consists of rest, ice, compression, and elevation (RICE). Once the initial swelling and pain has subsided, an exercise program is usually begun. This includes active range of motion of the knee, exercises for strengthening the quadriceps and hamstrings, and, for some patients, the use of a reinforced elastic brace. The return to a highly active lifestyle that includes sports is usually not allowed until range of motion is within normal limits and the strength in the affected extremity has returned to at least 90% of the unaffected extremity.

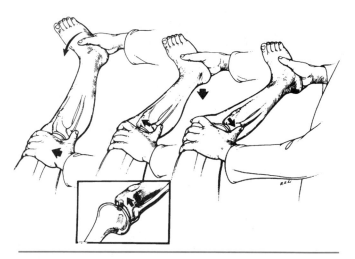

Figure 10–6 The pivot shift test of Galway and MacIntosh is performed with the knee in full extension. A valgus and internal stress is applied. *(Weinstein & Buckwalter (1994). Turek's Othropaedics: Principles and Their Application. 5th ed. Philadelphia: J.B. Lippincott-Raven.)*

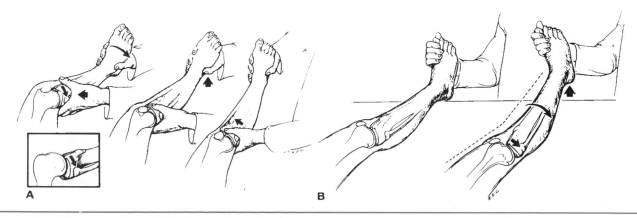

Figure 10–7 The reverse pivot shift test is done in flexion. An external rotation and valgus stress are applied. *(Weinstein & Buckwalter (1994). Turek's Othropaedics: Principles and Their Application. 5th ed. Philadelphia: J.B. Lippincott-Raven.)*

If there has been a complete disruption of the medial collateral ligament, a surgical repair may be necessary. Postoperative care following the surgical repair of the ligament usually involves the insertion of suction drainage before the surgical wound is closed; the leg is then placed in a long leg cast with the knee flexed approximately 60 degrees and the tibia internally rotated. The same is true for a lateral collateral ligament repair, except that the tibia is externally rotated.

NURSING PROCESS (Patient with Collateral Ligament Repair)

The following nursing process presents the care of a patient with a collateral ligament repair. The nursing process begins after the patient returns from surgery.

ASSESSMENT

The initial assessment for a patient following a repair of a collateral ligament involves taking vital signs and observing the patient's general color and warmth. Usually, the patient's skin feels cool and the patient appears pale. Determine the patient's level of consciousness and orientation. Have the patient cough and deep breathe, and auscultate the chest for clearness of the lungs and any cardiac abnormalities. Note that the patient's affected leg is in a long leg cast with the knee flexed 60 degrees and the tibia internally rotated (externally rotated for a lateral collateral ligament repair). Ensure that the leg is correctly positioned to reduce or prevent edema (and if the cast is plaster, to enhance cast drying). The leg can either be elevated on several pillows or be supported by a heavy canvas sling. Check to make sure that the canvas is sufficiently wide to distribute the weight and that it is not cutting into the wet cast. If the leg is on pillows, make sure that the pillows are positioned so that the leg is secure. Check the cast for tightness and the area at the top and bottom of the cast for possible skin irritation. See Chapter 5 for further assessment of a patient in a long leg cast. Note the neurovascular status of the affected extremity and any complaints of discomfort.

NURSING DIAGNOSIS

Based on all of the assessment data, the nursing diagnoses for a typical patient following a collateral ligament repair include:

- Pain and discomfort related to soft-tissue trauma
- Impaired physical mobility related to lack of joint mobility
- Anxiety related to knowledge deficit about the surgical procedure and the rehabilitation process

COLLABORATIVE PROBLEMS

- Circulatory impairment
- Musculoskeletal deficit
- Integumentary impairment

GOAL FORMULATION AND PLANNING

The goals are to have the patient experience (1) a decrease in the amount of pain in the knee through nursing measures and prescribed medications, (2) an increase in mobility through the use of exercises, (3) a decrease in anxiety through increased knowledge about the procedure and the rehabilitation process, and (4) an absence of complications.

INTERVENTIONS

ALLEVIATE PAIN

Note the type, severity, and location of pain to help determine the cause of the pain and thus the appropriate nursing measures. Pain relief measures following a collateral ligament repair involve keeping the leg elevated in extension for the first 24 to 48 hours postsurgery. Note the color and warmth of the toes, and verify that the cast is not too tight. Do neurovascular assessments of the affected leg (see Chapter 2). If circulatory impairment or swelling is noted, check the amount of elevation of the extremity. Elevate the leg (one pillow under the upper leg and two pillows under the lower leg) following the concept of "toes above the nose," but make sure that the elevation of the leg does not cause the patient low back discomfort Adjusting the level of elevation of the leg, lowering the head of the bed, or turning the patient onto one side helps to relieve back pain. Check the ice bags that are along the incision site, and refill as needed. They help to reduce swelling and thus prevent pain during the first 24 to 48 hours postsurgery. Muscle-setting exercises help to increase circulation and decrease pain. Administer prescribed pain medications as necessary.

INCREASE MOBILITY

Interventions to increase joint stability and eventual mobility are correct positioning, turning, exercises, ambulation, and immobilization with a long leg cast. For further information on casts, see Chapter 5.

Position The immobilized leg should be elevated in extension by the use of pillows, by elevating the foot of the bed, or by both means, depending on the size of the patient. Elevation is used to help prevent and reduce edema, and the foot should normally be higher than the nose. If there is increased swelling despite increases in the elevation of the leg, it may be necessary to lower the head of the bed. After 48 hours following surgery, the amount the leg is elevated may be decreased.

Turning After the patient returns from the postanesthesia room, turn the patient to their unaffected side. In most instances, the patient has been supine since the night before surgery. With assistance, the patient can turn to either side but will probably prefer the unaffected side. With the nurse providing support along the entire length of the operated leg, the patient is able to turn with the use of the trapeze and side rails. The nurse must make sure that the head of the bed is lowered and the leg does not twist as the patient turns. Once the patient has completed the turn, the operated leg is placed on one to three pillows (depending upon the patient's size) to keep the leg in correct alignment. Turning also assists in the drying of a plaster cast.

Exercises Exercises for the patient may begin the day of surgery. The exercise regime includes quadriceps and hamstring isometric exercises the first day, which are performed every 2 hours while the patient is awake. Assist the patient with leg lifts to strengthen the hip flexors and abductors as soon as the patient is able. (For further information on exercises, see Chapter 9.) Exercises may be incorporated into a home exercise program and are the key to a successful rehabilitation. The rehabilitation program for each patient should be individualized in terms of the patient's tolerance and rate of progression. Exercises may also be needed to build up muscles in the upper extremities for crutch walking. Refer to Chapter 4.

Ambulation

Ambulation is usually allowed as soon as the patient is able to lift the casted leg off the bed. Crutch walking is allowed with a three-point gait and no weight bearing on the affected leg. Refer to Chapter 4, and for further information on walking with a cast see Chapter 5.

PATIENT TEACHING AND HOME CARE CONSIDERATIONS

Two important aspects of patient teaching and home care are the care of the affected extremity with a cast (see Chapter 5) and safety procedures related to crutch walking. Refer to Chapter 4. The patient's length of hospital stay will be very short, though it will depend on the patient's rate of physical recovery. The emotional status of the patient, the family, and significant others affects how willing and able the patient is to do the exercises. As a whole, most patients are able to go home on crutches within 24 to 48 hours postsurgery, if they are hospitalized at all. The patient needs to understand the role of exercises in the rehabilitation of the knee and follow a home exercise program. The cast is usually changed about 2 weeks after surgery, and the new cast is left on for another 6 to 8 weeks. (For discussion of home care with a long leg cast, see Chapter 5.) It usually takes about 12 months for maximum strength and function to be attained after ligament repair.

MONITORING AND MANAGING POTENTIAL PROBLEMS

Postoperative nursing care for patients having a collateral ligament repair involves potential circulatory and integumentary complications.

CIRCULATORY

Circulatory complications include such problems as dehydration from blood and fluid loss, circulatory overload, venous stasis, and orthostatic hypotension. The most common complications are probably thrombophlebitis and compartmental syndrome.

Measures that help prevent these complications are bed exercises, especially the leg exercises discussed under mobility, and changing the patient's position. The patient should be kept as active as possible with exercises and with ambulation as tolerated. An elastic stocking, which extends from toes to groin, is usually applied to the unoperated leg before the patient returns to the nursing unit. The stocking should be checked for any creases, wrinkles, or pressure areas and should be removed for one-half hour twice a day. At that time, inspect the leg and the foot, especially the heel, for any redness. Patients are also placed on anticoagulant medications, such as aspirin, heparin, coumadin, and others. (For further information, see Chapter 4.)

A circulatory complication of special concern is known as compartmental syndrome, a condition in which progressive pressure within a confined space compromises the circulation and the function of tissues within that space. A compartment is enveloped by tough inelastic fascial tissue, and, when swelling of the muscles occurs, the fascia do not expand. In the lower leg, that can occur in the anterior, lateral, superficial posterior, or deep posterior compartments. The onset of the symptoms can vary from as little as 2 hours to as much as 6 days after the trauma or surgery. If the pressure is not relieved within approximately 12 hours of the onset of the syndrome (i.e., from the onset of excessive intracompartmental pressure), irreversible nerve and tissue damage is likely to result. For further discussion and nursing care measures related to compartmental syndrome, see Chapter 4 and Chapter 5.

INTEGUMENTARY

Following a collateral ligament repair and the application of a cast, the patient is susceptible to pressure sores related to the cast (see Chapter 5). An area of particular vulnerability is the heel of the casted leg because of the weight of the cast. Make sure that the patient's heel is "floating" (i.e., that the leg is given sufficient support to reduce the weight on the heel). That can be done by keeping the leg elevated on a pillow, a folded bath blanket, or 2 to 3 inches of foam.

Make sure there are no rough edges on the cast that can cause skin irritation (see Chapter 5). Petal the cast as necessary. Also verify that the cast is not too tight or too loose.

EVALUATION/OUTCOMES

In evaluating the goal of alleviating pain in the knee, determine whether the individual is having any pain by verbal responses and by the patient's outward appearance, including facial grimacing during activities, the position assumed, and restlessness or sleeplessness. If pain still exists, determine the location, duration, and intensity of the pain; what aggravates and intensifies it; and what measures have been able to relieve it.

When evaluating care to increase mobility, determine the patient's compliance with the exercise routine and utilization of assistive devices such as a walker or crutches. Determine whether or not the patient, the family, and significant others have been able to follow the rehabilitation regime, how useful the discharge plan appears to be, and how well they understand what the patient can and cannot do. Also determine their understanding of the care required for the casted leg and the patient's ability to ambulate.

CLINICAL PATHWAY (Patient with a Collateral Ligament Repair)

An example of a generic clinical pathway for a patient with a collateral ligament repair is presented in Figure 10–8.

Figure 10–8

Clinical Pathway: Lateral Collateral Ligament Repair of the Knee

Admission Date: _____   Discharge Plan: _____ Home _____ Skilled Nursing _____ Extended Care Facility

Pathway	Preadmission Office/OP clinic	Admission Day Op day	Discharge Postop 1	Postop 2	Postop 3	Postop 4	Outcomes Rehabilitation
Consultation	Primary Care/ Medical physician	Case Manager					Postoperative Appt with physician
		Anesthesia, PT	Cont.				Cont. with PT
Assessment	Nrsg database	Review & add					
	H & P Exam. by MD, NP or PA	Review H & P					
	Including normal Activity, History of Injury	Postop routine					
	Results of Posterior pivot shift test and reverse pivot shift test, and possibly ?? arthrometer	Check the CMST affected leg q 2 hrs					
Tests	ECG/blood/UA X-RAY knee—Anterior/posterior, lateral, intercondylar notch, & a patellar view, MRI						
Medications	D/C NSAIDS 3d. b/4 OR	✓ preadm meds					
	D/C ASA 10 d. b/4 OR	Routine meds					
	D/C anticoag. meds - MD	Local (bupivacaine) around the knee					Pain relieved by med or analgesics
		Intra-articular MS					States meds, when to take and purpose
		Oral pain meds	Cont. with oral pain meds or Analgesics As needed				

(continued)

Figure 10–8

Clinical Pathway: *(continued)*

Pathway	Preadmission Office/OP clinic	Admission Day Op day	Discharge Postop 1	Postop 2	Postop 3	Postop 4	Outcomes Rehabilitation
	Instruct on preop meds b/4 OR	Ice along incision area	Cont. If nec.				States the purpose of Cryotherapy
		Antibiotics	D/C antibiotics				
Diet	Assessment wt.	NPO b/4 OR (Min 8 hours)	Advance as tol				Tolerating diet
	Balanced diet						
Activity	Preop mobility	Crutch Walking with NWB per MD protocol	Cont.				Cont. CW with NWB
	Crutch walking	Elevate leg	Cont.				Cont with exc. @ home
		Straight Leg Lifts	Cont.				
		Quad & Glut	Cont.				
		Ankle Pumps	Cont.				
Treatments	Physical therapy	Exercises with PT	Cont.				
		Long Leg Cast					
Education	Teach pre & postoperative	Reinforce					Upon discharge, pt
	Teaching regarding surgical preparation	Review Cast Care & self-care with a cast					States the purpose of the cast and cast care
	Rev. hosp routine						Safe in doing CW
	Exercises, assistive device cane/crutches and WB						Upon discharge, pt states purpose and demonstrates exercises
	Pain management						
	Review hosp LOS (24–48 hrs)						
D/C Plan	Include exercise & activity level, signs of infection, & when to notify their physician						Knows when to contact physician
	DC when pain under controlled with meds/ cryotherapy						

CRUCIATE LIGAMENT INJURIES

The anterior and posterior cruciate ligaments crisscross in the center of the knee and provide for front to back and rotational stability of the knee. They are instrumental in preventing anterior and posterior dislocation of the tibia relative to the femur. These ligaments are intracapsular, originating on the tibia and inserting into the inner sides of the femoral condyles.

Violent injuries to the knee joint often rupture the anterior cruciate ligament (ACL). At the time of the injury, the patient has a great amount of pain, followed by hemarthrosis. The joint is usually in a slightly flexed position. In order to correctly determine the amount of injury, the swelling must subside or the blood must be aspirated from the knee joint. If not treated, the patient may later have symptoms of instability of the knee during activities such as walking down stairs.

An injury to the posterior cruciate ligament usually results from a direct blow on the head of the tibia while the knee is flexed. The signs are similar to those of an ACL injury.

POSTTRAUMA ASSESSMENT FOR CRUCIATE LIGAMENT INJURIES

To assess the integrity of the cruciate ligaments, there are a number of tests that may be done (e.g., the Lachman test and anterior and posterior drawer tests). To

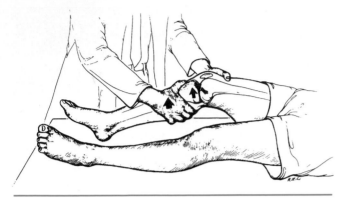

Figure 10–9   The Lachman test is performed with the knee flexed between 15 and 30 degrees. An anterior force is applied by the examiner.   *(Weinstein & Buckwalter (1994). Turek's Othropaedics: Principles and Their Application. 5th ed. Philadelphia: J.B. Lippincott-Raven.)*

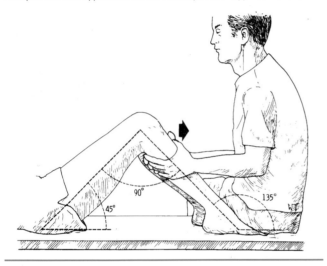

Figure 10–10   The anterior drawer test is performed with the patient supine and the affected knee bent 90 degrees. An anterior force is applied by the examiner.   *(Weinstein & Buckwalter (1994). Turek's Othropaedics: Principles and Their Application. 5th ed. Philadelphia: J.B. Lippincott-Raven.)*

perform the Lachman test, flex the patient's knee 15 to 30 degrees, stabilizing the femur, and pull the tibia anteriorly (Fig. 10–9). A positive Lachman test is when the tibia moves forward and the infrapatellar tendon slope disappears.

To perform the anterior drawer test (Fig. 10–10), the patient is supine with the affected knee flexed at 90 degrees and that foot flat on the table. Sit on the patient's foot to stabilize it. Cup your hands around the patient's knee, placing your fingers in the area of insertion of the medial and lateral hamstrings (in the popliteal fossa) and your thumbs along the lateral and medial line of the joint. To test the anterior cruciate ligament, pull the head of the tibia toward you so that it glides on the femoral condyles. If the tibia slides forward more than one cm, that is a positive anterior draw sign, and the anterior cruciate ligament may be torn. However, always check the other knee for comparison, because a few degrees of anterior draw may be normal if an equal amount occurs

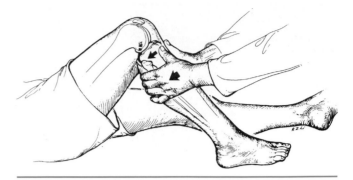

Figure 10–11   The posterior drawer test is done with the knee flexed 90 degrees. A posteriously directed force is supplied to the tibia.   *(Weinstein & Buckwalter (1994). Turek's Othropaedics: Principles and Their Application. 5th ed. Philadelphia: J.B. Lippincott-Raven.)*

in both knee joints. Because of the great amount of swelling that usually occurs initially with this injury, an aspiration of the fluid in the knee may be necessary before an adequate examination can be done.

To test the posterior cruciate ligament, utilizing the posterior drawer test (Fig. 10–11), assume the same position, but push the head of the tibia away from you. If the tibia slides backward on the femoral condyles, that is a positive posterior draw sign, indicating that the posterior cruciate ligament is damaged. Again, check the other knee for comparison. An isolated tear of the posterior cruciate ligament is rare.

TREATMENT
Immediate treatment of a torn cruciate ligament includes the application of ice, compression, and splinting. Controversy remains over the long-term treatment of ACL injuries (Whittington, 1998). Some physicians prefer to treat these patients conservatively with physical therapy and bracing (Fig. 10–12), while others treat with surgery. Macnicol (1992) proposes an exercise, endurance, movement, and proprioception plan in stages as follows: (1) gentle active range of motion and gentle isometric thigh contractions; (2) use of backshell or brace (allowing 20 to 120 degrees of flexion) for 2 weeks, accompanied by protected weight bearing with the use of crutches; (3) isometric exercises at various angles of knee flexion, isokinetic exercises, isotonic exercises, and pes anserinus and other rotational exercises; (4) 90 degrees to full squats, sit-ups, running in place, and stationary bicycling; and (5) running (straight line, sidestepping, and figures-of-8), wobble board, and cross-country running.

For surgical treatment, some prefer immediate reconstruction, while others delay reconstruction until after the swelling has dissipated. The repair surgeries sometimes include the use of the patellar tendon (Fig. 10–13) or the semitendinous ligament (Fig. 10–14). Today, the techniques involved in the reconstruction of the ACL vary in their use of operative procedures and different synthetic ligament graft materials (e.g., Gore Tex [Fig. 10–15], the Kennedy ligament augmentation device, or

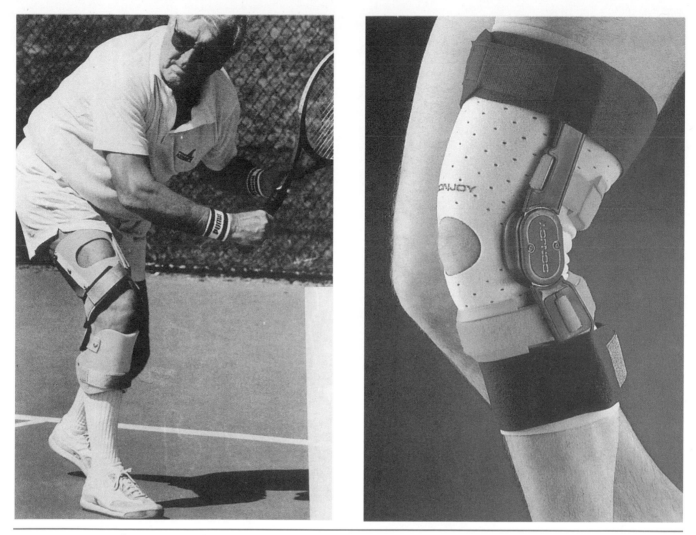

Figure 10–12 Knee braces. *(Aichroth, Cannon & Patel. Eds. (1992). Knee Surgery: Current Practice. New York: Raven Press.)*

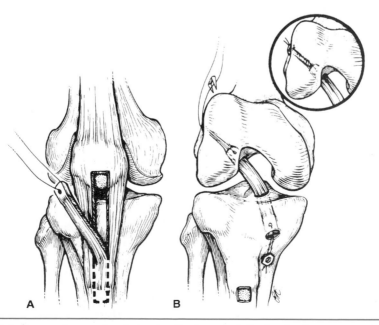

A   **B**

Figure 10–13 Anterior cruciate ligament reconstruction using the bone patellar tendon bone preparation. The middle third of the patellar tendon is used. *(Weinstein & Buckwalter (1994). Turek's Othropaedics: Principles and Their Application. 5th ed. Philadelphia: J.B. Lippincott-Raven.)*

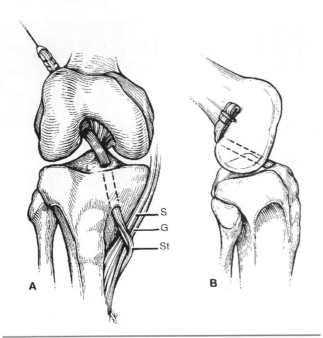

Figure 10–14   ACL reconstruction using the transfer of the semitendinosis tendon secured proximally with a staple. The gracilis tendon may also be used along with the semitendinosis tendons to add strength to the overall surgical construct. *(Weinstein & Buckwalter (1994). Turek's Orthopaedics: Principles and Their Application. 5th ed. Philadelphia: J.B. Lippincott-Raven.)*

carbon-Dacron composite prosthesis for chronic anterior cruciate instabilities). The length of hospital stay has changed from as long as 5 to 7 days in the past to as short as 3 days or no hospitalization at all, with the surgery being done on an outpatient basis.

Rehabilitation has also changed. For example, in the past a patient with an ACL repair using a carbon-Dacron composite prosthesis (Fig. 10–16) was immobilized in a long leg cast with 45 to 50 degrees of knee flexion and with the tibia slightly internally rotated. The cast was maintained for 6 weeks, and only after the cast was removed was an exercise program begun. Today, the knee is immediately mobilized using a continuous passive motion machine. A brace is applied 5 to 7 days after surgery with the range of motion restricted to between 20 to 80 degrees. The patient is non-weight bearing with crutches until the brace is removed and discarded at 6 weeks. Supervised quadriceps rehabilitation is started and full weight bearing is allowed. Between 3 and 6 months, fast walking, jogging, and swimming are encouraged. At 6 months, participation in mild recreational sporting activities is permitted; at 9 months, athletic training begins; and at 12 months, all contract sports are permitted (Patel, Aichroth, Jones, & Wand 1992).

NURSING PROCESS (Patient with an Endoscopic ACL Reconstruction)

The following nursing process presents the care of a patient following an endoscopic ACL reconstruction.

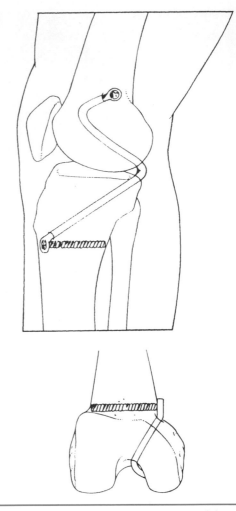

Figure 10–15   Diagrams showing the route of the Gore-Tex prosthetic ligament. The proximal and the distal ends of the prosthesis are fixed using screws.   *(Aichroth, Cannon & Patel. Eds. (1992). Knee Surgery: Current Practice. New York: Raven Press.)*

The nursing process begins after the patient returns from surgery.

ASSESSMENT

The initial postsurgical assessment of a patient following an endoscopic ACL reconstruction involves an assessment of the patient's general condition. The patient has a dressing and a knee immobilizer (Fig. 10–17) or a hinged brace in place on the operative leg. Check for any tightness, pain, or circulatory impairment that could be related to pressure from the dressing or immobilizing device. Do a neurovascular assessment of the affected leg (pulse, temperature, color, capillary filling, edema, and sensory and motor function) and check the position of the leg for proper alignment (e.g., that the leg is elevated on pillows, if ordered). Check that ice bags are placed along the incisional areas. Assess for any nausea or other reactions to the anesthesia. Note the amount and location of the patient's pain.

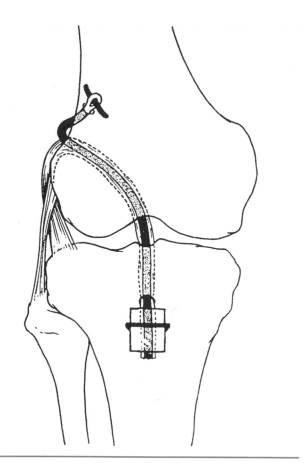

Figure 10–16   ACL reconstruction using carbon-Docron composite prosthesis   *(Aichroth, Cannon & Patel. Eds. (1992).* Knee Surgery: Current Practice. *New York: Raven Press.)*

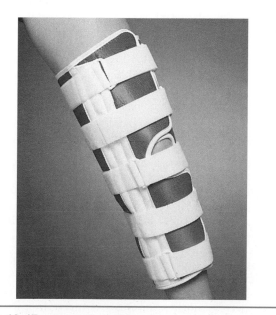

Figure 10–17   Knee immobilizer.   *(Courtesy of Zimmer, Inc.)*

NURSING DIAGNOSIS

Based on all of the assessment data, nursing diagnoses for a typical patient following an endoscopic ACL reconstruction include the following:

- Pain and discomfort related to soft-tissue trauma
- Impaired physical mobility related to the lack of joint mobility
- Increased anxiety related to knowledge deficit about the surgical procedure and the rehabilitation process

COLLABORATIVE PROBLEMS

- Infection

GOAL FORMULATION AND PLANNING

The goals are to have the patient experience (1) a decrease in pain through nursing measures and pre-scribed medications, (2) an increase in mobility through immobilization devices and controlled exer-cises, (3) a decrease in anxiety through patient educa-tion, and (4) an absence of complications. The long-term goal is a return in knee function without complications.

INTERVENTIONS

ALLEVIATE PAIN

Pain relief measures following an endoscopic ACL reconstruction involve keeping the leg elevated for the first 24 to 48 hours postsurgery. Ice bags applied to the incisional areas (but not directly over the incisions) help to prevent pain by their local anesthetic effect and by reducing edema. Check ice bags for positioning and refill as needed. Muscle-setting exercises help to increase circulation and decrease pain.

Mild aches and pains are not unusual and can usu-ally be relieved by acetaminophen. Moderate to severe pain will require a prescription medication for relief. Severe pain is not usual, and if it persists after medica-tion (when the patient is at home), it needs to be reported to the physician. To help reduce the potential for severe pain following surgery, a number of different procedures can be done in the operating room. One way to help reduce pain for the first 2 to 4 hours post-surgery is to inject a local anesthetic (e.g., bupivacaine) in and around the joint. A second is to administer an intramuscular injection of a nonsteroidal anti-inflam-matory medication (e.g., Ketorolac) before the patient leaves the operating room. A third, although newer and more controversial, is an intra-articular injection of morphine, which reduces pain in the knee for 3 to 6 hours. A fourth procedure is cryotherapy, where a cooling pad is incorporated within the layers of the incisional dressing and connected to a container that holds ice water. Some units are electrical and pump the cold water through the cooling pad, while others work by gravity (Fig. 10–18) to circulate the ice water (Brown, 1996).

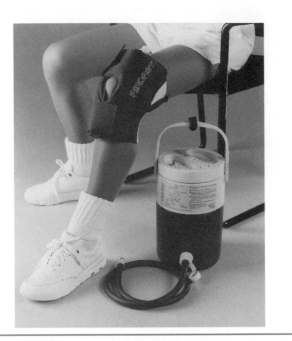

Figure 10–18   Cryo-Cuff applied to the knee. Cryotheraphy units work by gravity.   *(Courtesy of Aircast, Inc.)*

INCREASE MOBILITY

To increase knee joint stability and thus increase the patient's mobility, the nursing focus is on correct positioning of the leg, having the patient do specific exercises for specific periods of time, maintaining the immobilization device, and ambulation.

Position   The leg is usually kept in extension for 10 to 14 days and elevated during the first 24 to 48 hours following surgery to relieve pain and to prevent any swelling. The leg should also be elevated when sitting or lying.

Exercises   The patient begins a program of quadriceps- and gluteal-setting exercises (see Chapter 6 and 9) either the afternoon of surgery or on the first postoperative day. It is better if the patient has learned the exercise program presurgery, even if he or she needs to use the unaffected leg to practice. Some physicians will start immediate mobilization using a CPM machine (see Fig. 10–26 a & b). As soon as physically possible, some patients may also begin straight leg raises. In the beginning, the nurse or the physical therapist may have to lift the patient's leg to a position of 50 or more degrees of hip flexion and let the patient lower the leg to the bed. The nurse or the therapist still needs to assist the patient so that the leg does not drop to the bed. The quadriceps-setting exercises and straight leg lifts should be carried out every 2 hours while the patient is awake. The goal is five repetitions (later 10 repetitions) of the leg exercises each time. The patient may need a lot of emotional and physical support and encouragement with the straight leg raises.

Immobilization Device   Patients will wear a knee immobilizer or brace following surgery. If the patient is to wear a brace, some physicians will give the patient the brace before surgery so they can get accustomed to wearing the brace before surgery. The degrees of flexion allowed (usually between 20 and 80 degrees) will be set by the patient's physician before the brace is applied. For some patients, the brace is applied immediately after surgery, while others will have the brace applied 5 to 7 days post-surgery.

Ambulation   With the knee immobilizer or brace in place, the patient is allowed up with the use of a walker or crutches (see Chapter 4). Using an assistive device, the patient is usually allowed toe-touch weight bearing, weight bearing as tolerated, or non-weight bearing, depending upon the physician's rehabilitation protocol.

PATIENT TEACHING AND HOME CARE CONSIDERATIONS

The patient is usually discharged from the hospital 1 to 3 days following surgery, if admitted to the hospital at all. Some physicians encourage a home exercise program, whereas others require that the patient come into the physical therapy department and work with a therapist. The patient, the family, and significant others need to understand the importance of carefully following each step in the rehabilitation program. The premature use of heavy weights can produce pain and effusion and retard the healing process.

At discharge, ambulation with the use of crutches must be stressed. Even though the patient may not feel that crutches are required, they are needed until sufficient strength in the quadriceps has returned. The return function in the knee joint is directly proportional to the return of strength and muscle tone to the muscles of the knee and hip. Supervised quadriceps rehabilitation is started and full weight bearing is then allowed. Fast walking, jogging, and swimming are encouraged between 3 and 6 months after surgery. By 6 months, mild recreational sporting activities are permitted, at 9 months athletic training is allowed, and at 12 months all contact sports are allowed (Patel, Aichroth, Jones, & Wand, 1992).

MONITORING AND MANAGING POTENTIAL PROBLEMS

The nursing measures discussed in the care of a patient following a total knee replacement apply here, although complications are much less frequent. Infection is the most typical complication of the ACL reconstruction surgery. The potential for infection typically can come from a number of sources. First, there is a potential for infection due to a break in skin integrity from the surgical incisions. There is also the possibility of a break in sterile technique during surgery or in the care of the incisions following surgery. Another possible source is the knee immobilizer or brace. If either of these devices is not fitting properly, it can cause irritation to the patient's skin and a route for infection. The final possible source is the patient, who can develop an undetected systemic infection.

Teach the patient the signs and symptoms of infection and how to assess their skin for a potential break in skin integrity. The patient may also be placed on prophylactic antibiotics for a short period of time.

EVALUATION/OUTCOMES

For a typical patient recovering from an endoscopic ACL reconstruction, the evaluation includes an assessment of pain, signs and symptoms of infection,

and the patient's ability to follow the rehabilitation regime. Special emphasis should be given to evaluating the patient's compliance with the exercise regime and the patient's understanding of the mobility restrictions that will apply after discharge from the hospital.

CLINICAL PATHWAY (Patient with an Endoscopic ACL Reconstruction)

An example of a generic clinical pathway for a patient having an arthroscopic ACL reconstruction is presented in Figure 10–19.

Figure 10–19

Clinical Pathway: Arthroscopic Anterior Cruciate Ligament Reconstruction

Admission Date: _____   **Discharge Plan:** _____ Home   _____ Skilled Nursing   _____ Extended Care Facility

Pathway	Preadmission Office/OP clinic	Admission Day Op day	Discharge Postop 1	Postop 2	Postop 3	Postop 4	Outcomes Rehabilitation
Consultation	Primary Care/ Medical physician	Case Manager					PostOperative Appt with physician
		Anesthesia, PT	Cont.				Cont. with PT
Assessment	Nrsg database H & P Exam. by MD, NB or PA	Review & add Review H & P					
	Including normal Activity, History of Injury	Postop routine					
	Results of Lachman, Anterior drawer, Pivot shift maneuver, or arthrometer						
Tests	ECG/blood/UA/ X-ray knee— Anterior/posteri or, lateral, intercondylar notch, & a patellar view, MRI						
Medications	D/C NSAIDS 3d. b/4 OR	✓ preadm meds					
	D/C ASA 10 d. b/4 OR	Routine meds					
	D/C anticoag. meds - with MD	Local (bupivacaine) around the knee					Pain relieved by med or analgesics
		Intra-articular MS					
		Ketorolac (Toradol)	Cont. with oral pain meds or Analgesics As needed				States meds, when to take, and purpose

(continued)

Figure 10–19

Clinical Pathway: *(continued)*

Pathway	Preadmission Office/OP clinic	Admission Day Op day	Discharge Postop 1	Postop 2	Postop 3	Postop 4	Outcomes Rehabilitation
	Instruct on preop meds b/4 OR	Cryotherapy	Cont. If nec.				States the purpose of Cryotherapy
		Antibiotics	D/C antibiotics				
Diet	Assessment wt.	NPO b/4 OR (Min. 8 hours)	Advance as tol				Tolerating diet
	Balanced diet						
Activity	Preop mobility	Crutch Walking with NWB per MD protocol	Cont.				Cont. CW with NWB for 6 wks
	Crutch walking	Knee CPM	Cont.				Day 5 to 7 the Brace is applied for 6 wks
		Quad & Glut	Cont.				Brace compliance
		Ankle Pumps	Cont.				
Treatments	Physical therapy	Exercises with PT	Cont.				
Education	Teach pre & postoperative	Reinforce					
	Teaching regarding surgical preparation Rev. hosp routine						
	Exercises, assistive device cane/crutches and WB						Upon discharge, pt states purpose and demonstrates exercises
	Pain management						Pain controlled with meds
	Review hosp LOS						
D/C Plan	Include exercises & activity level, signs of infection, & when to notify their physician						Knows activity level
	DC when recovered from anesthesia & pain under control with meds/cryotherapy, usually same day as surgery						Knows when to contact physician

INJURY TO THE QUADRICEPS EXTENSOR APPARATUS

The extensor apparatus of the knee begins with the quadriceps muscle, which blends into the quadriceps tendon. That tendon surrounds the patella, becoming the patellar tendon, which inserts into the tibial tubercle. When that apparatus is shortened, such as by a rupture of the quadriceps tendon, a displaced fracture of the patella, a dislocation of the patella, a rupture of the patellar ligament, or an avulsion of the tibial tubercle, an inability to adequately extend and stabilize the knee can result (Fig. 10–20).

Disruption of the quadriceps extensor mechanism can occur due to direct or indirect trauma. Direct trauma usually results from a blow to the quadriceps muscle when it is contracted while the knee is slightly flexed. In an older person, a sudden violent contraction of the quadriceps muscle may also cause the extensor apparatus to rupture. The result is usually a separation of the tendon from the patella. The history given by

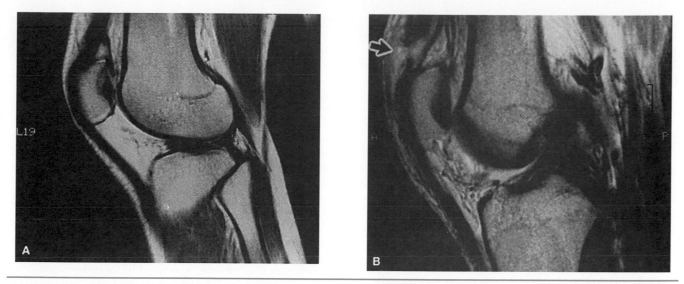

Figure 10–20   (**A**) Sagittal view of the knee through patellar ligaments. Note the quadriceps tendon, which has a normal low signal intensity throughout its length. (**B**) Sagittal view of the knee through the patellar tendon. The arrow points to rupture of the quadriceps tendon near its attachment to the patella. There is increased signal through the tendon as well as loss of continuity of the fibers. In addition, edema is in the surrounding soft tissue.   *(Weinstein & Buckwalter (1994). Turek's Othropaedics: Principles and Their Application. 5th ed. Philadelphia: J.B. Lippincott-Raven.)*

aged, overweight, or poorly conditioned individuals frequently involves jumping from a chair or short height, which resulted in a severe pain in the anterior knee area, a felt or heard snapping of the knee, and a buckling of the knee joint. Examination of the leg reveals swelling and tenderness of the quadriceps tendon, and a sulcus (a furrow or depression) may be palpable. The patient is usually unable to extend the knee, although when the tear is incomplete, quadriceps function is present but diminished. In a younger person, the injury is usually from athletic activities, and the avulsion is at the tendotubercle insertion. There is acute pain, tenderness, swelling, and impaired knee extension. A gap is usually palpable, and the patella is situated higher than normal. Such injuries can also occur from indirect trauma, such as when a running athlete is accelerating or decelerating (usually the latter).

PATELLAR FRACTURES

Patellar fractures occur frequently because of the patella's exposed position and the severe stresses that can be imposed upon it. The trauma can be either direct or indirect by means of a powerful force generated by the quadriceps muscle that produces enough energy to fracture one of the poles of the patella (Fig. 10–21). The patient may give a history that includes a blow to the knee, a fall, or some other direct stress. In older, obese, or poorly conditioned individuals, indirect injury can occur from a jump, descending the stairs, or a forceful squat. An audible and painful snap frequently occurs, followed by a fall or loss of balance, and the individual is usually unable to extend the knee.

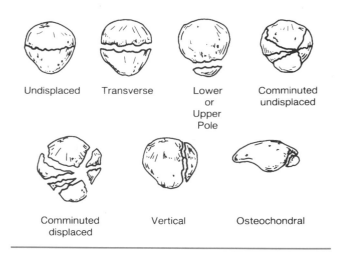

| Undisplaced | Transverse | Lower or Upper Pole | Comminuted undisplaced |
| Comminuted displaced | Vertical | Osteochondral | |

Figure 10–21   Patellar fracture classification.   *(Rockwood, C.A., et al. (1996). Rockwood & Green's Fractures in Adults. 4th ed. Philadelphia: Lippincott-Raven.)*

UNDISPLACED FRACTURES

Fractures may be displaced or undisplaced. With undisplaced fractures, upon examination there is swelling about the patella, tenderness, and generally some effusion. The patella may reveal deformity, and occasionally fragments of the patella may be movable. Nonoperative treatment will usually produce acceptable results in fractures that have no more than 1 to 2 mm of fragment displacement, a smooth articular surface, and a quadriceps mechanism capable of extending the knee against gravity. The initial treatment of these fractures includes the application of a compressive bandage and ice to minimize swelling. An aspiration of the hemarthrosis may be necessary later to relieve swelling and pain and to reduce the intra-articular tension.

These fractures will usually heal well by immobilizing the knee in a cylinder cast, groin to toe (see Chapter 5), with the knee in full extension but not hyperextended. After 3 to 6 weeks, the cast is replaced by an elastic compressive bandage. Weight bearing and straight-leg raising exercises are begun early and continued throughout cast immobilization. For patients with little pain, a knee immobilizer may be used instead of a cast, with knee motion beginning almost immediately. The immobilizer is worn for all active functions but is removed for personal care and controlled physical therapy. Vertical or nondisplaced marginal fractures of the lateral or medial facet may be managed by reduced activity and active and passive range-of-motion exercises for 3 to 6 weeks. No cast immobilization is required for these fractures.

DISPLACED FRACTURES

Displaced fractures of the patella must be surgically corrected. A physical examination often elicits significant anterior knee pain on direct palpation. The patient is unable to actively extend the knee against resistance, and there is often a palpable defect over the patella. The optimal time for surgery is as soon as the patient's condition and skin permit, usually within several days of the injury. Skin abrasions may occur with the original injury. If the abrasions are clean and the injury is less than 4 to 8 hours old, operative repair can be undertaken with minimal postoperative risks. However, extensive abrasions may necessitate waiting until the skin heals to reduce the risk of wound complications.

A transverse patellar fracture is usually best treated by open reduction and internal fixation with cancellous screws or with cerclage wiring utilizing a combination of Kirschner wires and lag-screws for fixation (Fig. 10–22). The fracture fragments are united by wire passed through the insertions of the quadriceps tendon and secured onto the anterior aspect of the patella. Two Kirschner wires or 4-mm cancellous lag-screws are used both to provide rotation control of the fragments and to facilitate anchorage of the cerclage wire. Closure of the wounds over large drains and short-term postoperative use of intravenous antibiotics are routine.

Postoperative care for patients with internal fixation includes splinting for 3 to 6 days until wound healing has begun. Physical therapy is then started with active assisted range-of-motion exercises, and partial weight bearing is allowed. Using a CPM machine (see Fig. 10–26 a & b) helps patients regain knee motion and is started in the early postoperative period. Passive range of motion is utilized with patients with low pain thresholds who require additional help in attaining knee flexion. If the fracture is severely comminuted or the fixation is marginal, immobilization may be required for 3 to 6 weeks after repair. Quadriceps isometric exercises and active movements may be used to prevent adhesions and retain quadriceps muscle tone. Full weight bearing is initiated when roentgenograms indicate progressive fracture healing, usually 6 weeks from stabilization.

Displaced apical fractures are best managed by doing a partial patellectomy (excision of the small fragments of the patella) and repairing the extensor mechanism by direct suturing of the quadriceps or patellar tendon to the remaining large bone fragment. Comminuted fractures of the patella that result in many small fragments, none large enough for attaching tendons, indicate a total patellectomy. The multiple fracture fragments are removed, and the continuity between the quadriceps and patellar tendons is provided either by imbrication or direct suture. Patients with a partial patellectomy with tendon repair requiring healing to bone and those with a total patellectomy need to be immobilized for at least 4 weeks. After that period, progressive rehabilitation of the knee is initiated with protective immobilization between exercise sessions. Passive stretching does not help to restore mobility and may harm the repair. Several months of continuous effort are necessary to produce maximum range of motion and strength. However, significant flexion limitations that remain after 8 to 12 weeks may

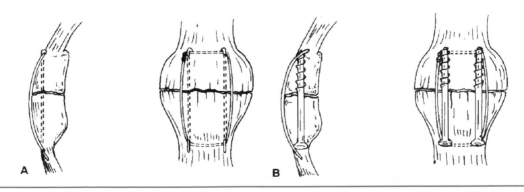

Figure 10–22   (A) Schematic drawing of the modified AO/ASIF anterior tension band writing using two Kirschner wires. The cerclage wire is placed through the quadriceps and patellar soft-tissue attachments and across the anterior half of the patella. It provides conversion of the distraction forces of the quadriceps mechanism into compression forces at the articular surface.
(B) Another modification using two 4-mm AO/ASIF cancellous lag screws to provide additional rotation and compression of the fracture.   *(Rockwood, C.A., et al. (1996). Rockwood & Green's Fractures in Adults. 4th ed. Philadelphia: Lippincott-Raven.)*

require gentle closed manipulation under anesthesia to increase flexion and an arthroscopic lysis of knee adhesions.

Patients with a patellar fracture need to be aware that although the patella heals, some crepitus and pain may still remain. Patellar arthritis may also result, depending on the severity of the fracture.

PATELLAR DISLOCATION

A dislocation in which the patella leaves the femoral groove can occur for various reasons, including severe falls, automobile accidents, and athletic injuries. The patient usually complains of the knee buckling and causing a fall and of pain in the anterior knee area. Effusion may occur, but usually it is not as severe as in an internal knee injury. There may be difficulty in extending the knee, but when the knee is extended the patella returns to its normal position. In chronic dislocations of the patella, examination reveals an excessive laxity of the extensor mechanism and excessive movement of the patella, generally in the lateral direction. The vastus medialis may be atrophic. Crepitation is felt and heard between the patella and its femoral groove. A recurrent dislocation of the patella is frequently associated with other knee pathology that impairs the extensor mechanism.

Treatment seeks to restore the continuity of the extensor mechanism and usually involves surgery. Ruptures of the quadriceps tendon and patellar ligament are usually repaired surgically, and the knee is protected in extension for at least 3 weeks. Early range-of-motion exercises are then begun to prevent knee stiffness. Surgical repair for a dislocation is aimed at changing the quadriceps pull, restoring the depth of the femoral sulcus, or decreasing the quadriceps laxity. The knee is protected for a period, and then gentle exercises are started.

OTHER TRAUMATIC INJURIES TO THE KNEE

FRACTURES OF THE TIBIAL CONDYLES

A fracture through one of the tibial condyles is one of the most common fractures involving the knee joint. This injury may be produced by direct compression, such as by jumping down, or by a forceful abduction or adduction of the knee joint. Fractures of the lateral tibial condyle (Fig. 10–23) occur more often than those of the medial tibial condyle because the lateral side of the knee is more exposed to trauma. A lateral force applied to the leg can cause both a fracture of the tibial condyle and a rupture of the medial collateral ligament.

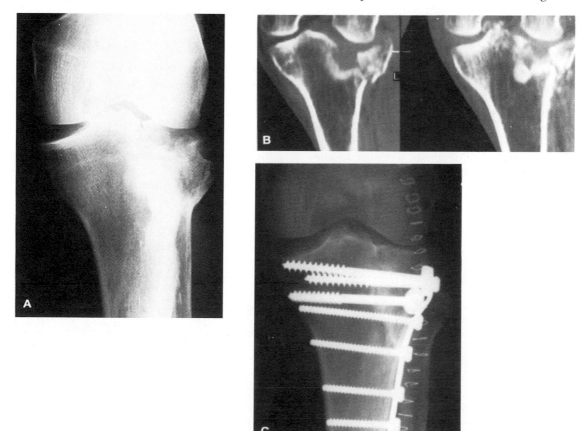

Figure 10–23   (A) AP radiograph showing a split-compression fracture of the tibia. (B) AP CT scan showing the depressed articular surface of the tibia. (C) A postoperative radiograph showing reduction and fixation of the fracture with a buttress plate. Iliac crest bone graft should be used.   *(Weinstein & Buckwalter (1994). Turek's Othropaedics: Principles and Their Application. 5th ed. Philadelphia: J.B. Lippincott-Raven.)*

Some tibial condyle fractures may be treated by closed reduction and the use of a long leg cast (see Chapter 5). Others may be treated by skeletal traction (see Chapter 6) or by open reduction with internal fixation and a long leg cast. The use of crutches without weight bearing on the affected leg is generally allowed after surgery, but full weight bearing is not usually allowed for 10 to 12 weeks.

DISLOCATIONS OF THE KNEE

A dislocation of the knee joint in an adult is usually produced by trauma and can be either anterior, posterior, medial, or lateral, depending upon the position of the tibia in relation to the femur. Anterior dislocations are the most common. Most physicians accept closed reduction under general anesthesia and immobilization as the treatment of choice for most dislocations, but some physicians prefer open reduction in order to repair soft-tissue damage. One serious potential complication is an injury to the popliteal artery, which may necessitate an amputation. Look for signs of vascular insufficiency or severe and increasing pain after reduction, which may indicate the possibility of vascular injury.

TRAUMATIC SYNOVITIS

A jarring or twisting injury to the knee may irritate the synovial membrane and cause an outpouring of normal appearing synovial fluid into the joint in the hours following the injury. Fluid distention of the joint and the suprapatellar pouch may cause pain, limitation of motion, and a limping gait. Traumatic synovitis may be suspected if injury to the joint surfaces, supporting ligaments, and menisci have been ruled out. Roentgenographic examination of the knee joint probably will be negative, except for possible capsular swelling due to the accumulation of fluid. The treatment of traumatic synovitis usually consists of rest and support to the joint. Joint distension may be relieved by aspiration of the excess joint fluid.

PREPATELLAR BURSITIS

The prepatellar bursa lies superficial to the distal end of the patella and the upper half of the patellar tendon. It may become acutely inflamed and swollen from local trauma or may be chronically irritated by repeated or prolonged kneeling. For that reason, the condition has been called "housemaid's knee" or "nun's knee." Clinically, a localized well-circumscribed fluctuant mass may be palpated over the anterior aspect of the knee. The knee joint itself is not involved. Treatment usually consists of aspirating the fluid, a local injection of corticosteroids, and the application of a pressure dressing. If the cause of the inflammatory response is infection, incision and drainage with proper antibiotic coverage are indicated. Occasionally, chronic recurrent enlargement justifies surgical excision of the bursal sac.

CHONDROMALACIA PATELLAE

Chondromalacia patellae or degenerative arthritis of the patellofemoral joint is frequent and can be as painfully disabling as degenerative arthritis of the femorotibial joint. Chondromalacia patellae frequently is a complication of other knee lesions, such as degenerative arthritis of the femorotibial joint or lesions of the cruciate or collateral ligaments. Its etiology is unclear, with possible causes including abnormal ridges on the femoral condyle, incongruity of the femoropatellar articulation, abnormal length of the infrapatella tendon, and malalignment of the patella. Signs of chondromalacia include retropatellar aching, a feeling of crepitation, a feeling of the knee "giving way," and pain on descending stairs or rising from a chair. Upon examination of the knee, one finds a normal knee with tenderness over the medial aspect of the patella. When pressure is applied on the patella with simultaneous quadriceps contraction, crepitation and pain are elicited. Roentgenographic findings are negative until the condition is advanced.

Nonsurgical treatment usually consists of avoiding any irritating activity such as deep knee bends or squats. If pain persists, brief immobilization in a cylindrical cast or retropatellar steroid injections may be used. Surgical intervention varies from arthroscopy and shaving the involved patella to a total patellectomy. One frequent approach is a combination of a patellar realignment and an excision of cartilage that modifies the **Q** angle (i.e., the lateral or medial patella deviation).

BAKER'S (OR POPLITEAL) CYST

Baker's cyst is the name given to a firm, tense cystic mass occasionally found along the medial border of the popliteal space. The patient is usually a child, but popliteal cysts may also be seen in adults, particularly in patients with RA. Although the condition may represent herniation through the posterior capsule of the knee joint, most popliteal cysts are believed to be a fluid distention of the bursal sac associated with the gastrocnemius and semimembranous muscles. No symptoms other than swelling may be noted, though the cyst may cause vague pain and discomfort associated with a sensation of weakness and "giving way." The cyst may be aspirated and injected with corticosteroids. Surgical excision may be required based on the intensity of the symptoms, or repeated aspiration and injection may be performed.

LOOSE BODIES

Loose bodies are fragments of cartilage, bone, or calcified tissue that lie free within a joint causing pain, joint irritation, and locking. Loose bodies have been discovered in practically every joint in the body, but occur most frequently in the knee joint. The fragments may be pieces of bone broken from the articular surface, such as a piece of tibial spine, a detached bone spur in an osteoarthritic knee joint, or a torn portion of a meniscus, or they may result from osteochondritis dissecans or osteochondromatosis. Locking occurs if a loose body becomes wedged between the bones, thereby forming a mechanical obstruction to complete extension.

Whereas loose bodies containing bone or calcified cartilage are visible on roentgenographic examination, loose bodies that are fragments of cartilage are not but may be visualized by arthrography. They are removed from the joint by a surgical procedure known as an arthrotomy or arthroscopy.

SURGICAL PROCEDURES

SYNOVECTOMY

A synovectomy is the surgical removal of the synovium. Persistent, unrelieved synovitis, usually related to RA, is the primary reason for a synovectomy, and the primary goal is to relieve pain. To be beneficial to the arthritic patient, the surgery must be done early in the course of the disease, prior to the onset of joint destruction. A late synovectomy may relieve pain, but it does not help restore functional effectiveness to the joint.

Nursing care following a synovectomy is similar to the care of a patient with a compression bandage and knee immobilizer. The leg is kept in extension with lateral rotation. The patient should do quadriceps-setting exercises and ambulate with partial weight bearing, using crutches.

PROXIMAL TIBIAL OSTEOTOMY

A proximal tibial osteotomy is done to correct varus or valgus deformities of the knee. The procedure realigns the articular surfaces and thus distributes the weight more evenly within the knee joint, which relieves pain (Fig 10–24).

The nursing care for a patient following an osteotomy is similar to that for a patient with an open reduction and a long leg cast (see Chapter 5). Healing is rapid because the surgery is performed through cancellous bone just proximal to the tibial tubercle. Postoperatively, the affected knee is placed in a knee immobilizer or cylinder cast. The patient is allowed partial weight bearing with the use of a walker or crutches. Because the affected leg will be slightly shorter after surgery, careful leg measurements need to be made so that the patient's shoes can be prepared with the proper amount of elevation. Potential complications include peroneal palsy, compartmental syndrome, and nonunion or delayed union.

TOTAL KNEE REPLACEMENT

A total knee replacement or total knee arthroplasty is surgery on an injured or diseased knee to reestablish a movable joint. The knee joint, like the hip joint, may be partially replaced (a hemiarthroplasty) or totally replaced. According to Altizer (1998), there are several types of knee replacements: unicompartmental replacement, constrained implants, semiconstrained implants, and totally constrained implants. An arthroplasty of the knee consists of the replacement of the femoral condyles and the tibial plateau and, possibly, the patella. The arthritic or diseased surfaces are removed and replaced by durable prosthetic components (Fig. 10–25) that are fixed firmly into place. The porous coated implants require no cement and press fit into place. The non-porous coated implants are cemented into place with a methyl methacrylate cement. The patella is checked for continued usability, and, if not usable, the patella is resurfaced and a polyethylene button is utilized. The stability of the unit or prosthesis is totally dependent upon good musculature and intact ligaments. Once the implants are securely placed, the incision is closed and wound catheters are inserted.

NURSING PROCESS (Patient with a Total Knee Replacement)

The following nursing process presents the care of a patient with a total knee replacement. The nursing process begins after the patient returns from surgery.

ASSESSMENT

The immediate postoperative assessment of a patient following a total knee replacement involves taking vital signs (pulse, respiration, and blood pressure) and observing the patient's general color and warmth. Usually, the patient's skin feels cool and the patient appears pale. The patient's level of consciousness and orientation should be determined. Have the patient cough and deep breathe, and auscultate the chest for clearness of the lungs and any cardiac abnormalities. A neurovascular assessment of the affected leg (pulse, temperature, color, capillary filling, edema, and sensory and motor function) should be made and the position of the leg checked for proper alignment and elevation on pillows. The patient may have a compression dressing and the knee immobilized in extension with a knee immobilizer, a posterior plaster splint, or nothing at all. The incisional dressing and the area posterior to the knee should be checked for drainage. If the patient has wound catheters in place, note the color and amount of drainage and whether the suction is working. The patient may also have a cell saver in place (see Chapter 9, total hip arthroplasty), since patients following a knee arthroplasty tend to have a large amount of drainage (500 to 1,000 cc). Assess the type, severity, and location of pain, and note whether the patient received pain medication in surgery or while in the postanesthesia room. Note the type of intravenous solution, the rate of flow, and the amount left in the bag. Obtain from the anesthesia and postanesthesia room records (or personnel) the amount of blood loss in surgery and the kind and amount of fluid replacement. Check the patient for bladder distention, urgency, or the need to void if the patient does not have a catheter.

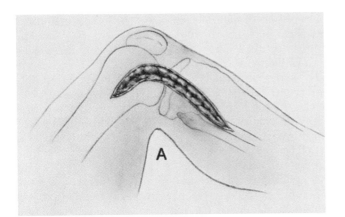

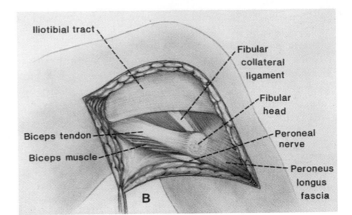

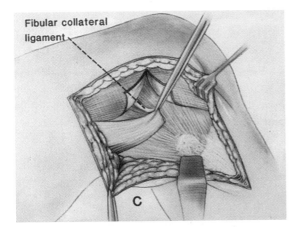

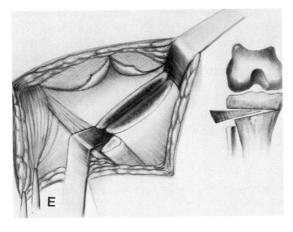

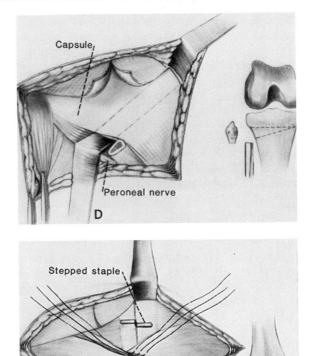

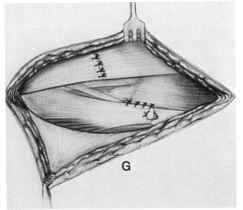

Figure 10–24   Proximal tibial osteotomy is performed by removal of a laterally based wedge of bone from the proximal tibia, which in turn creates a valgus alignment to restore the normal mechanical axis to the leg. The tibiofibular joint must be released or the proximal fibular head should be resected to allow closure of the osteotomy.   *(Weinstein & Buckwalter (1994). Turek's Othropaedics: Principles and Their Application. 5th ed. Philadelphia: J.B. Lippincott-Raven.)*

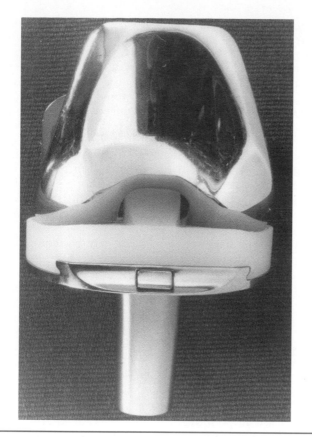

Figure 10–25   The posteriorly stabilized condylar total knee prosthesis. The design allows for up to 130 degrees of flexion.   *(Weinstein & Buckwalter (1994). Turek's Othropaedics: Principles and Their Application. 5th ed. Philadelphia: J.B. Lippincott-Raven.)*

NURSING DIAGNOSIS

Based on all of the assessment data, the nursing diagnoses for a typical patient following a total knee replacement include:

- Pain and discomfort related to soft-tissue and bone trauma from surgery
- Impaired physical mobility related to lack of joint mobility
- Potential infection related to the surgical procedure
- Increased anxiety related to knowledge deficit about the procedure and rehabilitation process

COLLABORATIVE PROBLEMS

- Respiratory complications
- Circulatory impairment
- Gastrointestinal disturbances
- Genitourinary complications
- Musculoskeletal complications
- Integumentary impairment

GOAL FORMULATION AND PLANNING

The goals are to have the patient experience (1) a decrease in the level of pain in the knee through nursing

measures and prescribed medications, (2) an increase in mobility through the use of exercises and assistive devices, (3) no signs of infection, (4) a decrease in anxiety through increased knowledge about the procedure and the rehabilitation process, and (5) an absence of complications. Long-term goals are to have the patient free of pain and able to walk without discomfort, initially using a four-point gait and crutches, and without assistive devices within 6 months to a year.

INTERVENTIONS

ALLEVIATE PAIN

Note the type, severity, and location of pain to help determine the cause of the pain and thus the appropriate nursing measures. The patient who has had a total knee replacement will probably have more pain for a longer period of time than will a patient who has had a total hip replacement. Following a total knee replacement, a typical patient will complain of severe to moderate pain for at least the first 24 to 48 hours and some patients even longer. Note the color and warmth of the toes, and check to see if the dressing, knee immobilizer, or splint is too tight. Do a neurovascular assessment of the affected leg (see Chapter 2). If circulatory impairment or swelling is noted, check to ensure that the extremity is elevated. To prevent back discomfort, adjust the level of elevation, lower the head of the bed, or turn the patient onto one side. Check the ice bags that are along the incision site, and refill as needed. They help to reduce swelling and thus prevent pain.

Sometimes the patient becomes anxious and tense and tightens their muscles. This increases the discomfort, which leads to even more muscle tightening. After reassuring the patient and getting the patient to relax the affected leg in your hands, use both hands and gently lift the leg and move it through its range of motion of the hip several times before repositioning it. Frequently the pain will go away or at least be reduced. In general, muscle-setting exercises, which increase circulation, help to relieve pain and should be encouraged.

Patients having a total knee replacement may complain of pain in the back of the knee. If they had a knee flexion contracture before the surgery, it will be painful postoperatively because the contracted muscles are extended when the leg is held in extension. These patients may try to get out of the knee immobilizer or try to talk the nurse into not putting the knee immobilizer back on, because they feel more comfortable when the knee is slightly flexed. It is important that they understand that keeping the knee flexed can impede their ambulation by causing another knee flexion contracture.

The nurse must be alert to any complaints of pain in the calf of the affected leg, as that may not be a result of the surgery but an indication of thrombophlebitis. Patients may also complain of pain after each exercise session. This is to be expected but can be prevented to some extent by giving the patient pain medications before they exercise. The pain needs to be relieved or it will interfere with the patient's program of rehabilitation, as he or she will not want to do the needed exercises.

Some patients ask for pain medications, others need to be encouraged to ask, and still others will not ask but will need to receive medication based on the nursing assessment. Following a total knee replacement, never let the patient go without pain medications just because he or she does not ask. For severe to moderate pain during the first 24 to 48 hours, most patients receive intramuscular injections of narcotics or are placed on a PCA machine where they administer their own medications. For lesser pain, patients usually are on oral medications. Patients should know what medications are available, how often they are available, and that they are expected to ask for medications when they are needed. Some individuals are more willing to ask for medication if they know that it is not going to be a shot.

INCREASE MOBILITY

Interventions to increase mobility are correct positioning, exercises, an immobilization device, a CPM machine, ambulation, and sitting.

Position The patient having a total knee replacement will return from the postanesthesia room lying supine with the operated leg in an immobilizing device to keep it extended and elevated on pillows. The knee is usually kept in extension with a knee immobilizer, but some physicians may use a posterior splint. Knee immobilizers are not ideal for every patient, because even though they come in a variety of sizes and styles, they do not fit the circumference and length of every leg, and some tend to slip when the patient gets out of bed. Some patients complain that the immobilizer is too warm to wear; others dislike wearing it and continually take it off. In some instances, the nurse may need to use sheet wadding or Webril on the leg to improve fit, or even get another size immobilizer after the compression dressing is off and the swelling is reduced. The knee immobilizer may be worn 24 hours a day (except during exercises) for 5 to 7 days, and is then worn only at night or while ambulating.

Turning One of the first procedures is to turn the patient to the side. With assistance, the patient can turn to either side but would probably prefer the unaffected side. The patient is able to turn with the nurse providing support along the entire length of the operated leg. The nurse must make sure that the head of the bed is lowered and that the leg does not twist as the patient turns. Once the patient has completed the turn, the operated leg is placed on one to three pillows (depending upon the patient's size) to keep the leg in correct alignment.

Patients are usually able to assist in changing their own position while supine with the use of a trapeze and side rails. That helps to make the patient feel more independent and less uncomfortable and assists the nurse in providing personal care.

Exercises Exercises for the patient who has had a total knee replacement may begin from the day of surgery to several days postoperatively. If the patient has had preoperative teaching about the exercises and has practiced them, the patient will be able to do the exercises in the postanesthesia room. However, some physicians may not want exercises to begin that quickly.

Most patients will be doing quadriceps- and gluteal-setting exercises, range-of-motion exercises for the ankle, plantar and dorsiflexion (ankle pump) exercises of the affected leg, and range of motion to all unaffected joints (as discussed in Chapter 9 for a patient following a total hip replacement). Normally, the patient will be asked to exercise 5 minutes out of every waking hour.

Additional exercises the patient may be required to do are straight leg raises, knee flexion exercises, restorator exercises, and CPM exercises. Initially, the patient may find it hard to do straight leg raises, and the help of a nurse or a physical therapist may be needed before the patient is able to do them alone. Some physicians will also have the patient do side-lying straight leg exercises or lie prone and do knee flexion exercises. Some physicians wait until the second or third postoperative day (after the wound catheters and the initial dressing have been removed) and then have the patient do knee flexion exercises using a knee sling. Some patients receive a whirlpool treatment before doing knee flexion exercises. The warm circulating water in the whirlpool increases the blood supply to the knee area and helps to relax the muscles in and around the knee joint. These patients probably still need oral pain medications before exercising.

Another exercise to increase flexion for the patient with a total knee replacement is the use of a restorator. A restorator is a set of bicycle-like pedals at the end of a pair of rods that attach to and extend forward from a chair. In a restorator exercise, the patient sits in the chair to which the restorator is attached, and the patient's feet are strapped onto the pedals. In the beginning, the patient is able to sit and pedal with a minimum of knee flexion. As the patient's rehabilitation progresses, the pedals are moved closer to the chair, thus forcing the knees to flex more. The restorator exercise may be done for 30 minutes twice a day.

Continuous Passive Motion *Continuous passive motion (CPM)* was first employed in the early 1960s. The involved extremity is placed in an electrically driven apparatus that continuously moves the involved joint through flexion and extension (Fig. 10–26). Since first described, the principle of CPM has been applied to several joints, including the knee. Passive motion, particularly if used continuously, accelerates healing, increases range of motion, and maintains a higher level of muscle strength. Postoperative patients who experience CPM progress more rapidly, use fewer analgesics, and are discharged earlier with greater function than those patients whose joint is kept immobilized postoperatively.

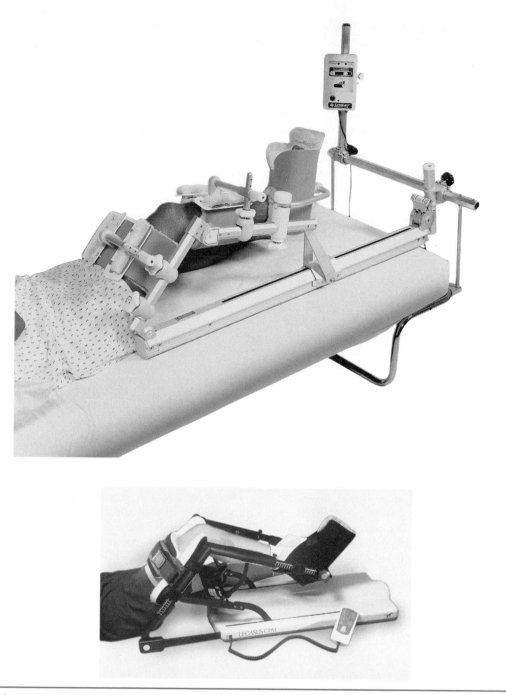

Figure 10–26   Continuous passive motion machine. (A) Lite lift CPM for hospital use. (B) Legasus CPM for home use.   *(Courtesy of OrthoLogic, Inc.)*

Patients following a total knee arthroplasty may be started on the CPM machine as early as 24 to 36 hours postsurgery, depending on the amount of drainage. To gain the most advantage from passive motion, it should be as continuous as possible, preferably 20 or more hours a day. Some physicians, however, may have the patient utilize CPM 4 hours once a day or 2 hours twice a day. The head of the bed can be elevated for comfort, but the patient must remain supine. The patient is prone to develop pressure areas, circulatory stasis, pulmonary stasis, and all the other sequelae of limited mobility.

Exercises like the ones discussed or variations of them may be incorporated into a home exercise program. The objective is to restore the knee to at least 90 degrees of flexion, but the rehabilitation program for each patient should be individualized in terms of the patient's tolerance and rate of progression.

Ambulation   The patient with a total knee replacement may start ambulating as soon as the wound catheters are discontinued and the initial dressing is removed. The patient is assisted out of bed with the knee immobilizer still in place. In the beginning, walking may be done only with the assistance of health personnel or the use of a walker. The patient usually uses a four-point gait as it is a safe, slow gait and allows for partial weight bearing on the affected leg. (For a discussion of ambulation with a walker or crutches using a four-point gait, see Chapter 4.) It makes no real difference which side of bed the patient gets out on, but the patient may find it easier to get out on the unaffected side and return on the affected side. By getting out on the unaffected side, the patient can use the overhead trapeze to support the upper body and slip the foot of the unaffected leg under the ankle of the operated leg to assist it to the floor. The same procedure can be done when getting back into bed on the other side. The patient should be encouraged to ambulate several times a day.

Sitting Sitting is not usually a problem for the patient following a total knee replacement, but sometimes getting into and out of a chair or on and off the toilet can present difficulties. A patient using crutches should be taught to back up until the back of the unaffected leg touches the seat and then grip both crutches in the hand on the unaffected side. The patient should next bend at the waist, place their hand on the affected side onto the seat, then move the affected leg forward, and gradually lower themselves onto the seat. To rise from the seat, the patient should reverse the procedure, pushing off against the seat with the hand on the affected side, and pulling the body upward with the other hand, which is holding both crutches.

Patients wearing a knee immobilizer are cautioned against bearing a lot of weight on a flexed knee, and should not sit in "overstuffed" living room furniture. When sitting in such furniture, the patient's bottom is much lower than their knees, and thus it may be very difficult for them to get out of the chair without assistance.

PATIENT TEACHING AND HOME CARE CONSIDERATIONS

Postoperative patient teaching for a patient having a total knee replacement emphasizes the rehabilitation program. An exercise program is developed with the physical therapist before the patient leaves the hospital. The exercises will gradually increase in the level of exertion required, as weights will be added and the number of repetitions increased. It is a good idea for the patient to set aside specific times for exercise. One of the best times to exercise is after showering.

The patient should be encouraged to return to nearly full activity after discharge, as restrictions are few. The patient should avoid twisting the knee, walking on rough terrain, sitting for long periods, and applying unauthorized weight to a flexed knee, such as in scrubbing floors or kneeling in prayer.

Immediately after discharge, the patient will need assistance at home because he or she is walking on crutches and tends to tire easily. Until the patient is quite ambulatory, elastic stockings have to be worn on both legs, and the patient usually needs help in getting them on, at least in the beginning. Crutch safety should be stressed. Pets or loose rugs could cause the patient to fall. It may be advisable to practice walking up and down stairs before discharge. No special chairs are necessary, but the patient should practice getting in and out of chairs. The patient should be encouraged to take showers instead of baths, as he or she will find it too difficult and even painful to get into and out of a tub. The patient can use a stool in the shower for safety. If the patient has to step into a tub to shower, assistance may be needed initially to prevent falling. The patient, the family, and significant others must be taught the signs of infection as discussed under potential complications of the integumentary system.

MONITORING AND MANAGING POTENTIAL PROBLEMS

Postoperative care for patients having a total knee replacement should recognize that most of these patients are not only weak from surgery but are elderly and have arthritis involving other joints in their body. In administering care and preventing complications, therefore, both orthopaedic and gerontologic nursing concepts should be considered.

A total knee replacement is a major reconstructive procedure and therefore subject to the same local and systemic postoperative complications as other major surgical procedures. The likelihood of local complications is increased by the implantation of a large amount of foreign material on the joint surfaces and by the poor tissue tolerance to injury and stress common to older patients. The more commonly occurring complications are discussed here, along with measures to prevent them.

RESPIRATORY

Recumbency, the drugs used for pain relief that depress respiration, a decrease in the body's need for oxygen due to inactivity, and the resistance of the bed against the chest wall with bed rest are some of the factors that can lead to such respiratory complications as pneumonia and pulmonary embolism. Nursing measures should stress the prevention and quick observation of abnormalities. The patient is asked to do turning, coughing, and deep breathing exercises on a regular basis and may also be asked to use an incentive respiratory device or other devices to facilitate respiratory hygiene. (For further discussion, see Chapter 4.)

CIRCULATORY

Circulatory complications include such problems as dehydration from blood and fluid loss, circulatory overload, venous stasis, and orthostatic hypotension. The most common complications are probably pulmonary embolism and thrombophlebitis because of the age of the patient, the immobility following surgery, and the use of a leg tourniquet during the operation.

Measures that help prevent these complications are bed exercises, especially the leg exercises discussed under mobility, and changing the position of the patient. The patient should be kept as active as possible with exercises and ambulation, as tolerated. An elastic stocking, which extends from toes to groin, is usually applied to the unoperated leg before the patient returns to the unit and to the operated leg after the initial compression dressing is removed. The stockings should be checked for any creases, wrinkles, or pressure areas and should be removed for one-half hour twice a day. At that time, inspect the legs and the feet, especially the heels, for any redness. Patients are frequently given anticoagulant medications such as aspirin, heparin, or coumadin. (For further information, see Chapter 4.)

A circulatory complication of special concern is known as compartmental syndrome, a condition in which progressive pressure within a confined space compromises the circulation and the function of tissues within that space. A compartment is enveloped by tough inelastic fascial tissue, and, when swelling of the muscles occurs, the fascia do not expand. In the lower leg, that can occur in the anterior, lateral, superficial posterior, or deep posterior compartments. Such ischemic conditions can occur after knee surgery with the onset of the symptoms from as little as 2 hours to as long as 6 days. If the pressure is not relieved within approximately 12 hours of the onset of the syndrome, irreversible nerve and tissue damage is likely to result. For further discussion and nursing care measures related to compartmental syndrome, see Chapter 5.

GASTROINTESTINAL

Immediately after surgery, the most common gastrointestinal problems are nausea and vomiting. They occur frequently but are usually self-limiting. Parenteral fluids are usually administered for 36 to 48 hours following surgery, primarily to administer antibiotics, but they can be used to help combat dehydration if nausea or vomiting persists.

Following a total knee replacement, the patient usually is able to tolerate fluids immediately after recovering from anesthesia, and a regular diet is tolerated quickly thereafter. Measures needed to assist with good nutrition should be stressed with additional fluids and fiber in the diet as needed to combat the constipation that can occur as a result of immobility, pain medication, and the patient's age. Note if any of the patient's oral medications, especially aspirin, are causing any digestive disorders. Other measures that help combat constipation are exercises and ambulation.

GENITOURINARY

Because of the anesthesia and the severe pain experienced immediately after surgery, some patients, especially elderly ones, may have difficulty voiding at first. Nursing measures should be directed toward relieving pain and relaxing the patient. It is helpful to get the patient in as near to a normal voiding position as possible. A Foley catheter is usually not necessary following a total knee replacement.

In the first 24 to 48 hours following surgery, some patients may have diuresis as a result of the intravenous fluids administered during surgery to maintain circulating volume. As a result, the patient may develop an electrolyte deficiency of sodium and potassium, and those electrolytes must be replaced.

MUSCULOSKELETAL

Nursing measures for patients following a total knee replacement should include measures to increase knee flexion. The goal is to have the patient regain as much active flexion in the knee as possible. Some patients will do the knee flexion exercises but stop flexing when it begins to hurt. The patient should be encouraged to gradually increase the amount of flexion so that they will regain the desired 90 degrees of flexion. If, despite such efforts, the patient is unable to regain 90 degrees of flexion, the physician may order a roentgenogram to determine if there is anything wrong with the prosthesis or the joint. If the roentgenogram is negative, the patient may be taken to surgery and the knee flexed 90 or more degrees under anesthesia. Immediately after the procedure, the patient will probably have pain and swelling in the knee, and the postoperative care for a patient following a total knee replacement should be reinstituted.

INTEGUMENTARY

Following a total knee replacement, a patient is susceptible to pressure sores in the usual areas and is particularly vulnerable on the heel because of the weight of the immobilized leg. Make sure that the patient's heel is "floating" (i.e., that the leg is given sufficient support to reduce the weight on the heel). That can be done by keeping the leg elevated on a pillow, a folded bath blanket, or 2 to 3 inches of foam.

To enhance wound healing and avoid or control infection, physicians use wound catheters connected to continuous suction to remove blood from between layers of muscle and thus prevent any subcutaneous pooling of blood or fluid. Catheters are usually removed 36 to 48 hours postoperatively, after having removed an average of 300 to 500 cc of fluid. Because an effusion in the knee may occur, firm pressure on the bursae should be maintained. For that reason, a Jones pressure bandage, which extends from midcalf to midthigh (hence, well below and well above the bursae), may be applied.

Once the catheters and the initial dressing are removed, the incision line requires special care. It may just be left open to the air, but that is rare because the line is usually covered by a knee immobilizer. Most patients will have a small dressing over the suture line, with the incision cleansed daily with betadine, alcohol, or a similar solution. Observe the incision and the stab wounds left by the catheters for signs of infection (e.g., heat, swelling, redness, drainage, and hardness).

Problems such as marginal wound necrosis, skin sloughs, hematoma formation, or wound dehiscence can usually be detected easily. If the wound appears to be healing but the patient complains of unrelieved pain, there is a possibility of a local deep infection in the joint (Fig. 10–27). This is a devastating complication that can led to an arthrodesis or even an above the knee amputation. Such infections may not be observed for several weeks or even years postoperatively.

EVALUATION/OUTCOMES

In evaluating the goal of alleviating pain in the knee, determine whether the individual is having any pain by verbal responses and by the patient's outward appearance, including facial grimacing during activities, the position assumed, and restlessness or sleeplessness. If pain still exists, determine the location, duration, and intensity of the pain; what aggravates and intensifies it; and what measures have been able to relieve it.

When evaluating care to increase mobility, determine the patient's compliance with the exercise routine and utilization of assistive devices such as a trapeze, knee immobilizer, and walker or crutches. Evaluate the degree to which the patient has regained flexion in the affected knee and the steadiness of the partial-weight-bearing gait. Determine whether or not the patient, the family, and significant others have been able to follow the rehabilitation regime, how useful the discharge plan appears to be, and how well they understand what the patient can and cannot do. Regarding complications, look for the absence of contractures, pressure areas, decubiti, an elevated temperature, and other problem signs. If the goals have not been met, both the goals and the plan of care must be reassessed and the nursing process begun again.

CLINICAL PATHWAY (Patient with a Total Knee Replacement)

An example of a generic pathway for a patient having a total knee replacement is presented in Figure 10–28.

ARTHRODESIS

An arthrodesis of the knee is a surgical fusion of the joint. It is indicated in infected knee joints, when the articular surfaces are so severely damaged that satisfactory function cannot be expected, or if the patient is a poor candidate for joint replacement. Arthrodesis also remains the salvage procedure of choice for failed reconstructive joint surgery. The goals of a knee arthrodesis are to decrease pain and allow mobility. However, the patient is left with a stiff knee and an extremity that is approximately 0.5 inches shorter.

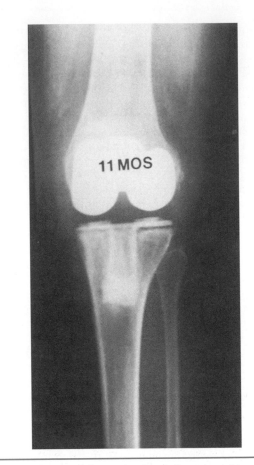

Figure 10–27 AP radiograph of an infected total knee replacement showing a radiolucency at the cement-bone interface beneath the medial plateau of the tibial component. *(Weinstein & Buckwalter (1994). Turek's Orthopaedics: Principles and Their Application. 5th ed. Philadelphia: J.B. Lippincott-Raven.)*

Because of the mobility limitations, the surgery is generally performed only if a single knee is involved.

A U incision is usually made on the anterior portion of the knee, and the articular cartilage is excised. A thin layer of subcortical bone is removed from the tibia and the femur to produce two flat surfaces, and the two bones are joined. (For an adult, 10 degrees of flexion and 10 degrees of external rotation of the tibia on the femur is considered the most useful position for walking or sitting.) Some form of fixation is then used to stabilize the joint for bone fusion, such as an intramedullary nail (Fig. 10–29). Immobilization can be accomplished with the use of external clamps attached to pins inserted through the proximal tibia and distal femur. Some prefer internal fixation using Steinmann pins with Charnley compression clamps. If the compression method is not used, Knowles pins, a graft, or other methods of internal fixation are used, because the position of the bone for fusion is difficult to maintain with external casting alone. Generally, knee fusion requires 3 months or more of immobilization postsurgery. The patient is allowed partial weight bearing with the use of a walker or crutches until there is a successful fusion.

Figure 10–28

Clinical Pathway: Total Knee Arthroplasty (Replacement)

Admission Date: _____   **Discharge Plan:** _____ **Home** _____ **Skilled Nursing** _____ **Extended Care Facility**

Pathway	Preadmission Office/OP clinic	Admission Day Op day	Hosp Day 2 Postop 1	Hosp Day 3 Postop 2	Hosp Day 4 Postop 3	Hosp Day 5 Postop 4	Outcomes
Consultation	Primary Care/ Rheumatologist or Medical	Case Manager	Social Work				Cont. @ Home or ECF
		Anesthesia, Dietitian	PT, OT if nec.				
		Acute Pain Service					
Assessment	Nrsg database	Review & add					Home Care Nurse ECF
	H & P Exam. by MD, NP, or PA Rehab/ECF/ home	Review H & P					
	Home equipment	Postop routine	Referral if nec.			Resolved	
	Home environment		Referral if nec.		✓ if obtained		Will have nec. equipment @ home
Tests	ECG/UA/CXR/ 1–2 units autol. blood	X-ray in OR	✓ CBC	✓ CBC			
	Coag. studies		Transfuse per protocol	Transfuse per protocol			
	Standing & Lateral Knee	H & H in PACU & repeat @ PM					
Medications	D/C NSAIDS 3d. b/4 OR	✓ preadm meds					States meds, when to take and purpose
	D/C ASA 10 d. b/4 OR	Routine meds					States purpose
	D/C anticoag. meds—MD	Anticoagulant	Cont. Anticoag.				
	Instruct on preop meds b/4 OR	Antibiotics	D/C antibiotics	D/C begin oral pain meds			Pain managed with oral medications
	Analgesics as nec.	PCA/Epidural		Analgesics			Analgesics @ home
		Bowel protocol					Normal bowel function
Diet	Assessment wt.	NPO @ MN b/4 OR	Liquids/soft	Advance as tol			Tolerating diet
	Overweight— lose weight slowly & sensibly						
	Underweight— eat balanced diet						
Activity	Preop mobility cane/walker	Ankle Pumps	Cont.				Use cane/ walker Safely
	Fatigue level	Turn Protocol q 2	Turn q 2hrs				Cont. @ home if nec.
	ADLs & upper arm strength	CPM per protocol	Cont.	Cont.	Cont.	Cont.	
		Quad & Glut q 2	Cont.				Cont.
		Straight Leg Raises	Cont.	Cont.	Cont.	Cont.	Cont.
		Bed rest/ to Chair	CW—NWB/WB as tol	Cont.	Cont.	Cont.	Cont.
		B RP with assist	CW to BRP with assist				

(continued)

Figure 10–28
Clinical Pathway: *(continued)*

Pathway	Preadmission Office/OP clinic	Admission Day Op day	Hosp Day 2 Postop 1	Hosp Day 3 Postop 2	Hosp Day 4 Postop 3	Hosp Day 5 Postop 4	Outcomes
Treatments	Set blood donation dates, 1 wk between units & 14 days between last unit and OR day	IV fluids/blood if necessary, I&O TEDs, IPCD, or foot pumps/CPM Hemovac/out put IS/TCDB q hr w/a Foley to drain		D/C PRN D/C			Cont. TEDS @ home Continue with exc No infection Normal bladder Function No infection
		Dressing	Do Not Change	Change PRN			States reason to Contact MD
Education	Teach postoperative Exercises	Reinforce	Reviews Rehab Process			Reinforce	
	View TKA video Rev. TKA booklet Attends gp ed class Pain management Review hosp LOS	Rev. hosp routine				View Postop TKA Video	Understands purpose of Exercise Regime
D/C Plan	Identify discharge plan			Notify Social Worker Or Home Health Care as appropriate			Discharged to home
	Caregivers & home situation (LOS 4–6 days)						

NURSING PROCESS (Patient with an Arthrodesis)

The following nursing process presents the care of a patient with an arthrodesis. The nursing process begins after the patient returns from surgery.

ASSESSMENT

Following an arthrodesis, the patient will typically have a long leg cast (groin to toes) and external Charnley clamps laterally and medially that extend above and below the knee. The immediate postoperative assessment involves taking vital signs (pulse, respiration, and blood pressure) and observing the patient's general color and warmth. Usually, the patient's skin feels cool and the patient appears pale. Determine the patient's level of consciousness and orientation. Have the patient cough and deep breathe, and auscultate the chest for clearness of the lungs and any cardiac abnormalities. Do a neurovascular assessment of the affected leg, and check the leg for proper alignment and elevation. Check the cast for dryness and for signs of drainage in the posterior area and the front of the leg. If the patient has wound catheters in place, note the color and amount of drainage and whether the suction is working. Assess the

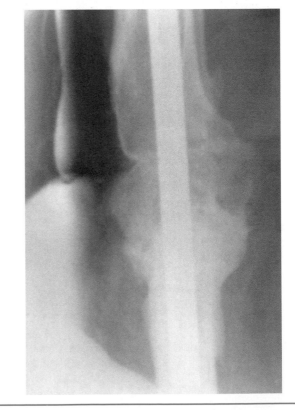

Figure 10–29 Knee arthrodesis using an intramedullary rod. *(Weinstein & Buckwalter (1994). Turek's Othropaedics: Principles and Their Application. 5th ed. Philadelphia: J.B. Lippincott-Raven.)*

type, severity, and location of pain, and note whether the patient received pain medication in surgery or while in the postanesthesia room. Note the type of intravenous solution, the rate of flow, and the amount left in the bag. Obtain from the anesthesia and postanesthesia room records (or personnel) the amount of blood loss in surgery and the kind and amount of replacement. Check the patient for bladder distention, urgency, or the need to void if the patient does not have a catheter.

NURSING DIAGNOSES

Based on all of the assessment data, the nursing diagnoses for a typical patient following an arthrodesis include:

* Pain and discomfort related to soft-tissue and bone trauma from surgery
* Impaired physical mobility related to lack of joint mobility
* Anxiety related to knowledge deficit about the procedure and rehabilitation process

COLLABORATIVE PROBLEMS

* Respiratory complications
* Circulatory impairment
* Gastrointestinal disturbances
* Genitourinary complications
* Integumentary impairment

GOAL FORMULATION AND PLANNING

The goals are to have the patient experience (1) a decrease in the amount of pain in the knee through nursing measures and prescribed medications, (2) an increase in mobility through the use of exercises and assistive devices, (3) a decrease in anxiety through increased knowledge about the procedure and the rehabilitation process, and (4) an absence of complications. Long-term goals are to have the patient free of pain and able to walk with a stiff knee within 3 to 6 months.

INTERVENTIONS

ALLEVIATE PAIN

Note the type, severity, and location of the pain to help determine the cause of the pain and thus the appropriate nursing measures. The patient who has had an arthrodesis will probably have a fair amount of pain over a longer period of time than patients following a total joint replacement. A typical patient will complain of severe to moderate pain for at least the first 24 to 48 hours and some patients even longer.

Sometimes the patient becomes anxious and tense and tightens their muscles. This increases the amount of pain. Help the patient to relax their muscles by lifting and moving the extremity. Some patients will ask for pain medications, others need to be encouraged to ask, and still others will not ask but will need to receive medications based on the nursing assessment of the patient. For further discussion, see the preceeding section on total knee replacements.

INCREASE MOBILITY

Interventions to increase mobility are correct positioning, exercises, immobilization, and ambulation.

Position The patient having an arthrodesis will return from the postanesthesia room lying supine with the operated leg immobilized with a cast and external clamps. The knee is extended, and the leg is elevated on pillows. The immobilized leg may be elevated in extension by the use of pillows, by elevating the foot of the bed, or by both, depending on the size of the patient. Elevation is used to help prevent and reduce edema, and the toes should normally be higher than the nose. If the patient is having increased swelling despite increases in the elevation of the leg, it may be necessary to lower the head of the bed. After 48 hours following surgery, the amount of leg elevation may be decreased. *Do not utilize the clamps or other external fixation devices in changing the patient's position.*

Exercises Exercises for the patient who has had an arthrodesis may begin from the day of surgery to several days postsurgery. If the patient has had preoperative teaching about the exercises and has practiced them, the patient will be able to exercise in the postanesthesia room. However, some physicians may not want exercises to begin that quickly. Most patients will be doing quadriceps- and gluteal-setting exercises. Normally, the patient will be asked to exercise 5 minutes out of every waking hour. Because the patient will be using a walker or crutches, exercises to build up the muscles in the upper extremities are important (see Chapter 4).

Ambulation Initially, the patient will be ambulating with crutches using a three-point gait with no weight bearing on the affected leg for 2 to 4 weeks. After that time, the patient is usually allowed partial weight bearing using crutches and a walking heel on the cast. (For a discussion of using a walker or crutches with a four-point gait, see Chapter 4) The patient will need assistance in getting out of bed with the immobilizing device in place. It makes no difference which side of bed the patient gets out on, but the patient may find it easier to get out on the unaffected side and return on the affected side. By getting out on the unaffected side, the patient can use the overhead trapeze to support the upper body and slip the foot of the unaffected leg under the ankle of the operated leg to assist it to the floor. The same procedure can be done when getting back into bed on the other side. The patient should be encouraged to ambulate several times a day.

PATIENT TEACHING AND HOME CARE CONSIDERATIONS

The patient, the family, and significant others need to understand that a period of immobilization after surgery is necessary for the knee joint to fuse. The patient will be in a cast from the toes to the groin with a window over the knee for 2 to 4 weeks postsurgery, until the tendency for swelling subsides. The cast is then changed, and the new cast is left in place for another 10 to 12 weeks or until substantial fusion has taken place. After that cast is removed, the leg is encased in a molded brace of suitable plaster or stiff leather with metal reinforcements that extends from groin to ankle. This brace is worn by the patient night and day until the fusion is solid, approximately 6 months.

Even after support is removed from the leg, the patient needs to take special care of the leg when walking. The affected leg should be carried through normally, rather than swung out to the side. When going up steps, the good leg should always lead, because the knee with the arthrodesis does not bend. The patient would otherwise have to tilt to the unaffected side and swing the affected leg out to the side. When going down steps, similar considerations make it best for the patient to lead with the affected leg. When the surgical procedure entails the removal of a larger than normal amount of bone, the affected leg may be significantly shorter than the other leg; therefore, an elevated shoe is needed on the affected side.

Immediately after discharge, the patient will need assistance at home because he or she will be walking on crutches with a long leg cast and will tend to tire easily. Crutch safety should be stressed, as pets or loose rugs could cause a fall. It is advisable to have the patient practice walking up and down stairs before discharge. No special chairs are necessary, but the patient should be aware that it is difficult to get out of some living room chairs with their leg in a long leg cast (or other knee immobilizing device).

The patient should be instructed to do sponge baths and only try to take a shower (with the affected leg covered in plastic) once a week. The patient can use a stool in the shower for safety. To step into a tub to shower, assistance may be needed initially to prevent falling. The patient, the family, and significant others must be taught the signs of infection and other potential complications.

MONITORING AND MANAGING POTENTIAL PROBLEMS

Postoperative care for patients having an arthrodesis should recognize that these patients may be weak from surgery. If they are elderly, they may also have arthritis or other physical conditions that affect their ability to ambulate. An arthrodesis is a major surgical procedure and therefore subject to the same local and systemic postoperative complications as other major surgical procedures. The potential complications following an arthrodesis are the same as those discussed following a total knee replacement (e.g., respiratory complications, circulatory impairment, gastrointestinal disturbances, and genitourinary complications). Make sure the patient's skin is protected from any rough edges of the cast (see Chapter 5).

EVALUATION/OUTCOMES

For a typical patient recovering from an arthrodesis of the knee, the evaluation is similar to that discussed for a patient following a total knee replacement. Special emphasis should be given to evaluating the patient's response to long-term immobilization of the knee in the initial stage and their ability to walk in the later stage. Check that the patient understands the extent of ambulation possible and how to care for the casted leg. Determine the patient's compliance with the exercise regime and understanding of the rehabilitation program.

CLINICAL PATHWAY (PATIENT WITH AN ARTHRODESIS)

An example of a generic clinical pathway for a patient having an arthrodesis is presented in Figure 10–30.

FRACTURES OF THE TIBIA AND FIBULA

Trauma to the shin area is often sufficient to simultaneously fracture both bones of the lower leg. A direct blow to the anterior lower leg may cause a transverse fracture through the proximal, midshaft, or distal portions of the tibia and the fibula. The fractures are frequently comminuted, but torsional injuries to the leg occur, causing a spiral or long oblique fracture. Because the fibula is a non-weight-bearing bone, fractures of the fibula alone are rare. A fracture of the fibula alone usually remains in good alignment and requires no reduction, but the leg is immobilized in a cast. The tibia is exposed to frequent injury, and because one-third of the surface is just below the skin, open fractures are more common in the tibia than in any other major bone. The blood supply of the tibia is also relatively vulnerable because its blood vessels are not enclosed in heavy muscles.

There are three methods for repairing fractures of the tibia: (1) closed reduction and cast, (2) internal fixation, and (3) use of an external fixation device. The choice of method depends primarily on the type and the location of the fracture.

CLOSED REDUCTION WITH CAST

Tibial fractures may be repaired using a closed method of reduction followed by the application of a leg cast in two ways. One is to use a long leg cast until the bone calcifies, that is, for approximately 8 to 10 weeks. The second method is to apply a long leg cast for 2 to

Figure 10–30

Clinical Pathway: Knee Arthrodesis

Admission Date: _____   **Discharge Plan:** _____ **Home** _____ **Skilled Nursing** _____ **Extended Care Facility**

Pathway	Preadmission Office/OP clinic	Admission Day Op day	Hosp Day 2 Postop 1	Hosp Day 3 Postop 2	Hosp Day 4 Postop 3	Hosp Day 5 Postop 4	Outcomes
Consultation	Primary Care/or medical Physician	Case Manager	Social Work				
		Anesthesia, Dietitian AcutePain Service	PT, OT if nec.				Cont. @ Home or ECF
Assessment	Nrsg database	Review & add					Home Care Nurse ECF
	H & P Exam. by MD, NP, or PA Rehab/ECF/ home	Review H & P					
			Referral if nec.			Resolved	
	Home equipment	Postop routine	Referral if nec.		✓ if obtained		Will have nec. equipment @ home
Tests	ECG/UA/CXR/ 1–2 units autol. blood	X-ray in OR	✓ CBC	✓ CBC			
	Coag. studies		Transfuse per protocol	Transfuse per protocol			
	Standing & Lateral Knee	H & H in PACU & repeat @ PM					
Medications	D/C NSAIDS 3d. b/4 OR	✓ preadm meds Routine meds					States meds, when to take, and purpose
	D/C ASA 10 d. b/4 OR						
	D/C anticoag. meds—MD	Anticoagulant	Cont. Anticoag.				States purpose
	Instruct on preop meds b/4 OR	Antibiotics	D/C antibiotics				Pain managed with oral medications
		PCA/Epidural		D/C begin oral pain meds			
	Analgesics as nec.			Analgesics			
		Bowel protocol					Normal bowel function
Diet	Assessment wt.	NPO @ MN b/4 OR	Liquids/soft	Advance as tol			Tolerating diet
	Overweight— lose weight slowly & sensibly						
Activity	Preop mobility cane/walker	Ankle Pumps	Cont.				Use cane/ walker Safely
	Fatigue level	Turn Protocol q 2	Turn q 2 hrs		Cont.		
	ADLs & upper arm strength	Quad & Glut q 2	Cont.	Cont.	Cont.	Cont.	Cont. when in bed or Sitting
		Elevate leg on pillow	Cont.	Cont.		Cont.	Cont.
		If Clamps in place Do Not use to move pt.	CW—NWB	CW to BRP c̄ assist			
		Bed rest/ to Chair	BRP/NWB c̄ assist				

(continued)

Figure 10–30

Clinical Pathway: *(continued)*

Pathway	Preadmission Office/OP clinic	Admission Day Op day	Hosp Day 2 Postop 1	Hosp Day 3 Postop 2	Hosp Day 4 Postop 3	Hosp Day 5 Postop 4	Outcomes
Treatments	Set blood donation dates, 1 wk between units & 14 days between last unit and OR day	IV fluids/blood if necessary, I&O TEDs, IPCD, or foot pump					Cont. TEDS @ home on unaffected leg
		Hemovac/output IS/TCDB q hr w/a		D/C PRN			Continue with exc
		Foley to drain		D/C			Normal bladder elim
Education	Teach postoperative Exercises & Care	Reinforce	Reviews Rehab Process			Reinforce	
	Attends preoperative education class	Rev. hosp routine				View Cast Video if casted	Understands purpose cast & exercises
	Pain management						States reasons to Contact physician
D/C Plan	Review hosp LOS Identify discharge plan		Notify Social Worker Or Home Health Care as appropriate				Discharged to home
	Caregivers & home situation (LOS 3–5 days)						Knows when to contact physician

4 weeks and then change to a below-knee patellar-tendon–weight-bearing cast until calcification is complete. In instances of delayed union, calcification may take 4 months or longer. See Chapter 5 for a discussion of the nursing care of a patient following a closed reduction of the tibia with a long leg cast.

INTERNAL FIXATION

A second method of treatment for fractures of the shaft of the tibia is internal fixation. With closed internal fixation, an intramedullary nail (e.g., a Lottes nail, a Küntscher nail, or an AO slotted nail) is driven down the medullary canal of the tibia. The patient is usually placed in a long leg cast with weight bearing for 4 to 6 weeks. Three complications can commonly occur: (1) infection, (2) nonunion of the fracture site, and (3) migration of the nail. The nursing care is similar to that for a patient with a fractured tibia who has a long leg cast (see Chapter 5).

In an open reduction internal fixation, plates and screws are used, and the leg is usually placed in a long leg cast for 4 to 6 weeks with partial or full weight bearing. Complications following this procedure include infection, nonunion, breakage of the plate or screws, and loss of fixation. The nursing care is similar to that for a patient with a fractured tibia who has a long leg cast (see Chapter 5).

EXTERNAL FIXATION

External fixation devices can be used for many fractures and are widely used for open fractures of the tibia and the fibula where there is also marked soft-tissue damage and skin loss. Normally, two or more heavy Steinmann pins are inserted proximal to the fracture and two distal to the fracture, and they are held in place by external devices such as Hoffman or Wagner devices. With the use of a single or double frame mounting and universal joint clamps, segmental fracture fragments can be aligned. In open fractures needing that type of repair, instability, malalignment, and soft-tissue complications with skin necrosis and deep infection are common. In many instances, these patients may return repeatedly for skin grafts. For a discussion of nursing care, see Chapter 7.

EXTERNAL FIXATION WITH PLASTER

Another external fixation technique has been used in the treatment of closed tibial shaft fractures and in open fractures without extensive soft-tissue damage or skin loss. Two pins are inserted in the tibia proximal and one distal to the fracture, and the pins are then incorporated in a plaster cast.

The initial cast is worn for 3 to 6 weeks. In stable transverse fractures with good opposition, the pins can be removed after 3 to 4 weeks, and in comminuted and oblique fractures, after approximately 6 weeks. A long leg walking cast is then applied, and weight bearing on crutches is allowed. Eight to ten weeks after surgery, the cast may be changed to a below-knee patellar-tendon–weight-bearing cast until calcification is complete. The nursing care is similar to that for a patient with a fractured tibia and a long leg cast (see Chapter 5).

RUPTURE OF THE ACHILLES TENDON

Traumatic rupture of the Achilles tendon is not uncommon, particularly among middle-aged men. Sudden contraction of the calf muscle with the foot fixed to the floor may cause the Achilles tendon to be pulled apart. The tendon rupture usually occurs within the sheath, leaving the sheath intact. The patient immediately notes sharp pain in the area and an inability to plantar flex the foot. On examination, a gap continuity of the tendon can be palpated. An immediate surgical repair of the Achilles tendon is usually done. The major complication is skin necrosis during the healing process.

It is possible to treat this injury by the application of a walking cast with the foot held in marked plantar flexion. This position allows the ruptured tendon fragments to come together and reunite within the cast. This process usually takes between 6 and 8 weeks, but recurrence of the rupture following cast removal is not uncommon.

RUPTURE OF THE PLANTARIS TENDON

The plantaris is a long, thin muscle in the calf that lies between the gastrocnemius and soleus muscles. Rupture may occur with vigorous use of the legs, causing the patient to experience a sharp, stinging pain in the calf. Plantar flexion is unaffected, and surgical treatment is not required. Rest, support to the calf, and the use of a heel lift are the only supportive measures needed.

References

Aichroth, P. M. (1992). Total knee replacement arthroplasty. In P. M. Aichroth, W. D. Cannon, & D. V. Patel (Eds.), *Knee surgery: Current practice* (pp. 639–641). New York: Raven Press.

Altizer, L. L. (1998). Degenerative disorders. In A. B. Maher, S. W. Salmond, & T. A. Pellino (Eds.), *Orthopaedic nursing* (2nd ed., pp. 480–545). Philadelphia: W. B. Saunders.

Altizer, T. J. (1997). Radiology review: Patellar complications in total knee replacement. *Orthopaedic Nursing, 16*(3), 58–60.

Berg, E. E. (1996). Radiology review: Osteochondritis dissecans of the medial femoral condyle. *Orthopaedic Nursing, 15*(3), 55–56.

Brown, F., Jr. (1996). Anterior cruciate ligament reconstruction as an outpatient procedure. *Orthopaedic Nursing, 15*(1), 15–20.

Buckwalter, J. A. (1994). Musculoskeletal tissues and the musculoskeletal system. In S. L. Weinstein & J. A. Buckwalter (Eds.), *Turek's orthopaedics: Principles and their application* (pp. 585–614). Philadelphia: J. B. Lippincott.

Crutchfield, J., Zimmerman, L., Nieveen, J., Barnason, S., & Pozehl, B. (1996). Preoperative and postoperative pain in total knee replacement patients. *Orthopaedic Nursing, 15*(2), 65–72.

Funk, J. R., MacBriar, B. R., & Peterson, A. F. (1990). Tibial osteotomy. *Orthopaedic Nursing, 9*(2), 29–34.

Garth, W. P., & Fagan, K. M. (1996). Knee injuries in sports. In V. R. Masear (Ed.), *Primary care othopaedics* (pp. 88–100). Philadelphia: W. B. Saunders.

Indelicato, P. A., & Brown, H. R. (1992). Gore-Tex prosthetic ligament in anterior cruciate deficient knees. In P. M. Aichroth, W. D. Cannon, & D. V. Patel (Eds.), *Knee surgery: Current practice* (pp. 281–298). New York: Raven Press.

Leininger, S. M. (1997). *Building clinical pathways.* Pitman, NJ: National Association of Orthopaedic Nursing.

Lichtenstein, R., Semaan, S., & Marmar, E. C. (1993). Development and impact of a hospital-based perioperative patient education program in a joint replacement center. *Orthopaedic Nursing, 12*(6), 17–25.

Macnicol, M. F. (1992). The conservative management of the anterior cruciate ligament deficient knee. In P. M. Aichroth, W. D. Cannon, & D. V. Patel (Eds.), *Knee surgery: Current practice* (pp. 206–217). New York: Raven Press.

Neal, L. J. (1996). Outpatient ACL surgery: The role of the home health nurse. *Orthopaedic Nursing, 15*(4), 9–13.

Patel, D. V., Aichroth, P. M., Jones, C. B., & Wand, J. S. (1992). A combined intra- and extra-articular reconstruction using carbon-Dacron composite prosthesis for chronic anterior cruciate instability: A two to six year follow-up study. In P. M. Aichroth, W. D. Cannon, & D. V. Patel (Eds.), *Knee surgery: Current practice* (pp. 222–225). New York: Raven Press.

Rothenberg, J. R. (1991). Innovations in treating anterior cruciate ligament deficiency. *Orthopaedic Nursing, 10*(2), 17–24.

Scuderi, G. R., Scott, W. N., & Insall, J. N. (1996) Injuries of the knee. In C. A. Rockwood, D. P. Green, R. W. Bucholz, & J. D. Hickman (Eds.), *Rockwood and Green's Fractures in Adults* (2001–2126). Philadelphia: Lippincott-Raven

Smith, J. E. (1990). Applying the continuous passive motion device. *Orthopaedic Nursing, 9*(3), 54–56.

Whittington, C. F. (1998). Exercises and sports related disorders. In A. B. Maher, S. W. Salmond, & T. A. Pellino (Eds.), *Orthopaedic nursing* (2nd ed., pp. 746–768). Philadelphia: W. B. Saunders.

Windsor, R. E. (1994). The adult knee. In S. L. Weinstein & J. A. Buckwalter (Eds.), *Turek's orthopaedics: Principles and their application* (pp. 585–614). Philadelphia: J. B. Lippincott.

This chapter focuses on the treatment and associated care of traumatic and pathologic conditions of the ankle and the foot. Conditions ranging from common ankle and foot problems, such as corns, calluses, sprains, and fractures, to fusion and reconstructive surgical procedures are discussed. The chapter begins with a review of the anatomy of the ankle and foot.

ANATOMY

BONES

The talocrural or ankle joint is a uniaxial joint. It is formed by the talus, the tibia, and the fibula and is stable because of its mechanical configuration and ligamentous supports (Fig. 11–1). The lower end of the tibia and its medial malleolus, the lateral malleolus of the fibula, and the inferior transverse tibiofibular ligament together form a deep recess in which the body of the talus is embraced. The ankle bones are connected by a fibrous capsule and by several ligaments, specifically the deltoid, anterior and posterior talofibular, and calcaneofibular ligaments.

The skeleton of the foot has three parts: the tarsus (or hindfoot), the metatarsus (or midfoot), and the phalanges (or forefoot). The seven tarsal bones make up the skeleton of the posterior half of the foot. The tarsal bones are arranged in proximal and distal rows with an additional bone interposed between the two rows on the medial side. The proximal row is comprised of the talus and the calcaneus. The distal row, from medial to lateral, is composed of the medial

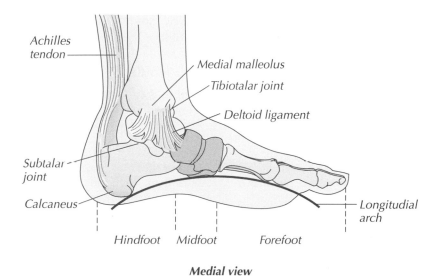

Medial view

Figure 11–1   The *heads of the metatarsals* are palpable in the ball of the foot. These and the associated *metatarsophalangeal joints* are proximal to the webs of the toes. An imaginary line along the foot bones extending from the heads of the metatarsals to the calcaneus is called the *longitudinal arch.*   *(Bates, B. (1995). A Guide to Physical Examination and History Taking. 6th ed. Philadelphia: J.B. Lippincott Company.)*

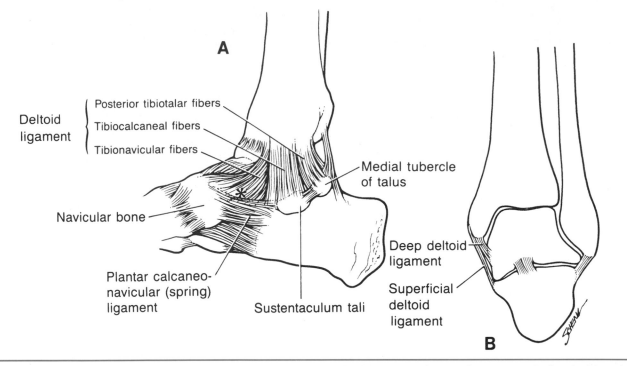

Figure 11–2   Medial collateral ligaments. (A) Bands of the superficial deltoid ligament. The asterik represents the head of the talus. (B) Position of the deep deltoid ligament.   *(Rockwood, C.A., et al. (1996). Rockwood & Green's Fractures in Adults. 4th ed. Philadelphia: Lippincott-Raven.)*

cuneiform, intermediate cuneiform, lateral cuneiform, and cuboid bones. On the medial side, the navicular bone is interposed between the head of the talus and the cuneiforms. Laterally, the calcaneus articulates directly with the cuboid.

The five metatarsal bones are situated in the distal part of the foot, connecting the tarsus to the phalanges. They are numbered 1 through 5 from the medial side. The metatarsals are miniature long bones possessing a shaft, a base or proximal end, and a head or distal end. The bases articulate with the distal row of the tarsus and with one another. The heads articulate with the proximal phalanges of their respective digits.

The 14 phalanges correspond in number and general arrangement to the phalanges of the hand. There are two phalanx bones in the big toe and three in each of the other toes. The terminal phalanx of the big toe normally shows a small degree of valgus (lateral) deviation. Such a deviation is also seen in the proximal phalanx of persons who have never worn shoes.

ANKLE MOVEMENT

When the foot is dorsiflexed, the talus is forced between the two malleoli and no lateral rotation is possible, but when the foot is plantarflexed, some lateral motion is allowed. The neutral or plantarflexed positions are thus more vulnerable to possible injury. The lateral and medial collateral ligaments stabilize the ankle, yet per-

mit plantar and dorsiflexion. The medial ligaments are taut in the neutral position, but the posterior strands relax in plantarflexion and the anterior fibers relax in dorsiflexion. The lateral collateral ligaments have a central axis and remain taut in all ranges of plantar and dorsiflexion. The ligaments run from the malleoli to the talus, calcaneus, and navicular bones. They are supplied with sensory nerves that, when stretched, evoke a reflex muscle spasm that protects the joint from further motion.

THE FIBROUS CAPSULE

A fibrous capsule surrounds the ankle joint. It is thin in front and in back and attaches to the borders of the articular surfaces of the tibia and the malleoli and, below, to the talus close to the margins of the trochlear surface (except in front, where it is attached to the dorsum of the neck of the talus). The fibrous capsule is supported on each side by strong collateral ligaments. A synovial membrane lines the capsule, and the joint cavity ascends for a short distance between the tibia and the fibula.

LIGAMENTS OF THE ANKLE

Stabilizing the medial side of the ankle both anteriorly and posteriorly is the strong, flat, triangular deltoid ligament, which consists of five components (Fig. 11–2). The deep component attaches to the undersurface of

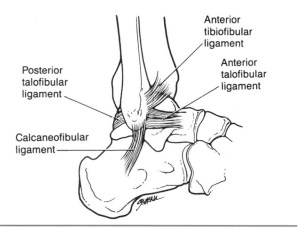

Figure 11–3 Lateral collateral ligaments with adjacent tibiofibular ligament. *(Rockwood, C.A., et al. (1996). Rockwood & Green's Fractures in Adults. 4th ed. Philadelphia: Lippincott-Raven.)*

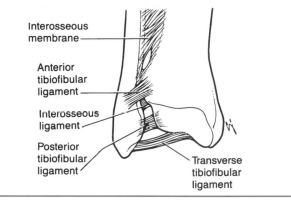

Figure 11–4 The syndesmotic ligaments of the ankle. *(Rockwood, C.A., et al. (1996). Rockwood & Green's Fractures in Adults. 4th ed. Philadelphia: Lippincott-Raven.)*

the medial malleolus and the body of the talus. The four superficial components are the tibionavicular and anterior talotibial components anteriorly, the calcaneotibial component centrally, and the posterior talotibial component posteriorly.

Laterally, there are three ligaments that help to stabilize the ankle (Fig. 11–3). The anterior talofibular ligament, which is 2 to 2.5 mm thick, attaches anteriorly to the border of the lateral malleolus and anteriorly to the neck of the talus. The calcaneofibular ligament, which is stronger than the anterior talofibular ligament, attaches superiorly to the tip of the lateral malleolus and inferiorly to the lateral surface of the calcaneus. It is the only lateral ligament that is extracapsular. The posterior talofibular ligament, which is the strongest lateral ligament, attaches anteriorly to the digital fossa of the fibula and posteriorly to the lateral tubercle on the posterior aspect of the talus. A fourth ligament, the lateral talocalcaneal ligament, supports the subtalar joint and lies between the anterior talofibular ligament and the calcaneofibular ligament, blending with both.

The ligaments that bind the distal tibia and the fibula together (Fig. 11–4) are (1) the anterior and posterior inferior tibiofibular ligaments, which attach superiorly and medially to the tibia and inferiorly and laterally to the fibula; (2) the inferior transverse ligament, which attaches laterally to the lateral malleolus and medially to the posterior border of the distal articular surface of the tibia; and (3) the interosseous ligament, the strongest bond between the bones, which attaches to the contiguous rough surfaces of the tibia and the fibula.

TENDONS, VESSELS, AND NERVES

Starting from the medial side, the tendons, vessels, and nerves of the ankle (Fig. 11–5) are, in front, the tibialis anterior tendon, the extensor hallucis longus tendon,

the anterior tibial vessels, the deep peroneal nerve, the extensor digitorum longus tendon, and the peroneus tertius tendon. From behind, there are the tibialis posterior tendon, the flexor digitorum longus tendon, the posterior tibial vessels, the tibial nerve, and the flexor hallucis longus tendon. In the groove behind the fibular malleolus, there are the peroneus longus and peroneus brevis tendons.

Arteries supplying the joint are derived from the malleolar branches of the anterior tibial artery and from the peroneal arteries. The nerves are derived from the deep peroneal and tibial nerves.

MUSCLES OF THE ANKLE JOINT

When the body is in an erect position, the foot is at right angles to the leg (see Fig. 11–5). The active movements of the ankle joint are those of dorsiflexion and plantarflexion. In dorsiflexion, the angle between the front of the leg and the dorsum of the foot is diminished; whereas in plantarflexion, that angle is increased. Slight amounts of side-to-side gliding movement and rotation, abduction, and adduction are permitted when the foot is in plantarflexion. To obtain dorsiflexion, the muscles used are the tibialis anterior muscle, assisted by the extensor digitorum longus, extensor hallucis longus, and peroneus tertius muscles. For plantarflexion, the muscles used are the gastrocnemius and soleus, assisted to a lesser degree by the plantaris, tibialis posterior, flexor hallucis longus, and flexor digitorum longus muscles.

THE ANKLE

A force applied to the ankle joint may cause a strain, a sprain, a ligamentous rupture, a dislocation, a fracture, or a combination of injuries, depending on the nature and the amount of force applied. The most severe injury to the ankle is the fracture dislocation, the least severe is the strain, and the most common is the sprain.

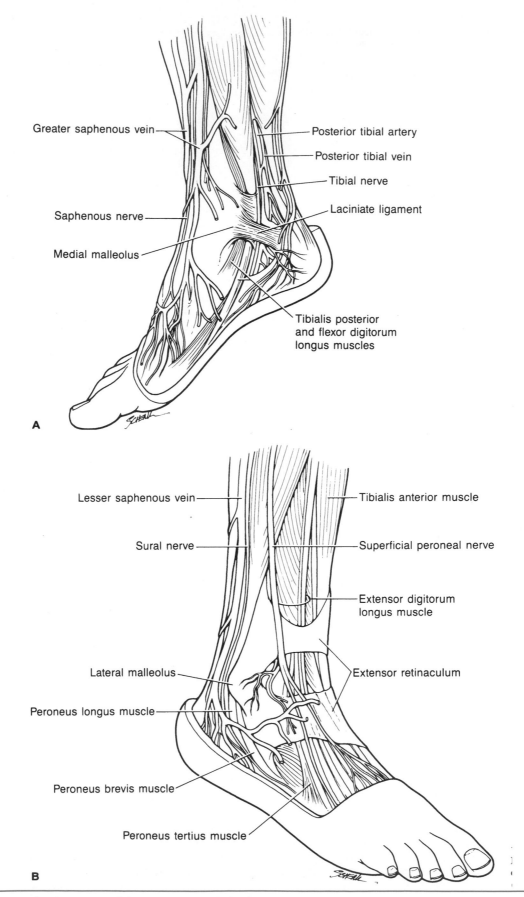

Greater saphenous vein

Saphenous nerve

Medial malleolus

Posterior tibial artery

Posterior tibial vein

Tibial nerve

Laciniate ligament

Tibialis posterior
and flexor digitorum
longus muscles

A

Lesser saphenous vein

Sural nerve

Lateral malleolus

Peroneus longus muscle

Peroneus brevis muscle

Peroneus tertius muscle

Tibialis anterior muscle

Superficial peroneal nerve

Extensor digitorum
longus muscle

Extensor retinaculum

B

Figure 11–5   Superficial anatomy of the ankle. (A) Medial side. (B) Lateral side.   *(Rockwood, C.A., et al. (1996).* Rockwood & Green's
Fractures in Adults. *4th ed. Philadelphia: Lippincott-Raven.)*

STRAIN

A strain to the ankle is an overstretching of the ligaments without disrupting the integrity of their fibers or avulsing them from their bony attachments. The strained ankle retains normal joint stability, and a strain is usually considered a minor injury that heals within a few weeks with minimal care.

SPRAIN

A sprain of the ankle joint is a stretching injury of the joint capsule and supporting ligaments by a twisting force. It occurs most frequently when a stress is applied to an ankle in an unstable position. The ankle is most unstable when plantarflexed, and it is in that position that forceful inversion or eversion will stretch the ligaments. This action can occur when running, walking over uneven ground, or even from unaccustomed walking in high-heeled shoes.

Sprains may be classified according to the amount of soft-tissue injury. *Type I sprains* involve trauma with minor ligamentous injuries, *type II sprains* involve incomplete ligamentous injuries, and *type III sprains* involve complete disruption of the ligament. Doctor Watson-Jones is credited for saying, "It is worse to sprain an ankle than to break it," because a fracture will receive treatment whereas a sprain may be neglected or receive inappropriate care. Eversion and abduction of the foot may result in disruption of the deltoid ligament, whereas inversion stress may cause ligamentous disruption on the lateral side of the ankle. Diagnosis and treatment are dependent on an understanding of the ligamentous structure about the ankle. The most common sprain occurs from inversion stress while the foot is slightly plantarflexed and results in stretching the lateral collateral ligaments. The lateral ligaments are much weaker than the medial ligaments and most frequently injured during the inversion of the ankle (DiChristina & Garth, 1996). The anterior talofibular ligament is the most commonly affected. If the inversion stress occurs with the ankle at a right angle, the calcaneofibular ligament receives the stretch force.

POSTTRAUMA ASSESSMENT

When assessing a patient who has an ankle injury with a possible sprain of the ankle joint, obtain information on how the injury occurred, what position the foot was in, what the person heard or felt, and how long ago the injury occurred. With a sprain, you would expect to find that there was a forced inversion with the foot plantarflexed and that a short time after injury there was a great amount of swelling, tenderness, and stiffness of the joint. The tenderness is localized mostly along the stretched ligament (e.g., to the tissues immediately below the lateral malleolus). When walking, there is instability of the ankle and severe discomfort. Within a few days, an area of ecchymosis develops, caused by blood seeping beneath the deep fascia. The discoloration may even go as far as the toes.

Roentgenograms are usually negative, and arthrograms for ligamentous injuries of the ankle are of limited value. Upon physical examination of a possible sprained ankle, look for evidence of ligamentous injury and test the ankle for instability. Because the anterior talofibular ligament is the ligament most often involved in ankle sprains, tenderness elicited along its course may indicate such damage. To test that ligament, do an inversion stress test (talar tilt test) by turning the patient's foot into plantarflexion and inversion. If inversion stress increases the pain, there is a distinct possibility that the ligament is sprained or torn. The inversion stress test indicates the condition of the talofibular ligament and calcaneofibular ligaments but does not give evidence of joint stability. Usually, a tear in that ligament allows the talus to slide forward on the tibia because the anterior talofibular ligament is the only structure preventing subluxation of the talus. Therefore, test for anterior instability between the tibia and the talus using the anterior drawer sign.

In performing the anterior drawer sign test, the patient sits on the edge of the table or bed with their legs dangling and their feet in a few degrees of plantarflexion. Place one hand on the anterior aspect of the lower tibia and grip the calcaneus in the palm of your other hand. Then, draw (pull) the calcaneus and talus anteriorly, while pushing the tibia posteriorly. Normally, the anterior talofibular ligament is tight in all positions of the ankle joint, and there should be no forward movement of the talus on the tibia. Under abnormal conditions, the talus slides anteriorly from under the cover of the ankle joint (positive drawer sign); you may even feel a "clunk" as it moves.

To test the stability of the deltoid ligament on the medial side, stabilize the patient's leg around the tibia and the calcaneus and evert the foot. If the deltoid ligament is torn, you may feel a gross gapping at the joint. The posterior talofibular ligament can be torn only in conjunction with the other lateral ligaments. It takes a massive trauma to the ankle joint, such as a dislocation, to damage the posterior talofibular ligament. After the tests are completed on the involved foot, test the normal one as a means of comparison to determine the extent of abnormal gapping. Stress roentgenograms are usually the best way to confirm the physical findings described.

MEDICAL TREATMENT

The treatment of ankle sprains has evolved over the years to the current standard of aggressive functional rehabilitation. The initial steps include modalities such as cold therapy (Fig. 11–6), compressive dressings, and nonsteroidal anti-inflammatory medication to reduce the pain and swelling. The majority of type I or II sprains or ligamentous injuries can usually be treated by rest, ice, compression support, and elevation (RICE) with excellent prognosis for return of normal function. In a type III sprain, where a complete dissolution of fibers has occurred, the initial steps of RICE are initiated, with range-of-motion exercises and weight bearing as tolerated, utilizing crutches if necessary. Strengthening

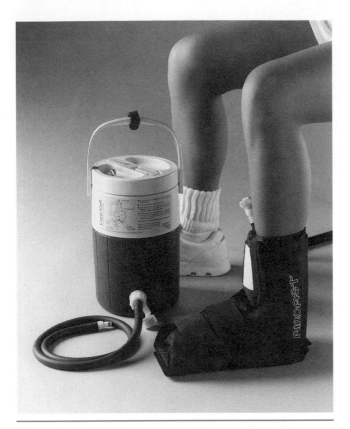

Figure 11–6 Cold therapy or cryotherapy-utilizing the cryo cuff. (*Courtesy of Aircast, Inc.*)

exercises, particularly of the peroneal musculature for inversion sprains, and proprioceptive exercises should begin as soon as possible (DiChristina & Garth, 1996). Usually, the acute symptoms subside over a period of weeks, but some tenderness and swelling may persist about the lateral aspect of the ankle. The average duration of discomfort has been reported to be anywhere from 4½ to 26 weeks, or even longer, depending on the severity of the sprain. The return of activities largely depends on the severity of the initial injury and the patient's diligence in following treatment protocols. The major potential complication is talar instability. Patients with ankle sprains are treated on an outpatient basis.

FRACTURE-DISLOCATIONS

It is extremely rare to dislocate the ankle without fracturing either the medial or lateral malleolus or the anterior or posterior lip of the distal articular surface of the tibia. Usually, any ankle dislocations that do occur are easily reduced by closed methods, but posterior dislocation of the fibula behind the tibia can contribute to difficulty with closed reduction and thus may require open reduction.

FRACTURES

Besides ligamentous and soft-tissue injures, trauma to the ankle joint can cause bone injuries. Ankle fractures

may be classified along anatomical lines, such as mono-malleolar, bimalleolar (Pott's), or trimalleolar (Cotton) fractures, or by the mechanism of injury. An explosion fracture of the ankle, that is, a malleolar fracture with a comminuted fracture of the distal tibial articular surface and the distal third of the tibia, is usually produced by a fall from a height. Sometimes an immediate open reduction may be extremely difficult or impractical. In such cases, a closed reduction of the fracture may be possible using traction through a transverse calcaneal pin or manipulation with a tibial pin proximal to the fracture in addition to the calcaneal pin. Both require a cast with pins incorporated. If there are difficulties in reduction or healing, an arthrodesis of the ankle joint may be required later.

MONOMALLEOLAR FRACTURES

Most monomalleolar fractures fall into one of three categories. First, there are supination-eversion fractures, where eversion is defined as an external or lateral rotation. The supination-eversion fracture is a spiral oblique fracture of the distal fibula associated with a rupture of the deltoid ligament or a fracture of the medial malleolus. Second, there are pronation-abduction fractures, which produce a transverse fracture of the medial malleolus associated with an oblique fracture of the tibia. Third, there are pronation-eversion fractures, which are characterized by a deltoid tear or a fracture of the medial malleolus associated with a spiral oblique fracture of the tibia. In all cases, closed reduction with a short leg cast is usually the treatment of choice (see Chapter 5 for nursing care of a patient with a short leg cast).

BIMALLEOLAR OR POTT'S FRACTURES

Bimalleolar or Pott's fractures can be reduced by either open or closed methods. Closed reduction frequently can be accomplished once the swelling has been reduced, but often the anatomical position of the ankle is not maintained. In up to 20% of bimalleolar fractures, intra-articular injuries to the talus and tibia are present and are untreated when closed reduction is utilized. For most displaced bimalleolar fractures, treatment by open reduction and internal fixation of both malleoli is essential to restore the ankle joint. To repair the joint, various methods are used, such as oblique pins, screws, Kirschner wires, or even a small plate (Fig. 11–7). See Chapter 5 for the nursing care of a patient with a Pott's fracture and cast.

TRIMALLEOLAR OR COTTON FRACTURES

Trimalleolar or Cotton fractures usually require open reduction. In addition to fractures of the medial malleolus and fibula, the posterior lip of the articular surface of the tibia is fractured and displaced, allowing posterior and lateral displacement and external rotation with supination of the foot. Each fracture is repaired by first reducing the fracture to anatomical position and then fixating it with mechanical devices such as screws or pins. Once the fractures are repaired, the leg is placed in

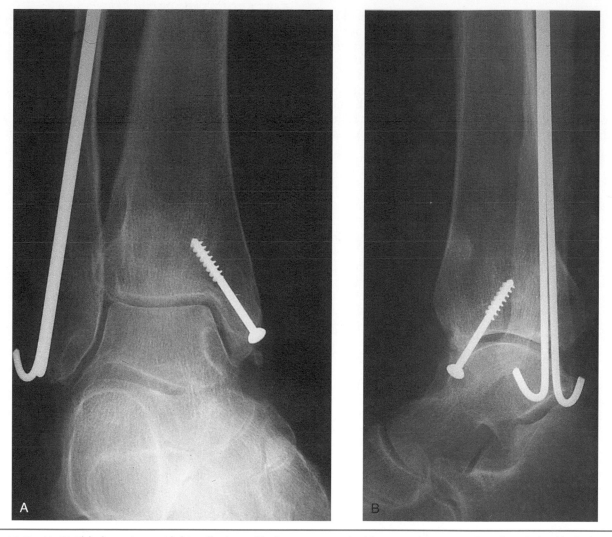

Figure 11–7   (A, B) Elderly patient with bimalleolar ankle fracture treated with retrograde-inserted Rush rods for fibula fixation. *(Koval & Zuckerman (1998). Fractures in the Elderly. Philadelphia: Lippincott-Raven.)*

a short leg cast (see Chapter 5, nursing care of a patient with a Pott's fracture and cast). As a rule, malleolar fractures require 10 to 12 weeks to calcify.

SURGICAL PROCEDURES

ARTHRODESIS

An ankle arthrodesis (fusion) is an operation to induce bony ankylosis in the ankle joint in order to (1) relieve pain, (2) halt disease, or (3) provide stability. The operative technique for fusion may be (1) intra-articular, (2) intra-articular and extra-articular, or (3) extra-articular. The choice of technique for any given patient depends on the patient's age, the pathologic process involving the joint, and the presence or absence of a gross deformity in the joint. With the intra-articular method, the articular surfaces are denuded to permit the approximation of cancellous bony surfaces and to allow for a more satisfactory correction of any deformity. Grafts of autogenous cancellous bone help to achieve more rapid and certain fusion. This method is used if there is a need

to remove diseased tissue, as is often the case in tubercular and arthritis.

A combination of intra-articular and extra-articular techniques is useful in many different circumstances, including tubercular, infected, and arthritic joints. The joint capsule is incised, as much of the synovium as possible is excised, the articular surfaces are denuded, and bone grafts are placed across the joint. An extra-articular arthrodesis is a method of obtaining a union between normal bony surfaces entirely outside the joint capsule. Many of the extra-articular techniques devised for tubercular joints are now used in conjunction with intra-articular techniques.

Indications for an arthrodesis are pain and disability due to rheumatoid, traumatic, or degenerative arthritis or due to a malunited fracture of the ankle. In a typical ankle fusion procedure, the first step is to denude the surfaces of the talus, the tibia, and both malleoli and correct any deviations from correct alignment. A bone graft (e.g., a sliding graft from the anterior distal tibia, the proximal tibia, or the iliac crest) is then placed across the joint line of the anterior distal tibia and the talus. Steinmann pins can then be placed across the talus and the tibia where Charnley compression clamps are applied to them. Additional bone chips may then be added to fill in any space between the malleoli and the talus. The procedure may also be done utilizing bone grafts alone or utilizing Steinmann pins and Charnley clamps without a sliding bone graft. The patient is then placed in a short leg cast.

NURSING PROCESS (Patient with an Ankle Arthrodesis)

The following nursing process demonstrates the nursing care of a typical patient following an ankle arthrodesis and the application of a cast. The nursing process begins when the patient returns to the nursing unit.

ASSESSMENT

The initial assessment is of the patient's total body, as for any patient recovering from anesthesia. After the initial assessment, special emphasis should be given to the fused ankle. The patient will be in a short leg cast with or without Steinmann pins and Charnley compression clamps. Check the neurovascular status of the involved foot (see Chapter 2). Note any bleeding into the cast. The foot, elevated on pillows, should be free of any pressure areas, especially around the heel. The Steinmann pins and Charnley compression clamps should be free of any entanglement with the linen, and, in most instances, sterile corks or other protective devices are placed over the sharp ends of the pins. Check the cast for pressure areas and dryness. Assess the patient for pain due to surgery. Correct the positioning of the involved leg, and make certain that the total body is in correct alignment. With an ankle fusion, most surgical procedures involve a bone graft. The most common donor site is the iliac crest. Check the dressing for any bleeding, and assess for pain at the donor site.

NURSING DIAGNOSIS

Based on all of the assessment data, the major nursing diagnoses for a typical patient with an ankle fusion and immobilization in a short leg cast may include the following:

- Pain and discomfort related to bone and soft-tissue trauma
- Impaired physical mobility related to immobilization of the ankle joint
- Impaired skin integrity related to the immobilization device
- Increased anxiety related to knowledge deficit about the surgical procedure and prognosis

COLLABORATIVE PROBLEMS

- Infection
- Nonunion
- Malunion

GOAL FORMULATION AND PLANNING

The goals are to have the patient experience (1) an absence of pain in the ankle; (2) a return of mobility using assistive devices, with the ankle immobilized in a cast; (3) a decrease in anxiety through an understanding of the surgical treatment and the prognosis; and (4) an absence of complications from surgery and decreased activity. Long-term goals are to have the ankle free of pain and to have a stable ankle joint that permits walking with a safe gait.

INTERVENTIONS

ALLEVIATE PAIN

Nursing measures that focus on pain relief are elevating the leg to prevent or reduce swelling, using ice bags, and placing the leg in correct anatomical alignment. The patient can help keep the affected leg in alignment and should be advised to look down along the leg periodically to see that it is properly positioned. Normally, a line from the anterior superior spine to the second toe should pass over the mid-patella. If the position is incorrect, pain is likely to result. To allow for swelling, a rectangular window is sometimes cut in the cast over the dorsum of the foot and ankle. The window is then held loosely in place with bandages.

INCREASE MOBILITY

To increase mobility, the focus of nursing care is to help the patient develop arm strength for crutch walking, maintain immobilization of the ankle, and assist with ambulation on crutches without weight bearing.

Exercises. The goal of exercise is to develop the patient's arms for crutch walking and to maintain range of motion and strength in all unaffected extremities. Exercises to regain mobility for walking with a fused ankle will follow cast removal.

Immobilization. The period of immobilization depends on the type of fusion and the results of roentgenograms. For postsurgical patients with a short leg cast and Steinmann pins, the cast is worn for 4 to 6 weeks with nonweight bearing. The pins are then removed, and a walking boot cast is applied and worn for another 4 to 6 weeks until the fusion is solid. Other patients may receive a boot or walking cast 4 weeks after surgery, and partial weight bearing may be cautiously resumed. Full weight bearing is usually delayed for 8 to 12 weeks after the operation. Cast immobilization is continued until the ankle joint is solidly fused. Some patients have cast walking delayed for 2 or 3 months after surgery and after an additional 3 to 4 months in a walking cast go into a short leg brace with a rigid ankle joint. The short leg brace is worn until roentgenograms show a solid fusion.

Ambulation. Many of these patients have been on crutches previously, but with a different gait. In every case, it is necessary to check the correctness and safety of gait. At first, ambulation on crutches is while wearing a short leg cast and uses a three-point non-weight-bearing gait. See the previous paragraph for guidance on weight bearing.

MAINTAIN SKIN INTEGRITY

Skin complications can easily occur with a patient in a cast. Patients who have casts following a surgical procedure may not have a stockinette under the cast, increasing the need for measures to prevent skin breakdown. The edges of the cast may be rough and need to be petaled when the cast is dry to protect the skin from irritation. (For discussion on how to petal a cast and the care of a cast, see Chapter 5). When a window is made in the cast to change a dressing or to remove sutures, make sure the cast window is replaced and secured with tape so there will not be swelling at the site of the window.

PATIENT TEACHING AND HOME CARE CONSIDERATIONS

Patient teaching plays a vital role in helping the patient and the family adjust to the long rehabilitation period. The patient needs answers to questions concerning the postoperative course of treatment, the length of time before weight bearing, and the length of time of immobilization. The amount of time off from work depends on the patient's condition, the type of work, and the health and safety policies of their employer.

Make sure the patient has a clear understanding of crutch walking (see Chapter 4). When weight bearing is allowed, the patient must remember that the position of the fused ankle and the condition of the other joints of the foot influence how well the patient is able to walk. Instruct the patient how to detect complications related to the cast and how to perform personal hygiene with a cast in place. Emphasize cast care as discussed in Chapter 5. Give the patient a copy of home care instructions. One thing some patients want to do is drive their car. Driving may not be feasible unless the patient's right leg is unaffected and the patient has a car with an automatic transmission.

Have the patient contact the physician if any of the following occur: (1) increasing pain; (2) pain unrelieved by prescribed medication; (3) swelling unrelieved by elevating the leg for at least an hour; (4) a change of sensation in the toes (e.g., numbness, tingling, or burning); (5) decreased movement or loss of movement in the toes; (6) a change in skin color above or below the cast; (7) a bad smell coming from inside the cast; (8) a warm area or fresh stain on the cast; (9) a foreign object dropped into or stuck in the cast; and (10) a weakened, cracked, loose, or tight cast.

Discuss the observations necessary to ensure comfort and prevent complications. For example, show the patient how to move their toes to assess motion. Because the leg will be in the cast for some time, explain the importance of exercise in preventing complications. Also, demonstrate how to perform any special exercises ordered.

MONITORING AND MANAGING POTENTIAL PROBLEMS

To prevent complications from decreased activity, the nurse needs to focus on the total patient. Exercises for all uninvolved joints, to be done at least twice a day, should be encouraged. In the absence of other pathology, the patient is able to do most of the activities of daily living. Work with the patient and the occupational therapist in developing activities to help stimulate both the patient's mind and body. Following an ankle arthrodesis, the most common potential complications are infection, nonunion, and malunion.

INFECTION

An infection at an orthopaedic surgical site can cause poor healing, nonunion, or malunion. However, since an infection of the bone is hard to eradicate, having an infection is very serious and could eventually lead to an amputation. Preventive measures must be instituted from the beginning. Keep the surgical site dry. Watch for any signs of infection and educate the patient about the signs and symptoms of infection, both local and general. Make sure the patient eats a well-balanced diet and gets adequate rest.

NONUNION

Nonunion is where there is insufficient calcification of the bone to form a solid union. Some of the reasons for a nonunion are inadequate blood supply to the bones to be fused, movement of the fusion that breaks or tears the calcifying bridge between the bones, infection at the fusion site, and marked dietary deficiency. Make sure the patient understands the need to eat a well-balanced diet and get plenty of rest. Determine that the patient understands the reasons for the exercises and avoiding bearing weight on the fusion site until approved by their physician. Check the immobilizing device for proper fit to prevent movement in the ankle.

MALUNION

Malunion occurs when the bones fuse in a deformed or angulated position. In most instances, malunion occurs as the result of inadequate reduction and immobilization. Check the fit of the immobilizing device, and teach the patient how to assess proper fit. For example, the cast may become too loose due to the reduction of swelling in the ankle, muscle atrophy, or a break in the cast. Make sure the patient knows to keep their weight off the foot until approved by the physician.

EVALUATION/OUTCOMES

Determine whether the patient has been provided with sufficient data to feel confident about going home with a cast and ambulating on crutches. If not, ask specific questions to determine what the patient does not understand and explain it again. Evaluation of the nursing care of a patient following an ankle arthrodesis concentrates on the type and the amount of pain and the effective measures taken to relieve the pain. Postoperative pain should have been reduced by nursing measures and medication and the overall pain in the ankle decreased. If not, consider the possibility of requesting a change in pain medications. The neurovascular status in the affected leg should be good, without signs of irritation on the patient's skin or complaints of discomfort related to the cast. There should be no signs or symptoms of infection.

Determine that the patient, the patient's family, and significant others have been provided with data to cope with the long rehabilitation and the potential of a permanent change in gait. If not, review the content area that is unclear. Support persons, such as clergy, psychiatric nurses, or support services personnel, may be useful in helping the patient adjust to the change in body image.

CLINICAL PATHWAY (Patient with an Ankle Arthrodesis)

An example of a generic clinical pathway for a patient with an ankle arthrodesis is presented if Figure 11–8.

Figure 11–8
Clinical Pathway: Ankle Arthrodesis

Admission Date: _____ Discharge Plan: _____ Home _____ Skilled Nursing _____ Extended Care Facility

Pathway	Preadmission Office/OP clinic	Admission Day Op day	Hosp Day 2 Post-op 1	Hosp Day 3 Post-op 2	Hosp Day 4 Post-op 3	Hosp Day 5 Post-op 4	Outcomes
Consultation	Primary Care/ Medical Physician	Case Manager Anesthesia, Acute Pain Service	Social Work PT,OT if nec.				Cont. @ Home or ECF
Assessment	Nrsg database H & P Exam. by MD, NP, or PA Rehab/ECF/home Home equipment	Review & add Review H & P Postop routine	Referral if nec. Referral if nec.		Resolved ✓ if obtained		Will have nec. equipment @ home
Tests	ECG/UA/CXR/ Chem7 Coag.studies	H & H in PACU & repeat @ pm					
Medications	D/C NSAIDs/ASA b/4 OR	✓ preadm meds Routine meds					States meds, when to take, and purpose
	Instruct on preop meds b/4 OR	Anticoagulant Antibiotics	Cont. Anticoag. D/C antibiotics				States purpose
	Analgesics as nec.	PCA/Epidural		D/C—oral meds			Pain managed with oral medications
		Bowel protocol					Normal bowel function
Diet	Assessment wt. & presurgery diet	NPO @ MN b/4 OR	Liquids/soft	Advance as tol			Tolerating diet
Activity	Preop mobility cane/walker	Ankle Pumps Turn Protocol q 2	Cont. Turn q 2hrs			Cont.	Use cane/ walker Safely
	Fatigue level	Quad & Glut q 2	Cont.		Cont.		
	ADLs & upper arm strength	Elevate leg on pillow	Cont.	Cont.			Cont. when in bed or Sitting
		If Clamps in place Do Not use to move pt.			Cont. Cont.		
		Bed rest/to Chair	CW—NWB B RP/NWB CW	Cont. CW—NWB to BRP			Safe in doing NWB—3- Point crutch walking

(continued)

Figure 11–8
Clinical Pathway: (continued)

Pathway	Preadmission Office/OP clinic	Admission Day Op day	Hosp Day 2 Post-op 1	Hosp Day 3 Post-op 2	Hosp Day 4 Post-op 3	Hosp Day 5 Post-op 4	Outcomes
Treatments		IV fluids/blood if necessary, I&O		D/C			Cont. TEDS @ home on unaffected leg
		TEDs on unaffected leg	Off 1/2 h. 2×d	Cont.	Cont.		
		Short leg cast	Cast care	Cont.	Cont.		Cast on for 4–6 wks
		Hemovac/output		D/C			No infection
		IS/TCDB q hr w/a		PRN			Lungs clear
		Foley to drain, if nec		D/C			Normal bladder Function
Education	Teach postoperative Exercises & care	Reinforce	Reviews Rehab Process		Reinforce		
					View Cast Video if casted		Understands purpose cast & exercises
	Attends preoperative education class	Rev. hosp routine					States reasons to Contact physician
	Pain management						
	Review hosp LOS						
	Teach care of cast and how to live with short leg cast						
				Review cast care			Knows care for cast
D/C Plan	Identify discharge plan		Notify Social Worker Or Home Health Care as appropriate				Discharged to home
	Caregivers & home situation (LOS 2–4 days)						Patient knows when to contact physician

THE FOOT

FRACTURES

HEEL FRACTURES

A fracture is suspected when a patient has pain in the heel following trauma. The calcaneus is the most frequently fractured of the tarsal bones (Fig. 11–9). Fractures may be caused by a powerful contraction of the gastrocnemius and soleus muscles or by direct trauma to the heel (e.g., when a falling person lands on their feet). As a rule, two general types of fractures occur, avulsion fractures through the posterior portion of the bone, and comminuted or crush fractures involving the talocalcaneal joint. A fracture of the calcaneus may also be accompanied by a compression fracture of a vertebra or an avulsion of the Achilles tendon from its insertion. Characteristic signs of a fractured calcaneus bone are that the heel is broadened and that the hollows beneath the malleoli are obliterated because of exudate. Later, ecchymosis appears around the heel. All movements of the calcaneus are painful and markedly restricted. Roentgenograms help to confirm the presence, site, and extent of the fracture.

Medical treatment is focused on restoring the contour of the bone, particularly the plantar surface and the talocalcaneal joint, while maintaining joint motion. Many of the fractures are treated not with attempted reduction, but by compression dressings, nonweight bearing, and early joint motion. Fractures with substantial widening of the calcaneus, however, are usually reduced by manual compression and are immobilized using a short leg cast. (For nursing care of a patient with a short leg cast, see Chapter 5.) Some fractures may require surgical intervention. Depending on the location of the fracture and the degree of comminution, the fracture may be repaired by skeletal traction, pin or screw fixation, or open reduction with bone graft.

Fractures of the calcaneus may result in prolonged incapacity and, in some cases, permanent disability and pain. The major complication is the development of traumatic arthritis at the talocalcaneal joint. If this occurs, the patient will have pain on weight bearing, particularly with motions requiring eversion and inversion of the foot. If the pain persists despite nonoperative methods, a triple arthrodesis may be done.

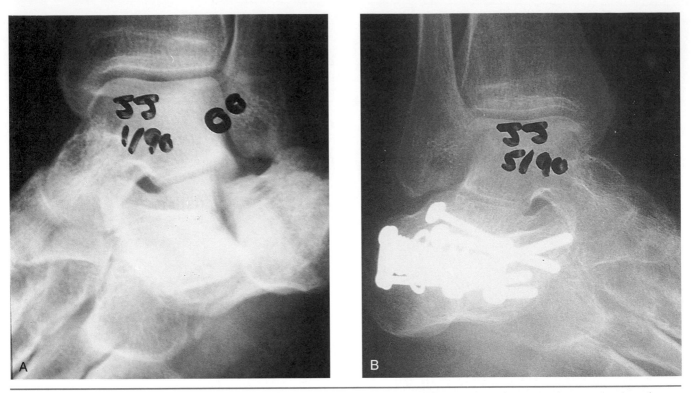

Figure 11–9   (A) Displaced intra-articular calcaneus fracture. (B) stabilized with lag screws and a cervical reconstruction plate. *(Koval & Zuckerman (1998).* Fractures in the Elderly. *Philadelphia:* Lippincott-Raven.)

METATARSAL FRACTURES

Fractures of the metatarsal bones are common (Fig. 11–10 and Fig. 11–11) and may be caused by twisting injuries of the forefoot or by heavy objects falling on the foot. A fracture through the neck of the metatarsal may allow the metatarsal head to displace toward the sole of the foot. Repairs are directed at restoring and maintaining the normal alignment of the longitudinal arch and preventing the subsequent development of a painful plantar callus.

Many displaced metatarsal fractures can be treated by closed reduction and immobilization in a short leg cast. If that is unsuccessful, skeletal traction, percutaneous pinning, or open reduction with internal metallic fixation (using Kirschner wires) may be done. If an open reduction with internal fixation is done, a short leg cast is usually applied (see Chapter 5). After 3 weeks, the Kirschner wires are removed and a walking boot cast is applied for another 3 to 5 weeks until the fracture is well healed.

March Fractures. A march fracture is a stress fracture of a metatarsal shaft, often involving minimal or no trauma. Such fractures can occur during a long march, hence the name. Roentgenograms may be negative initially because the fracture is hairline with no displacement of fragments. Later, as callus forms around the fracture, roentgenography reveals that a fracture existed. Clinically, there is a tenderness at the middle of the involved metatarsal shaft, and flexion or extension of the toes may be painful. Treatment usually consists of avoidance of weight bearing or walking,

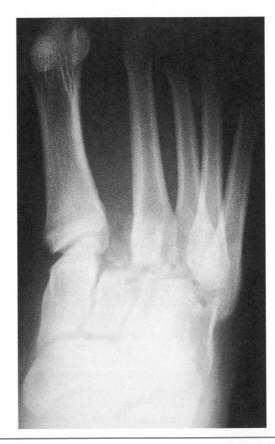

Figure 11–10   Lisfranc's fracture dislocation of the left foot with flecks of bone at the base of the second metatarsal. *(Koval & Zuckerman (1998).* Fractures in the Elderly. *Philadelphia: Lippincott-Raven.)*

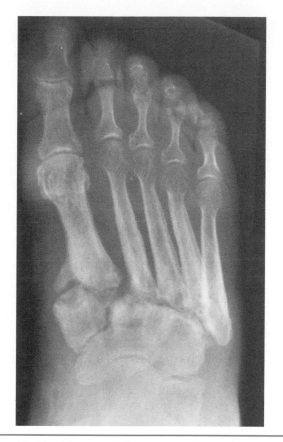

Figure 11–11   Charcot midfoot fracture dislocation.   *(Koval & Zuckerman. (1998). Fractures in the Elderly. Lippincott-Raven.)*

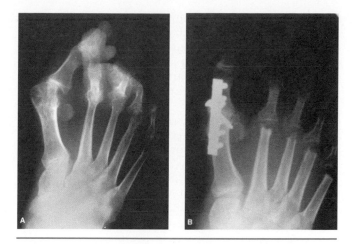

Figure 11–12   A rheumatoid foot. (A) Preoperative radiograph of typical rheumatoid changes with a severe hallux valgus deformity and subluxation and dislocation of the lesser metatarsophalangeal joints. (B) Reconstruction using an arthrodesis of the first metatarsophalangeal joint and arthroplasties of the lesser metatarsophalangeal joints. *(Weinstein & Buckwalter (1994).* Turek's Othopaedic: Principles and Their Applications: *Philadelphia: J.B. Lippincott Company.)*

depending upon the severity of the symptoms. When symptoms are severe, a walking cast may be applied for 3 to 4 weeks.

FRACTURES OF THE TOES

A toe fracture is usually caused by trauma, such as by a weight falling on a toe or by stubbing a toe while barefoot. As a rule, these are painful but not serious injuries. The objective of treatment is to maintain the alignment of the toes so that overlapping or hammertoe does not occur. Frequently, this can be accomplished by strapping the broken toe to its neighbor or simply by wearing a sock. If multiple toe fractures are present, a walking cast may be applied for immobilization. (For nursing care of a patient with a short leg cast, scc Chapter 5.)

ARTHRODESIS

ARTHRODESIS OF THE FOOT

An arthrodesis of the foot may be done by a number of procedures. One is the Dunn arthrodesis, where the navicular bone is removed and the foot is displaced posteriorly and fused. Another is the Hoke arthrodesis where the talar head and neck are removed, reduced in size by resection of the bone, replaced, and fused. This procedure permits backward displacement of the foot but jeopardizes the blood supply to the talus. A third is the triple arthrodesis, which fuses the subtalar, the

talonavicular, and the calcaneocuboid joints to correct instability of the foot due to muscle imbalance. A triple arthrodesis is usually indicated when there is a deformity of the foot, with or without instability. After the surgery, the foot is placed in a long leg cast. (For nursing care, see Chapter 5, patient with a fractured tibia and long leg cast.)

At 10 to 14 days, the long leg cast is removed and roentgenography done. If necessary, manipulation to correct alignment is made and a boot cast is applied. (For nursing care, see Chapter 5, patient with a Pott's fracture and short leg cast.) Approximately 6 weeks after surgery, a walking cast is applied and controlled weight bearing begun. The cast is worn until solid bony union is demonstrated both clinically and roentgenographically, which is usually about 12 weeks after surgery. Once the cast is removed, the patient must learn to walk with a fused foot. Fusion of the calcaneus usually results in a stiff "peg leg" gait, with a lack of pushoff. Too much equinus produces a halting gait where the affected foot is kept in front of the body while walking. Thus the patient takes short steps with the arthrodesed foot being pushed ahead of the body and larger steps when the other foot is brought up from the rear. Potential complications are infection, pseudarthrosis, malunion (especially if the cast was applied with the foot in an improper position), nonunion (particularly if the cast was removed too soon), and avascular necrosis of the body of the talus.

ARTHRODESIS OF THE FIRST METATARSOPHALANGEAL JOINT

Arthrodesis of the MTP joint of the great toe is done to salvage the foot after failure of other operations for hallux valgus and rheumatoid arthritis (Fig. 11–12). It is especially useful for active young people who have a painful hallux rigidus. The procedure not only corrects the deformity of the MTP joint but also reduces the varus deformity of the first metatarsal. It involves the excision of the bursa, trimming down the distal end of the metatarsal, and reaming out a hole at the proximal base of the phalanx. The bones are then correctly positioned for fusion. The amount of toe extension for men is usually 15 to 20 degrees. For women who wear medium heels, it is 15 to 25 degrees, but for women who wear high heels at all times, 35 to 40 degrees of extension are usually needed. Some physicians recommend 15 degrees of extension for both men and women and thus limit their patients to a heel height of 3.8 cm. Once the toe is in the desired position, a long screw is inserted that extends almost the entire length of the metatarsal. After surgery, an elastic spica dressing or cast is applied. On the third or fourth postoperative day, weight bearing is permitted. If no cast was applied, a shoe that has been cut away over the toe is used. For 6 weeks, the patient is not allowed to push off with the end of the toe while walking.

GREAT TOE IMPLANT

Patients with rheumatoid arthritis, hallux valgus (Fig. 11–13), hallux rigidus (Fig. 11–14), or a painful or

unstable joint following a bunionectomy may be candidates for implants. The goal of a great toe implant is to relieve pain and provide stability. The procedure involves resection of the proximal third of the great toe. Any exostosis (bony growth) of the head is removed, providing a smooth articular surface. The proximal phalanx is then reamed to accept the stem of the implant, and the implant is put in place. After surgery, a bulky dressing is applied for 3 to 5 days. A dynamic splint is then applied to maintain alignment while allowing motion. The splint is worn constantly for 3 to 4 weeks and then only at night for 4 to 6 weeks. Guarded weight bearing is started at 3 weeks in a wooden-soled postoperative boot. Potential complications following the surgery are infection, dislocation, or breakage of the implant.

DISORDERS OF THE ARCH

FLATFOOT OR PES PLANUS

The Latin term *pes planus* and its English equivalent, *flatfoot*, are generally used to designate any deformity of the foot in which the longitudinal arch is depressed (Fig. 11–15). Clinically, different types of pes planus are distinguished based on whether the arch is relatively too

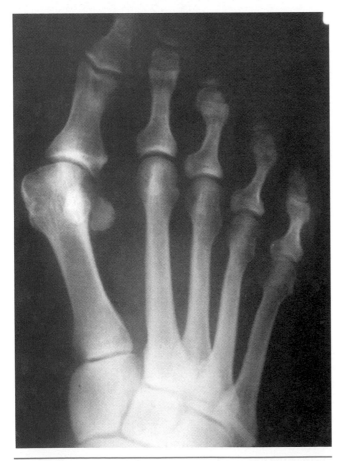

Figure 11–13   Radiograph of a hallux valgus deformity. Note the lateral deviation of the proximal phalanx on the metatarsal head, the medial deviation of the metatarsal head, and subluxation of the sesamoids.   *(Weinstein & Buckwalter (1994). Turek's Othopaedic: Principles and Their Applications: Philadelphia: J.B. Lippincott Company.)*

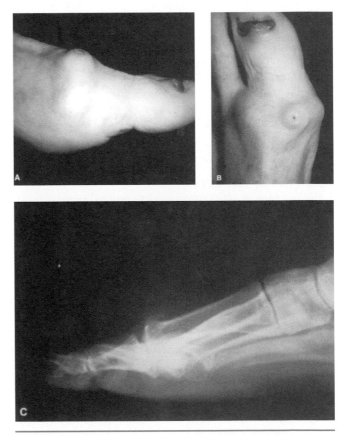

Figure 11–14   (A and B) First metatarsophalangeal joint in a patient with hallux rigidus. Note the increased bulk of the joint and marked osteophyte formation. (C) Lateral radiograph of a patient with hallux rigidus, with a large dorsal osteophyte that mechanically blocks dorsiflexion of the proximal phalanx.   *(Weinstein & Buckwalter (1994). Turek's Othopaedic: Principles and Their Applications: Philadelphia: J.B. Lippincott Company.)*

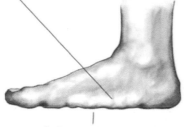

Medial border becomes convex

Sole touches floor

Figure 11–15   Signs of flatfoot may be apparent only when the patient stands, or they may become permanent. The longitudinal arch flattens so that the sole approaches or touches the floor. The normal concavity on the medial side of the foot becomes convex. Tenderness may be present from the medial malleolus down along the medial-plantar surface of the foot. Swelling may develop anterior to the malleoli. Inspect the shoes for excess wear on the inner side of the soles and heels.   *(Bates, B. (1995).* A Guide to Physical Examination and History Taking. *6th ed. Philadelphia: J.B. Lippincott Company.)*

flexible or too rigid and whether the peroneal muscles are spastic or normal. The three principal types are (1) the flexible type with normal peroneals (pronated flatfoot, the most common); (2) the rigid type with normal peroneals (structural flatfoot); and (3) the rigid type with spastic peroneals (spastic flatfoot; Fig. 11–16).

Exercises can be helpful. One is to have the patient stand with their feet and toes inverted (rotated inward along the longitudinal axes) so that the weight is borne on the outer border of the feet. The exercise should be repeated 30 times. Another exercise for the longitudinal arch is done by rising on the balls of the feet, raising the heels, and everting the ankles. The exercise is usually repeated 20 to 30 times. Painful feet in the adult caused by structural or spastic flatfeet may require operative fusion of the subtalar joints (a triple arthrodesis) for pain relief.

METATARSALGIA

If the bones forming the metatarsal arch bear a disproportionate amount of weight, thick calluses may form

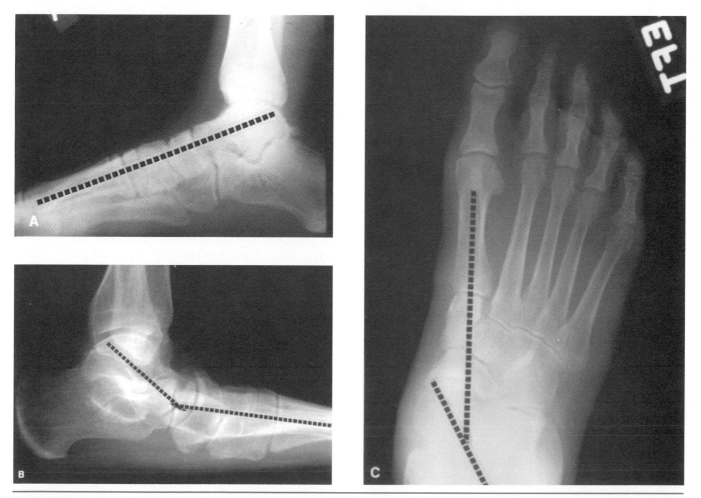

Figure 11–16   Radiographs of the flatfoot deformity. (A) Normal lateral radiograph demonstrating the relation between the long axis of the talus and first metatarsal. (B) In the flatfoot deformity, there is a sagging of the talonavicular joint. (C) In the AP view, there should be a straight line relation between the long axis of the talus and first metatarsal. In flatfoot, this line is disrupted, and there is medial deviation of the head of the talus.   *(Weinstein & Buckwalter (1994).* Turek's Othopaedic: Principles and Their Applications: *Philadelphia: J.B. Lippincott Company.)*

on the ball of the foot and the patient may experience a painful burning sensation in that area with weight bearing. That condition is known as metatarsalgia. It occurs primarily in adults and is more common in women. It may occur alone, but it is frequently seen in association with pronation of the foot. In addition to callus formation and burning pain in the front of the foot, tenderness to palpation is usually noted between the metatarsal heads on the dorsum of the foot. Severe cases may be associated with clawing of the toes.

Exercises that help to relieve symptoms are those that strengthen the muscles of the arch. One of them is the "towel" exercise. A towel is placed on the floor, and the feet are placed parallel to each other about an inch apart, with the heels just over the back edge of the towel. The toes of each foot are then contracted in succession so that the towel is gradually accumulated under the arch. Another exercise is the "marble" exercise. Ten to twelve marbles are placed on the floor and are picked up, moved, and released using the toes and the flexor tendons. Pencils may be used instead of marbles, or the toes may be contracted rhythmically over the edge of a step or a large book upon which the patient is standing.

DEFORMITIES OF THE TOES

HALLUX VALGUS (BUNION)

Hallux valgus (Fig. 11–17) is a deformity of the foot characterized by (1) a valgus deformity of the great toe at the MTP joint so that the base of the proximal phalanx is subluxed laterally, (2) a medial prominence of the first metatarsal head (the bunion), and (3) a varus deformity of the first metatarsal. Hallux valgus may occur with rheumatoid arthritis and osteoarthritis and may be bilateral or unilateral. As hallux valgus develops, the increase in the varus of the first metatarsal decreases the power of the great toe to push off in walking. Thus, the load carried by the second and third metatarsal heads increases, callosities develop beneath them, and the area becomes painful. Corns, calluses, hammertoes, subluxations of joints, and other afflictions of the foot are often associated with hallux valgus of long duration, and all must be treated if discomfort in the foot is to be relieved.

Surgical Treatment of Hallux Valgus (Bunionectomy).
Surgery is indicated in hallux valgus primarily to relieve pain. The surgical procedure should (1) correct the valgus deformity of the proximal phalanx; (2) remove any exostotic bone from medial and dorsal aspects of the first metatarsal head and remove the bursa when necessary; (3) correct the varus deformity of the first metatarsal; (4) correct any excessive tightness of the extensors of the great toe; and (5) correct any associated deformities of the forefoot, such as corns, hammertoes, and subluxations of joints. Six different operations have been devised to correct hallux valgus.

The McBride operation frees the adductor hallucis tendon from the proximal phalanx and attaches it to the first metatarsal so the proximal phalanx is no longer pulled into valgus position, which helps correct the varus deformity of the first metatarsal. That procedure is used in younger and middle-aged patients when the deformity is only moderate, and it only involves a revision of soft tissue.

The Keller operation resects the proximal half of the proximal phalanx of the great toe, which shortens the toe and relaxes the conjoined adductor tendon and the contracted lateral part of the joint capsule, correcting the deformity. A Kirschner wire is inserted longitudinally through the great toe and into the first metatarsal. The Keller procedure is used for most patients who require excision of bone, especially for those with hallux rigidus and with lesser degrees of degenerative arthritis of the first MTP joint. Patients should be advised that for several months after surgery the toe will be floppy and plump, that it will be permanently shortened, and that active control of it will be slightly impaired.

The Lapidus operation is designed to narrow the angle at the base of the first and second metatarsals, remove any exostotic bone from the head of the first metatarsal, and release the pull of the adductor hallucis. The first metatarsocuneiform joint and the adjacent bases of the first and second metatarsal are arthrodesed to hold the first metatarsal shaft in alignment. Weight bearing after surgery is delayed until fusion takes place, which requires some 2 to 3 weeks. The procedure is used in patients with hallux valgus where the primary deformity is congenital varus angulation of the first metatarsal and the associated valgus angulation of the great toe is secondary.

The Mitchell operation involves an osteotomy made through the first metatarsal, which displaces the metatarsal head laterally and slightly plantarward. Because the time required for healing after osteotomy is longer than for most other surgeries for hallux valgus, the Mitchell operation is usually more suitable for young and middle-aged patients who can calcify bone more rapidly and are better able to ambulate without weight bearing than are the elderly. Significant arthritic changes or limitations of motion in the MTP joint may make the Mitchell operation unsuitable.

The Stone operation consists of an incomplete resection of the first metatarsal head. It is used, though not frequently, in the treatment of hallux rigidus and hallux valgus. The Joplin operation was devised not only to correct hallux valgus but also to reduce splaying of the foot and varus deformities of the first metatarsal. The procedure is rarely used today.

NURSING PROCESS (Patient with a Bunionectomy)

The following nursing process demonstrates nursing care following a bunionectomy. The nursing process begins when the patient returns to the unit. (Note, some

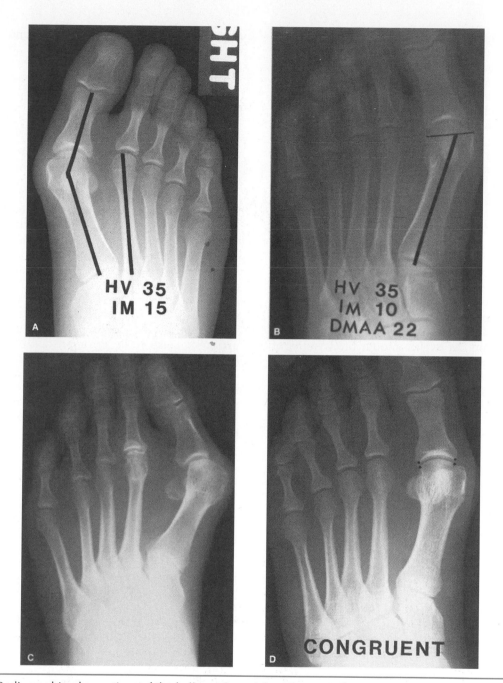

Figure 11–17   Radiographic observations of the hallux valgus deformity. (A) Hallux valgus angle: normal (less than 15 degrees). Intermetatarsal angle: normal (less than 9 degrees). (B) Distal metatarsal articular angle (DMAA): normal (less than 10 degrees lateral deviation). (C) Marked obliquity of the metatarsocuneiform joint should alert clinician to possible instability of this joint. (D) A congruent joint is one in which there is no lateral subluvation of the proximal phalanx on the articular surface of the metatarsal head.   *(Weinstein & Buckwalter (1994).* Turek's Othopaedic: Principles and Their Applications: *Philadelphia: J.B. Lippincott Company.)*

patients may have the surgery done as an outpatient and not be admitted to the hospital.)

ASSESSMENT

After a general assessment of the total patient, the focus is on the affected foot. On the patient's return from sur-

gery after a bunionectomy, check the neurovascular status of the toes at least every 2 hours for the first 24 hours, and then every 8 hours, even if the patient has no complaints. Note the temperature and skin color of the toes and if there is any swelling or drainage. To help determine the temperature of the affected foot, check the temperature of the other foot. There may be some discoloration of the toes from solutions used in the surgical preparation of the foot. Check the circulation of the toes by blanching; realize, however, that the ability to blanch may be impaired or incomplete because of the surgical procedure. For example, following a Keller procedure, which includes a correction of a hammertoe, pins, protective splints, or casts may extend over the end of the foot. Temperature may thus be the most important measure for assessing circulatory status. Bloody drainage is usually not present on the external dressing or cast.

Determine the motor function of the foot by evaluating the patient's ability to wiggle or move their toes. Check to make sure the swelling, cast, splints, or dressing are not impeding movement. Determine the sensory response as indicated by complaints of numbness, tingling, or lack of feeling in any toe when tested by a sharp or dull touch. Postoperative pain in the foot may make it difficult for the patient to distinguish between pain from the operation and pain due to nerve pressure or circulatory impairment. Determine the amount, kind, and location of pain. Note the amount of elevation of the foot and whether it is safely secured in that position with no pressure on the heel. There should be support under the full length of the leg and support along both sides of the leg to prevent rotation. No linen should be in contact with the elevated foot, and ice bags should be placed alongside the foot for the first 24 to 48 hours.

NURSING DIAGNOSIS

Based on all of the assessment data, the major nursing diagnoses for a typical patient following a bunionectomy may include the following:

- Pain and discomfort related to bone and soft-tissue trauma to the MTP joint of the great toe
- Impaired physical mobility related to lack of MTP joint stability
- Increased anxiety related to knowledge deficit about the ability to walk after surgery

COLLABORATIVE PROBLEMS

- Recurrence of the deformity
- Hallux varus deformity
- Clawing of the great toe
- Necrosis of the edges of the wound
- Numbness of the great toe
- Limitation of motion of the MTP joint
- Contractures of the web between the first and second toes.

GOAL FORMULATION AND PLANNING

The goal is for the patient to experience (1) an absence of pain in the foot and toes by elevation, immobilization, and medications; (2) an increase in mobility through immobilization of the toes and the use of crutches; (3) a decrease in anxiety through knowledge

of the surgery and the rehabilitation; and (4) an absence of complications. Long-term goals are to have the patient free of pain and to have return of toe and foot function with no residual complications.

INTERVENTIONS

ALLEVIATE PAIN

The foot is usually elevated higher than the heart for the first 72 hours to prevent or reduce swelling. With the foot elevated, the heel must be free of pressure. To promote comfort and prevent swelling after surgery, ice bags are placed along the side of the foot near the incision site. Ice bags should not be placed directly on swollen toes as that will only increase pain. The source of the swelling is in the area of the incision; thus, the ice is needed there. A surgical glove, a small plastic glove, or a small plastic bag filled with ice may be sufficient, and it can be secured alongside the foot by a roll of gauze or (if the patient has a cast) adhesive tape.

The linen needs to be kept off the foot to reduce pressure. This can be accomplished by a bed cradle, a footboard at the end of the bed, or rods attached to the bed frame that support the linen and thus prevent it from touching the foot. Such precautions are especially important for patients with a Kirschner wire, as the linen can catch on the wire and cause an increase in pain, bright red drainage, and a displacement of the wire.

During the first 24 to 48 hours, the patient may need pain medication every 3 hours, even with the preceding nursing measures. Once the patient starts to ambulate, there may be throbbing pain in the foot. The source of pain must be determined. It could be from the surgical procedure, the cast, or from a distorted or unnatural gait.

INCREASE MOBILITY

Interventions to increase mobility are correct positioning, exercises, and ambulation.

Position. For the first 24 to 48 hours, the patient has restricted ambulation or even bed rest, depending on the surgical procedure. If the patient is in bed, encourage them to turn and change position while still keeping the foot elevated. In the beginning, it is usually necessary to assist the patient in turning by holding and turning the affected foot, repositioning the pillows, and replacing the foot on the pillows. The patient can lie prone, but it is difficult to do so and still keep the foot elevated, the toes free of pressure, and the ice bags in place.

Exercises. Active range-of-motion exercises to all unaffected joints are usually started immediately after surgery. Encourage quadriceps-setting exercises and, if the foot is not in a cast, plantar and dorsiflexion exercises of the ankle for 5 minutes every hour the patient is awake. Exercises to build up strength in the upper extremities are started if the patient will be using crutches.

Ambulation. Different surgical procedures allow ambulation, with or without weight bearing, at different times. Following a McBride procedure, the patient is usually allowed up in a chair or wheelchair after 72 hours, and guarded weight bearing is started 12 to 14 days postsurgery. An elastoplast dressing is usually worn until the wound is healed and the sutures removed. An adhesive strapping to hold the toes in slight varus is then worn for 2 to 3 weeks before the patient is allowed to gradually resume activities. With a Keller procedure, the patient will have a Kirschner wire protruding from the end of the great toe; the wire may or may not be covered by a small cork. The Kirschner wire and dressing are usually removed at approximately 12 to 14 days after surgery, and walking is then begun. After a Mitchell procedure, the great toe is splinted in 5 degrees of flexion and in slight varus position, usually by means of tongue blades applied to the dorsal, medial, and plantar aspects of the foot and toe. The splint is removed after 10 days, and a walking boot cast is applied and worn until the osteotomy heals (approximately 4 to 8 weeks). Following a Stone procedure, full weight bearing is allowed as soon as the patient is comfortable, usually 2 or 3 days postsurgery. The dressing and sutures are usually removed 8 to 10 days after surgery, and a felt pad is placed between the great and second toes. The pad is usually worn for 2 to 3 weeks and then replaced with a smaller pad that is worn for 4 to 5 months. At about 4 weeks postsurgery, a normal, large, soft shoe can be worn by the patient.

Pain or throbbing in the foot may be experienced when the patient begins to ambulate, with or without crutches. Patients are usually very apprehensive about bumping their toes. They tend to distort their normal gait to avoid pressure on the toes and the forefoot and thus tend to walk on their heels, which usually causes pain in the ankles or calves.

PATIENT TEACHING AND HOME CARE CONSIDERATIONS
Efforts should focus on the specific type of surgical procedure and the rehabilitation process. If the patient is to ambulate on crutches, reinforce the instructions given by the therapist. Patients need encouragement and understanding to overcome their hesitancy to walk on the affected foot. In the beginning, patients will not want to walk on the foot at all. Then they tend to walk on the heel, before developing a flat-footed gait with no pushoff that can be used until healing is complete. Patients may need to be reminded that correct posture helps avoid fatigue. They should also be instructed as to the importance of frequent rest periods with the foot elevated during the convalescent period.

Patients need to understand that it is necessary for them to discard their old shoes, because they are shaped to their foot before surgery and therefore apply stress to the corrected foot. Following a Keller procedure, however, patients may use an old pair of shoes cut out over the great toes until the wire is removed. Following a McBride procedure, some patients may need properly placed metatarsal pads in their shoes for several months.

For patients who are discharged with a cast, information on cast care needs to be given (see Chapter 5). All patients should be instructed on the signs and symptoms of infection and what to do if an infection develops.

MONITORING AND MANAGING POTENTIAL PROBLEMS

The major complication following a bunionectomy is infection. Institute nursing measures to prevent infection, and discuss these measures with the patient since the hospital stay is very short if at all. Other complications from the procedure include (1) recurrence of the deformity, (2) a hallux varus deformity, (3) clawing of the great toe, (4) necrosis of the edges of the wound, (5) numbness of the great toe, (6) limitation of motion of the MTP joint, and (7) contractures of the web between the first and second toes.

EVALUATION/OUTCOMES

Determine whether postoperative pain in the foot has been relieved by nursing measures and pain medication. Evaluate the circulation and neurologic status of the foot. Check that the dressing or the cast is not too tight and that there is no swelling of the toes. The leg should be correctly aligned and elevated on pillows. When walking with crutches, the patient should have a safe, steady gait. If not, more instruction and work with the therapist may be needed. Determine whether the patient feels confident about going home with a dressing and pins or a cast. If not, ask questions to determine what the patient does not understand, and explain it again.

CLINICAL PATHWAY (Patient with a Bunionectomy)

An example of a generic clinical pathway for a patient with a bunionectomy is presented in Figure 11–18.

BUNIONETTE (TAILOR'S BUNION)
Bunionette, or tailor's bunion, is a varus angulation of the fifth toe at the MTP joint that tends to develop in splayed (or flat) feet. Pressure from poorly fitted shoes may then cause chronic inflammation of the bursa on the lateral aspect of the fifth metatarsal head and a hard corn on the dorsolateral aspect of the proximal interphalangeal joint of the fifth toe. When surgery is indicated by chronic pain, one of two procedures is generally done. In the first procedure, the lateral third of the fifth metatarsal head is resected, and in the second, the entire head of the fifth metatarsal is removed. The procedures shorten and realign the fifth toe, relieving pressure on any hard corn that may be present.

After surgery, a compression dressing is applied. Weight bearing is resumed approximately 10 days or less after surgery, using a cast shoe or shoes with the part over the fifth metatarsal head removed to prevent

Figure 11–18

Clinical Pathway: Bunionectomy

Admission Date: _____   Discharge Plan: _____ Home _____ Skilled Nursing _____ Extended Care Facility

Pathway	Preadmission Office/OP clinic	Admission Day Op day	Hosp Day 2 Post-op 1	Hosp Day 3 Post-op 2	Hosp Day 4 Post-op 3	Hosp Day 5 Post-op 4	Outcomes
Consultation	Primary Care/Medical physician	Case Manager Anesthesia Review & Add					Returns for MD appt
Assessment	Nrsg database H & P Exam. by MD, NP, or PA	Review H & P Postop routine	Resolved				
Tests	ECG/UA/Chem7 Coag. studies, if approp.						
Medications	D/C NSAIDs/ASA b/4 OR	✓ preadm meds Routine meds Oral Antibiotics					States meds, when to take and purpose
	Instruct on preop meds b/4 OR						Pain controlled with oral medications
	Analgesics as nec.	Oral pain meds					
Diet	Assessment wt. & presurgery diet	NPO @ MN b/4 OR	Diet as tolerated				Tolerating diet
Activity	Preop mobility cane/walker	Ankle Pumps	Cont.				Use cane/walker
		Elevate leg on pillow	Cont.when in bed				Cont.when sitting
		BR or Restricted amb for 24–48 hours	Up in Chair/WC				Limited activity/ WC PWB
Treatments		IV fluids, if nec. Drain	D/C				Returns for removal
		Dressing					Returns for change No infection
Education	Teach postoperative care	Reinforce	Reviews Rehab				
	Pain management Home care of foot						Knows when to Contact physician
	Review hosp LOS						
D/C Plan	Identify discharge plan LOS (0–1 day). The procedure is usually done as an outpatient, and then patient goes home when awake and pain under control						Knows activity level
							Knows when to contact physician

pressure. Wide shoes with medium or low heels should be worn for several months after surgery. A circular elastic metatarsal support that holds the metatarsal heads in close alignment during weight bearing is useful during the first few weeks after surgery to help prevent recurrence of the deformity.

HAMMERTOES

With a hammertoe deformity, the proximal interpha-
langeal joint is flexed and the distal interphalangeal joint is either flexed or extended (Fig. 11–19). The metatarsal head is depressed and prominent on the plantar surface of the foot, causing a painful callosity to develop. Irritation from shoes may cause corns to develop on the dorsum of the flexed proximal interphalangeal joint and on the end of the toe. The deformity may affect one or more toes and may either be congenital or acquired. When acquired, it is usually caused by wearing poorly fitted shoes and is often associated with hallux valgus. The second toe is most often affected.

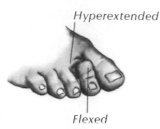

Figure 11–19   Most commonly involving the second toe, a hammertoe is characterized by hyperextension at the metatarsophalangeal joint with flexion at the proximal interphalangeal joint. A corn frequently develops at the pressure point over the proximal interphalangeal joint.
(Bates, B. (1995). A Guide to Physical Examination and History Taking. 6th ed. Philadelphia: J.B. Lippincott Company.)

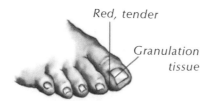

Figure 11–20   In an ingrown toenail, the sharp edge of a toenail may dig into and injure the lateral nail fold, resulting in inflammation and infection. A tender, reddened, overhanging nail fold, sometimes with granulation tissue and purulent discharge, results. The great toe is most often affected.   *(Bates, B. (1995). A Guide to Physical Examination and History Taking. 6th ed. Philadelphia: J.B. Lippincott Company.)*

A common surgical procedure to correct the deformity is the resection of bone from the middle phalanx and the head of the proximal phalanx to allow the toe to be straightened and the remaining osseous surfaces to be opposed. The bones are then fixed together with a longitudinal Kirschner wire to promote fusion. After surgery, the end of the wire is sealed with a collodion dressing and capped with a small sterile cork. If additional immobilization is required, the toe is strapped with adhesive tape to an adjacent toe. Weight bearing is allowed with a wooden-soled cast shoe, and the wire is removed 3 to 4 weeks after surgery. The patient needs to be aware that the affected toe will be straightened, but it will be shorter and the middle joint will be fused.

INGROWN TOENAIL

The term *ingrown toenail* is misleading. The nail does not grow in, but rather soft tissues overgrow and obliterate the medial and lateral side grooves of the nail. An ingrown toenail can be caused by an excessively short trimming of the nail or by a crowding of the toes in shoes or tight stockings. As the nail grows, its corner penetrates the overgrown soft tissue and infection with suppuration develops. Ingrown toenails almost always involve the great toe (Fig. 11–20).

Conservative measures are to control the infection by wet packs and rest and to try and allow the nail to grow out beyond the obliterated groove by elevating it using a small bit of cotton, a metal shield, or even a plastic

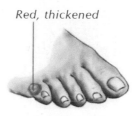

Figure 11–21   A corn is a painful conical thickening of skin that results from recurrent pressure on normally thin skin. The apex of the cone points inward and causes pain. Corns characteristically occur over bony prominences (e.g., the 5th toe). When indicated in moist areas (e.g., at pressure points between the 4th and 5th toes), they are called corns.
(Bates, B. (1995). A Guide to Physical Examination and History Taking. 6th ed. Philadelphia: J.B. Lippincott Company.)

strip. Once the nail has grown out, the toenail must always be trimmed squarely across the end so each corner always extends beyond the groove, or the condition will reoccur. If a conservative method is unsuccessful, surgery is done to remove all or a portion of the nail. A light elastic dressing is applied. The foot is elevated to help prevent swelling and reduce pain. The dressing is changed in 24 to 48 hours, and the patient is allowed to walk in a cast shoe or a shoe that has the top cut out over the toe. The nail grows back normally in 8 months.

COMMON FOOT PROBLEMS

HARD CORNS (CLAVUS DURUM)

A hard corn is a thickening of the soft tissue over a bony prominence and is usually caused by pressure over a period of time. The most common hard corn on the foot is on the dorsolateral aspect of the proximal interphalangeal joint of the fifth toe (Fig. 11–21). The hard corn is caused by a flexion-adduction deformity of the toe that causes the toe to press against the shoe. A corn in that location can be permanently cured only by shortening the fifth toe and removing the osseous deformity. Corns may also develop on the dorsum of the proximal interphalangeal joints of the other toes. One caused by a hammertoe or claw toe deformity spontaneously disappears after the toe has been shortened and the deformity has been corrected. A corn may be softened with hot water or preparations containing salicylic acid and then trimmed with a scalpel. Steps should also be taken to relieve pressure on bony prominences from tight-fitting shoes.

SOFT CORNS (CLAVUS MOLLUM)

Soft corns typically develop between the toes and are soft because of the moistness of the area. Although a soft corn may develop between any two toes, it develops most frequently on the lateral aspect of the base of the fourth toe, deep in the web between the fourth and fifth toes. There it is usually caused by pressure on the base of the phalanx of the fourth toe by the proximal interphalangeal joint or the distal metaphysis of the proximal phalanx of the fifth toe. The corn is painful and often disabling. It is rare to find a soft corn between the fourth and fifth toes without also finding a hard corn on the dorsolateral aspect of the fifth toe.

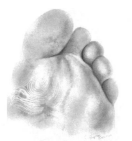

Figure 11–22   Like a corn, a callus is an area of greatly thickened skin that develops in a region of recurrent pressure. Unlike a corn, however, a callus involves skin that is normally thick, such as the sole, and is usually painless. If a callus is painful, suspect an underlying plantar wart.   *(Bates, B. (1995). A Guide to Physical Examination and History Taking. 6th ed. Philadelphia: J.B. Lippincott Company.)*

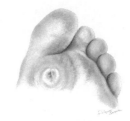

Figure 11–23   A plantar wart is a common wart (verruca vulgaris) located in the thickened skin of the sole. It may look somewhat like a callus or even be covered by one. Look for the characteristic small dark spots that give a stippled appearance to a wart. Normal skin lines stop at the wart's edge.   *(Bates, B. (1995). A Guide to Physical Examination and History Taking. 6th ed. Philadelphia: J.B. Lippincott Company.)*

CALLUS

A callus is a growth composed of a hypertrophied horny layer of squamous epithelium that occurs in response to excessive pressure (Fig. 11–22). It is similar to a corn, but generally larger in size. The usual sites are at the points of bony prominences, such as the plantar aspect of the first metatarsal head, the plantar surface of the second metatarsal head, the dorsal aspect and the tips of clawed toes, the dorsum of the foot at the base of the first metatarsal, the skin overlying a bunion, and over the os calcis at the insertion of the Achilles tendon.

The callus in itself is not painful. As a thickening over a bony prominence, it can increase pressure from the shoe on the tissues beneath, and, in response, a bursa is likely to form beneath it. Traumatic bursitis can then develop and is the most common cause of the discomfort associated with calluses. When a callus develops between the toes, perspiration softens it, and a soft corn results. Removal of pressure is the essence of treatment. Shoes of adequate width with low heels should be worn. A felt pad behind or surrounding (but not over) the bony prominence may relieve some pressure. The callus can be trimmed down to a flat surface. Hot soapy foot soaks are often prescribed, followed by applications of a keratolytic agent, such as a 20% solution of salicylic acid in collodion.

PLANTAR WARTS

A plantar wart is an extremely painful vascular papillomatous growth that may occur on any part of the skin of the sole of the foot (Fig. 11–23). Plantar warts usually occur on the ball of the foot but are situated independent of points of pressure. The surface of the wart is flat and continuous with the adjacent skin and is pressed inward by weight bearing. Usually a large "mother wart" is surrounded by several smaller warts. Callus may form completely over the surface of the wart, increasing the degree of local tenderness. Warts are believed to be caused by viruses and can appear, disappear, and reappear spontaneously. Some of the procedures that have been used to treat plantar warts are surgical removal by local excision with electrocoagulation and surgical excision with roentgenotherapy.

MORTON'S NEUROMA

The most common interdigital neuritis is Morton's neuroma, a painful fusiform swelling of a digital nerve. The most common site is the nerve between the third and fourth toes, but it can also occur between the second and third metatarsals. The neuroma is usually located where the interdigital nerve branches to the two neighboring toes. The condition occurs most often in middle-aged women. The patient usually gives a history of a desire to take off their shoes and massage the metatarsal area. Pain is produced by pressure between the metatarsal heads (in metatarsalgia, tenderness is found by pressure on the plantar surface of the metatarsal heads).

Adequately broad shoes that permit the forefoot to spread may be sufficient treatment. A metatarsal pad behind the heads to elevate the transverse arch can sometimes be of benefit as well. An injection of a local anesthetic with a steroid gives some relief. The injection is given from the dorsum of the foot directly into the interdigital area. Persistence of symptoms may warrant surgical excision of the neuroma.

References

Alonso, J. E. (1996). Ankle fractures. In V. R. Masear (Ed.), *Primary care orthopaedics* (pp. 117–121). Philadelphia: W. B. Saunders.

Bartlett, C. S., & Weiner, L. S. (1998). Tibia and pilon. In K. J. Koval & J. D. Zuckerman (Eds.), *Fractures in the elderly* (pp. 217–232). Philadelphia: Lippincott-Raven.

Bates, B. (1995). *A guide to physical examination and history taking* (6th ed.). Philadelphia: J. B. Lippincott Company.

Cummingham, M. E. (1994). Bursitis and tendinitis. *Orthopaedic Nursing, 13*(5), pp. 13–16.

DiChristina, D., & Garth, W. P. (1996). Ankle sprains. In V. R. Masear (Ed.), *Primary care orthopaedics* (pp. 117–121). Philadelphia: W. B. Saunders.

Folcik, M. A. (1998). Sport-related lower extremity fractures. In V. C. Williamson (Ed.), *NAON: Management of lower-extremity fractures*. Pitman, NJ: National Association of Orthopaedic Nurses.

Garth, W. P. (1996). Overuse syndromes of the upper and lower extremities. In V. R. Masear (Ed.), *Primary care orthopaedics* (pp. 236–245). Philadelphia: W. B. Saunders

Geissler, W. B., Tsao, A. K., & Hughes, J. L. (1996). Fractures and injuries of the ankle. In C. A. Rockwood, D. P. Green, R. W. Buchholz, & J. D. Heckman (Eds.), *Rockwood and Green's fractures in adults* (4th ed., pp. 2201–2266). Philadelphia: Lippincott-Raven.

Heckman, J. D. (1996). Fractures and dislocations of the foot. In C. A. Rockwood, D. P. Green, R. W. Buchholz, & J. D. Heckman (Eds.), *Rockwood and Green's fractures in adults* (4th ed., pp. 2227–2395). Philadelphia: Lippincott-Raven.

Leininger, S. M. (1997). *Building clinical pathways*. Pitman, NJ: National Association of Orthopaedic Nursing.

Mann, R. A. (1994). The adult ankle and foot. In S. L. Weinstein & J. A. Buckwalter (Eds.), *Turek's orthopaedics: Principles and their application* (5th ed., pp. 656–687). Philadelphia: J. B. Lippincott Company.

Masear, V. R. (1996). Fractures and dislocations of the foot. In V. R. Masear (Ed.), *Primary care orthopaedics*. (pp. 128–1141). Philadelphia: W. B. Saunders.

O'Malley, M. J., & DeLand, J. T. (1998). Foot and ankle. In K. J. Koval & J. D. Zuckerman (Eds.), *Fractures in the elderly* (pp. 233–246). Philadelphia: Lippincott-Raven.

Pepe, M., & Hoshowsky, V. M. (1995). Foot and ankle. In V. M. Hoshowsky (Ed.), *NAON: Orientation to the orthopaedic operating room*. Pitman, NJ: National Association of Orthopaedic Nurses.

Whittington, C. F. (1998). Exercise-and sport-related disorders. In A. B. Maher, S. W. Salmond, & T. A. Pellino (Eds.), *Orthopaedic Nursing* (2nd ed., pp. 746–768). Philadelphia: W. B. Saunders.

Chapter

12

Care of a Patient with Hand and Wrist Surgery

Chapter 12 focuses on the treatment and associated nursing care of patients with traumatic and pathologic conditions of the wrist and the hand, from minor sprains to amputations and reconstructive surgery. The chapter begins with a review of the anatomy of the wrist and the hand.

ANATOMY

BONES

The skeleton of the wrist and the hand has four main segments: (1) the distal radius and ulna, (2) the carpal or wrist bones, (3) the metacarpal bones of the palm, and (4) the phalanges or bones of the fingers (Fig. 12–1).

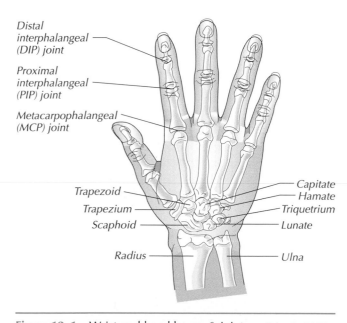

Figure 12–1 Wrist and hand bones & joints. *(Bates, B. (1995). A Guide to Physical Examination and History Taking. 6th ed. Philadelphia: J.B. Lippincott Company.)*

DISTAL RADIUS AND ULNA

The distal portion of the radius, its widest end, is four-sided. With the arm in pronation, the medial surface of the radius is slightly rough and projects downward beyond the rest of the bone to form a styloid process. Its lateral surface is the ulnar notch, a smooth strip, concave for articulation with the head of the ulna in the inferior radioulnar joint. The anterior surface is a thick, prominent ridge, and the posterior surface is marked by the dorsal tubercle. The most distal surface of the radius is smooth and articulates with the wrist bones.

The distal ulna is slightly enlarged and comprises a rounded head and a styloid process. With the arm in pronation, the head forms a surface elevation on the lateral part of the posterior aspect of the wrist. The styloid process is then a short, rounded projection from the lateral aspect of the distal ulna.

CARPAL BONES

The carpus (wrist) is composed of eight carpal bones that are arranged in proximal and distal rows, each containing four bones. With the arm in supination, the bones of the proximal row from lateral to medial are the scaphoid (navicular), the lunate, the triquetrium, and the pisiform. The bones of the distal row are the trapezium, the trapezoid, the capitate, and the hamate. In the proximal row, the pisiform is on the palmar surface of the triquetrium bone and is separated from the other carpal bones. The other bones of the proximal row form an arch that articulates with the radius and the articular disc of the distal radioulnar joint.

METACARPAL BONES

The metacarpus (palm) consists of five metacarpal bones, conventionally numbered from lateral to medial (with the arm in supination). The metacarpals are miniature long bones, each possessing a rounded head, a shaft, and an expanded base. The heads are the distal ends and articulate with the proximal phalanges. The prominence of the knuckles is produced by the metacarpal heads. The bases are the proximal ends and articulate with the distal row of the carpal bones and with one another, except that the first metacarpal bone (for the thumb) is isolated and does not articulate with the second metacarpal bone.

PHALANGEAL BONES

There are 14 phalanges, two in the thumb and three in each of the other digits. Each has a head, a shaft, and a base or proximal end. The bases of the proximal phalanges articulate with the heads of the metacarpal bones.

JOINTS OF THE WRIST AND HAND

THE DISTAL RADIOULNAR JOINT

The distal radioulnar joint is a uniaxial pivot joint between the distal end (head) of the ulna and the ulnar notch of the distal end of the radius. The joint surfaces are enclosed in an articular capsule and held together by an articular disc.

The movements that take place at the radioulnar joint result in pronation and supination of the hand. The muscle producing pronation is the pronator quadratus, which is aided during rapid movement and movement against resistance by the pronator teres. The muscle producing supination in slow unresisted movements and when the elbow is extended is the supinator. It is assisted by the biceps in fast movements with the elbow flexed, especially when resistance is encountered.

THE RADIOCARPAL OR WRIST JOINT

The radiocarpal or wrist joint is a biaxial joint. Proximally, it is formed by the distal end of the radius and the lower surface of the articular disc between the radius and the ulna, and distally by the scaphoid, the lunate, and the triquetral bones. The fibrous articular capsule of the radiocarpal joint is lined by a synovial membrane. The joint capsule is strengthened by a number of ligaments, specifically the palmar radiocarpal and ulnocarpal, the dorsal radiocarpal, and the radial and ulnar collateral. The movements of the radiocarpal joint are closely associated with those in the intercarpal joints. The arteries supplying the joint are the anterior interosseous, the anterior and posterior carpal branches of the radial and ulnar, the palmar and dorsal metacarpals, and some recurrent branches of the deep palmar arch. The nerves are derived from the anterior and posterior interosseous nerves.

INTERCARPAL JOINTS

The intercarpal joints connect the carpal bones to one another and may be subdivided into (1) joints between the bones of the proximal row of the carpus; (2) joints between the bones of the distal row; and (3) a somewhat complicated and extensive joint between the two rows, termed the midcarpal joint. The carpal bones are connected by an extensive system of ligaments.

CARPOMETACARPAL JOINTS

The five carpometacarpal joints connect the carpal bones to the metacarpal bones. The first is the carpometacarpal joint of the thumb, which is a saddle-shaped joint between the first metacarpal bone and the trapezium and which is held together by lateral, anterior, posterior, and capsular ligaments. The second through fifth are the joints between the carpus and the second, third, fourth, and fifth metacarpal bones. The bones of each of those four joints are united by articular capsules and are strengthened by dorsal, palmar, and interosseous ligaments.

METACARPOPHALANGEAL JOINTS

The five metacarpophalangeal (MCP) joints connect the articulating heads of the metacarpals with shallow concavities in the bases of the proximal phalanges. Each joint has a palmar, a deep transverse metacarpal, and two collateral ligaments.

INTERPHALANGEAL JOINTS

The interphalangeal joints in each digit are uniaxial hinge joints. In addition to a fibrous capsule, each has a palmar and two collateral ligaments. Extensor tendons take the place of dorsal ligaments.

CARPAL ARCH

The carpal bones form an arch that is concave on its palmar surface. The ligament that spans the arch and maintains it is called the flexor retinaculum or the transverse carpal ligament. The ligament is composed of a proximal and a distal band. The proximal band attaches from the tubercle of the scaphoid to the pisiform. The distal band connects the tubercle of the trapezium to the hook of the hamate.

The space between the arched carpal bones and the spanning transverse carpal ligament is termed the carpal tunnel. The tunnel contains the tendons of the flexor digitorum profundus, which lie upon the carpal bones, and the tendons of the flexor digitorum superficialis. Also within the tunnel are the flexor carpi radialis tendon, the flexor pollicis longus tendon, and the median nerve. The transverse carpal ligament protects the median nerve from external pressure.

THE WRIST

The wrist, because of its mobility and exposed position, is frequently subjected to trauma, including lacerating injuries, sprains, dislocations, and fractures.

LACERATIONS

The wrist is the narrowest part of the arm. The tendons, nerves, and blood vessels of the hand must all pass through that narrow neck. Lacerating injuries at the wrist, therefore, can sever tendons, arteries, and nerves and inflict serious damage to the hand. With prompt medical attention, a lacerated or severed artery can usually be repaired or ligated (sutured) without danger of compromising circulation. The repair of severed tendons and nerves is much more difficult, and successful restoration of the hand may depend upon sound surgical judgment and, frequently, the use of microsurgical techniques.

SPRAINS

Wrist sprains can give rise to pain, swelling, and loss of function in the hand. Most sprains of the wrist are momentary subluxations that spontaneously reduce. In a subluxation, as in a complete dislocation, the capsule and the collateral ligaments may be torn. Sprains are usually not detected on roentgenograms and thus tend to be ignored or minimized. Still, many authorities believe sprains of the wrist should be diagnosed as reduced subluxations. In the absence of complications, therefore, they should be treated by immobilization in a slightly flexed position for a period of 2 or 3 weeks, followed by the initiation of progressive active exercises. Despite treatment, limitation and swelling of the wrist may persist for months following a sprain. If pain and discomfort are not quickly reduced by immobilization, however, further investigation is required to eliminate more serious conditions, for example, a fracture of the scaphoid.

DISLOCATIONS

Dislocations of the wrist may occur at the radiocarpal joint or involve the bones of the carpus. Dislocations of the radiocarpal joint are commonly caused by a fall on the palm, which displaces the hand dorsally. Usually, a dislocation of the radiocarpal joint can readily be treated by closed manipulation followed by immobilization for 3 to 4 weeks. If a closed reduction is unsuccessful, an open reduction may be necessary (see Chapter 5).

A dislocation of the lunate bone of the carpus is common and may be caused by a fall on the palm that forces the wrist into sudden extension. In some instances there may not be any other damage to the wrist, but in others it may dislocate anteriorly and proximally, tearing the capsule and coming to rest in the carpal tunnel. In that position, the lunate bone presses against the flexor tendons and causes the hand to be held with the wrist and the fingers in semiflexion. Motion of the wrist and the fingers is painful. The dislocated lunate bone may also press against the median nerve, causing a median neuritis characterized by pain, paresthesia, atrophy, and weakness or paralysis of the muscles of opposition. The injury may be difficult to detect on a roentgenogram.

If diagnosis is made early, closed reduction may be successful. A closed reduction may be accomplished under general or regional anesthesia by prolonged heavy traction or by direct pressure upon the palmar aspect of the lunate with simultaneous traction to the thumb and the fingers. A cast is then applied, or the wrist is immobilized in a dorsal splint with the hand in a compression dressing for the first 24 to 72 hours. After 24 to 72 hours, active range-of-motion exercises of the fingers are begun. The wrist is usually immobilized for 4 to 6 weeks. If closed reduction is not successful, an open reduction is necessary to reduce the dislocated lunate and repair the capsular tear. Some

authorities favor excising a lunate bone if the bone is dislocated for a period longer than 3 weeks before reduction, because of the likelihood that avascular necrosis of the bone will develop. For further discussion and nursing care, see Chapter 5, patient with a dislocated lunate and a short arm cast.

FRACTURES

FRACTURES OF THE DISTAL RADIUS

Colles' Fracture. A Colles' fracture is a nonarticular fracture of the distal radius, with or without a fracture of the ulnar styloid. There is a volar angulation of the radius and a dorsal displacement of the distal fragment. Colles' fractures are commonly produced by a fall on an outstretched hand and may be accompanied by a fracture of the elbow or shoulder. They are often seen in elderly women. Clinically, the wrist appears puffy and deformed. The distal radial fragment gives rise to the characteristic hump ("silver fork" or "dinner fork") deformity seen when the wrist is viewed from the side. Backward displacement of the distal radial fragment causes shortening of the radius and an alteration in the normal position of the radial styloid in relation to the ulnar styloid. There is tenderness over the distal radius and over the ulnar styloid or medial ligament of the wrist. The normal volar concavity of the radius is lost, and the area feels distended to the touch. Roentgenographic examination confirms the diagnosis and also shows if impaction or comminution of the fragments is present. Many Colles' fractures can be adequately reduced by closed manipulation with or without anesthesia. After reduction, the wrist and elbow are immobilized to prevent pronation and supination, and a hand pressure dressing may be applied during the first 24 to 48 hours to help prevent swelling of the fingers. Immobilization can be achieved by the use of a forearm (sugar-tong) splint or a long arm cast (See Chapter 5, patient with a Colles' fracture and a long arm cast). Still other patients may be treated with an external fixation device (see Chapter 7).

Smith's Fracture. A Smith's fracture is a nonarticular fracture of the distal radius with a dorsal angulation of the radius and with the distal fragment and accompanying carpal row of bones displaced volarly (i.e., toward the palm). A Smith's fracture is also known as a reverse Colles' fracture. Smith's fracture is usually secondary to a blow on the dorsum of the wrist or distal radius with the forearm in pronation.

Treatment usually involves closed reduction under anesthesia. In that procedure, with the hand in pronation and flexion, longitudinal traction is applied in line with the deformity until any impacted fragments are dislodged. Supination of the hand and application of dorsal pressure on the distal fragment usually reduce the fracture. Immobilization is accomplished using a long arm cast with the forearm in supination and the wrist in extension. Follow-up care is the same as for a patient with a Colles' fracture in a long arm cast (see Chapter 5). If closed reduction is unsuccessful, open reduction with plate and screws may be used (Fig. 12–2).

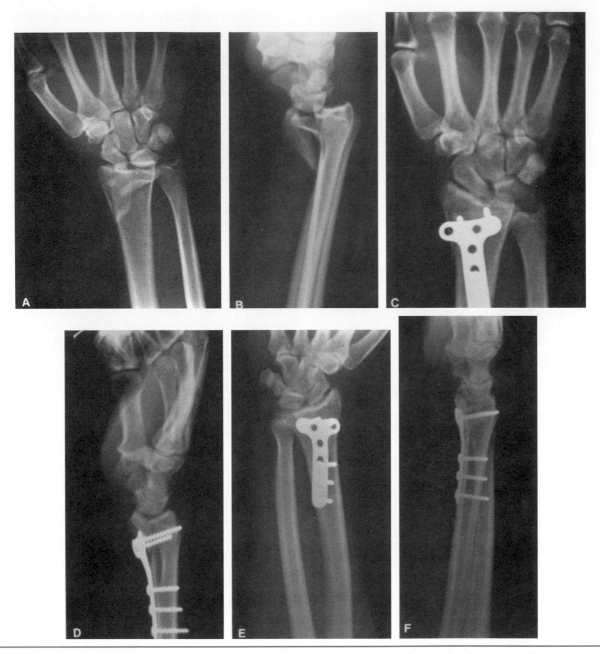

Figure 12–2   Smith's fracture. Palmar displacement of the carpus with a distal radius fracture in a 26-year-old plumber who fell forward from his motorcycle. (A) In the PA view there is an oblique fracture through the radius. Note the double shadow over the lunate, indicating volar displacement. (B) The lateral view shows a fracture of the distal radial articular surface with volar displacement of the carpus; a comminuted intra-articular fracture (Thomas type III). (C, D) Open reduction and volar buttress plate fixation Distal screws were used to hold reduction of the intra-articular fracture components. (E, F) Reduction well maintained (1 year later), with excellent alignment of the joint articular surface and a well-united fracture.   *(Rockwood, et al. (1996).* Rockwood & Green's Fractures in Adults. *Philadelphia: Lippincott-Raven.)*

Stabilizing Distal Radial Fractures.   Most nonarticular distal radial fractures can be successfully treated nonoperatively. When maintenance of the reduction of a Colles' or Smith's fracture requires prolonged immobilization in an extreme position (particularly if the patient is elderly with osteoarthritic changes in the joints of the hand), closed reduction followed by percutaneous pinning of the distal radius through the radial styloid is usually indicated. This method is particularly applicable when there is a large radial styloid fragment

but may be used for many comminuted fractures of the distal radius. After the fracture is manipulated and reduced, two large Kirschner wires are inserted through the radial styloid across the fracture and into the opposite metaphyseal cortex. The wires usually provide sufficient fixation to minimize radial collapse and radial shortening and allow immobilization in a cast with the wrist in a neutral position.

For fractures that are not suitable for percutaneous Kirschner wire stabilization through the radial styloid,

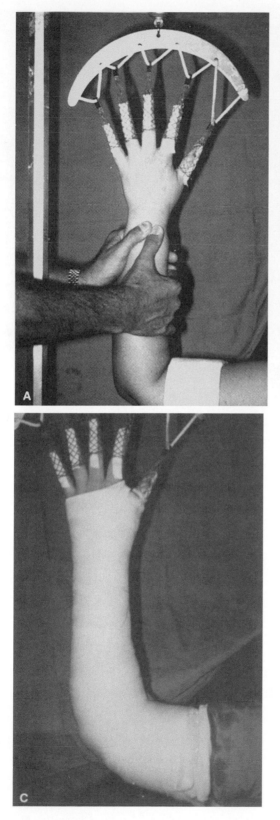

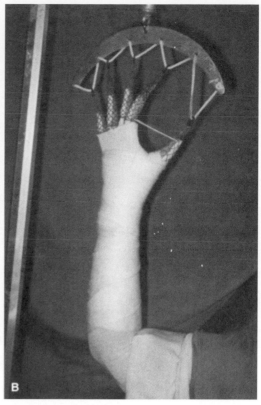

Figure 12–3 Preferred technique of closed reduction for fractures of the distal radius. Undisplaced fractures are treated in a short arm cast, while displaced fractures are treated in a long arm cast. Displaced fractures require (A) gentle manipulation and sustained traction, and (B, C) application of the long arm cast while maintaining traction. The finger traps are removed and the cast trimmed to allow for full finger and thumb motion.   *(Rockwood, et al. (1996). Rockwood & Green's Fractures in Adults. Philadelphia: Lippincott-Raven.)*

pins and plaster or a traction cast are often used and produce good results. Following anesthesia, those fractures are reduced by suspending the forearm from the fingers in Chinese finger traps (Fig. 12–3). After approximately 5 minutes of traction, gentle manipula-

tion helps to reduce the fracture. A Steinmann pin is then inserted transversely through the proximal ulna 7.5 to 10 cm distal to the olecranon, and a second pin is inserted transversely through the bases of the second and third metacarpals. A plaster cast is then applied

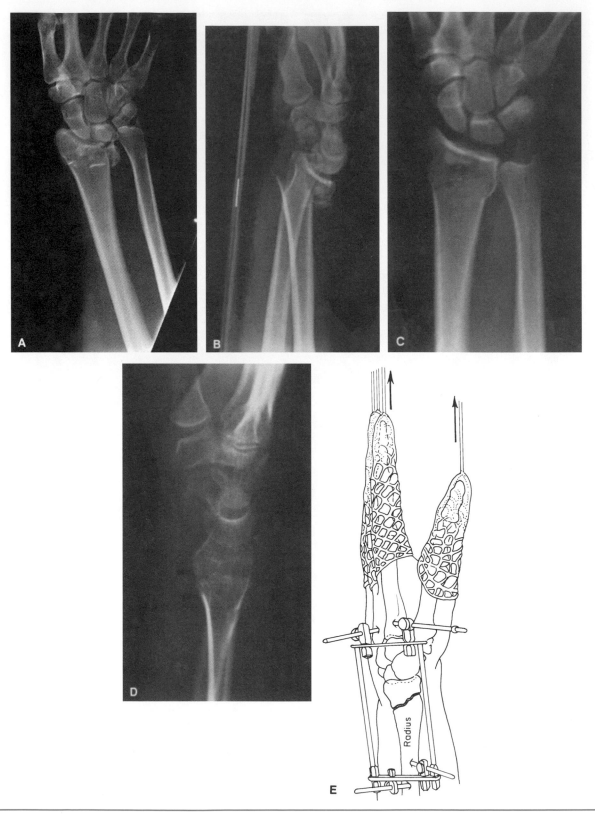

Figure 12–4   A 32-year-old teacher fell on ice and sustained this intra-articular distal radius fracture (type IV). (A) Her intra-articular fracture involved the lunate lossa of the distal radius. (B) Lateral view showing dorsal angulation of 65 degrees with dorsal comminution. (C) Traction view, with anatomical reduction achieved. (D) Anatomical alignment of the palmar cortex (buttress effect). (E) External fixation with a quadrilateral frame was used to maintain the reduction. *(continued)*   *(Rockwood, et al. (1996).* Rockwood & Green's Fractures in Adults. *Philadelphia: Lippincott-Raven.)*

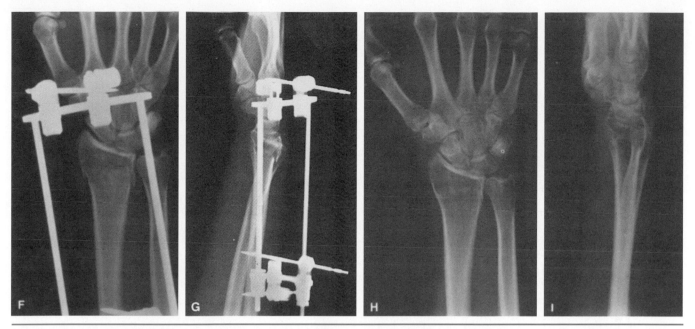

Figure 12–4 (F, G) Radiographic appearance (PA and lateral) at 4 weeks; reduction maintained, (H, I) End result with nearly normal anatomical alignment of the distal radius 7 months postinjury. *(Rockwood, et al. (1996). Rockwood & Green's Fractures in Adults. Philadelphia: Lippincott-Raven.)*

above the elbow, incorporating the two pins. The palm of the cast, once it is dry, is cut back proximal to the flexion crease in the hand to allow full active motion of the fingers. The cast and pins remain in place for a minimum of 8 weeks, as removing the pins earlier may allow the distal radius to shorten or reimpact. An open reduction of Colles' and Smith's fractures is almost never required.

INTRA-ARTICULAR FRACTURES OF THE DISTAL RADIUS

Barton's fractures are distal radial fractures into the joint that involve the dorsal or volar margins of the articular surface. They may be reduced by closed reduction and, when the marginal fracture is small, immobilized satisfactorily with a cast. Dorsal margin fractures are usually more stable when the wrist is dorsiflexed and the forearm pronated, whereas volar margin fractures are usually more stable with volar flexion of the wrist and supination of the forearm (Fig. 12–4). Stability is promoted by the intact carpal ligament opposite the fracture.

When the marginal fracture involves a large portion of the distal articular surface of the radius, closed reduction may be achieved but not maintained because of subluxation of the carpus. Accordingly, many authorities treat volar marginal Barton's fractures with a small buttress plate, and dorsal marginal Barton's fractures with Kirschner wires. The Kirschner wires are used for dorsal fractures instead of a plate and screws because of the location of the extensor tendons. Following the insertion of a small buttress plate and screws, immobilization may not be required, as simple limitation of activity until the fracture heals may be sufficient. In

other cases, however, a plaster sugar-tong splint (see Chapter 5) is used, with gentle active exercises performed 2 or 3 times a day for the following 2 weeks. The splint is removed after 4 weeks, and progressive exercises are continued until union is solid.

FRACTURES OF THE CARPALS

Fractures of the Scaphoid. A fracture of the carpal scaphoid bone is the most common fracture of the carpus and the most commonly undiagnosed fracture of the upper extremity. Acute fractures of the scaphoid are difficult to view on roentgenograms for the first 10 to 14 days after trauma. Fractures of the scaphoid occur in persons 10 years or older but most commonly occur in young adult males. The fracture usually occurs as a result of a fall on an outstretched palm, which causes severe hyperextension and slight radial deviation of the wrist. Limitation of extremes of wrist motion are usually present because of pain and tenderness in the wrist near the styloid process of the radius. Immediate closed reduction and immobilization in a cast for 6 to 12 weeks is the preferred treatment. For further discussion and nursing care, see Chapter 5, care of a patient with a scaphoid fracture in a thumb spica cast.

Other Carpal Fractures. Fractures of other carpal bones are less common but may occur when there is wrist trauma. Because they receive a good blood supply, most fractures of the other carpal bones heal satisfactorily with 6 to 8 weeks of immobilization. If there is significant displacement, reduction is indicated. Of special note is the fracture of the hook of the hamate, which can cause a neurologic deficit.

SURGICAL PROCEDURES

ARTHRODESIS

Arthrodesis of the wrist (fusion of the radiocarpal joint) is indicated when there is gross bone and cartilage destruction or when the carpal bones are markedly subluxed. Fusion of the wrist is most often utilized for tuberculosis, for nonunion or malunion fractures of the scaphoid with associated radiocarpal traumatic arthritis, and for severely comminuted fractures of the distal end of the radius. Less commonly, it is done for Volkmann's ischemic paralysis and for stabilization of the wrist in poliomyelitis and in spastic cerebral palsy of the wrist.

The wrist is fused in a position that will not be fatiguing and will allow maximum grasping strength in the hand. This position is usually neutral or in 10 to 20 degrees of extension, with the long axis of the third metacarpal shaft aligned with the long axis of the radial shaft. Clinically, it is the position that the wrist normally assumes with the fist strongly clenched.

The operative procedure involves denudation of the proximal row of carpals and the distal end of the radius by removing the dorsal aspect of cortical bone. The distal end of the ulna may or may not be removed, and Kirschner wires may or may not be used for internal fixation. Most of the many techniques used to obtain wrist fusion include the use of a bone graft from the ilium. In some, the graft extends from the radius to the proximal carpal bones, but in others it extends distally to the base of the third metacarpal. Some authorities recommend, however, that the second and third carpometacarpal joints always be included in the fusion to prevent the development of any painful motion in those joints, and because the underlying disease process frequently extends into them. At least some carpometacarpal joints will be preserved, and thus some motion in the wrist will be retained.

Once the arthrodesis is completed, a long arm cast is applied from the upper arm to the tips of the fingers and thumb, with the elbow at a right angle, the forearm in neutral position, the wrist at 10 to 15 degrees extension, and the fingers and thumb slightly flexed. To allow for swelling, the dorsum of the cast is windowed. Three weeks after surgery, a short arm cast (from below the elbow to just proximal to the metacarpophalangeal joints) is applied. Support to the wrist is continued until firm fusion is present, ordinarily 10 weeks. For nursing care, see Chapter 5, care of a patient with a dislocated lunate and a short arm cast.

RESECTION OF THE DISTAL ULNA

A resection of the distal ulna is done to relieve pain and restore motion in the wrist. It may be done in instances of malunion or nonunion following a Colles' fracture, pain and disability due to radioulnar arthritis, and dislocation or subluxation of the ulna. The distal ulna is resected approximately one inch from the end of the bone. The ulnar collateral ligament is then sutured to the periosteum to stabilize the end of the ulna. Postoperatively, no immobilization is usually required, and active exercises are allowed the following day. Complications include infection and diminished strength in the wrist.

JOINT IMPLANTS

A wrist implant of flexible silicone is utilized in patients with arthritic or traumatic disabilities resulting in wrist instability due to subluxation, severe deviation of the wrist, stiffness, or fusion of the wrist in a nonfunctional position. The procedure is to provide stability and restore painless motion to the wrist, and involves the removal of the scaphoid, the lunate, the proximal third of the capitate, and the medial portion of the triquestrum. The distal end of the radius is removed, and the intramedullary canal of the radius is reamed. The remaining portion of the capitate and the intramedullary canal of the third metacarpal are also reamed. The wrist joint implant is fitted into the radial canal and through the capitate into the third metacarpal canal. The distal portion of the ulna may or may not be excised and fitted with an ulnar head implant. The extensor tendons may be shortened or transferred as necessary for stabilization. Following closure, a bulky hand dressing is applied. In 3 to 5 days, a short arm cast is applied with the wrist in a neutral position. The cast is worn for 2 to 4 weeks. An outrigger device may be added to the cast if the extensor tendons have been repaired. The primary complications are infection and breakage or dislocation of the implant. Active exercises are begun after cast removal. Nursing measures are focused on prevention of complications and rehabilitation of the wrist.

An ulnar head implant is indicated where there is instability, pain, or weakness of the wrist due to rheumatoid, degenerative, or traumatic arthritis of the ulnar head. The goal of the procedure is to provide painless motion and improve stability in the wrist. The surgical procedure involves the removal of the ulnar head and the implantation of a flexible silicone head. After the initial incision, the ulnar head is excised at the neck and a complete synovectomy is done. The excised end of the ulna is then smoothed, and two holes are drilled into the bone. The ulnar canal is reamed to accept the stem of the ulnar head implant. Nonabsorbable retention sutures, attached to the implant, are then passed through the canal and out the drill holes. With the guidance of the retention sutures, the ulnar implant is inserted into the ulna. After skin closure, a bulky hand dressing and a palmar splint are applied. At approximately 3 to 5 days postoperatively, a short arm cast or splint is applied with the hand in slight dorsiflexion.

IMPLANTS OF CARPAL BONES

Implants of carpal bones significantly improve motion and reduce pain in the wrist for patients with a number of different pathologic conditions, including chronic wrist pain, instability of the joint, recurrent dislocation, avascular necrosis, traumatic arthritis, rheumatoid arthritis, degenerative arthritis, acute fractures, and pseudarthrosis following a fracture. After surgery, the arm is usually immobilized before rehabilitation with exercises is begun. The most common complications are infection and breakage or dislocation of the implant.

To replace the carpal lunate with an implant, the lunate is removed and a hole is drilled into the triquetrum to accept the stem of the implant. A small

Kirschner wire may or may not be used for added stability. If the wire is used, it is placed through the lunate implant and either the radius or an adjacent carpal bone. Postoperative care includes immobilizing the wrist in a short arm cast for 6 weeks. Progressive exercises are begun when the cast is removed. If a Kirschner wire is used, the wire is removed through a window in the cast at 3 weeks.

The installation of a scaphoid implant involves resecting the scaphoid and drilling a small hole in the trapezium to accept the stem of the scaphoid implant. Postoperative care includes the use of a bulky dressing and a volar splint for 3 to 5 days. A short arm cast is then applied and worn for 4 to 6 weeks.

The replacement of the trapezium involves removing that bone and drilling a hole in the proximal metacarpal of the thumb to accept the stem of the trapezium implant. Adjacent tendon reconstruction or a Kirschner wire through the first and second metacarpals may be necessary to achieve stability. Postoperatively, the patient will have a bulky dressing with a splint or a thumb spica for 3 to 5 days. A short arm cast is then applied for 4 to 6 weeks. If a Kirschner wire is used, it is removed at 4 to 6 weeks.

SPECIAL CONDITIONS

GANGLION

A ganglion is a cystic swelling overlying a joint or a tendon sheath (Fig. 12–5). One large main cyst develops and is either uniocular or multiocular. Multiple small accessory cysts usually lie adjacent to the large cyst. The cyst walls are dense fibrous capsules, and the cyst fluid is thick, sticky, clear, and colorless with the consistency of soft jelly. No communication with the joint or tendon sheath is apparent, but invariably the cyst is bound to those structures by dense tissue. A ganglion occurs most frequently about the wrist, but may appear adjacent to any joint or tendon sheath. At the wrist, the cyst's usual location is the dorsum between the long extensor of the thumb and the extensor to the index finger, and it may be traced down to the articulation between the scaphoid and the lunate. Over the volar aspect of the wrist, the swelling often appears between the brachioradialis and the flexor carpi radialis tendons, and it usually is closely adherent to the latter. In the palm of the hand, the ganglion develops from the deep pulley of the finger flexors over the metacarpal heads.

There are two theories to explain why ganglions develop. One is that the dense collagenous tissue of the wrist undergoes degeneration, which leads to the formation of multiple small cysts containing mucin. Over time, several small cysts may coalesce into one large cyst. The other theory postulates a defect in the joint capsule or tendon sheath, which permits a protrusion of synovial tissue. The communicating channel between the protruding tissue and the joint becomes obliterated, and a cyst remains as a nonpatent pedicle or adhesion. If the defect in the capsule or sheath persists, additional cysts may be formed.

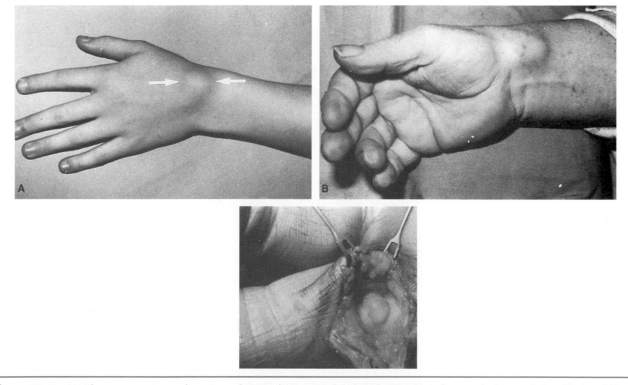

Figure 12–5 (A) The most common location of a ganglion is on the dorsal wrist over the scapholunate joint. (B) Another common location for a ganglion is on the radial aspect of the wrist anteriorly. Careful examination is necessary to distinguish a ganglion in this location from a radial artery aneurysm. (C) A ganglion at the base of the finger arises from the flexor tendon sheath. These are palpable but not visible on physical examination. *(Weinstein & Buckwalter (1994).* Turek's Orthopaedic: Principles and Their Applications: *Philadelphia: Lippincott-Raven.)*

A ganglion of the wrist can be treated by both nonoperative and operative procedures. Nonoperative procedures include (1) aspirating the cyst fluid and injecting the remaining tissue with cortisone, (2) rupturing the cyst by means of an external force; and (3) using roentgenographic therapy (e.g., a 1.5-erythema dose, repeated in one month). However, nonoperative methods are frequently unsuccessful, and surgical excision is required. After surgical removal, a splint is used to immobilize the wrist in a relaxed position for approximately 3 weeks. Once the splint is removed, active exercises are needed because the capsular tightening done at the time of surgery produces a temporary limitation of motion.

CARPAL TUNNEL SYNDROME

Carpal tunnel syndrome, also known as tardy median nerve palsy, results from a compression of the median nerve within the carpal tunnel (where the nerve passes under the transverse carpal ligament on the volar surface of the wrist). It occurs most often in patients between the ages of 30 to 60 years and is 5 times more frequent in women than in men. Any condition that reduces the capacity of the carpal tunnel may initiate the syndrome, for example a malaligned Colles' fracture, infection, trauma, tumor, or rheumatoid tenosynovitis. Systemic conditions such as obesity, diabetes mellitus, thyroid dysfunction, and Raynaud's disease can also produce the syndrome. However, many patients have no systemic condition but have engaged in repetitive motion activities of the wrist that could have initiated the syndrome.

Paresthesia over the sensory distribution of the median nerve is the most frequent symptom. Pain frequently causes the patient to awaken during the night with a burning and numbness of the hand that is relieved by exercise. Tinel's sign may also be demonstrated in most patients by percussing the median nerve at the wrist (Fig. 12–6). Some atrophy of the thenar muscles, which are innervated by the median nerve, is frequently reported. Acute flexion of the wrist for 60 seconds (Phalen's test) or strenuous use of the hand increases the paresthesia. Application of a blood pres-

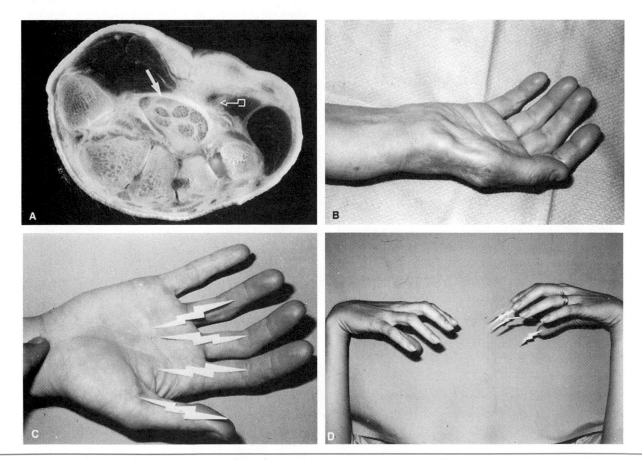

Figure 12–6   (A) At the level of the metacarpal bases, the median nerve (*closed arrow*) lies beneath the dense transverse carpal ligament. Tenosynovitis in the adjacent tendons can cause carpal tunnel syndrome. The ulnar nerve (*open arrow*) lies more superficially in a less well-defined tunnel. (B) Severe carpal tunnel syndrome causes wasting of the median innervated thenar musculature. Note the flattening of the normally convex thenar contour. (C) Tinel's sign is elicited by gently tapping over the median nerve just proximal to the carpal canal. A positive test elicits paresthesia in the thumb, index, middle finger, and radial half of the ring finger. (D) The Phalen wrist flexion test is positive for carpal tunnel syndrome when paresthesia appears or increases in the median nerve distribution within one minute.   *(Weinstein & Buckwalter (1994).* Turek's Orthopaedic: Principles and Their Applications: *Philadelphia: Lippincott-Raven.)*

sure cuff on the upper arm sufficient to produce venous distention may also initiate the symptoms.

Conservative management includes splinting the extremity at night in a neutral position to prevent hyperextension and prolonged flexion of the wrist. If mild symptoms exist and there is no thenar muscle atrophy, an injection of hydrocortisone into the carpal tunnel may give relief. When the symptoms are persistent and progressive and there is muscle atrophy, division of the deep carpal ligament is usually indicated. After a surgical division of the ligament, a compression dressing and a volar splint are usually applied. The hand is actively used as soon as possible after surgery, but care must be taken to prevent the hand from being in a dependent position. A smaller dressing may be applied after one week, and normal use of the hand is then encouraged. The sutures are removed after 10 to 14 days, and the splint is maintained for 14 to 21 days. Since first used, there is controversy between endoscopic surgery and open surgery. A bulky hand dressing or splint is applied post endoscopic surgery to immobilize the wrist. The arm is then elevated to reduce edema, range-of-motion exercises are started immediately, and oral pain medications are given (Ellwood, 1998).

ULNAR TUNNEL SYNDROME

Ulnar tunnel syndrome results from compression of the ulnar nerve within a tight, triangular fibroosseous tunnel, about 1.5 cm long, which is located at the wrist. The tunnel is formed by the superficial and deep transverse ligaments, the pisiform bone, and the pisohamate ligaments. Symptoms follow the distribution of the ulnar nerve, and the amount of nerve compression determines whether these symptoms are motor, sensory, or both. Usually a ganglion is the cause of the compression, but other causes may be an aneurysm of the ulnar artery, thromboses of the ulnar artery, hemorrhage from a fracture of the hamate, or a lipoma. Treatment consists of surgical exploration of the ulnar nerve at the wrist and removal of the cause of compression.

THE HAND

Because of its multifaceted activities, the hand is often injured. Lacerating and crushing injuries to the hand may sever tendons and nerves. Joint dislocations and fractures are common. Industrial accidents may result in traumatic amputations of fingers or even the entire hand. Treatment of hand trauma frequently poses perplexing problems that require specialized knowledge from orthopaedic surgeons, plastic surgeons, and microsurgeons.

TENDON INJURIES

FLEXOR TENDON INJURIES

Each finger contains two flexor tendons: the flexor sublimus, which inserts on the middle phalanx, and the flexor profundus, which inserts on the distal phalanx.

The thumb has only one long flexor tendon, inserting on the distal phalanx. These tendons are contained in dense fibrous tunnels or sheaths in the area from the distal flexion crease of the palm of the hand to the distal finger joints. Many common industrial and household accidents can result in lacerating injuries to the hand and fingers that sever one or more flexor tendons.

Flexor tendon injuries require surgical intervention, but the procedures involved depend upon the time elapsed between injury and treatment, the amount of contamination in the wound, and the location and extent of the damage. In many recently inflicted wounds without extensive contamination, the wound can be cleansed and the tendon(s) immediately repaired. In older wounds, or wounds with extensive contamination, tendon repair is often delayed. In the basic repair, the tendon ends are found, trimmed, and repaired by end-to-end suturing. In some immediate repairs and in most delayed repairs, the muscles have contracted and the end-to-end repair would probably result in too much tension on the tendon. In those cases, a transfer or tendon graft is required. Donor tendons for grafting, in order of preference, are usually the palmaris longus, the plantaris, the long extensors of the toes, the extensor indicis proprius, and the flexor digitorum sublimis. Artifical grafts are also used. After repair, a cast or splint is usually applied and worn for 4 to 6 weeks (see Chapter 5). Progressive range-of-motion exercises are begun following the removal of the immobilizing device.

Infection and adhesions may prevent the complete return of normal motion. In some areas of the hand and the fingers, a laceration may sever both the flexor sublimus and the flexor profundus tendons at the same level in the hand. If both tendons are repaired at the same level at the same time, they frequently will adhere to each other during the healing period with resulting finger stiffness. Many authorities believe that the proper treatment in such cases is to repair the profundus and excise the sublimus tendon. The profundus runs to the distal phalanx and has sufficient strength to flex the entire finger in the absence of the sublimus tendon. If a tendon becomes adherent to its fibrous sheath by scar formation, resulting in a loss of function in a finger, treatment may include complete excision of the tendon and the insertion of a tendon prosthesis around which a new sheath can form. Months later, the prosthesis can be removed and a flexor tendon graft inserted through the newly formed tendon sheath.

EXTENSOR TENDON RUPTURE (MALLET FINGER)

Mallet finger (or baseball finger) is a term applied to an extensor tendon rupture deformity that results when a direct blow on the tip of an extended finger forces the distal phalanx into sudden flexion and ruptures the extensor tendon at its insertion (Fig. 12–7). The injury may be a closed or open injury, and the extensor tendon may pull away from the distal phalanx cleanly or it may avulse (Fig. 12–8). The end of a mallet finger exhibits a characteristic "droop" into flexion, and the patient

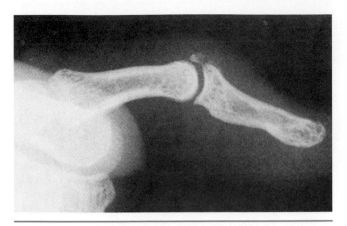

Figure 12–7   Mallet finger deformities with small fragments such as this should be treated as tendon injuries rather than as fractures.   *(Rockwood, et al. (1996)* Rockwood & Green's Fractures in Adults. *Philadelphia: Lippincott-Raven.)*

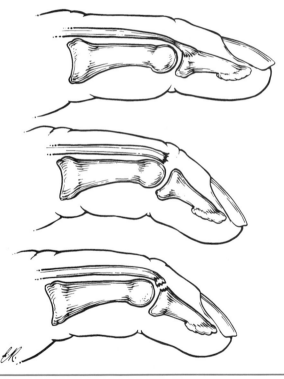

Figure 12–8   The three types of injury that cause a mallet finger of tendon origin. (*Top*) The extensor tendon fibers over the distal joint are stretched without complete division of the tendon. Although there is some drop of the distal phalanx, the patient retains weak active extension. (*Center*) The extensor tendon is ruptured from its insertion on the distal phalanx. There is a 30-degree to 60-degree extensor lag at the distal joint. (*Bottom*) A small fragment of the distal phalanx is avulsed with the extensor tendon. This injury has the same clinical findings as that shown in the center drawing.   *(Rockwood, et al. (1996).* Rockwood & Green's Fractures in Adults. *Philadelphia: Lippincott-Raven.)*

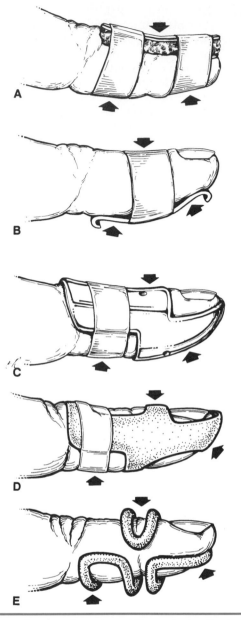

Figure 12–9   Some prefer to immobilize only the distal interphalangeal joint in treating mallet fingers. This may be done with a dorsal padded aluminum splint (A), a volar unpadded aluminum splint (B), a Stack splint (C), a modified Stack splint (D), or an Abouna splint (E). Note that each of these splints uses a three-point fixation principle.   *(Rockwood, et al. (1996).* Rockwood & Green's Fractures in Adults. *Philadelphia: Lippincott-Raven.)*

loses the ability to actively extend the fingertip. Initially, the distal interphalangeal joint is swollen and painful. Later, the deformity may only be annoying because of the tendency of the drooped finger to get in the way (e.g., catch on clothing or in pockets). If the injury is closed and treated soon after trauma, the distal phalanx may be splinted in hyperextension, with the proximal interphalangeal joint in flexion, for a period of 4 to 8 weeks (Fig. 12–9). Occasionally, there may be an associated avulsion fracture or an injury severe enough to warrant surgical intervention with the use of pin fixation for 3 weeks. In either instance, the tendon usually reattaches to the bone and there is a return of function. In patients with a deformity of long duration, surgical repair is often unsatisfactory. However, fusion of the distal interphalangeal joint in the position of function gives good results.

RUPTURE OF EXTENSOR POLLICIS LONGUS TENDON

The rupture of the extensor pollicis longus tendon of the thumb may follow a Colles' fracture. It may also be produced by degenerative changes in the tendon caused by the tendon rubbing against an irregular bony surface. Such ruptures are not uncommon in certain occupations, such as drummer and carpenter. Rupture causes a loss of extension of the distal thumb joint and a partial loss of extension in the proximal joint, with a consequent impairment of grasp. Direct suturing of the tendon through the ruptured area is frequently not feasible because the proximal segment retracts. By one month after injury, a fixed contracture of the muscle usually develops.

The preferred treatment is to repair the rupture by use of a tendon graft or tendon transfer. After surgery, a splint is applied with the wrist in near full extension and the thumb extended and abducted. The splint is begun distal to the elbow and extends to the thumb tip and to the distal palmar crease. That immobilizes the thumb but allows movement in the fingers. The splint is worn for 4 weeks, after which the thumb is gradually permitted to move while the wrist is kept splinted for another week.

DISLOCATIONS

Dislocations of finger joints (Fig. 12–10) can occur at the interphalangeal and metacarpophalangeal (MCP) joints. They are usually caused by hyperextension injuries and, as a rule, are reduced quite readily by the application of manual traction with simultaneous slight flexion. Following reduction, the joint is immobilized in a position of slight flexion for one week (Fig. 12–11). Occasionally, the end of a dislocating bone will "button-hole" through the capsule of the joint. When this occurs, the torn capsule may fold around the bone end, making closed manipulation reduction impossible. An open reduction and surgical capsular repair then become necessary.

A dislocation of the MCP thumb joint is the most common digit dislocation, and it frequently causes a capsular tear. The proximal phalanx usually displaces backward (dorsally), and the head of the metacarpal may protrude through the capsule, which can buttonhole the head of the metacarpal and maintain the dislocation. Occasionally, a metacarpal dislocation of the thumb is accompanied by a fracture of the hook of the first metacarpal. When a dislocation of the thumb occurs without a fracture or a capsular tear and is recognized early, it can be reduced and the joint immobilized for 4 to 6 weeks to prevent recurrent dislocations. Other instances require an open reduction and surgical capsular repair.

The fifth MCP joint is a saddle joint and resembles the first (thumb) MCP joint. Open reduction is usually necessary in a dislocation of the fifth MCP joint, with a wire inserted to maintain the reduction. Degenerative changes usually occur following such a dislocation. These changes impair the cupping of the hand and prevent the formation of a good grip.

FRACTURES

Fractures of the phalanges and the metacarpals may be spiral or transverse. Often there is no displacement of the fracture fragments, and simple immobilization suffices to ensure healing. Nondisplaced finger fractures are usually immobilized for approximately 10 to 14 days in a position of gentle flexion. Nondisplaced metacarpal fractures are immobilized for a 3- to 4-week period with the hand and wrist in a position of function.

Displacement of the fracture fragments leads to shortening and rotation of the involved finger. If the displacement cannot be reduced and maintained by

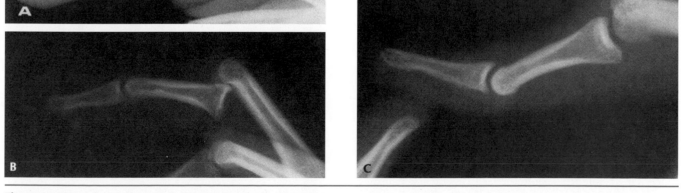

Figure 12–10 Dislocations of the proximal interphalangeal joints are of three types. Although the common dorsal dislocation (A) and the rare volar dislocation (B) are easy to reduce, the volar dislocation carries with it a greater likelihood for permanent impairment because of rupture of the central slip. (C) The most uncommon type of dislocation is rotatory subluxation. Note that the middle and distal phalanges are seen in true lateral profile, and the proximal phalanx has an oblique orientation. *(Rockwood, et al. (1996). Rockwood & Green's Fractures in Adults. Philadelphia: Lippincott-Raven.)*

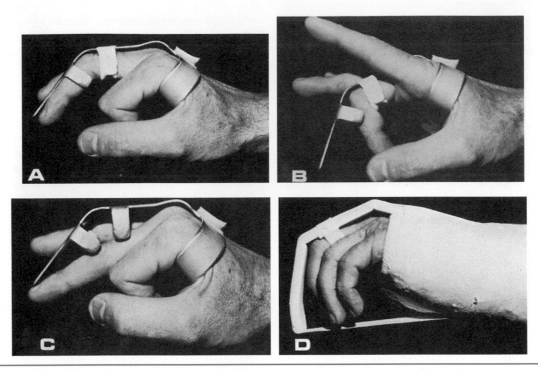

Figure 12–11 The dorsal extension block splint is useful in treating some unstable injuries of the proximal interphalangeal (PIP) joint. Extension of the PIP joint can be limited to a predetermined angle (A), while at the same time active flexion can be carried out by the patient (B). It is particularly important to secure the proximal phalanx to the splint because if this is not done, flexion of the MCP joint allows extension of the PIP joint, thereby negating the function of the splint (C). A custom-made orthosis is not necessary. The simplest way to construct the dorsal extension block splint is with a plaster (or fiberglass) gauntlet and a malleable outrigger that is firmly attached to the volar aspect of the cast to prevent bending: in extension (D). The tip of the outrigger should extend about 1/2" beyond the tip of the linger to allow unrestricted active flexion. *(Rockwood, et al. (1996). Rockwood & Green's Fractures in Adults. Philadelphia: Lippincott-Raven.)*

closed methods, surgical intervention is usually necessary. Surgical treatment consists of open or closed reduction and internal fixation, usually with a Kirschner wire. Internal fixation is indicated when (1) a displaced fracture with a fragment too small to manipulate involves a joint; (2) a fracture is displaced so severely that interposition of soft tissue prevents realignment by manipulation; (3) a fracture is so unstable that muscle contraction with joint motion will soon displace it; (4) fractures are multiple, and the hand cannot be maintained in a position of function without internal fixation; (5) a fracture is open; and (6) a fracture traps a tendon between the fragments. Internal fixation usually consists of one or two oblique or intramedullary Kirschner wires or two parallel or crossed wires.

BENNETT'S FRACTURE

Bennett's fracture is an intra-articular fracture through the base of the first metacarpal (Fig. 12–12). The shaft of the metacarpal is laterally dislocated (with the hand in supination) by the unopposed pull of the abductor pollicis longus, but the medial fragment remains in place or is slightly rotated because of its capsular attachment. The fracture is usually caused by a force applied to the end of the thumb, and if not properly reduced can result in a permanent disability. If the lateral displacement is minimal, reduction may be obtained by immobilizing the hand and the wrist in a

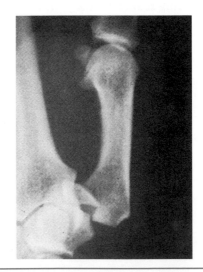

Figure 12–12 A typical Bennett's fracture dislocation. The small volar lip fragment remains attached to the anterior oblique ligament that anchors the fragment to the tubercle of the trapezium. *(Rockwood, et al. (1996). Rockwood & Green's Fractures in Adults. Philadelphia: Lippincott-Raven.)*

cast with the thumb in wide abduction. Nonetheless, the use of a cast to maintain reduction by pressure on the base of the metacarpal may be unsatisfactory, because too much pressure causes skin necrosis and too little allows loss of reduction.

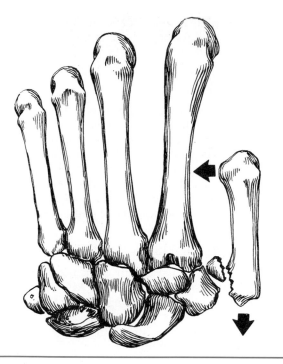

Figure 12–13 In a Bennett's fracture, the base of the metacarpal is pulled dorsally and radially by the abductor pollicis longus, and the adductor further levers the base into abduction. *(Rockwood, et al. (1996). Rockwood & Green's Fractures in Adults. Philadelphia: Lippincott-Raven.)*

Fractures with fragments that are displaced and unstable (Fig. 12–13) usually require skeletal traction, closed percutaneous pinning, or open reduction with pin fixation. Skeletal (rubber band) traction that employs a transverse pin through the proximal phalanx is usually not dependable, as immobilization may be incomplete. Closed percutaneous pinning is accomplished by first placing a Kirschner wire pin into the base of the metacarpal, across the joint, and into the trapezium; then applying manual traction to reduce the fracture; and finally applying a forearm cast to effect immobilization with the wrist in extension and the thumb in abduction. The distal joint of the thumb is kept free of the cast. If closed percutaneous pinning is unsatisfactory, an open reduction is necessary. In an open reduction, the fracture is exposed and then reduced and maintained with the use of Kirschner wires. After surgery, a forearm cast is applied as already described. The cast is removed for wound inspection at 2 to 3 weeks and then replaced until 4 weeks after surgery. The wires are then removed and the hand immobilized for another 2 to 4 weeks.

BOXER'S FRACTURE

The term *boxer's fracture* applies to a fracture of the neck of the fifth metacarpal, which can occur when an object is struck with a clenched fist. The head of the fifth metacarpal is displaced into the palm, and there is a flattening or loss of knuckle prominence. There is also a great tendency for the pull of the extensor carpi ulnaris to proximally displace the metacarpal shaft. It may be possible to restore the depressed metacarpal head to normal alignment by simultaneously pushing upward on the flexed proximal phalanx of the finger and downward on the metacarpal shaft. Once reduction is accomplished, it is difficult to maintain that position, and percutaneous pinning of the fracture fragments may be necessary to maintain the reduction. If manual reduction is impossible, the fracture may be reduced by mechanical traction or percutaneous pinning, followed by the application of a cast for immobilization. Boxer's fractures that are healing in a displaced position may need either correction of the malunion by osteotomy or a resection arthroplasty.

SURGICAL PROCEDURES

ARTHRODESIS

Arthrodesis of a joint of a finger or a thumb may be indicated when the joint has been so damaged by injury or disease that pain, deformity, or instability prevent useful motion. Occasionally, a joint must be arthrodesed because the muscles that control the digit are not strong enough to both stabilize and move all joints. Of the three finger joints, arthrodesis is most often indicated for the proximal interphalangeal joint. The distal interphalangeal joint can frequently be stabilized by tenodesis. Arthrodesis is indicated least often for the MCP joint because of the importance of motion in that joint. Thus when muscle power is sufficient, an arthroplasty is usually indicated; and when it is not, procedures to limit muscle function to the MCP joint are usually indicated. Of the joints of the thumb, arthrodesis is indicated most often for the MCP joint, because it results in little loss of function, and then for the interphalangeal joint, because fusion only results in a partial loss of the ability to pinch. Arthrodesis is indicated least often for the carpometacarpal joint because that joint is the most useful joint in the thumb. If the carpometacarpal joint of the thumb is to be arthrodesed, the function of the two distal joints should be satisfactory.

The following are the degrees of flexion at which joints are usually arthrodesed: (1) in the fingers, the MCP joints are usually at 20 to 30 degrees of flexion, the proximal interphalangeal (PIP) joints are usually at 40 to 50 degrees, and the distal interphalangeal joints at 15 to 20 degrees; and (2) in the thumb, the interphalangeal joint is usually at 20 degrees, the MCP joint at 25 degrees, and the carpometacarpal joint at 0 degrees.

Arthrodesis of the Interphalangeal Joints. In an arthrodesis of a PIP joint, the joint is incised and the proximal end of the middle phalanx is squared off. The distal end of the proximal phalanx is shaped by resecting its condyles until the proper angle for arthrodesis is obtained. The volar cartilaginous plate in a flexion contracture is not disturbed. (The plate stabilizes and compresses the ends of the bones anteriorly as the joint is forced into extension.) With the bones compressed, the joint is stabilized with parallel or crossed Kirschner wires. Resected bone fragments used as bone grafts are placed about the joint. The joint is then immobilized in a splint until roentgenograms show solid fusion. A similar procedure is used to fuse distal interphalangeal joints.

Arthrodesis of the Metacarpophalangeal Joint of the Thumb. Arthrodesis of the MCP joint of the thumb is usually indicated for degenerative arthritis after a malunited Bennett's fracture, for subluxation of the joint, for osteoarthritis, and for rheumatoid arthritis. The surgical procedure involves resecting the proximal phalanx and the distal end of the first metacarpal. The ends are then positioned together and held by Kirschner wires. After the surgery, the thumb is maintained in a thumb spica cast for 2 weeks. The skin sutures are then removed and the thumb spica cast reapplied and kept in place until roentgenograms demonstrate that bone fusion is obtained, usually at 12 weeks postsurgery.

ARTHROPLASTY

The goal of an arthroplasty is to provide stability, relieve pain, and increase mobility. Of the finger joints, the MCPs are the most likely to be treated by arthroplasty. The operation is usually indicated when degenerative changes in an otherwise useful finger joint result in less than 30 degrees of motion. The muscles that control the joint must have functional strength, or an arthroplasty will be of no value. Arthroplasty of a PIP joint is usually indicated only when a joint has lateral instability of 30 degrees or more and when flexion and extension of 60 degrees or more is preferable to a fused joint. Again, the muscles that control the joint must have functional strength. Arthroplasty of the distal interphalangeal joint of a finger and the interphalangeal, joint of the thumb is rarely indicated.

An arthroplasty for the joints of the fingers and the thumb is indicated when rheumatoid or degenerative arthritis causes pain, deformity, or disability in the MCP or interphalangeal joints. In the procedure, the proximal and distal portions of the involved joints are cut away and the canals reamed. The implant is then fitted into the canals. Tendon or ligament repairs are done as necessary for improved stability. With finger implants, a bulky hand dressing and volar splint are applied postoperatively. They are removed in 3 to 5 days, and a dynamic brace is applied to the splint so that active finger motion can be started. After a carpometacarpal arthroplasty of the thumb, there is usually sufficient pain to require protection and immobilization for several weeks. When movement is started, the ability to pinch will be extremely weak and possibly painful for several months, until a buildup of heavy scar tissue takes place. Activities such as opening car doors, cutting with scissors, putting on socks, and winding watches will eventually be possible, but will require practice and patience.

NURSING PROCESS (Patient with an Metacarpophalangeal Joint Arthroplasty)

The following nursing process demonstrates the nursing care for a typical patient following an MCP joint arthroplasty with a bulky dressing and volar splint. The nursing process begins when the patient returns to the nursing unit.

ASSESSMENT

The initial step in the assessment of a patient with an MPC joint implant is to determine the neurovascular status of the hand (see Chapter 2). In many instances, it may be very difficult to do a complete neurovascular assessment because of the bulky dressing and volar splint. Check that the hand is properly elevated. Look for any drainage on the dressing, and determine the location, duration, and severity of pain.

NURSING DIAGNOSIS

Based on all of the assessment data, the nursing diagnoses for a typical patient with an MCP joint arthroplasty may include the following:

* Pain and discomfort related to the surgery
* Impaired physical mobility related to joint instability and the bulky dressing and volar splint
* Increased anxiety related to knowledge deficit about the procedure and rehabilitation

COLLABORATIVE PROBLEMS

* Infection
* Breakage or dislocation of the implant
* Failure to fully reduce the joint deviation

GOAL FORMULATION AND PLANNING

The goal is to have the patient experience (1) a decrease in the amount of pain through nursing measures and prescribed medications, (2) an increase in mobility through the use of controlled exercises, (3) a decrease in anxiety through increased knowledge, and (4) an absence of complications from surgery and decreased activity in the hand. Long-term goals are to have the patient free of pain and to have return of function in the hand.

INTERVENTIONS

ALLEVIATE PAIN

Nursing measures that help reduce pain are to elevate the hand to prevent swelling and to give prescribed medications. The hand can be elevated on one or more pillows, or it can be elevated by placing the affected hand and arm in a special sling and attaching it to an intravenous pole. Make sure the sling does not produce pressure on the patient's elbow. It is important that the patient keep the affected hand elevated at all times during the first few weeks, even during exercises, so that the swelling will decrease.

Patients with MCP joint implants have a reduction in pain after the first few days following surgery. The pain level may increase, however, after they start their exercise program. Pain is used as a guide to the amount and vigor of the exercises. If pain lasts more than 2 hours following an activity, look at how and for how long the activity was performed, and adjust accordingly to avoid excessive strain.

INCREASE MOBILITY

The bulky dressing and volar splint are left on until the postoperative swelling has decreased, usually 3 to 5 days. For patients with MCP joint replacements, the initial dressing is removed and a dynamic brace is applied over a lightly padded dressing. The brace supports the patient's fingers in the desired position and allows movement in the artificial joint. If a brace is not available, guided early motion may still be obtained by applying a lightweight short arm cast fitted with outriggers and rubber band slings.

The brace, with extension slings, is usually worn day and night for the first 3 weeks and then worn part time. If there is severe flexor weakness and good extension, the extension slings may be removed 1 to 2 hours a day during the second and third weeks to achieve greater active flexion of the MCP joints. After 3 weeks, a flexion cuff may be attached to the brace and worn for 1 to 2 hours twice a day so that the MCP joints may be flexed passively. Beginning with the fourth postoperative week, the extension slings are usually worn at night for another 3 weeks.

Even though the patient's fingers may be sore, it is necessary that they be bent and straightened in the brace frequently during the day. The goal of the exercise program is to obtain full extension and 70 degrees of flexion. The reconstructed joints start tightening during the second postoperative week and will usually be quite tight after 3 weeks. If the desired range of motion has not been obtained by then, it will be difficult to achieve it. The patient needs to continue the exercise program for 3 months or more after surgery to maintain movement and increase strength. The patient should also exercise the neck, shoulder, elbow, and wrist twice a day so that they do not become stiff.

PATIENT TEACHING AND HOME CARE CONSIDERATIONS

Patient teaching and home care instruction are started before surgery, as the hospital stay will be short, if at all. Make sure the patient understands their exercise regime and is able to follow the program. Before the patient goes home, the occupational therapist should go over an outline of the patient's exercise program. The patient must return for check-ups to make sure that there are no problems, to adjust the brace or splint, and to modify the exercise program. Six weeks after surgery, patients are able to use their hand for light activities and for most personal care. It is advisable to caution the patient about doing heavy work for at least several months and then only with the approval of the physician.

Stress that the new joint should be used but not abused. To reduce stress on the MCP joints, the patient should remember (1) to hold heavy objects in the palm of the hand instead of with the thumb and fingers (i.e., to grasp instead of pinch; (2) to use three points, the thumb, the index, and the middle finger, when it is necessary to pinch; (3) to try to avoid movements that push the fingers toward the ulnar side of the hand; (4) to transfer the weight to the wrist and forearm when picking up heavy objects; (5) to slide rather than lift, and push instead of pull when moving heavy objects; (6) to use assistive devices in grasping to prevent strain on the fingers and the hand; and (7) to move fingers through their range of motion frequently and avoid prolonged resting positions.

Daily exercises are necessary to maintain range of motion. The patient needs to (1) move the wrist up and down and to each side; (2) roll the fingertips into the palm; (3) oppose each finger with the thumb to form a letter O; (4) place the palm of the hand on a flat surface and then raise each finger individually; and (5) do a finger walk with the hand; that is, with the palm of the hand flat, adduct the index finger toward the thumb, then move the middle finger to meet the index finger, and so on.

MONITORING AND MANAGING POTENTIAL PROBLEMS

The major complications that may occur following an MCP joint implant are infection, breakage or dislocation of the implant, and failure to correct the deviation totally. Nursing interventions to prevent infection are instituted from the very beginning. Breakage or dislocation of the implant usually can be controlled by educating the patient about the rehabilitation process. Failure to correct the deviation totally may be due to an inability to obtain the desired surgical result or a failure to follow the exercise program.

EVALUATION/OUTCOMES

Following an MCP joint implant, the patient should have increased movement in the joint. Pain should be controlled by mild analgesics. The patient should be able to demonstrate the required exercises, have the motivation to do them without supervision, and be able to verbalize an understanding of potential complications and activity reductions.

CLINICAL PATHWAY (Patient with a Metacarpophlangeal Arthroplasty)

An example of a generic clinical pathway for a patient with a metacarpophalangeal joint arthroplasty is presented in Figure 12–14.

Figure 12–14

CLINICAL PATHWAY: Metacarpophalangeal Joint Arthroplasty

Admission Date: _____   **Discharge Plan:** _____ **Home** _____ **Skilled Nursing** _____ **Extended Care Facility**

Pathway	Preadmission Office/OP clinic	Admission Day Op day	Discharge Postop 1	Postop 2	Postop 3	Postop 4	Outcomes Rehabilitation
Consultation	Primary Care/ Meidcal physician/ Rheumatologist	Case Manager Anesthesia, OT PT, if necessary	Cont. Cont.				Postoperative Appt with physician Cont. with OT
Assessment	Nrsg database H & P Exam. by MD, NP, or PA	Review & add Review H & P Postop routine					
	Including normal Activity	Assess arm postop.	Cont.				
Tests	ECG/blood/UA/ Hand x-ray						
Medications	D/C NS AIDs/ ASA 10 days b/4 OR	✓ preadm meds Routine meds					
	Analgesics as needed	Oral narcotic meds/ analgesics as needed	Cont.				Minimal amt of pain relieved with meds
	Instruct on preop meds b/4 OR	Antibiotics	D/C antibiotics				
Diet	Assessment wt. Balanced diet	NPO b/4 OR (Min. 8 hours)	Advance as tol				Tolerating diet
Activity	Preop mobility	ROM exercises to unaffected joints HOB elevated BRP					Exercises begin once dressing is romoved
Treatments		Bulky dressing and Volar splint					Drsg removed in 3–5 Days— Dynamic Brace applied and exercises begin
Education	Teach pre & postoperative Teaching regarding surgical preparation Rev. hosp routine	Reinforce					Knows exc. regime
	Exercises with and without Brace Review hosp LOS	Demonstrate exercises					Cont. exc. at home
D/C Plan	Include exercises & activity level, signs of infection, & when to notify their physician DC when recovered from anesthesia, usually one day or the same day as surgery	Rev. restricted activities Rev. signs of infection					Knows when to contact physician

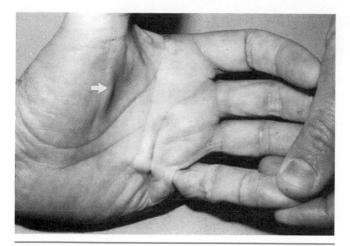

Figure 12–15 Dupuytren fasciitis commonly causes contracture in the ring and little fingers. Bands in the first web area are common but rarely limit motion.   *(Weinstein & Buckwalter (1994). Turek's Orthopaedic: Principles and Their Applications: Philadelphia: Lippincott-Raven.)*

SPECIAL CONDITIONS

DUPUYTREN'S CONTRACTURE

Dupuytren's contracture (Fig. 12–15) arises from a chronic hyperplasia of the palmar fascia of the hand. Contractures that pull the fingers into a position of fixed flexion are caused by a proliferative fibroplasia of the subcutaneous palmar tissue, which occurs in the form of nodules and cords. Other changes include a thinning of the overlying subcutaneous fat; adhesions of the skin to the lesion; and, later, a pitting or dimpling of the skin. "Knucklepads" are also common on the dorsum of the PIP joints.

The fingers most frequently affected are the ring finger and the little finger. The contracture occurs more commonly in men, affects one percent of Caucasian men over 40, and is usually bilateral (Ellwood, 1998). The exact cause is unknown, but a hereditary pattern has been noted. Trauma is thought not to play a significant role, because the condition occurs frequently in those who do not do heavy manual labor. A high incidence has been observed in patients with gout and diabetes. As a rule, the condition is painless, but it does impair the function of the hand.

Surgery is usually the treatment of choice, as no conservative treatment has been effective. The surgical procedure is to resect the palmar fascia. Some physicians do a conservative resection, whereas others favor a more radical resection, which necessitates skin grafting. Postoperatively, a bulky hand dressing with or without a volar splint is usually applied for 5 to 7 days. Finger and hand exercises are begun after 24 to 48 hours, but maximum rehabilitation may not be obtained for several months. Potential complications are infection, incomplete release of the contracture, scarring if exercise is not instituted early, and recurrence of the contracture.

TRIGGER FINGER

A trigger or snapping finger is one that locks in a flexed position and can be extended only with some difficulty

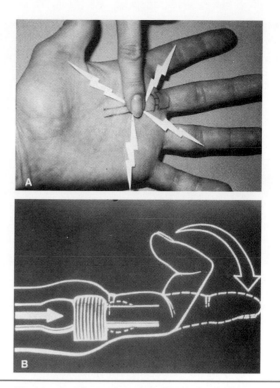

Figure 12–16 (A) Physical examination of a digit with stenosing tenosynovitis (trigger finger) reveals tenderness over the flexor tendon sheath at the level of the metacarpal head. Often, a small nodule can be palpated. (B) In trigger finger, the enlarged area of the tendon does not glide smoothly within the flexor tendon sheath. A snapping is noted as the digit pops from a fully extended to a fully flexed position. *(Weinstein & Buckwalter (1994). Turek's Orthopaedic: Principles and Their Applications: Philadelphia: Lippincott-Raven.)*

and an associated "snap" or "pop" (Fig. 12–16). That condition is due to a narrowing or constricting of the flexor sheath at the level of the metacarpal neck. There is usually an accompanying nodular enlargement of the tendon that is probably secondary to the constriction. The "trigger mechanism," which is almost always located at the level of the metacarpal head, blocks free passage of the tendon, and if the tendon passes the point of obstruction, a click or snap is produced.

Occasionally the condition is relatively painless, but in most instances there is an aching pain as a mechanical tenosynovitis develops. Treatment often consists of (1) rest of the involved digit by splinting to limit motion and decrease activity and (2) an injection of hydrocortisone into the sheath at the level of the trigger mechanism to reduce local edema and allow the tendon to glide freely. If that is not successful, surgical excision of the constricted portion of the sheath is necessary.

BUTTONHOLE OR BOUTONNIÈRE DEFORMITY

The so-called buttonhole or boutonnière deformity is commonly seen in patients with rheumatoid arthritis (RA), although the tendon imbalance that causes the deformity is not unique to that condition (Fig. 12–17). The names (boutonnière is French for buttonhole) arise because the extensor tendon splits around a joint,

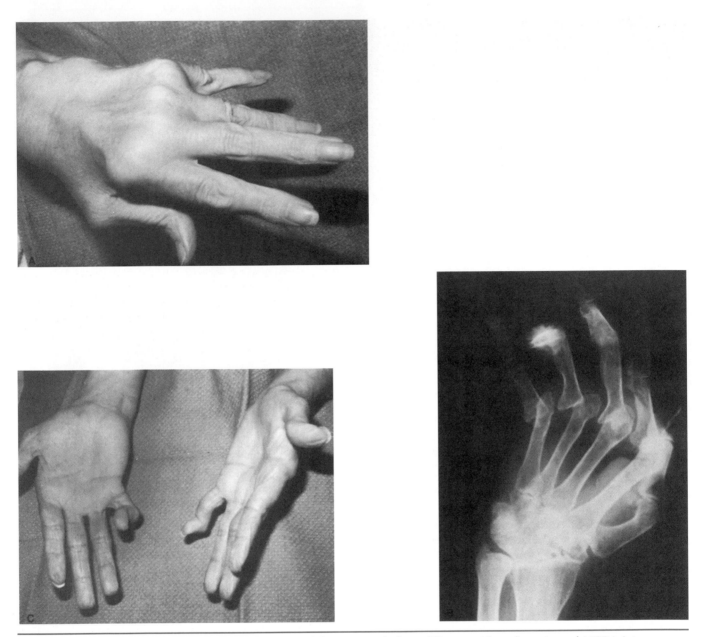

Figure 12–17   (A) Characteristic rheumatoid soft-tissue deformities include prolific synovitis at the wrist and MCP joints, Z-collapse of the thumb- and extensor tendon ruptures to the ring and small fingers. (B) Collapse deformities in RA often form a Z-collapse pattern. Note the ulnar shift of the carpal bones, radial deviation of the wrist, intercarpal fusions, and MCP joint subluxations with ulnar drift of the digits. (C) Although rheumatoid changes in the hand are often symmetric, a boutonnière deformity is noted in the right little finger, and a swan-neck deformity in the left little finger.   *(Weinstein & Buckwalter (1994).* Turek's Orthopaedic: Principles and Their Applications: *Philadelphia: Lippincott-Raven.)*

which then pokes through it, and the split tendon resembles a buttonhole. The deformity is caused by a synovitis of the PIP joint, which causes a rupture of the central portion of the extensor and forces the lateral bands of the extensor to subluxate volarward. As the deformity progresses, the lateral bands of the extensor are forced farther over the condyles of the PIP joint, become tightened by their new course and by pressure from the underlying swollen joint, and finally become fixed in a subluxated position volar to the transverse axis of the joint. The result is a secondary hyperexten-

sion contracture of the distal interphalangeal joint and a flexion contracture of the PIP joint. The MCP joint is usually in a position of extension, but joint motion is not lost.

The operative procedure to be used for reconstruction depends on the extent of the deformity. A mild flexion deformity (approximately 15 degrees) may be treatable by releasing the lateral tendons near their insertion in the distal phalanx. A moderate flexion contracture (approximately 40 degrees) usually requires a functional restoration of the central portion of the extensor and correction

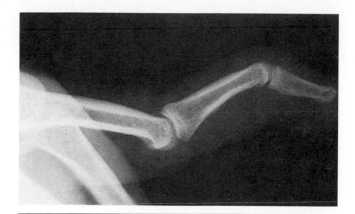

Figure 12–18 With severe flexion deformity of the distal joint in mallet finger injury, a secondary hyperextension deformity of the PIP joint may occur because of imbalance of the extensor mechanism. This produces the typical swan-neck deformity. *(Rockwood, et al. (1996). Rockwood & Green's Fractures in Adults. Philadelphia: Lippincott-Raven.)*

of the subluxation of the lateral bands. A severe buttonhole deformity usually requires an arthrodesis or possibly an interphalangeal joint arthroplasty.

SWAN-NECK DEFORMITY

A swan-neck deformity is usually caused by RA (see Fig. 12–17) but may also be related to cerebral palsy. Several fingers may be involved, and the condition may be quite disabling. The swan-neck deformity is characterized by flexion of the distal interphalangeal joint, hyperextension of the PIP joint, and flexion of the MCP joint. It is caused by muscle imbalance and by secondary ligamentous and capsular relaxation at the PIP joint that allow that joint to hyperextend (Fig. 12–18).

There are a number of surgical treatments that may improve function. One is a tenodesis of the PIP joint. Another is a synovectomy, possibly with the release of intrinsic muscle contractures. If there is marked PIP joint extension associated with joint destruction, an arthrodesis may be the procedure of choice if there is a near normal MCP joint or if an MCP joint arthroplasty is anticipated. An arthroplasty of the PIP joint may be done when there is a near normal MCP joint. Most authorities would not favor an arthroplasty of both the MCP joint and the PIP joint of the same finger because of concerns about joint strength and stability.

ULNAR DEVIATION OF THE FINGERS

The deformity of ulnar drift, or a marked deviation of the fingers toward the ulnar side of the hand, may be found in patients with RA and a few other conditions. Although the pathogenesis is not completely understood, ulnar deviation is thought to be caused by a combination of (1) stretching of the collateral ligaments of the MCP joints by the volarly directed forces of the flexor tendons, which permits volar displacement of the proximal phalanges; (2) stretching of the

accessory collateral ligaments, which permits ulnar displacement of the flexor tendons within their tunnels; (3) stretching of the flexor tunnels, which permits additional ulnar displacement of the long flexor tendons; (4) ulnar displacement of the long flexor tendons caused by surgical procedures to release their sheaths for multiple trigger fingers or for improving strength of grasp to the fingers; (5) contractures of the interosseous muscles that cause hyperextension of the PIP joints, flexion of the MCP joints, and eventually subluxation of the MCP joints; and (6) rupturing of the long extensor tendons.

In the surgical treatment of ulnar drift, a mild to moderate ulnar drift may be improved by extensor tendon realignment and MCP joint synovectomy. Presently, there is no procedure available to realign ulnarly displaced flexor tendons. In severe ulnar drift with a dislocation of one or more MCP joints, the function of the dislocated joints may be improved by arthroplasty (i.e., a flexible silicon implant). An arthroplasty of the MCP joint usually relieves pain, maintains stability and alignment, and permits acceptable motion.

References

Bomar, K. S., & Calandruccio, J. H. (1996). Crush injuries to the hand and forearm. *Orthopaedic Nursing, 15*(6), 56–65.

Bonatz, E. (1996a). Bone and soft-tissue injuries of the hand. In V. R. Masear (Ed.), *Primary care orthopaedics* (pp. 185–198). Philadelphia: W. B. Saunders.

Bonatz, E. (1996b). Overuse syndromes of the hand and wrist. In V. R. Masear (Ed.), *Primary care orthopaedics* (pp. 246–249). Philadelphia: W. B. Saunders.

Cooney, W. P., Linscheid, R. L., & Dobyns, J. H. (1996). Fractures and dislocations of the wrist. In C. A. Rockwood, D. P. Green, R. W. Bucholz, & J. D. Heckman (Eds.), *Rockwood and Green's fractures in adults* (4th ed., pp. 744–868). Philadelphia: Lippincott-Raven.

Dinowitz, M. I., Koval, K. J., & Meadows, S. (1998). Distal radius. In K. J. Koval & J. D. Zuckerman (Eds.), *Fractures in the elderly* (pp. 127–142). Philadelphia: Lippincott-Raven.

Doheny, M., Linden, P., & Sedlak, C. (1995). Reducing orthopaedic hazards of the computer work environment. *Orthopaedic Nursing, 14*(1), 7–15.

Ellwood, L. (1998). Disorders of the hand and replantation. In A. B. Maher, S. W. Salmond, & T. A. Pellino (Eds.), *Orthopaedic nursing* (2nd ed., pp 859–898). Philadelphia: W. B. Saunders.

Fierro, R., Savoie-Ball, S., & Stone, E. (1995). Wrist, hand, and microvascular. In V. M. Hoshowsky (Ed.), *NAON: Orientation to the orthopaedic operating room* (pp. 117–144). Pitman, NJ: National Association of Orthopaedic Nurses.

Green, D. P., & Butler, T. E. (1996). Fractures and dislocations in the hand. In C. A. Rockwood, D. P. Green, R. W. Bucholz, & J. D. Heckman (Eds.), *Rockwood and Green's fractures in adults* (4th ed., pp. 607–744). Philadelphia: Lippincott-Raven.

Hekmat, N., Burke, M., & Howell, S. J. (1994). Preventive pain management in the postoperative hand surgery patient. *Orthopaedic Nursing, 13*(3), 37–42.

Jonas, G., & Masear, V. R. (1996). Fractures and ligament injuries of the wrist. In V. R. Masear (Ed.), *Primary care orthopaedics* (pp. 169–184). Philadelphia: W. B. Saunders.

Lee, D. H. (1996). Fractures of the forearm. In V. R. Masear (Ed.), *Primary care orthopaedics* (pp. 165–168). Philadelphia: W. B. Saunders.

Leininger, S. M. (1997). *Building clinical pathways.* Pitman, NJ: National Association of Orthopaedic Nurses.

Meals, R. A. (1994). The wrist and hand. In S. L. Weinstein & J. A. Buckwalter (Eds.), *Turek's orthopaedics: Principles and their application* (5th ed., pp. 417–446). Philadelphia: J. B. Lippincott Company.

Richards, R. R., & Corley, F. G. (1996). Fractures of the shafts of the radius and ulna. In C. A. Rockwood, D. P. Green, R. W. Bucholz, & J. D. Heckman (Eds.), *Rockwood and Green's fractures in adults* (4th ed., pp. 870–910). Philadelphia: Lippincott-Raven.

Salmond, S. W., Mooney, N. E., & Verdisco, L. A. (Eds.). (1995). *NAON: Core curriculum for orthopaedic nursing* (3rd ed.). Pitman, NJ: National Association of Orthopaedic Nurses.

Sipos, D. A. (1993). MP implants for rheumatoid arthritis in the hand. *Orthopaedic Nursing, 12*(5), 7–14.

Sipos, D. A. (1995). Carpal tunnel syndrome. *Orthopaedic Nursing, 14*(1), 17–20.

Chapter

13

Care of a Patient with Shoulder and Elbow Injury

Chapter 13 focuses on the treatment and associated nursing care of conditions of the shoulder and elbow, including the upper and lower arm and the clavicle. Common surgical procedures, such as repairs for recurrent dislocations of the shoulder and torn rotator cuffs, and less-common procedures, such as arthrodesis and arthroplasty, are presented. The chapter also discusses minor limiting conditions like tennis elbow and major trauma of the elbow, including dislocations and fractures. The chapter begins with a review of the relevant anatomy.

ANATOMY

BONES

The bones of the shoulder and elbow include the scapula, the clavicle, the humerus, the ulna, and the radius.

SCAPULA

The scapula (or "shoulder blade") is a large, flattened, triangular bone on the posterolateral aspect of the thorax, overlapping parts of the second to the seventh ribs. It has costal and dorsal surfaces; upper, lateral, and medial borders; inferior, superior, and lateral angles; and three bony processes, the scapular spine, the acromion, and the coracoid process. The dorsal surface is divided by the scapular spine, a horizontal bony ridge that extends laterally past the glenoid fossa and ends in the bulbous acromial process. This process overhangs the head of the humerus, is the site where the clavicle attaches (the acromioclavicular joint), and contains the attachment of the coracoacromial ligament. The acromion and the coracoacromial ligament form part of the arch overlying the suprahumeral joint.

The scapula moves in a gliding manner in conjunction with the motion and the rotation of the clavicle. The motions of the scapula and the clavicle are primarily produced by two muscles, the trapezium and the serratus anterior. The upper fibers of the trapezium originate from the nuchal ligament in the lower

cervical region, the posterior spinous process of the cervical spine, and the upper thoracic spine. They attach to the upper margin of the medial and central scapular spine, act to pull the scapula upward, and cause inward pivoting of the acromioclavicular joint. The middle fibers, which originate from the spinous processes of the upper thoracic vertebrae, attach to the medial border of the scapular spine and "fix" the scapula during abduction of the arm. The lower fibers, which originate from the spinous processes of the lower thoracic vertebrae, attach to the medial portion of the spine of the scapula and act to pull the medial border of the spine of the scapula down and in. The serratus anterior muscle, which originates from the upper eight ribs, attaches to the medial (vertebral) and inferior borders of the scapula and acts to pull the scapula forward.

The trapezium muscle is supplied by the spinal accessory nerve (XI). The serratus is innervated by the long thoracic nerve formed by the anterior branches of the roots of C5, C6, and C7 (primarily C6) before entering the brachial plexus.

CLAVICLE

The clavicle (or "collarbone") extends almost horizontally across the root of the neck laterally toward the point of the shoulder. The lateral or acromial end of the bone is flattened and articulates with the medial side of the acromion, whereas the medial or sternal end is enlarged and articulates with the clavicular notch of the manubrium of the sternum. The shaft is gently curved with a shape that resembles the italic letter *f*.

HUMERUS

The humerus is the longest and largest bone of the upper extremity. The upper (proximal) end consists of a greater and lesser tuberosity and a rounded "head" that articulates with the glenoid cavity of the scapula to form a ball-and-socket joint (Fig. 13–1). The lower (distal) end is condylar and adapted to the forearm bones (the ulna and the radius) to form the elbow joint.

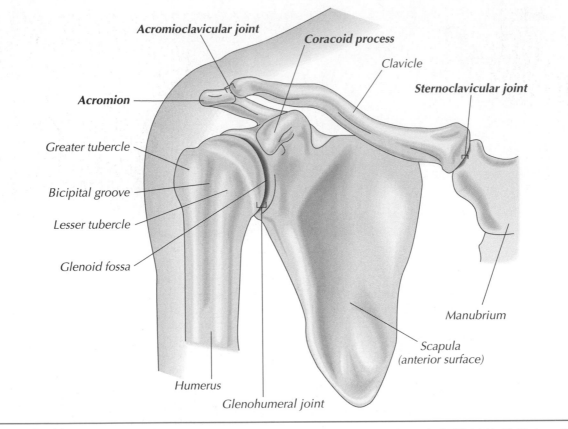

Figure 13–1   Shoulder structures.   *(Bates, B. (1995). A Guide to Physical Examination and History Taking. 6th ed. Philadelphia: J.B. Lippincott Company.)*

The lower end of the humerus is basically a broad condyle with articular and nonarticular parts. The articular parts adjoin the radius and the ulna at the elbow joint. The humerus is divided by a faint groove into a lateral, convex surface, the capitellum, and a medial, pulley-shaped surface, the trochlea. The capitellum is a rounded, convex projection formed by the anterior or inferior surfaces of the lateral part of the condyle of the humerus. It articulates with the disc-like head of the radius, which lies in contact with its inferior surface when the elbow is in full extension. The trochlea is a grooved surface that covers the anterior and posterior surface of the condyle of the humerus. The trochlea of the humerus articulates with the trochlear notch of the ulna.

The nonarticular part of the condyle of the humerus includes the medial and lateral epicondyles, together with the olecranon, coronoid, and radial fossae. The medial epicondyle is a blunt projection on the medial side of the condyle. Its posterior surface is smooth and crossed by the ulnar nerve, which runs down into the forearm; and its anterior surface has the attachment of the superficial group of the forearm flexor muscles. The lateral epicondyle is the lateral part of the condyle, and its anterior surface has the origin of the superficial group of forearm extensor muscles. A deep hollow situated on the posterior surface of the condyle, immediately above the trochlea, is the olecranon fossa. The olecranon fossa contains the tip of the olecranon of the ulna when the elbow is extended. A similar but smaller hollow, the coronoid

fossa, lies immediately above the trochlea on the anterior surface of the condyle. A very slight depression situated above the capitellum on the lateral side of the coronoid fossa is the radial fossa, which articulates with the head of the radius when the elbow is fully flexed.

RADIUS

The radius is the lateral bone of the forearm. It is wider at its proximal and distal ends, especially the latter. The proximal end of the radius includes a head, a neck, and a tuberosity. The head is disc-shaped, and its upper surface is a shallow cup for articulation with the capitellum of the humerus. The articular circumference of the radial head is smooth and deepest medially where it articulates with the radial notch of the ulna. The neck of the radius is the constricted part below the head, and the tuberosity is located just below the medial part of the neck.

ULNA

The ulna is the medial bone of the forearm and is parallel to the radius when the forearm is supine. Its proximal end is thick, strong, and hook-like, with the concavity of the hook directed forward. The proximal end of the ulna has two substantial processes, the olecranon and the coronoid, and two articular areas, termed the trochlear and the radial notches, which articulate with the humerus and the radius.

The olecranon is the uppermost part of the ulna. It forms a prominent beak that projects into the olecranon fossa of the humerus when the forearm is extended. The coronoid process is a bracket-like projection from the front of the ulna immediately below the olecranon. The upper part of the lateral surface contains the shallow radial notch that articulates with the side of the head of the radius, and the bone below it is indented to make room for the tuberosity of the radius during movements of pronation and supination. The anterior surface of the coronoid process is triangular in shape, and its lower part becomes the rough tuberosity of the ulna. The trochlear notch, formed by the anterior surface of the olecranon and the superior surface of the coronoid process, articulates with the trochlea of the humerus.

JOINTS

STERNOCLAVICULAR JOINT

The sternoclavicular joint is formed by the sternal end of the clavicle articulating with the superior lateral portion of the manubrium of the sternum and the cartilage of the first rib. The articular surface of the clavicle is covered with a layer of fibrocartilage. The ligaments that surround the joint are the anterior and posterior sternoclavicular, the interclavicular, and the costoclavicular ligaments. The anterior and posterior sternoclavicular ligaments reinforce the loose fibrous capsule of the joint, and the interclavicular ligament connects the two clavicles. The costoclavicular ligament, which originates from the medial portion of the first rib and attaches into the undersurface of the clavicle, acts as a fulcrum for all motion of the shoulder girdle and stabilizes the clavicle.

The arteries supplying the joint are branches of the internal thoracic and supracapsular arteries. The nerves are from the anterior supraclavicular nerve and the nerve to the subclavius.

ACROMIOCLAVICULAR JOINT

The acromioclavicular joint articulates between the lateral (acromial) end of the clavicle and the anterior medial portion of the acromial process of the scapula. Both articular surfaces are covered with fibrocartilage. On the acromial end of the clavicle is a narrow, oval area that is directed downward and laterally to overlap a corresponding area on the medial border of the acromion. The acromioclavicular joint has a weak, relaxed fibrous capsule that is reinforced by strong superior and inferior acromioclavicular ligaments that prevent posterior displacement of the clavicle upon the acromion. The clavicle is attached to the scapula by the coracoclavicular ligament, formed by the lateral trapezoid and the medial coronoid ligaments.

The arterial supply to the acromioclavicular joint is derived from the supracapsular and thoracoacromial arteries (Fig. 13–2). The nerve supply is from the supracapsular and lateral pectoral nerves

GLENOHUMERAL JOINT

The glenohumeral or shoulder joint (Fig. 13–3), the pivotal joint of the upper extremity, is a type of ball-and-socket joint. The ball, the humeral head, has only a small

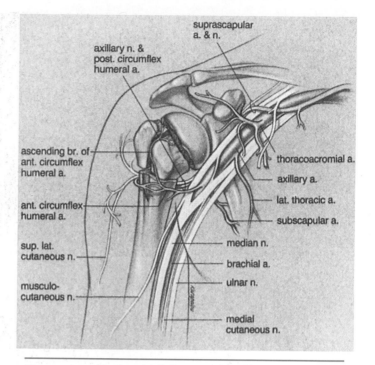

Figure 13–2 The brachial plexus and axillary artery lie adjacent to the coracoid process and can be injured with fractures of the proximal humerus. The major blood supply to the humeral head is through the ascending branch of the anterior humeral circumflex artery, which penetrates the head at the superior aspect of the bicipital groove and becomes the arcuate artery. There are three important nerves about the shoulder: the axillary, suprascapular, and musculocutaneous. *(Rockwood, et al. (1996). Rockwood & Green's Fractures in Adults. Philadelphia: Lippincott-Raven.)*

area of bony contact with the glenoid fossa, a shallow, ovoid socket that faces anteriorly, laterally, and upward. Both articular surfaces are covered with a layer of hyaline cartilage. The cartilage on the head of the humerus is thickest in the center and becomes thinner peripherally, whereas the reverse is true for the glenoid cavity. Surrounding the perimeter of the fossa, to deepen the cup, is a fibrous lip known as the glenoid labrum. Compared to the ball-and-socket joint of the hip, the construction of the shoulder joint permits greater movement but provides less stability. Structurally the joint is weak because it depends on the support given by the surrounding muscles, not on its bone structure or the presence of strong ligaments.

The capsule of the glenohumeral joint is an extremely thin-walled, loose container that attaches to the entire perimeter of the glenoid rim. The capsule is attached medially to the glenoid cavity beyond the glenoid labrum, laterally to the anatomical neck of the humerus close to the articular margin, and superiorly to the root of the coracoid process so as to include the origin of the long head of the biceps. Throughout the joint, there is a synovial lining that blends with the hyaline cartilage of the head of the humerus but fails to reach the cartilage of the glenoid fossa.

Rotation of the arm around its longitudinal axis has an effect on the tautness and laxity of the capsule. The

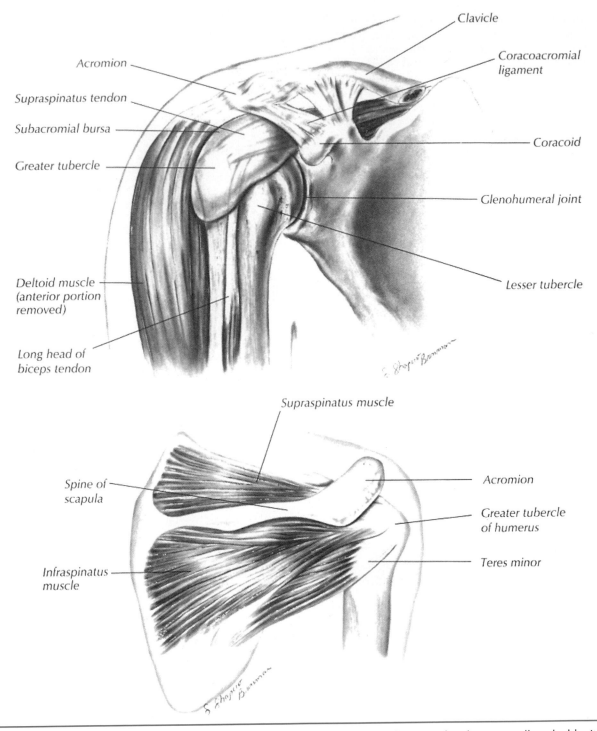

Figure 13–3   The *glenohumeral joint,* between the scapula and the humerus, is deeply situated and not normally palpable. Its fibrous capsule is reinforced by the tendons of four muscles, which together are called the *rotator cuff.* The supraspinatus, which runs above the joint, and the infraspinatus and teres minor, which cross it posteriorly, all insert on the greater tubercle of the humerus.   *(Bates, B. (1995). A Guide to Physical Examination and History Taking. 6th ed. Philadelphia: J.B. Lippincott Company.)*

anterior portion of the capsule is reinforced by the superior, middle, and inferior glenohumeral ligaments. They are attached on the humerus and converge toward the glenoid rim to attach on the anterior superior portion of the glenoid and adjacent scapular bone. The external rotation of the humerus upon the glenoid fossa is limited by the coracohumeral ligament. The coracohumeral ligament originates at the coracoid process of the scapula and attaches to the front of the greater tubercle of the humerus, blending with the tendon of supraspinatus. The transverse humeral ligament functions as a retinaculum for the tendon of the long head of the biceps. It passes from the lesser to the greater tubercle of the humerus and attaches above the epiphysis line. The

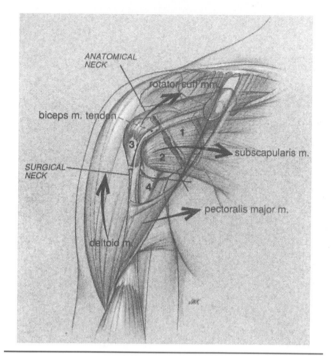

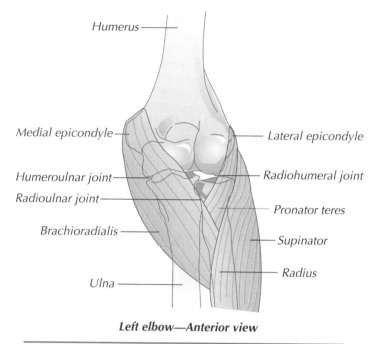

Humerus

Medial epicondyle — — Lateral epicondyle

Humeroulnar joint — — Radiohumeral joint

Radioulnar joint —

Brachioradialis — — Pronator teres

— Supinator

— Radius

Ulna —

Left elbow—Anterior view

Figure 13–4   The anatomy of the shoulder is complex, and shoulder function depends on proper alignment and interaction of anatomical structures. Displacement of fracture fragments is due to the pull of muscles attaching to the various bony components. The four anatomical components of the proximal humerus are the head, lesser tuberosity, greater tuberosity, and shaft. The anatomical neck is at the junction of the head and tuberosities, and the surgical neck is below the greater and lesser tuberosities. The subscapularis inserts on the lesser tuberosity, causing medial displacement, whereas the supraspinatus and infraspinatus insert on the greater tuberosity, causing superior and posterior displacement. The pectoralis major inserts on the humeral shaft and displaces it medially.   (Rockwood, et al. (1996). Rockwood & Green's Fractures in Adults. Philadelphia: Lippincott-Raven.)

Figure 13–5   Left-elbow—Posterior view.   (Bates, B. (1995). A Guide to Physical Examination and History Taking. 6th ed. Philadelphia: J.B. Lippincott Company.)

fibrous capsule is strengthened above by the tendon of supraspinatus, below by the long head of the triceps, behind by the tendons of the infraspinatus and teres minor, and in front by the tendon of the subscapularis. The muscles and tendons of the subscapularis, the supraspinatus, the infraspinatus, and the teres minor are all intimately blended with the fibrous capsule forming a cuff, termed the rotator cuff. They reinforce the capsule and provide active support for the joint. Besides the muscles of the rotator cuff, the deltoid muscle is also important in joint movement (Fig. 13–4). In conjunction with the muscles of the rotator cuff, contraction of the deltoid muscle elevates the humerus.

ELBOW JOINT

The elbow (Fig. 13–5) is a compound hinge joint that includes the humeroulnar joint between the trochlea of the humerus and the trochlear notch of the ulna, the humeroradial joint between the capitellum of the humerus and the head of the radius, and the radioulnar joint between the head of the radius and the radial notch of the ulna. Flexion is produced by the brachialis,

biceps, and brachioradialis muscles. Extension is accomplished by the triceps and the anconeus muscles. The joint has a fibrous articular capsule and ulnar and radial collateral ligaments.

BURSAE

There are numerous bursae in the neighborhood of the shoulder. The subscapularis bursa is between the tendon of the subscapularis and the joint capsule, communicating with the joint through an opening between the superior and the middle glenohumeral ligaments. There is a bursa that separates the tendon of infraspinatus and the capsule. The subacromial bursa lies between the deltoid muscle and the capsule. There is a bursa on the upper surface of the acromion, one between the teres major and the long head of the triceps, and one in front of, and another behind, the tendon of the latissimus dorsi. In addition, one is frequently found between the coracoid process and the capsule and another is sometimes found behind the coracobrachialis.

Two bursae of the elbow lie in relation to the triceps insertion. One lies between the triceps tendon and the upper surface of the olecranon. The other, the larger and more important one, lies between the skin and the dorsal surface of the olecranon. Another bursa lies between the neck of the radius and the biceps tendon, as the latter approaches the bicipital tuberosity. Other bursae are located about the lateral collateral ligament.

ARTICULAR CAPSULE OF THE ELBOW

The anterior portion of the fibrous capsule is a broad and thin layer. The proximal part is attached to the front of the medial epicondyle of the humerus, and the distal portion is attached above the coronoid and radial fossae of the ulna and to the annular ligament. Posteriorly, the fibrous capsule is very thin. The proximal portion is attached to the humerus behind the capitellum and to the lateral margins of the trochlea. The distal portion is attached to the rim of the olecranon fossa and to the medial epicondyle of the ulna. The capsule is supported laterally by the ulnar and radial collateral ligaments. A synovial membrane surrounds the articular surfaces of the humerus, the radius, and the ulna.

LIGAMENTS OF THE ELBOW

The ulnar collateral ligament of the elbow is a thick triangular band that consists of an anterior and a posterior portion. The anterior part is attached above to the medial epicondyle of the humerus and below to a tubercle on the upper part of the medial margin of the coronoid process of the ulna. The posterior part is attached above to the lower and back part of the medial epicondyle of the humerus and below to the medial margin of the olecranon. The ulnar collateral ligament is related to the triceps and flexor carpi ulnaris muscles and to the ulnar nerve.

The radial collateral ligament of the elbow is attached above to the lower part of the lateral epicondyle of the humerus and below to the annular ligament. The radial collateral ligament is related to the brachialis, the triceps, and the anconeus muscles. Laterally, it is related to the common tendon of the extensor muscles and medially to the common tendon of the flexor muscles and the flexor carpi ulnaris.

The annular ligament is composed of transversely disposed fibers that encircle the radial head, and it attaches distally to the radial neck and medially to the anterior and posterior margins of the lesser sigmoid fossa of the ulna. The major artery of the elbow is the brachial artery, which divides just below the elbow into the radial and ulnar arteries. The veins are laterally the cephalic and medially the basilic veins. The articular nerves are mainly from the musculocutaneous and radial nerves, but the ulnar, the median, and sometimes the anterior interosseous nerves also contribute to the articular branches.

THE SHOULDER

The term *shoulder* is used clinically to encompass the entire shoulder girdle, which comprises the upper humerus, the scapula, the clavicle, and the sternum. These bones articulate through the glenohumeral, the acromioclavicular, and the sternoclavicular joints. The clavicle acts to hold the arm and the scapula outward and backward. Elevation of the arm is forward flexion, and abduction takes place through the glenohumeral joint, accompanied by rotation of the scapula on the thorax. Rotation of the scapula involves movement in the acromioclavicular joint and the rotation of the clav-

icle in the sternoclavicular joint. Thus, the active range of motion of the arm involves the complete shoulder girdle.

SCAPULA

A fracture of a portion of the scapula is an unusual injury. It is usually caused by a direct blow and is often associated with bruising of muscles, fractures of underlying ribs, or other injuries in patients sustaining severe trauma. Persons with a fractured scapula tend to hold their arm in adduction. Although painful, displacement of the fragments is rare because the scapula is encased in a heavy muscular envelope. Fractures of the scapula are almost always treated symptomatically. The arm is rested in a sling until the pain has disappeared. As a general rule, there is a full restoration of movement and function.

CLAVICLE

Fractures of the clavicle (collarbone) are one of the most common bony injuries and are encountered much more frequently in children than in adults. The injury commonly occurs because of a fall on an outstretched hand or a fall on the arm or shoulder, though it may be due to a direct injury. The clinical picture is of a patient who has a drooping of the shoulder, a hematoma over the site of the clavicle, an obvious protrusion of the inner half of the bone, and pain. The patient usually holds the arm against the chest in a protective manner. In some instances, an undisplaced clavicular fracture may be overlooked. The fracture is usually self-healing and does not require elaborate splinting.

ACROMIOCLAVICULAR JOINT

The acromioclavicular (AC) joint, where the clavicle joins the scapula, is a synovial joint that has relatively weak capsular ligaments. The joint is usually injured by a direct fall on the point of the shoulder (i.e., a force applied to the lateral or superior aspect of the acromion), which is not uncommon in athletic and industrial accidents. Such an injury may tear the supporting ligaments and cause varying degrees of disruption of the AC joint. Depending on the force, the capsule and the ligaments around the AC joint may be stretched, sprained, or torn, with the degree of injury ranging from a sprain to a dislocation of the joint. That dislocation has been termed a *shoulder separation*, but it does not indicate any injury to the glenohumeral ("shoulder") joint.

A *first-degree AC sprain* (shoulder pointer) is an incomplete tear of the AC ligament without subluxation of the joint. A *second-degree sprain* is a more severe disruption of the joint capsule that allows subluxation (partial separation) of the AC joint, but with the coracoclavicular ligaments remaining intact. With these sprains, the deformity is usually small and the swelling minimal. A *third-degree sprain*, which is a complete dislocation of the AC joint, occurs when the injury ruptures the joint capsule and overlying musculature along with the coronoid and trapezoid ligaments. Dislocations that do not disrupt the AC joint surfaces are usually treated with some type of encircling bandage designed to reduce the dislocation and hold the parts together until healing occurs. A common procedure is to use a figure-of-eight bandage splint with adhesive strapping from the chest to the back together with a pad over both clavicles, or an easy-to-apply commercial splint. Immobilization must be maintained long enough to allow complete healing.

On the other hand, better anatomical and functional results may be obtained with operative methods. Those methods are (1) open reduction with internal fixation using two Kirschner-wires that usually pass through the AC joint; (2) fixation of the distal clavicle to the coracoid process with a screw (which has the disadvantage of requiring synchronous motion of the clavicle and scapula); (3) fixation by cerclage of the clavicle and coracoid process with fascia, nonabsorbable sutures, wires, or nails; (4) internal fixation of the AC joint itself using a heavy nonabsorbable suture; and (5) lateral clavicular resection arthroplasty. After the repair of the AC joint is completed, the patient will have a Velpeau dressing or a sling and swathe. In chronic painful dislocations, the resection of the outer inch of the clavicle usually leads to relief of symptoms and restoration of function. Recovery occurs in about 3 weeks.

NURSING PROCESS (Patient with an Open Reduction of an AC Joint Separation)

The following nursing process demonstrates the care of a typical patient with an open reduction of an AC joint separation and the application of a Velpeau bandage. The nursing process begins after the patient returns to the unit.

ASSESSMENT

The initial nursing assessment of a patient following the open reduction of an AC separation and the application of a Velpeau bandage, a sling and swathe, or a shoulder immobilizer is to check the neurovascular status of the affected arm. Pulse, color, temperature, movement, and sensation in the involved extremity are determined and compared with those of the uninvolved side. (For further information on assessment, see Chapter 2.) If a commercially available Velpeau-type support is used, there should be no problem in completing every step of the neurovascular assessment. If a physician-made Velpeau bandage is used, however, the bandage may prevent a complete motor assessment by immobilizing the wrist. Record specifically what assessments were made. With a Velpeau bandage or a sling and swathe, the neurovascular assessment of the involved arm is vital, because the flexion of the elbow means that there is an added potential for neurovascular impairment. For a patient with a sling and swathe, also check that the hand is higher than the elbow.

Assess the patient's respiratory status for rate, depth, and rhythm, and determine whether they are affected by a change in position. Does the patient need to be in a sitting or semi-Fowler position to breathe comfortably? Determine if the Velpeau bandage is too tight or if it prevents the patient from taking deep breaths. Determine the amount, location, and severity of pain. Check the upper trunk, affected arm, and immobilizing device for position and comfort. Note if there is any undue pressure or tautness to the skin from the immobilizing device.

NURSING DIAGNOSIS

Based on all of the assessment data, the major nursing diagnoses for a typical patient with an open reduction for an AC separation and a Velpeau bandage, a sling and swathe, or a shoulder immobilizer may include the following:

- Pain and discomfort related to soft-tissue trauma
- Impaired physical mobility related to lack of AC joint stability and an immobilized arm
- Increased anxiety related to knowledge deficit about the surgery and rehabilitation

COLLABORATIVE PROBLEMS

- Incomplete reduction
- Inadequate maintenance of immobilization
- Infection

GOAL FORMULATION AND PLANNING

The goals are to have the patient experience (1) a decrease in the amount of pain through the use of surgery, nursing measures, and prescribed medications; (2) an increase in mobility through exercise; (3) a decrease in anxiety through increased knowledge about the surgery and the rehabilitation process; and (4) an absence of complications from surgery and decreased activities. The long-term goals are to have the patient pain free and to have full return of motion and function in the involved arm.

INTERVENTIONS

ALLEVIATE PAIN
AC joint pain may be due to muscle spasms, the surgical repair of the joint, incorrect positioning of the immobilizing device, neurovascular impairment, or skin impairment. The assessment must determine the source, location, and severity of the pain.

For muscle spasms, repositioning and muscle-setting exercises that increase circulation to the area may help reduce pain, but medications may still be necessary.

Position the patient so as to maintain the trunk of the body in correct alignment. Verify that the shoulders are level. Check the position and neurovascular status of the arm. If a patient is in a sling, the arm may have moved to the side of the chest. Repositioning the arm to the front of the chest reduces discomfort. When the patient is lying supine, a small support at the side of the chest may be needed to keep the arm in the correct position. Verify that the hand of the involved arm is level with or higher than the elbow, and readjust the sling accordingly. For patients in a commercial Velpeau bandage (or shoulder immobilizer), periodic readjustment of the immobilizer may be necessary. For instance, if the hand is not positioned properly, the edge of the strap may cut into the wrist. If the strap over the upper arm is slipping down, circulation may be impaired at the elbow. The chest strap of a shoulder immobilizer can be another source of discomfort to the patient if it is fastened too tight.

If swollen fingers occur, the patient must do finger exercises to increase circulation and reduce swelling. Excessive pain and swelling at the AC joint may be reduced by applications of ice. If ice is utilized, make sure the ice bags are not placed directly over the AC joint, as that would cause pressure and add to the pain.

INCREASE MOBILITY

After the surgical repair of a separated AC joint, the amount of activity in the affected arm depends on the type of surgical procedure. Some allow the patient to use the arm immediately, whereas others require the arm to have a period of immobilization. When a patient has the end of the clavicle resected, the arm may have minimal or no immobilization and the patient is encouraged to use the arm immediately after surgery. Patients with an AC separation repaired by the use of a screw usually have their arm immobilized in a sling. Patients with a Kirschner inserted for repair usually have the involved arm immobilized in a Velpeau bandage or shoulder immobilizer for at least 2 weeks.

Velpeau Bandage.   The Velpeau bandage (Fig. 13–6) is a comfortable, effective method of bandaging the arm to the trunk of the body and immobilizing the shoulder girdle. It may be used in the treatment of a fracture of the surgical neck or shaft of the humerus; a fracture of the scapula or clavicle; and following the reduction of a dislocated glenohumeral, sternoclavicular, or AC joint. There are a number of commercially developed Velpeau bandages, sometimes called Velpeau slings. Alternatively, a physician-made Velpeau bandage can be used.

To apply such a bandage, the patient should sit on an examining table or stool with someone supporting the affected arm in the position of immobilization. The axilla on the affected side should be clean and dry, and for female patients the area beneath the breasts should also be clean and dry. Padding is then placed in the axilla (and beneath the breasts of a woman) to prevent the skin of the arm from being pressed against the skin of the trunk. The arm is then placed across the patient's chest so that the fingers lie just below the shoulder. Padding

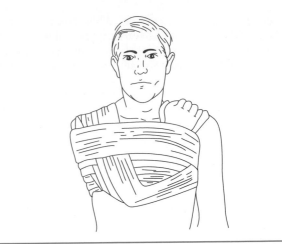

Figure 13–6   The Velpeau bandage.

may also be placed under the hand. Some 10 to 12 layers of rolled gauze bandage are applied smoothly around the chest to hold the arm against the trunk. The bandage may or may not be encased in a single layer of plaster of Paris. If the plaster is applied, care is taken to make sure that it does not come in contact with the patient's skin.

Position.   Patients with a reduced AC separation will find the supine, with slight elevation of the head of the bed, the most comfortable position in bed. The patient is not allowed to turn to the affected side or lie prone and will probably find lying on the unaffected side uncomfortable.

Exercise.   The surgical repair determines the type of exercises allowed and when they should be started. If the end of the clavicle was resected, the use of the arm is encouraged immediately after surgery. Raising the arm above the horizontal is not permitted for 3 to 4 weeks, however. For patients whose AC separation was surgically repaired by the use of a screw, gentle active exercises are permitted and usually encouraged in the first week postsurgery. Motion above 90 degrees of abduction, heavy lifting, and strenuous exercises are avoided until the screw is removed (about 6 or 8 weeks after the surgery). Once the screw is removed, more vigorous exercises are permitted, and full activities may be resumed 10 weeks after surgery. Patients who have had Kirschner wires inserted as the method of repair have active-motion exercises begun 2 weeks postsurgery. The wires are usually not removed until approximately 8 weeks after surgery, and then more vigorous exercises are begun.

The patient with a Velpeau bandage or with an arm in a sling must do finger exercises to increase circulation and maintain joint mobility. The more swollen the fingers, the greater the need for finger exercises. Recommended finger exercises include the following:

1. Fully extend the fingers and spread them into abduction.
2. Flex the fingers by touching the palm with the fingertips.

3. Flex the metacarpophalangeal joints by attempting to touch the front of the wrist.
4. Approximate the tip of the thumb to each finger in turn. The thumb must also be exercised.

Ambulation. The patient is usually allowed up the first day following surgery but will probably need help initially. Once the patient is out of bed, make sure he or she is steady before starting to walk. With one arm immobilized across the chest, the patient may become unsteady when walking because of the change in balance and lack of arm swing.

PATIENT TEACHING AND HOME CARE CONSIDERATIONS

Discuss the rehabilitation regime with the patient, the family, and significant others. Make sure the patient understands the surgical procedure, the need for an immobilizing device, the exercises that are allowed or encouraged, and the limitations that have been imposed. Teach the patient how to assess for neurovascular status in the affected arm by using the unaffected arm. Explain the importance of notifying the physician immediately if there is a change in neurovascular status. Include a discussion of the signs and symptoms of infection, the potential for developing an infection, and what to do if one seems to be developing.

Have an open discussion with the patient on activities of daily living, what the patient will realistically be able to do for him or herself, and what others will need to do. Stress that the immobilizing device must not be removed. If the patient feels moisture from perspiration under the immobilizer or feels that he or she has body odor, the skin under the immobilizer can be washed and dried by lifting part of the immobilizer off the body and cleansing under it. The patient will not be able to do this alone. Cleansing under the affected arm with a washcloth and soap may be difficult or impossible. Other ways to cleanse the body include the use of products like "Handi-wipes," alcohol swabs, or "Tucks." Antiperspirants are suggested whenever possible. The patient will usually be taking a sponge bath but may also sit in a bathtub that has only a couple of inches of water to prevent the bandage from getting wet. Help will probably be needed for safety even though the water should be drained from the tub before the patient starts to get out. Help may also be needed in washing hair, shaving, and eating.

Discuss with the patient what clothing to wear when the Velpeau bandage is on. Clothing may be modified by letting out seams, and Velcro straps may be used for closure. Clothing should not be tight over the chest and arm as that would add to discomfort.

MONITORING AND MANAGING POTENTIAL PROBLEMS

The major complications following reduction of an AC separation are incomplete reduction, inadequate maintenance of immobilization, and infection.

INCOMPLETE REDUCTION

To help prevent an incomplete reduction from occurring, make sure the immobilizing device is maintained in proper position to prevent stress on the repair site.

INADEQUATE MAINTENANCE OF IMMOBILIZATION

To help prevent complications, make sure the immobilization device is secured in place and properly positioned. The patient should not do exercises beyond those stipulated or use the arm in activities that cause stress to the site. For some patients, there may be long-range reduced range of motion postsurgery if the patient is not diligent in doing the required exercises.

INFECTION

There is also the potential for infection at the surgical site. Utilize preventive measures, and be alert to the early signs and symptoms of infection. An infection may also occur as a secondary complication of skin irritation from the immobilizing device. The arm, which is supported by a sling supplemented by a modified Velpeau bandage, needs a soft pad placed in the axilla to help prevent skin excoriation. Verify that the shoulder immobilizer straps do not cut into the skin of the patient's arm. Assess and implement nursing measures to prevent skin irritation.

EVALUATION/OUTCOMES

The interventions to relieve pain are effectively reducing the patient's pain. The patient understands the limits of activities and that trying to do too much on his or her own can lead to added stress and discomfort. The patient understands and follows the required exercise program. The patient should be free of any neurovascular impairment or infection.

CLINICAL PATHWAY (Patient with a Surgical Repair of AC Joint Separation)

A generic clinical pathway for a patient with a surgical repair of an AC joint separation is shown in Figure 13–7.

GLENOHUMERAL (SHOULDER) JOINT

The glenohumeral joint is a ball-and-socket joint that allows greater range of motion but less stability than the ball-and-socket joint of the hip. Stability is augmented by the glenoid labrum, the rotator cuff, the coracoacromial arch, and the long heads of the biceps and triceps muscles. The branches of the brachial plexus nerve lie just anterior to the glenohumeral joint, and the axillary nerve is immediately inferior to the joint.

Figure 13–7

Clinical Pathway: Surgical Repair of AC Joint Separation

Admission Date: _____   **Discharge Plan:** _____ **Home**   _____ **Skilled Nursing**   _____ **Extended Care Facility**

Pathway	Preadmission Office/OP clinic	Admission Day Op day	Discharge Postop 1	Postop 2	Postop 3	Postop 4	Outcomes Rehabilitation
Consultation	Primary Care/ Medical physician	Case Manager					Postoperative appt. with physician
		Anesthesia, OT	Cont.				Return for OT appts.
		PT, if necessary	Cont.				
Assessment	Nrsg database	Review & add					
	H & P Exam. by MD, NP, or PA	Review H & P					
	Including normal activity	Postop routine					
		N/V status affected arm	Cont.	Cont.			
Tests	ECG/blood/UA/ shoulder x-rays						
Medications	D/C NSAIDs/ASA 10 days b/4 OR	✓ preadm meds					
	Analgesics as needed	Routine meds					
	Instruct on preop meds b/4 OR	Oral narcotic meds/ analgesics as needed	Cont.	Cont.			Minimal amt. of pain relieved with meds then ice
		Antibiotics	D/C antibiotics				
Diet	Assessment wt.	NPO b/4 OR (Min. 8 hours)	Advance as tol.				Tolerating diet
	Balanced diet						
Activity	Preop mobility	ROM exercises to unaffected joints					Exercises begin once dressing is removed
		Arm use, if allowed					
		HOB elevated					
Treatments		Screws in place, sling	Cont.	Cont.			Vig. exc. screws out
		K-wire immobilized with Velpeau bandage	Cont.	Cont.			Active exc. 2 wks postsurgery
		Exercises— Finger	Cont.	Cont.			Cont. finger exercises @ home
		Wound catheters	D/C				No infection
		Dressing	Cont.	Cont.			Change when return for MD appt.
Education	Teach pre & postoperative teaching regarding surgical preparation Rev. hosp routine	Reinforce					Follows teaching protocol
	Finger exercises	Demonstrate exercises					
	Review hosp LOS						

(continued)

Figure 13–7

Clinical Pathway: *(continued)*

Pathway	Preadmission Office/OP clinic	Admission Day Op day	Discharge Postop 1	Postop 2	Postop 3	Postop 4	Outcomes Rehabilitation
D/C Plan	Include exercises & activity level, signs of infection, & when to notify their physician	Rev. restricted activities					Knows activity level
	DC when recovered from anesthesia, usually 1–2 days or the same day as surgery	Rev. signs of infection					Knows when to contact physician

DISLOCATION

A dislocation of the glenohumeral joint is one of the most common upper-extremity injuries and accounts for approximately 50% of all major joint dislocations. Of all shoulder dislocations, 95% are anterior. Of all anterior dislocations, 50% to 70% are in patients under 30 years of age. After a primary anterior dislocation, recurrent dislocations appear in 90% to 95% of patients under 20 years of age, but with appropriate immediate care that risk may be reduced to 25% to 35%. For patients over 40 years of age, the recurrence rate is to 10% to 15%. With anterior dislocations, damage to the major nerves of the arm or to the axillary nerve occurs some 5% to 14% of the time, and bony lesions (fractures of the humeral head or greater tuberosity in conjunction with the dislocation) occur some 38% of the time. With axillary nerve injury, the disability varies from slight weakness of the deltoid muscle and hypesthesia over the upper outer aspect of the arm to complete paralysis of the muscle and anesthesia in the same area. Both usually clear up within a few weeks to several months.

Posttrauma Assessment.   The patient with an anterior dislocation seeks medical attention because of shoulder pain and severe disability. The patient usually resists any attempt at passive movement or active abduction of the arm. Clinical observation reveals a loss of symmetry of the shoulder. There is a flattening of the normally rounded shoulder contour when compared to the uninvolved side. The acromion is inordinately prominent, there is fullness anteriorly, and the humeral head can be palpated anteriorly in the subcoracoid region. (In very obese patients, however, those signs may be difficult to elicit.) Check the integrity of the axillary, radial, median, and ulnar nerves and the arterial circulation to the arm. If the axillary nerve is involved, there will be paralysis of the deltoid muscle and an area of anesthesia on the lateral aspect of the arm. Locating an area of anesthesia is important in assessing the axillary nerve function because the dislocation itself is so painful that

active abduction; that is, voluntary contraction of the deltoid, might be impossible. Roentgenography is an essential part of the assessment and demonstrates whether the head of the humerus has been displaced forward or backward in relation to the glenoid fossa.

Medical Treatment.   Treatment for a dislocated shoulder is to reduce the dislocation as soon as possible, immobilize the joint long enough for the damaged tissues to heal, and mobilize the joint soon enough to prevent permanent limitation of motion. Immediate reduction provides the patient with a great deal of relief. Reduction may be accomplished with or without general anesthesia. A reduction without general anesthesia requires muscle relaxation, possibly by means of 5 mg of diazepam intravenously, along with meperidine or morphine to reduce pain. The following are two of the numerous maneuvers that are utilized to reduce a dislocated shoulder. First, after medication, the patient is placed prone with the involved arm and shoulder hanging over the edge of the stretcher or table. A weight (approximately 10 pounds) is secured to the patient's hand. The patient is reassured and placed in a quiet area to let the medication relax the muscles. In about 20 to 30 minutes, the combination of muscle relaxation and the weighted pull on the arm should bring about reduction. If not, the physician may then place a hand in the axilla and lift the humerus laterally, using 5 to 10 pounds of force with gentle internal and external rotation. If successful, the shoulder will snap quickly into position.

Reduction under general anesthesia may be the method of choice, or it may be used if the first method fails. Once the shoulder is reduced, the timing of immobilization varies with the age of the patient. In young people, the risk of habitual or recurrent dislocation is fairly high, so the shoulder is usually immobilized either by a collar and cuff or by binding the arm to the side by means of a Velpeau bandage. Immobilization is usually maintained for 3 to 6 weeks to allow soft tissues and muscles to heal and to minimize the danger of permanent stiffness. In patients over 50, the risk of recurrent dislocation is minimal but the risk of permanent shoulder stiffness is considerable, so the shoulder is immobilized for much less time, if at all. These patients are usually started on gentle active and assisted movements as soon as they can tolerate them. In the older patient, it may be difficult to restore full movement, and for such patients a course of treatment for a stiff shoulder may be necessary. Complications following a dislocated shoulder include (1) damage to the nerves originating in the brachial plexus, (2) tears of the rotator cuff, (3) avulsion fractures of the greater tuberosity, and (4) recurrent dislocations of the shoulder.

Recurrent Dislocation. Dislocation of the shoulder joint in a young patient carries with it a high rate of recurrence. Recurrence is not nearly as frequent in middle-aged or elderly patients because of the normal tendency of the subscapularis muscle to tighten with age, thereby limiting the external rotation of the joint. Some persons experience multiple shoulder dislocations following unguarded movements of the arm (e.g., abduction and external rotation), and many become adept at reducing their own dislocations. Recurrence can become so frequent as to preclude vigorous physical activity in an otherwise healthy person, and no amount of immobilization will prevent that tendency. Operative repair is necessary for permanent correction of recurrent dislocations, and many different surgical techniques are performed to tighten the soft-tissue components of the joint. Some of these procedures are

1. The Bankart operation, in which the detached anterior structures of the glenoid labrum and the anterior part of the capsule are reattached to the rim of the glenoid cavity using sutures passed through holes in the glenoid rim
2. The staple capsulorrhaphy of du Toit and Roux, in which the detached capsule and labrum are stapled with no reconstruction of the muscles
3. The Putti-Platt operation, in which the subscapularis tendon is overlapped and shortened and the capsule is overlapped and tightened
4. The Manson and Stack operation, in which the anterior capsulomuscular wall is tightened by advancing the tendon of the subscapularis laterally on the humerus
5. The Eden-Hybbinette operation, in which a bone graft is placed against the anterior aspect of the neck of the scapula and the rim of the glenoid cavity so that it blocks anterior displacement of the humeral head
6. The Bristow procedure, in which the coracoid process is transplanted, with the attached conjoined tendons of the short head of the biceps and the coracobrachialis, to the anterior rim of the glenoid

The choice of repair depends upon the patient's age and activity level, and the degree of damage to the glenoid. The most common are the Putti-Platt and the Bristow repairs; the latter is preferred for athletic individuals who want as much external rotation as possible.

NURSING PROCESS (Patient with a Surgical Repair of a Recurrent Shoulder Dislocation)

The following nursing process demonstrates the nursing care of a patient with a surgical repair of a recurrent shoulder dislocation with a Velpeau bandage, a sling and swathe, or a shoulder immobilizer. The nursing process begins after the patient returns to the nursing unit.

ASSESSMENT

The first step in the nursing assessment of a typical patient following surgical repair of a recurrent dislocated shoulder and the application of a Velpeau bandage, a sling and swathe, or a shoulder immobilizer is to check the neurovascular status of the affected arm (see Chapter 2). Assess the respiratory status and the position of the upper trunk, affected arm, shoulder, and immobilizing device. Note if there is any undue pressure or tautness of the skin due to the immobilizing device. Assess the location, type, and severity of pain, and note if there is any drainage.

NURSING DIAGNOSIS

Based on all of the assessment data, the major nursing diagnoses for a typical patient with a surgical repair of a recurrent dislocated shoulder may include the following:

- Pain and discomfort related to the surgical procedure
- Impaired physical mobility related to a lack of glenohumeral joint stability
- Increased anxiety related to knowledge deficit about the surgery and rehabilitation

COLLABORATIVE PROBLEMS

- Circulatory impairment
- Shoulder joint stiffness
- Reduced range of motion
- Infection

GOAL FORMULATION AND PLANNING

The goals are to have the patient experience (1) a decrease in the amount of pain through nursing measures and prescribed medications, (2) an increase in joint mobility and stability based on the surgical procedure, (3) a decrease in anxiety through increased knowledge about the surgery and the rehabilitation process, and (4) an absence of complications from surgery and decreased activities. The long-term goals are to have the patient pain free and to have full return of joint motion without dislocation.

INTERVENTIONS

ALLEVIATE PAIN

The amount of pain the patient has is related to the extent of the procedure and the physical condition of the shoulder before surgery. A patient with a very large shoulder and arm usually has more postoperative pain because more soft tissue is incised. A patient with an internal fixation usually has more postoperative pain than a patient with soft-tissue suturing. Correct positioning, immobilization, and the application of ice around the incisional area may be helpful in reducing pain. The ice also helps to reduce any swelling that may occur postsurgery. Make sure the ice bags are not placed on the incision line.

Pain at the surgical site may be caused by stress from incorrect positioning or immobilization. Check to make sure that the patient is in correct body alignment and that the immobilizing device is properly applied. The immobilizer can cause a pull on the skin, which leads to discomfort. Because of the awkwardness of having the arm and the shoulder immobilized, patients may suffer a painful "jar" to the shoulder when they first try to get out of bed alone. Give the patient pain medications as needed.

INCREASE MOBILITY

The focus of nursing care to increase mobility is on correct positioning, exercises, and ambulation.

Position. The appropriate position for the shoulder following a surgical repair of a recurrent dislocation depends upon the surgical procedure. Patients who have had the Bankart, the Putti-Platt, the Manson and Stack, or the Eden-Hybbinette operation have their shoulder immobilized for the first 2 to 4 weeks in a Velpeau bandage (see NURSING PROCESS for a patient with an AC separation in this chapter). The Velpeau bandage is then removed and gentle exercises started, but the shoulder and arm may still need to be supported in a sling until approximately 6 weeks postsurgery. With the Bankart procedure, the sling is worn at night only, whereas with the Manson and Stack operation it is worn all the time.

The Bristow and du Toit and Roux procedures usually require a sling and a swathe dressing. Patients having the du Toit and Roux procedure may be placed in a simple triangular sling the day following surgery, and that sling is worn for approximately one week. With the Bristow procedure, the sling is usually worn for 4 to 5 weeks postsurgery.

Sling. A sling is used to support the arm with the hand level to or about the elbow and the hand and the wrist in a functional position. Such support is often desirable if there is edema in the hand, the wrist, or the elbow; shoulder pain; or an excessive pull on the shoulder. The use of a sling promotes comfort and, in some cases, helps to protect the extremity.

Many commercial slings are available, or a properly fitting sling can be made (Fig. 13–8). Obtain a triangular piece of cloth or bandage. Place the top corner of the

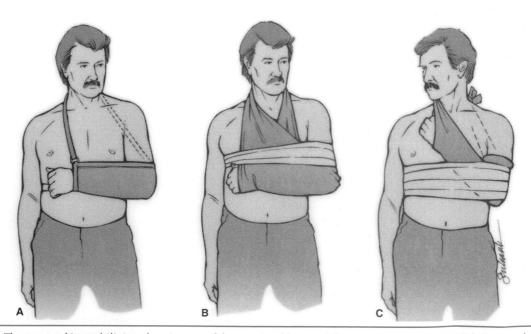

Figure 13–8   The types of immobilizing dressings used for proximal humeral fractures. (A) A commercial sling and swathe that permit easy removal of the arm for hygiene and are comfortable on the neck. (B) A conventional sling and swathe. (C) A stockinette Velpeau and swathe are used when there is an unstable surgical neck component, because this position relaxes the pectoralis major.   *(Smelzer & Bare (1996). Brunner & Suddarth's Textbook of Medical-Surgical Nursing. 8th ed. Philadelphia: Lippincott. p. 1921.)*

triangular cloth sling over the front of the patient's affected shoulder with the sling hanging between the patient's body and affected arm and the point of the triangle toward the patient's affected elbow. Bring the bottom corner of the triangle over the affected arm, up and over the unaffected shoulder, and behind the neck to the affected shoulder. Tie the sling at the side of the patient's neck, and fold the point of the triangle over the front of the patient's elbow, securing it with a safety pin. Check to make sure the patient's forearm and hand are level with or slightly higher than the elbow. Make sure that the hand is well supported. Assess the patient for comfort and support of the affected arm. Monitor for adequate circulation every 2 hours.

A sling should not be used continuously. The position of the extremity should be changed frequently to prevent tightness and discomfort in the muscles of the arm and the shoulder. Check the sling to ensure that (1) no pull is exerted on the shoulder joint, (2) the patient is not trying to protect the muscles of the neck and upper torso by contracting them, (3) excessive pressure is not exerted on the neck, and (4) the shoulder does not droop forward. The weight of the arm should be evenly distributed across the back of the neck.

Exercises. The type of exercises and when they are begun depend upon the type of surgical repair. Following a du Toit and Roux procedure, pendulum exercises without weights are usually begun at the end of the first week after surgery. At approximately 3 weeks postsurgery, gentle range-of-motion exercises with active abduction and external rotation are begun and are increased gradually over the next 3 weeks. By the sixth week postsurgery, all motion except external rotation has usually returned to normal. Increasingly active exercises for the shoulders are continued without weights so that by the end of 3 months normal motion has returned, except for some slight restriction of external rotation. Patients are not permitted to exercise with weights or return to vigorous manual labor and competitive athletics for 3 or more months.

The patient having a Bristow operation usually begins circumduction exercises between the third and sixth week postsurgery. After 6 weeks, increasing range-of-motion exercises without weights are started. Passive elbow extension is allowed at 4 to 5 weeks, but active extension is not allowed for at least 6 weeks after surgery.

With the Bankart, Putti-Platt, Eden-Hybbinette, and Manson and Stack operations, active exercises are begun when the Velpeau bandage is removed. The exercises are very gentle and are increased gradually, with the patient being instructed to avoid external rotation. Pendulum exercises are used, at first passively and later actively. With the Bankart procedure, rehabilitative exercises that allow the shoulder joint to be abducted to 90 degrees are begun approximately 6 weeks postsurgery. At 8 to 12 weeks, there is a full return of shoulder function, except that abduction and external rotation may be somewhat limited. The Putti-Platt and Manson and Stack procedures usually allow the patient to begin an exercise program 3 to 4 weeks after surgery. At 6 weeks postsurgery, a vigorous rehabilitation program is begun to restore motion in the joint and strengthen the muscles of the shoulder girdle and arm. For patients having a Manson and Stack procedure, external rotation of the shoulder will always be limited to about 50% of normal.

Ambulation. Because of the awkwardness resulting from not having the use of the involved arm, patients need assistance when first getting out of bed. In the beginning, they may also have problems in walking because of the lack of arm swing.

PATIENT TEACHING AND HOME CARE CONSIDERATIONS
Tell the patient that some skin irritation under the immobilizer is probably inevitable, especially in hot weather or under heavy wool clothing. The immobilizer must be kept in place, but the skin underneath can be cleansed and dried. If possible, antiperspirants should be used under the affected arm to reduce body odor. Discuss sponge bathing and taking a tub bath with a minimal amount of water to maintain overall hygiene.

To help the patient reduce discomfort at home, reinforce techniques utilized in the hospital. Discuss the types of chairs that are best for the patient to sit in. The patient needs to evaluate how stressful to the shoulder it will be to get out of a comfortable living room chair before sitting in one. Long, uninterrupted car rides should be avoided because the motion of the car affects the shoulder. Discuss with the patient, the family, and significant others the goals of the rehabilitation process.

In the beginning, the patient is usually taught to do pendulum or gentle range-of-motion exercises without weights or external rotation. The exercises are then gradually increased over time. Pendulum exercises are carried out by having the patient (1) lean forward, (2) allowing the arm to hang down and away from the body, and (3) slowly swinging the arm from side to side. In the beginning there may be very little pendulum swing, but it will gradually increase. Teach the patient what range of motion is, and provide a routine to follow. Tell the patient not to do internal or external rotation movements until allowed to so by the physician. Joint movements help to maintain and increase muscle strength as well as to regain full joint motion. Later, internal rotation may be regained by having the patient place the hand behind the lower back and then reach upward toward the scapula.

There are a number of exercises that will help the patient regain external rotation. The following four exercises are done with the patient lying supine:

1. With the arms parallel to the body, the palms are alternately pronated and supinated.
2. With the hands clasped behind the head, the elbows are alternately raised and flattened against the bed.

3. With the shoulders abducted to a right angle, the top of the bed is touched with each hand.
4. The patient reaches over their head to touch the opposite ear.

These four exercises can also be performed with the patient standing with their back to a wall. Another exercise is to have the patient stand sideways to a wall and have the fingers "climb" up the wall as far as possible. It is encouraging for the patient to mark the level reached each time so that the amount of progress can be observed.

MONITORING AND MANAGING POTENTIAL PROBLEMS

Patients with a surgical repair of a recurrent shoulder dislocation are at potential risk for infection, circulatory impairment, stiffness of the shoulder joint, and reduced range of motion of the glenohumeral joint, especially for external rotation.

INFECTION
Infection is a potential threat following surgery because of the break in skin integrity. Nursing procedures aimed at prevention should be implemented. Check the dressing for drainage. Keep the dressing dry. Do not allow the patient to shower or get the incision wet until after the sutures/staples are removed and the incision shows no sign of infection.

CIRCULATORY IMPAIRMENT
The surgical procedure and the position of the immobilized arm both put the patient at risk for circulatory impairment. Check the neurovascular status of the affected arm every 2 hours for the first 24 hours after surgery. Note any swelling, discoloration, or temperature change, and make comparisons with the unaffected arm. Have the patient do finger exercises to maintain circulation in their fingers.

SHOULDER JOINT STIFFNESS
Having the shoulder immobilized for a period of time will cause a certain degree of shoulder stiffness. Periodic roentgenograms are required following the Bristow procedure to note any change of position of the transferred coracoid or of the screw utilized in the repair. To prevent further complications, a loose screw is usually removed. An osseous union only occurs in approximately 50% to 75% of the patients and is difficult to determine even by roentgenograms. A fibrous union occurs in the remaining 25% to 50%. Following the prescribed exercise program rigorously helps to prevent complications.

EVALUATION/OUTCOMES

Determine the level of pain and whether nursing measures and drug therapy are effective in relieving it. Note whether the patient is able to maintain correct positioning in bed and when ambulating. Determine whether the immobilizing device is effectively immobilizing the shoulder and the arm. In discussions with the patient, the family, and significant others, determine the level of understanding about the exercise program and the total rehabilitation process. Supply information or correct misconceptions as needed. If the patient lives alone, make sure help is available. Discuss potential problems with the patient (and social worker) if indicated. Make sure the patient understands the importance of adhering to the physician's orders regarding follow-up visits and what to do if problems arise.

CLINICAL PATHWAY (Patient with a Surgical Repair Recurrent Shoulder Dislocation)

A generic clinical pathway for a patient with a surgical repair of a recurrent shoulder dislocation is shown in Figure 13–9.

PROXIMAL HUMERAL FRACTURES
Fractures of the proximal humerus in adults may be classified as (1) avulsion fractures of the tuberosities, (2) impacted fractures of the surgical or anatomical neck, (3) fracture dislocations, and (4) displaced fractures of the neck. Avulsion fractures of the tuberosities may result from a variety of mechanisms, but they frequently occur as a result of seizures or secondary to glenohumeral dislocations. Impacted fractures occur almost exclusively in older people. In most cases, the use of a sling to support the arm and progressive arm exercises are all that is required for repair. Fracture-dislocations of the shoulder are common injuries and occur in all age groups. They usually require only closed reduction, but occasionally open reduction and internal fixation are necessary.

A fracture of the surgical neck of the humerus with a slight displacement is one of the most common fractures of the elderly. The fracture occurs when the elderly person falls directly against the shoulder with the arm against the chest. In a displaced fracture, the pectoral muscles pull the distal fragment inward and forward, and the deltoid pulls it upward. These fractures are usually treated symptomatically with guided, active, assisted range-of-motion and pendulum exercises to prevent stiffness of the shoulders. In some cases, the arm and the shoulder are immobilized in a Velpeau bandage for 3 weeks (see care of a patient with an AC separation earlier in this chapter), in a hanging arm cast (see Chapter 6, nursing care of a patient with a fractured humerus and a hanging arm cast), or in a lateral traction apparatus that maintains forward flexion and traction until a soft callus forms (see Chapter 6). If displacement of the fragments is too severe to expect return of function, an open reduction to replace the fragments is performed.

Figure 13–9

Clinical Pathway: Surgical Repair of a Recurrent Shoulder Dislocation

Admission Date: _____   Discharge Plan: _____ Home   _____ Skilled Nursing   _____ Extended Care Facility

Pathway	Preadmission Office/OP clinic	Admission Day Op day	Discharge Postop 1	Postop 2	Postop 3	Postop 4	Outcomes Rehabilitation
Consultation	Primary care/ Medical physician	Case Manager					Postoperative appt. with physician
		Anesthesia, OT	Cont.				Return for OT appts.
		PT, if necessary	Cont.				
Assessment	Nrsg database	Review & add					
	H & P exam. by MD, NP, or PA	Review H & P					
	Including normal activity	Postop routine N/V status affected arm	Cont.	Cont.			No deficit
Tests	ECG/blood/UA/ Shoulder x-rays						
Medications	D/C NSAIDs/ASA 10 days b/4 OR	✓ preadmn meds					
	Analgesics as needed	Routine meds					
	Instruct on preop meds b/4 OR	Oral narcotic meds/analgesics as needed	Cont.	Cont.			Minimal amt. of pain relieved with meds
		Antibiotics	D/C antibiotics				
Diet	Assessment wt.	NPO b/4 OR (min. 8 hours)	Advance as tol.				Tolerating diet
	Balanced diet						
Activity	Preop mobility	ROM exercises to unaffected joints					Exercises begin once dressing is removed
		HOB elevated					
		Sling support for arm or shoulder immobilizer					
Treatments		Exercises— Finger	Cont.	Cont.			Cont. exc @ home
							Pendulum exercises 1 wk P.O.
							See physician orders for exercises based on specific procedure
Education	Teach pre & postoperative teaching regarding surgical preparation Rev. hosp routine	Dressing Reinforce	Cont.	Cont.			Change when return for MD appt.
	Discuss exercises	Demonstrate finger exc					
	Review hosp LOS						

(continued)

Figure 13–9
Clinical Pathway: *(continued)*

Pathway	Preadmission Office/OP clinic	Admission Day Op day	Discharge Postop 1	Postop 2	Postop 3	Postop 4	Outcomes Rehabilitation
D/C Plan	Include exercises & activity level, signs of infection, & when to notify their physician	Rev. restricted activities					Knows activity level
	LOS usually 2–3 days	Rev. signs of infection					Knows signs and symptoms of infect.
							Knows when to contact physician.

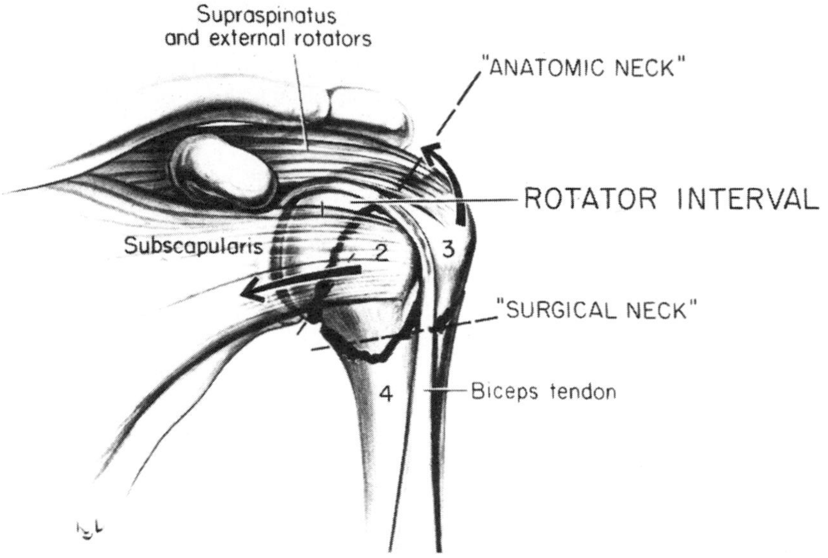

Figure 13–10   Drawing showing the rotator interval, a ligamentous area between the tendons of the supraspinatus and subscapularis, and the four major fragments of proximal humerus fractures: (1) head, (2) lesser tuberosity, (3) greater tuberosity, and (4) shaft.   *(Koval & Zuckerman (1998).* Fractures in the Elderly. *Philadelphia: Lippincott-Raven.)*

ROTATOR CUFF TEARS

The rotator cuff is a musculotendinous cuff that stabilizes the humeral head as it moves against the glenoid labrum and acts a fulcrum, allowing the deltoid to elevate (abduct) the arm without impingement between the superior humeral head and the acromion process of the scapula (Fig. 13–10). The four muscles and their tendons that make up the rotator cuff are (1) the subscapularis (anterior); (2) the supraspinatous (posterior); (3) the infraspinatous (posterior, superior); and (4) the teres minor (posterior, inferior) (Heveron & Kaempffe, 1995). The rotator cuff of the shoulder normally undergoes some degenerative changes with advancing age. Asymptomatic "worn out" spots may appear in the cuff. A rupture of the rotator cuff can then occur if a sudden adduction force is applied to the cuff while the arm is being held in abduction. Traumatic tears of the cuff can also result from a fall on the shoulder, from throwing, from heavy lifting, or in conjunction with a glenohumeral dislocation. Such a tear in younger patients is usually the consequence of substantial trauma.

Patients with a tear of the rotator cuff have shoulder pain where the tear comes in contact with the coracoacromial ligament when the arm is in abduction or externally rotated (Fig. 13–11). Local tenderness may be noted over the cuff, and the patient may be unable to initiate or maintain active abduction of the arm at the shoulder joint (Fig. 13–12). The arm can be passively abducted at the shoulder, but the patient may be unable to sustain that position and the arm will drop to the side. Full mobility of the shoulder joint is not lost because the scapula is not affected. Atrophy of the cuff muscles (i.e., the supraspinatus, infraspinatus, and teres

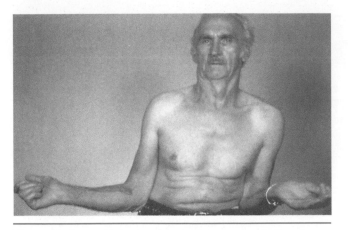

Figure 13–11   Full-thickness tear of the rotator cuff in the left shoulder of a patient. Although active external rotation on the right appears normal, there is inability to initiate external rotation on the left, owing to the involvement of the infraspinatus and teres minor with the tear.   *(Weinstein & Buckwalter (1994).* Turek's Orthopaedic: Principles and Their Applications. *Philadelphia: Lippincott-Raven.)*

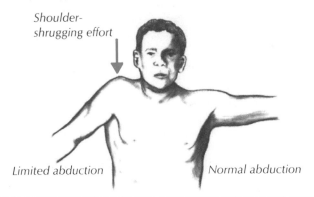

Figure 13–12   Repeated impingement (or other conditions) may weaken the rotator cuff and eventually cause partial or complete tears in it, usually after the age of 40 years. Injury, such as falling, may precipitate a tear. Manifestations include weakness, atrophy of the supraspinatus and infraspinatus muscles, pain, and tenderness. In a complete tear of the supraspinatus tendon (illustrated), active abduction at the glenohumeral joint is several impaired. Effort to abduct the arm produce a characteristic shoulders shrugging instead. *(Bates, B. (1995).* A Guide to Physical Examination and History Taking. *6th ed. Philadelphia: J.B. Lippincott Company.)*

minor) may be palpated. Roentgenographic examination is often normal but can show spur formation along the anterior edge of the acromion or a displaced fracture of the tuberosity. MRI examination can be more definitive (Fig. 13–13). The diagnosis of a ruptured rotator cuff can also be confirmed by an arthrogram that demonstrates leakage of the contrast material from the shoulder joint capsule into the subacromial bursa.

Treatment of rotator cuff tears depends on the age of the patient and the size of the tear. A young patient with an ordinary or large tear is usually treated with immediate surgical repair. In an older patient or one with a small tear, the treatment is symptomatic, with the emphasis on maintaining good passive range of motion and on the return of abduction strength. Later surgical

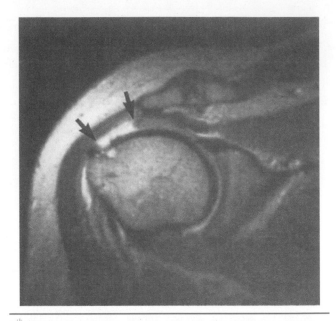

Figure 13–13   MRI scan showing a full-thickness tear of the rotator cuff. The arrows outline the extent of tear, and high-signal intensity indicates fluid, which tracks from the glenohumeral joint into the subacromial space. This is a tear in the supraspinatus and is easily identifiable between two arrows.   *(Weinstein & Buckwalter (1994).* Turek's Orthopaedic: Principles and Their Applications. *Philadelphia: Lippincott-Raven.)*

repair might be indicated if satisfactory abduction strength does not return after at least 6 weeks of physical therapy. Because many patients sustain only an incomplete rupture and gradually recover strength and motion spontaneously, initial treatment of a torn rotator cuff is usually conservative. The arm is supported in a sling, and hot applications may be used on the shoulder after the initial bleeding stops.

Surgical treatment of the rotator cuff area (Fig. 13–14) is used for patients who do not respond to a conservative program, usually after 6 to 8 months (Heveron & Kaempffe, 1995). Those patients have usually sustained massive tears or complete ruptures of the rotator cuff. An acromioplasty (Fig. 13–15) is performed by resecting one half of the thickness of the anterior acromion and tapering the resection posteriorly. The rotator cuff is mobilized and repaired, the technique depending upon the location and size of the tear. Every effort is made to obtain a repair that is tension free with the patient's arm at their side and internally rotated to about 30 degrees. If a massive, full-thickness tear cannot be repaired, which occurs occasionally, then the surgical option is to do a subacromial decompression (acromioplasty) and a débridement of nonviable rotator cuff tissue without attempting a direct repair. The use of autogenous or allograft tendon grafts or the use of active tendon transfers is implemented. Other procedures that involve massive tears have involved suturing together the edges with heavy nonabsorbable suture or attaching the torn edges to the humeral head through drill holes or a wedge-shaped osteotomy. Postoperatively, simple repairs are

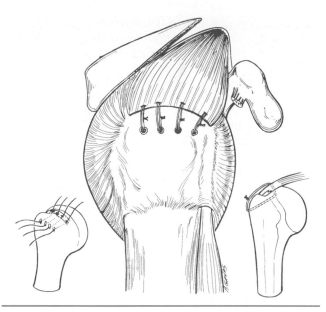

Figure 13–14 Method of rotator cuff repair. The torn edges of the rotator cuff tendon are advanced into the bone and anchored with sutures, which go through the bone. *(Weinstein & Buckwalter (1994). Turek's Orthopaedic: Principles and Their Applications. Philadelphia: Lippincott-Raven.)*

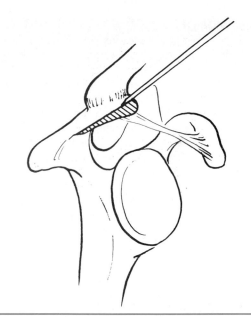

Figure 13–15 An anterior acromioplasty removes the undersurface of anterior acromion (and the overhanging anterior acromial spur). In addition, the coracoacromial ligament is removed. This removes the impingement wear. *(Weinstein & Buckwalter (1994). Turek's Orthopaedic: Principles and Their Applications. Philadelphia: Lippincott-Raven.)*

treated with a sling. Pendulum exercises are started on the third or fourth postsurgical day, and progressive active exercises are started after 2 weeks. More extensive repairs may require side arm suspension and restriction of abduction for 4 to 6 weeks. Aggressive exercises are begun after that period.

NURSING PROCESS (Patient with a Rotator Cuff Repair)

The following nursing process demonstrates the nursing care for a typical patient following the surgical repair of a torn rotator cuff. The nursing process begins when the patient returns to the nursing unit.

ASSESSMENT

The first step in the nursing assessment of a patient with a surgical repair of the rotator cuff and a shoulder immobilizer is to assess the neurovascular status of the affected arm (see Chapter 2). Check the position of the arm and the position of the shoulder immobilizer. Verify that the immobilizing straps are not too tight or irritating to the patient's skin. It is important to check the arm where there is direct skin-to-skin contact between the arm and chest. Elicit information on the location, duration, and severity of pain.

NURSING DIAGNOSIS

Based on all of the assessment data, the major nursing diagnoses for a typical patient with a surgical repair of a torn rotator cuff may include the following:

- Pain and discomfort related to soft-tissue trauma from the surgery
- Impaired physical mobility related to immobilization of the affected shoulder and arm
- Increased anxiety related to knowledge deficit about the surgical procedure and rehabilitation

COLLABORATIVE PROBLEMS

- Reduced function at the shoulder and elbow joint
- Infection

GOAL FORMULATION AND PLANNING

The goals are to have the patient experience (1) a decrease in the amount of pain through the immobilization of the shoulder and prescribed medications, (2) an increase in physical mobility through stabilization of the shoulder joint, (3) a decrease in anxiety through increased knowledge about the surgery and rehabilitation, and (4) an absence of complications. Long-term goals are to have the patient obtain full recovery within one year.

INTERVENTIONS

ALLEVIATE PAIN
Nursing measures that help to reduce pain are applying ice to reduce swelling, correct positioning, and having the patient do exercises as allowed. Medicate for pain as needed. (For further interventions, see the NURSING PROCESS for a patient with an AC joint repair earlier in this chapter.)

INCREASE MOBILITY

The focus of nursing care interventions to increase mobility is on correct positioning, exercises, and ambulation.

Position.   The patient usually finds that the most comfortable position in bed is the supine position with the head of the bed slightly elevated. The patient can turn from their back to the unaffected side but will usually find just tilting onto their side is the most comfortable. However, they will probably not find lying on their side for any period of time comfortable as it is more comfortable to keep the shoulder and arm in a position of reduced stress, even with the shoulder immobilizer in place. The patient should be encouraged to use the trapeze with the unaffected arm to readjust and change position in bed and to help with daily care.

Exercises.   The patient should do finger exercises and muscle-setting or isometric exercises with the affected arm immediately after surgery. By the afternoon following a morning surgery, the patient may start pendulum exercises and then do them twice a day thereafter. It is also important at that time and during every pendulum exercise period that the patient exercise the elbow. Because the repair is likely to be weakest at 3 weeks, a structured therapy program of shoulder motion is not initiated until 4 weeks postoperatively (Heveron & Kaempffe, 1995). Resistive exercises are begun 8 weeks after surgery, and the patient continues with a physical therapy exercise session twice weekly to gain strength and motion for another 12 to 16 weeks postsurgery. The patient will continue doing exercises at home until full recovery, which may take up to one year.

Shoulder Immobilizer.   Most institutions use commercial shoulder immobilizers as they are usually easier for the patient to remove and reapply. In a number of hospitals, the physical therapist teaches the patient how to remove and reapply the shoulder immobilizer when they teach them about their exercises. During the 2 to 3 days of hospitalization, the immobilizer is removed to allow the patient to do pendulum exercises twice a day.

Ambulation.   The patient is usually allowed up shortly after the application of the shoulder immobilizer but needs assistance in getting out of bed the first few times. Do not support the patient under the affected elbow or put pressure on the patient's affected shoulder. Have the patient get out of bed on the unaffected side.

PATIENT TEACHING AND HOME CARE CONSIDERATIONS

Teach the patient how to do the prescribed exercises. Try to work out a schedule that fits into the patient's daily activities. After week 4, the patient will begin a more structured therapy program of shoulder motion. Resistive exercises are begun 8 weeks after surgery, and the patient will continue with physical therapy twice a week for 12 to 16 weeks. Make sure the patient understands that he or she has the responsibility for doing the exercises to regain function in the shoulder. Although the patient may be able to return to work in 3 months, the rotator cuff repair may take from 6 months to a year before complete function is regained.

Help the patient, the family, and significant others learn the required care. Make sure the patient understands the purpose and objectives of the shoulder immobilizer. The patient may need help in dressing and doing activities of daily living.

MONITORING AND MANAGING POTENTIAL PROBLEMS

Potential complications for a patient with a rotator cuff repair and shoulder immobilizer are contractures of the elbow and shoulder and infection. Contractures of the shoulder and elbow can occur if the patient does not follow the exercise and rehabilitation regime. It is important that the patient understands, before surgery, their responsibility in doing the exercises in order to regain full range of motion and function within the shoulder joint with no reduction in function at the elbow.

INFECTION

Infection is a risk following any open surgery. Keep the dressing dry and intact. Most patients will be on antibiotics for the first 24 to 48 hours. Check the patient's skin at the edges of the immobilizer. If the immobilizer is too loose or too tight, it can irritate the patient's skin. Make sure the patient's clothing/hospital gown is between the patient's chest and the immobilizer, as the immobilizer will sometimes irritate the patient's skin along the chest wall. Teach the patient the signs of infection and how to prevent skin irritation from the immobilizer.

EVALUATION/OUTCOMES

A patient with a surgical repair of the rotator cuff should have a decrease in pain. If pain persists, nursing measures and medication should relieve it. The patient should be free of any skin irritation from the immobilizer. Determine how comfortable the patient is in administering self-care and whether he or she needs help when returning home.

CLINICAL PATHWAY (Patient with Surgical Repair of a Rotator Cuff)

A generic clinical pathway for a patient with surgical repair of a rotator cuff is shown in Figure 13–16.

ARTHROPLASTY

Lesions about the shoulder requiring arthroplasty are much less common than those of weight-bearing joints such as the hip and the knee. An arthroplasty of the shoulder may be a prosthetic humeral head replacement (hemiarthroplasty) or a total shoulder arthroplasty,

Figure 13–16

Clinical Pathway: Surgical Repair of a Rotator Cuff

Admission Date: _____   **Discharge Plan:** _____ **Home**   _____ **Skilled Nursing**   _____ **Extended Care Facility**

Pathway	Preadmission Office/OP clinic	Admission Day Op day	Discharge Postop 1	Postop 2	Postop 3	Postop 4	Outcomes Rehabilitation
Consultation	Primary Care/ Medical physician	Case Manager Anesthesia,					Postoperative appt. with physician
		OT	Cont.				Return for OT appts.
		PT, if necessary	Cont.				
Assessment	Nrsg database	Review & add					
	H & P exam. by MD, NB, or PA	Review H & P					
	Including normal activity	Postop routine					No N/V deficit
		N/V status affected arm	Cont.	Cont.			
Tests	ECG/blood /UA/ Shoulder x-rays	✓ preadm meds					
Medications	D/C NSAIDs/ASA 10 days b/4 OR						
	Analgesics as needed	Routine meds					
	Instruct on preop meds b/4 OR	Oral narcotic meds/ analgesics as needed	Cont.	Cont.			Minimal amt of pain relieved with meds
		Antibiotics	D/C antibiotics				
Diet	Assessment wt.	NPO b/4 OR (Min. 8 hours)	Advance as tol				Tolerating diet
	Balanced diet						
Activity	Preop mobility	ROM exercises to unaffected joints					
		HOB elevated					
		Shoulder immobilizer					
Treatments		Exercises— Finger	Cont.	Cont.			Cont. exc @ home
		Shoulder immobilizer removed for pendulum exercises 2 × da	Cont.	Cont.			Pendulum exercises and stress elbow motion
							Structured shoulder exc. for 4 wks—1 year for recovery
		Wound catheters	D/C				No infection
		Dressing	Cont.	Cont.			Change when return for MD appt.
Education	Teach pre & postoperative	Reinforce					Able to follow exc. regime
	Teaching regarding surgical preparation Rev. hosp routine						
	Discuss exercises	Demonstrate finger exc					
	Review hosp LOS						

(continued)

Figure 13–16

Clinical Pathway: *(continued)*

Pathway	Preadmission Office/OP clinic	Admission Day Op day	Discharge Postop 1	Postop 2	Postop 3	Postop 4	Outcomes Rehabilitation
D/C Plan	Include exercises & activity level, signs of infection, & when to notify their physician	Rev. restricted activities					Knows activity level
	LOS usually 2–3 days	Rev. signs of infection					Knows signs and symptoms of infect
							Knows when to contact physician

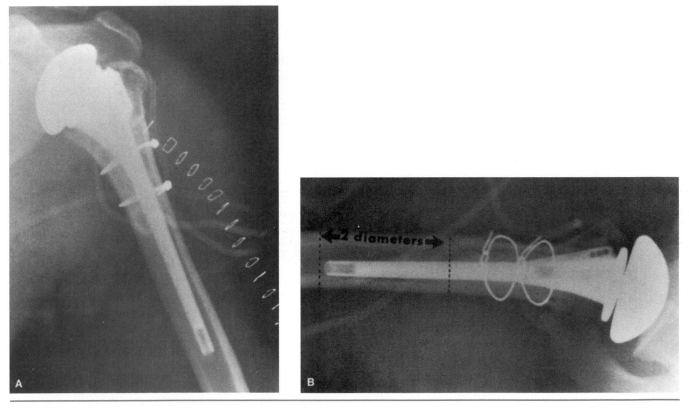

Figure 13–17   (A) This patient sustained a comminuted three-part fracture dislocation of the proximal humerus that extended distally for several centimeters. Treatment consisted of a cemented hemiarthroplasty augmented with cerelage wires. (B) Note that the humeral stem bypasses the distal extent of the fracture by about two cortical diameters.   *(Rockwood, et al. (1996).* Rockwood & Green's Fractures in Adults. *Philadelphia: Lippincott-Raven.)*

where the humeral head is replaced and the glenoid cavity resurfaced. A hemiarthroplasty (Fig. 13–17) is usually indicated for the treatment of certain acute fractures of the proximal humerus or painful, chronic glenohumeral incongruities. Replacement of the proximal humerus is done for fracture-dislocations and for the treatment of fractures in which reduction is almost impossible and the articular fragment is likely to undergo avascular necrosis. These patients usually need

surgery as soon as possible after the injury. A delay of 10 to 14 days or longer results in increased scarring, contractures of the muscles and other soft-tissue structures, and increased osteoporosis of the bone fragments.

A total shoulder arthroplasty is indicated when there is severe destruction of the joint from trauma or a disease process such as rheumatoid arthritis, avascular necrosis, or arthritis after instability surgery. The total shoulder arthroplasty replaces the humeral head with a metallic

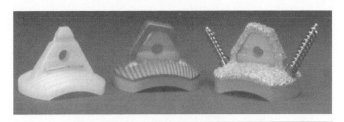

Figure 13–18 A matching glenoid component for total shoulder system. Various types of glenoids are available, depending on the particular need of the patient. *(Weinstein & Buckwalter (1994).* Turek's Orthopaedic: Principles and Their Applications. *Philadelphia: Lippincott-Raven.)*

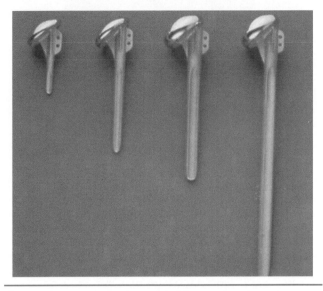

Figure 13–19 A typical proximal humeral replacement consists of a ball that articulates with a plastic glenoid. An intermedullary stem aids in fixation. *(Weinstein & Buckwalter (1994).* Turek's Orthopaedic Principles and Their Applications. *Philadelphia: Lippincott-Raven.)*

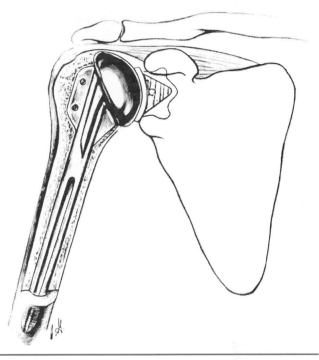

Figure 13–20 A total shoulder arthroplasty (humerus and glenoid in place). With elimination of the pain through resurfacing of the arthritic joint, the muscles providing motion for the glenohumeral joint can be rehabilitated successfully. *(Weinstein & Buckwalter (1994).* Turek's Orthopaedic: Principles and Their Applications. *Philadelphia: Lippincott-Raven.)*

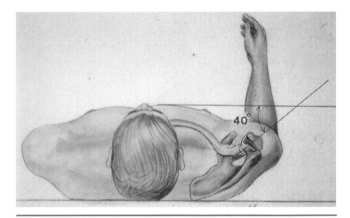

Figure 13–21 A total shoulder replacement in place, showing the position of the glenoid and the humeral head viewed from above. *(Weinstein & Buckwalter (1994).* Turek's Orthopaedic: Principles and Their Applications. *Philadelphia: Lippincott-Raven.)*

component (Fig. 13–18) and resurfaces the glenoid cavity. Prostheses for the humerus (Fig. 13–19) are available in a range of stem lengths, neck lengths, and head diameters that allow the normal anatomy of the shoulder to be closely approximated. Developmental work is continuing.

During a total shoulder replacement procedure, the tip of the coracoid may be resected, and the subscapularis muscle and capsule are divided to expose the glenohumeral joint. The humerus is then dislocated, and the humeral head is resected. The glenoid cavity and the humeral canal are reamed in preparation for the prosthesis. The humeral and glenoid components are then cemented into place with methyl methacrylate cement as press-fit glenoid components are still experimental at this time. The glenohumeral joint is reduced, and the capsule and subscapularis are closed (Fig. 13–20 and Fig. 13–21). Once the procedure is completed and the wound closed, the physician tries to make the repair of the incision as cosmetically pleasing as possible since the incision is located on the front of the patient's shoulder. A sling and swathe bandage is applied. If the musculo-tendinous (rotator) cuff has required reconstruction, an abduction humeral splint may be used.

NURSING PROCESS (Patient with a Shoulder Arthroplasty)

The following nursing process demonstrates the nursing care of a patient with a shoulder arthroplasty and the application of a splint or a sling and swathe. The nursing process begins after the patient returns to the nursing unit.

ASSESSMENT

The first step in the nursing assessment of a typical patient following a shoulder arthroplasty with a splint or a sling and swathe is a neurovascular assessment of the affected arm to check the brachial plexus of the affected extremity (see Chapter 2). Continue to do a neurovascular assessment every 2 hours for the first 24 hours or according to the institution's policy. Check vital signs every 4 hours. Check the depth, rate, and rhythm of respirations, and auscultate the patient's chest for clearness of their lungs and for any heart abnormalities. Assess the wound dressing for any signs of bleeding, and note the amount of drainage. If wound catheters are in place, check the amount and color of the drainage every 8 hours. Make sure the patient is in correct body alignment and that the immobilizing device is supporting the arm and relieving the pull on the shoulder. The arm may be placed on a pillow. Determine the location, type, and severity of pain.

NURSING DIAGNOSIS

Based on all of the assessment data, the major nursing diagnoses for a typical patient following a shoulder arthroplasty may include the following:

- Pain and discomfort related to bone and soft-tissue trauma from the surgical procedure
- Impaired physical mobility related to a lack of shoulder joint stability and decreased muscle strength
- Increased anxiety related to knowledge deficit about the surgery and rehabilitation

COLLABORATIVE PROBLEMS

- Instability of the glenohumeral joint
- Infection
- Impingement syndrome
- Nerve injuries
- Loosening or failure of the prosthesis

GOAL FORMULATION AND PLANNING

The goals are to have the patient experience (1) a decrease in shoulder pain, (2) an increase in joint mobility through controlled exercise, (3) a decrease in anxiety through increased knowledge about the surgical procedure and the rehabilitation process, and (4) an absence of complications from surgery and decreased mobility. Long-term goals are to have the patient free of pain and able to have full function in the glenohumeral joint (Fig. 13–22).

INTERVENTIONS

ALLEVIATE PAIN
Following a shoulder arthroplasty, the patient may have pain during the first few days after surgery even though

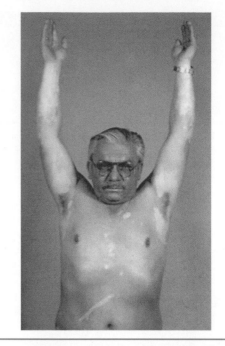

Figure 13–22   A patient who has primary osteoarthritis of the shoulder after bilateral total shoulder replacements. Because the rotator cuff and deltoid muscles are typically normal in primary osteoarthritis, the potential exists for near full range of motion of the shoulder.   *(Weinstein & Buckwalter (1994).* Turek's Orthopaedic: Principles and Their Applications. *Philadelphia: Lippincott-Raven.)*

the arm is immobilized. The patient recognizes the post-surgery shoulder pain as distinctly different from the preoperative pain. Some physicians may use a regional block to provide effective pain relief for approximately the first 12 hours postsurgery. Other patients may use a patient controlled analgesic (PCA) pump, or intramuscular (IM) morphine or meperidine every 3 to 4 hours which may be supplemented with IM ketorolac (Toradol) every 6 hours for the first 24 hours. After the first 24 hours, oral analgesics (i.e., Vicodin or Tylenol #3) are given as needed for pain (Deuschle & Romeo, 1998).

Check the patient for correct body alignment to reduce the stress on the shoulder. Elevating the head of the bed and positioning the affected arm on a pillow may be necessary to help keep the shoulder aligned while the patient is in bed. Ice may be applied near the incision to reduce swelling and discomfort.

Pain medications are administered after nursing interventions for specific problems. Do not wait until the patient asks for medications, but assess and intervene before the pain becomes severe. When the patient begins a shoulder exercise program, give medication before beginning the exercise.

INCREASE MOBILITY
Measures to increase the patient's mobility focus on correct positioning, exercises, and ambulation.

Position.   Nursing interventions after a shoulder arthroplasty are based on maintaining the proper position of the affected arm to reduce pain, promote healing, and prevent complications. A sling, a sling and swathe bandage, or a shoulder immobilizer is usually employed to immobilize the arm unless the musculo-tendinous rotator cuff required reconstruction during the arthroplasty. If so, an adduction humeral splint or cast shell may be used. If the arm is immobilized in a sling, a sling and swathe, or a shoulder immobilizer, the arm should be in the immobilizing device at all times, except when exercising. The head of the bed is elevated for comfort, usually 30 degrees. The patient usually lies supine but may turn onto the uninvolved side. After the turn, pillows are necessary to help support the affected arm. The patient may use the trapeze to help readjust their position, but only with the unaffected arm.

Exercises. Exercises of all the joints, except those of the involved arm, are encouraged from the day of surgery. Finger and thumb exercises with the involved arm may also be started immediately. Under supervision, the patient begins gentle passive exercises consisting mainly of forward flexion and external rotation shoulder exercises. For many patients, pendulum type exercises are not started until approximately 10 days postsurgery. The gentle passive and active assisted exercises progress according to the patient's pain tolerance. Passive exercises may be instituted on the day of surgery using a continuous passive motion (CPM) machine. (See Chapter 8 for a discussion of the CPM machine and its utilization in the rehabilitation of a patient following a total knee arthroplasty.) The shoulder CPM can provide passive motion in all three planes of the shoulder, although only forward flexion and external rotation are used initially. Motion in other planes may be added as the patient continues to use the CPM machine at home (Johnson, 1993).

To a great degree, functional recovery depends on implementing a comprehensive postoperative rehabilitation regime. The patient needs to do the exercise program for up to a year after surgery. The prescribed exercises may vary with the patient's condition and the type of prosthesis. For example, a patient with a hemi-arthroplasty prosthesis who has had few muscles severed and a fully functional rotator cuff has more muscle power than a patient who has undergone a total gleno-humeral replacement. Both have had their deltoid muscles cut, so neither should attempt to actively elevate their arm to the side until the deltoid muscle has healed, usually 6 to 8 weeks after surgery. Other patients may begin the pendulum exercises as early as the second postoperative day. Because that would be the first time the affected arm has been extended and lowered in some time, the patient will usually complain of tingling. Once the exercise program is begun, the role of the nurse includes encouraging the patient and reinforcing the instructions.

Ambulation. In the beginning, the patient will need assistance in getting out of bed. Because of the lack of arm swing with their arm held close to their chest, the patient will need to adjust quickly to a change in balance. Make sure they have a steady gait to prevent falls

or injury to the affected shoulder and that they do not try to pull their arm out of the shoulder immobilizer for balance or to protect themselves from falling.

PATIENT TEACHING AND HOME CARE CONSIDERATIONS
Patients with uncomplicated osteoarthritis of the glenohumeral joint have the best success with a total shoulder arthroplasty, but patient education is a must. Complete and optimal recovery from a total shoulder arthroplasty is a lengthy, therapy-intense process. The patient must be willing to do the exercises, as they are as important in recovering mobility as what the physician did. The family must understand the importance of the exercise regime so they can encourage and motivate the patient. Individual initiative must be consistently solicited and praised. The outpatient/home therapy program will continue for 6 months or more. Pain relief is usually not accomplished for at least 2 months.

The patient must understand not only the need for the exercises but how to protect the immobilized arm until healing of soft tissue occurs. Make sure the patient understands that they are not to move the shoulder joint in planes not approved by their physician. Once the patient is home, most patients will be allowed to shower and cleanse the incision with mild soap and water.

MONITORING AND MANAGING POTENTIAL PROBLEMS

Potential complications following a total shoulder arthroplasty are similar to those encountered with other joint arthroplasties and consist of prosthetic loosening or failure, contractures (due to lack of follow-through with the exercise regime), dislocation and/or subluxation, tuberosity nonunion in proximal humeral fractures, and ectopic ossification. Total shoulder arthroplasty patients have a higher risk of joint instability, infection, nerve injuries, impingement syndrome, and continued pain. In spite of the surgical procedure and follow-through with exercises, the patient may continue to have pain in the shoulder area.

INSTABILITY OF THE GLENOHUMERAL JOINT
The instability of the glenohumeral joint following a total shoulder arthroplasty is a major concern. To help prevent this from occurring, the patient must understand the importance of the exercises, how to do them correctly, and how often to do them. They must then rigidly follow the exercise program.

INFECTION
Infection is always a major concern for patients having a total joint arthroplasty. Make sure the dressing is dry and intact. Verify that the suction drains, if used, are working correctly. Note if there is any redness, hardness, or drainage from the incisional area. Assess the patient's general condition for any signs or symptoms of infection. Teach the patient how to

assess for infection before they go home. The patient will be on antibiotic therapy.

IMPINGEMENT SYNDROME

Bones and ligaments provide coverage and protection for the top of the rotator cuff, effectively deepening and stabilizing the shoulder joint. However, this limits the space available to the rotator cuff for its movements during shoulder motion. Specifically, when the shoulder is elevated 90 degrees and moved forward into 45 degrees of abduction from the sagittal plane, the rotator cuff is pushed against—impinged—by the greater tuberosity of the humerus and the undersurface of the coracoacromial arch. Any condition that limits this space can result in chronic irritation and can ultimately precipitate a rupture of the rotator cuff. This process has become known as the "impingement syndrome." The impingement syndrome is usually treated with an acromioplasty performed either arthroscopically or as an open procedure.

NERVE INJURIES

A risk particular to the total shoulder arthroplasty is neurologic injury or nerve palsy related to the proximity of the brachial plexus to the surgical field. The risk may be minimized by careful surgical technique during the total shoulder procedure.

EVALUATION/OUTCOMES

Determine the patient's ability to understand and accomplish the required exercises. The amount of pain at the incisional site should decrease over time, but there should still be some pain after exercising as the patient continues to regain joint function. The patient should be free of any complications from the surgery and decreased mobility.

CLINICAL PATHWAY (Patient with a Shoulder Arthroplasty)

A generic clinical pathway for a patient with a shoulder arthroplasty is shown in Figure 13–23.

THE PAINFUL SHOULDER

Pain in the shoulder may be caused by various conditions. Apart from traumatic lesions, 85% to 90% of painful disabilities of the shoulder are due to nonarticular disorders of tendons, bursae, tendon sheaths, and the musculotendinous cuff.

Calcific Tendonitis (Subacromial Bursitis). Bursitis is an inflammation of the sac (bursa) covering a bony prominence. When the underlying tendon is also inflamed,

---

Figure 13–23
Clinical Pathway: Shoulder Arthroplasty

Admission Date: _____ **Discharge Plan:** _____ **Home** _____ **Skilled Nursing** _____ **Extended Care Facility**

Pathway	Preadmission Office/OP clinic	Admission Day Op day	Discharge Postop 1	Postop 2	Postop 3	Postop 4	Outcomes Rehabilitation
Consultation	Primary care/ Medical physician/ Rheumatologist	Case manager Anesthesia, OT	Cont.				Postoperative appt. with physician Return for OT appts.
		PT, if necessary Review & add	Cont.				
Assessment	Nrsg database H & P exam. by MD, NP, or PA Including normal activity and strength measures	Review H & P Postop routine N/V status affected arm X-ray in OR	Cont.	Cont.			No complications
Tests	ECG/blood/UA/ Shoulder x-rays	✓ preadm meds					
Medications	D/C NSAIDs/ASA 10 days b/4 OR	Routine meds Regional block for 12 hr pain control					
	Analgesics as needed	PCA/IV pain meds	Cont.	DC and oral narcotic meds/ analgesics as needed		Cont.	Oral pain meds @ home

(continued)

Figure 13–23

Clinical Pathway: *(continued)*

Pathway	Preadmission Office/OP clinic	Admission Day Op day	Discharge Postop 1	Postop 2	Postop 3	Postop 4	Outcomes Rehabilitation
	Instruct on preop meds b/4 OR	IV Antibiotics	Cont.	D/C antibiotics			
Diet	Assessment wt.	NPO b/4 OR (Min. 8 hours)	Advance as tol.				Tolerating diet
	Balance diet						
Activity	Preop mobility	ROM exercises to unaffected joints					Exercises begin once dressing is removed
		HOB elevated					
		Shoulder immobilizer or sling & swathe					
Treatments		IS/TCDB q 2 hr w/a		Postsurgery			
		Exercises— Finger	Cont.	Cont.			Cont. finger exercises @ home
		IV fluids	Cont.	D/C			
		Wounds catheters	Cont.	D/C			
		Dressing dry	Changed	Changed PRN			No signs of infection
			ROM shoulder exc.	Cont.			Cont exc program @ home and appts with physical therapists 6 wks b/4 pulling, pushing, & lifting 3 mo b/f weight lifting
			Exc elbow & wrist				
				Pendulum exc.	Cont.		
Education	Teach pre & postoperative teaching regarding surgical preparation	Reinforce					Reduced anxiety to follow exc. regime
	Rev. hosp routine						
	Finger exercises	Demonstrate exercises					
	Review hosp LOS						
D/C Plan	Include exercises & activity level, signs of infection, & when to notify their physician	Rev. restricted activities					Knows activity level
		Rev. signs of infection					Knows sign & symptom of infect
	LOS usually 2–3 days						Knows when to contact physician.

tendonitis is combined with bursitis (Fig. 13–24). There tends to be an increase in calcium content with degenerative changes in the tendon, and calcific deposits in and about the rotator tendon are the most frequent abnormality encountered in the subacute or acutely painful shoulder. The patient complains of pain, tenderness, and limitation of motion. The onset may be sudden, without known injury, and the pain severe and agonizing. The patient may complain of pain at the upper humerus and in the subacromial area, which may radiate to the insertion of the deltoid, and in severe cases up to the neck and down to the fingertips. Pain is

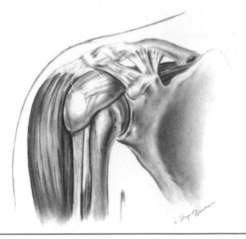

Figure 13–24   Calcific tendonitis refers to a degenerative process in the tendon that is associated with the deposition of calcium salts. Like rotator cuff tendonitis, it usually involves the supraspinatus tendon. Acute, disabling attacks of shoulder pain may occur, usually in patients over 30 years of age and more often in women. The arm is held close to the side, and all motions are severely limited by pain. Tenderness is maximal below the tip of the acromion. The subacromial bursa, which overlies the supraspinatus tendon, may become involved in the inflammation. Chronic, less severe pain may also occur.   *(Bates, B. (1995). A Guide to Physical Examination and History Taking. 6th ed. Philadelphia: J.B. Lippincott Company.)*

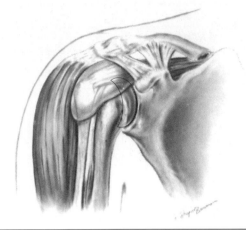

Figure 13–25   Adhesive capsulitis refers to a mysterious fibrosis of the glenohumeral joint capsule, manifested by diffuse, dull, aching pain in the shoulder and progressive restriction of motion, but usually no localized tenderness. The condition is usually unilateral and occurs in persons aged 50 to 70. There is often an antecedent painful disorder of the shoulder or possibly another condition (such as myocardial infarction) that has decreased shoulder movements. The course is chronic, lasting months to years, but the disorder often resolves spontaneously, at least partially.   *(Bates, B. (1995). A Guide to Physical Examination and History Taking. 6th ed. Philadelphia: J.B. Lippincott Company.)*

increased with motion, particularly abduction and external rotation. Extreme tenderness is felt at the lateral area of the humeral head, below the acromion, and above at the insertion of the deltoid. Acute symptoms may persist for several days and then diminish abruptly or gradually.

Treatment usually consists of resting the shoulder with a sling, with complete or partial immobilization if necessary. Ice bags are applied during the acute stage, which lasts approximately 2 days, and then heat applications are used. Anti-inflammatory and pain-relieving drugs are usually prescribed, and, in some instances, a local anesthetic and corticosteroids are injected into the bursa. As the pain subsides, physical therapy and exercises are started to restore function as rapidly as possible to prevent residual subacute or chronic progression. In the beginning, exercises may be the Codman or pendular passive exercises that add traction to the glenohumeral joint, stretch the capsule, avoid active abduction, and minimize scapular shrugging.

Adhesive Capsulitis (Frozen Shoulder).   Adhesive capsulitis (Fig. 13–25), also known as frozen shoulder, is a condition in which fibrous tissues develop in the shoulder joint capsule, causing progressive loss of movement and pain, particularly during abduction and rotation. The pain can become constant and disabling and may radiate down the arm and the back to the scapula. Motion in abduction and external rotation is limited (Fig. 13–26), and atrophy of the muscles of the shoulder

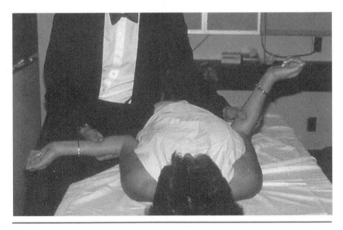

Figure 13–26   A patient with frozen shoulder with limited passive range of motion in external rotation, measured with the arm near the side.   *(Weinstein & Buckwalter (1994). Turek's Orthopaedic: Principles and Their Applications Philadelphia: Lippincott-Raven.)*

girdle may occur. There is an obliteration of the subdeltoid bursa and adhesive inflammation between the joint capsule and the peripheral articular cartilage. Adhesive capsulitis is distinct from calcific tendonitis in that adhesive capsulitis has a gradual onset, slowly increasing pain and stiffness, little or no localized tenderness, and progressive limitation of motion (Fig. 13–27). No specific cause is known, but prolonged bed rest or immobilization of the shoulder joint appear to be predisposing factors. Secondary causes tend to include

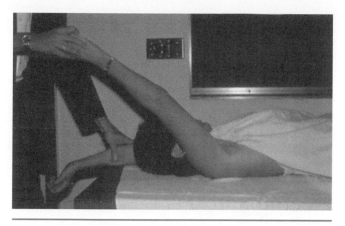

Figure 13–27 Frozen shoulder syndrome with limitation of passive forward flexion. *(Weinstein & Buckwalter (1994).* Turek's Orthopaedic: Principles and Their Applications. *Philadelphia: Lippincott-Raven.)*

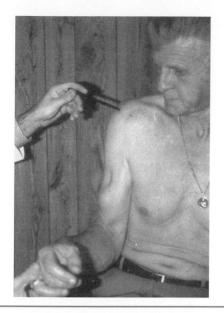

Figure 13–28 A patient with a spontaneous rupture of the long head of biceps. This most often results from subacromial impingement and is frequently accompanied by a full-thickness tear of the rotator cuff. In this patient, the clinician points to the area of pain, suggesting that the rotator cuff is involved. A spontaneous rupture of the long head of biceps should make the clinician focus on the area of the rotator cuff as the source of pathology. *(Weinstein & Buckwalter (1994).* Turek's Orthopaedic: Principles and Their Applications. *Philadelphia: Lippincott-Raven.)*

fracture-dislocations and arthritic conditions. Physical therapy with heat and assistive exercises and analgesics and anti-inflammatory drugs help to relieve pain and joint inflammation.

THE UPPER ARM

The upper arm region includes the shaft of the humerus and its covering muscles, principally the biceps brachii and the triceps brachii. In this chapter, the proximal end of the humerus is included with the shoulder and the distal end with the elbow.

FRACTURES OF THE HUMERAL SHAFT

Fractures of the shaft of the humerus may be due to a direct force, such as a blow to the side of the arm; an indirect force, such as a fall on an outstretched hand; or pathology, such as a secondary malignancy. Fractures of the shaft of the humerus do not produce as much overriding of the fragments as do fractures of the femur, because the muscles of the arm are not as powerful as those in the leg, and their retraction is inhibited by the weight of the arm. The possibility of overriding is greatest in humeral fractures when the fracture is above the attachment of the deltoid muscle.

Humeral shaft fractures are usually easily corrected by manipulation and treated nonoperatively with a sugar-tong splint and a Velpeau bandage, an arm cylinder cast with a collar and cuff sling, or an abductor splint. In some instances, an open reduction and an internal fixation with plates and screws, medullary nails, or external fixation devices are indicated. Methods of repair are usually (1) for transverse or short oblique fractures, a compression plate with the arm supported in a sling for 3 to 4 weeks postoperatively; (2) for long oblique and spiral fractures, transfixation lag screws with external support, such as an abduction humeral splint, until the fracture heals; (3) for open fractures of the humerus in which the insertion of inter-nal fixation is inappropriate, external fixation (see Chapter 7); and (4) for pathologic fractures secondary to malignant tumors (see Chapter 3), medullary fixation, possibly in conjunction with methyl methacrylate cement for increased stability. The two major complications of fractures of the humeral shaft are nonunion of the bone and radial nerve palsy.

RUPTURE OF THE BICEPS BRACHII

A rupture of the biceps brachii muscle (Fig. 13–28) can occur in the tendon of the long head of the muscle, in the muscle itself, or in the distal tendon. Usually a rupture is preceded by degenerative changes in the tendon and the tendon sheath and occurs as a result of chronic bicipital tenosynovitis or acute stress to the arm, such as from lifting a heavy weight. A sudden force to the weakened tendon may cause it to fray apart, with resulting pain and weakness. The distal fragment, with the attached muscle belly, retracts toward the elbow, giving a ball-like appearance to the arm muscle. When the patient "makes a muscle," the biceps bunches up closer to the elbow than normal because the long head at the upper end has pulled loose. The lower shoulder and upper arm area is tender to palpation, and a muscular gap can be felt. There is soft-tissue swelling, and the overlying skin becomes ecchymosed. In an elderly patient or one not involved with heavy lifting, the treatment for a rupture of the biceps brachii long head tendon may be conservative, using a Velpeau bandage with the elbow held at more than 90 degrees of flexion. For others, surgical

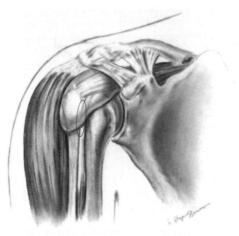

Figure 13–29   Inflammation of the long head of the biceps tendon and its sheath causes anterior shoulder pain that may resemble rotator cuff tendonitis and may coexist with it. This tendon, like the cuff, may suffer impingement injury. Tenderness is maximal in the bicipital groove. By externally rotating and abducting the arm, you can more easily separate this area from the subacromial tenderness of supraspinatus tendonitis. With the patient's arm at the side, elbow flexed to 90 degrees, ask the patient to supinate the forearm against your resistance. Increased pain in the bicipital groove confirms this condition.   *(Bates, B. (1995). A Guide to Physical Examination and History Taking. 6th ed. Philadelphia: J.B. Lippincott Company.)*

attachment of the ruptured tendon to the bicipital groove or to the coracoid process is indicated.

BICIPITAL TENOSYNOVITIS

Tenosynovitis involves an inflammation of the tendon and the tendon sheath (Fig. 13–29). Irritation produced by the mechanical gliding mechanism of the tendon of the long head of the biceps in the bicipital groove of the humerus is a common cause of shoulder pain. The smoothness of the gliding is readily disturbed by excessive activity of the arm, particularly under stress, or by direct trauma to the area of the bicipital groove. Once the gliding mechanism is disturbed, abduction and external rotation, as well as internal rotation and extension (e.g., the motions involved in combing hair, putting on a shirt or jacket, fastening a bra, reaching for a telephone, or shoveling snow), are likely to irritate the biceps tendon and cause pain. The patient is usually a woman 45 to 65 years old who has a history of either gradual onset of pain or acute onset following vigorous arm activities. The pain usually originates in the anterior and medial aspects of the shoulder and may radiate down the biceps muscle and on to the fingers or up to the shoulder and neck. Pain in the bicipital groove may be elicited by a combination of abduction, external rotation, and extension of the arm at the shoulder. Forced flexion of the elbow against resistance and forced supination of the forearm against resistance with the elbow flexed will also cause pain in the bicipital groove. Treatment usually includes resting the arm and shoulder in a sling, moist heat applications, diathermy

and ultrasound treatments, oral anti-inflammatory drugs, and a hydrocortisone injection into the tendon sheath. In some patients, however, a hydrocortisone injection may cause degenerative lesions in and eventual rupture of the biceps tendon.

THE ELBOW

The elbow is a uniaxial or hinge joint that permits flexion and extension between the lower end of the humerus and the upper ends of the radius and the ulna.

DISLOCATION

A dislocation of the elbow occurs when the humerus, the ulna, and the radius are forced out of correct anatomical position. A fall on an outstretched hand is the usual cause of a traumatic dislocation. An anterior dislocation of the elbow is quite rare. A posterior dislocation typically involves the lower end of the humerus being driven over the coronoid process of the ulna and out through the torn anterior capsule. The ulna and the radius are then forced backward, and the ulna ends up being lodged behind the lower end of the displaced humerus (Fig. 13–30). There is usually an avulsion of the anterior brachialis muscle from the coronoid process, a stripping of the periosteum, and the development of a subperiosteal hematoma. There may also be an injury to the median and radial nerves or damage to the brachial artery. The dislocation results in a painful deformity of the elbow that is marked by swelling. The olecranon process is unusually prominent. The patient's arm assumes an attitude of 40 degrees of flexion, and the joint is immovable, either actively or passively.

Closed manipulative reduction under anesthesia is carried out as soon as possible. In adults, if reduction is delayed for several hours, permanent limitation of movement usually results. Once muscle relaxation has been achieved, reduction of the elbow may be accomplished by the elbow being flexed over the physician's knee. The elbow is then immobilized in a hinged elbow splint (Fig. 13–31) or in a posterior splint at a safe degree of flexion for 3 weeks. The elbow joint has poor tolerance for injury and immobilization, and it may be months before full motion returns.

FRACTURES

SUPRACONDYLAR FRACTURE OF THE HUMERUS

The supracondylar area of the humerus is the lower flared end of that bone just above the elbow joint. Fractures in this area occur more commonly in children and the elderly, but they can occur at any age. The mechanism of injury is trauma when the elbow is in either extension or flexion. The extension injury is produced by a fall on the extended elbow, and before repair the arm is stable only in significant flexion. (Such fractures may also be accompanied by intracondylar or intracapsular injuries.) The flexion injury is produced by a fall on the flexed elbow, and the arm is relatively stable in

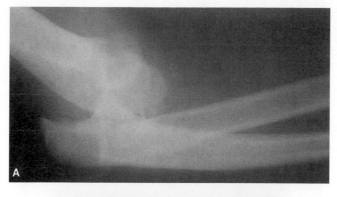

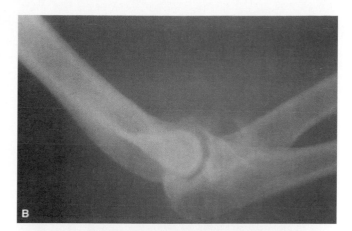

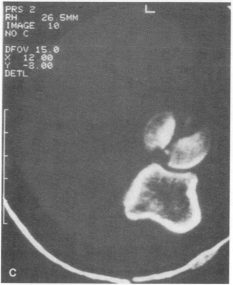

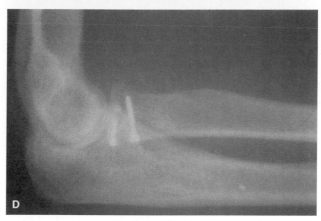

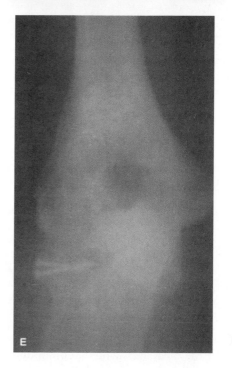

Figure 13–30   (A) A fracture dislocation with displaced fracture of the radial head. (B) Reduction of elbow dislocation. (C) CT scan of the radial head demonstrating the size of the fragments. (D and E) Appearance alter internal fixation using minifragment screws in the sale zone.
(Rockwood, et al. (1996). Rockwood & Green's Fractures in Adults. Philadelphia: Lippincott-Raven.)

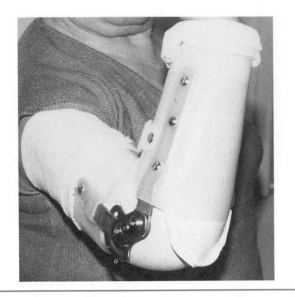

Figure 13–31   A hinged elbow splint can provide support after a stable reduction of a dislocated elbow. *(Koval & Zuckerman (1998).* Fractures in the Elderly. *Philadelphia: Lippincott-Raven.)*

extension. (For nursing care, see the Chapter 6 section on a patient with a supracondylar fracture of the humerus and side arm traction.)

INTERCONDYLAR FRACTURES

Intercondylar fractures are usually due to direct violence. There is considerable comminution of the bony fragments and damage to the articular surface. The most common are T- or Y-type fractures of the lower end of the humerus with a vertical component running into the elbow joint, but any combination of fractures may be involved. The elbow is often grossly swollen and painful and can look like a "bag of bones." The treatment of intercondylar fractures varies with the extent of the damage. If the fracture is one in which reduction and firm fixation can be achieved by open reduction and internal fixation, that may be done. Movements of the hand and the fingers are usually begun immediately, but shoulder movement is not allowed for 2 to 3 weeks. If it appears that the bony fragments cannot be restored to their proper positions, the aim is to develop what joint movements are possible by putting the arm in a splint or a collar and cuff and beginning gentle, early, active exercises.

OLECRANON FRACTURES

Fractures of the olecranon (Fig. 13–32) are more common in adults than in children. They are usually caused by direct violence from a fall on the elbow or by muscular violence from a contraction of the triceps muscle following a fall on the hand with the elbow flexed. Associated laceration of the lateral aponeurosis of the triceps tendon often allows marked separation of the fragments. The patient is unable to extend the elbow actively, and a gap can be felt between the olecranon and the rest of the shaft of the ulna. Undisplaced olecranon fractures are

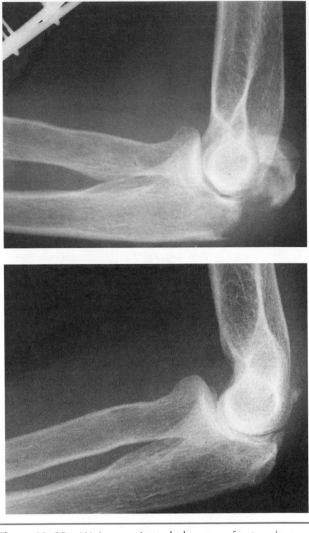

Figure 13–32   (A) A comminuted olecranon fracture in a 74-year-old woman with multiple medical problems, (B) treated with proximal fragment excision and reattachment of the triceps. *(Koval & Zuckerman. (1998).* Fractures in the Elderly. *Philadelphia: Lippincott-Raven.)*

usually treated in a posterior splint with the elbow flexed 90 degrees. Pronation and supination movements are then started 2 or 3 days after splinting, and flexion-extension movements are started 2 weeks after splinting. The protective splinting is continued until there is evidence of union (usually about 6 weeks).

Displaced fractures are generally reduced and internally fixed. The procedure usually used is either (1) open reduction and fixation with a figure-of-eight (Kirschner) wire loop (Fig. 13–33), used when the fracture is not comminuted and is proximal to the coronoid process; (2) medullary fixation when the olecranon is comminuted and its distal fragments and the head of the radius are dislocated anteriorly; or (3) excision of the proximal fragment of the olecranon when a comminuted fracture extends as far distally as the coronoid process. When the olecranon is excised, the triceps muscle is resutured to

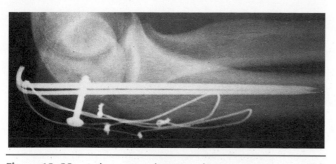

Figure 13–33 A three-part olecranon fracture in a 64-year-old; physician treated using a tension-band technique. *(Koval & Zuckerman (1998).* Fractures in the Elderly. *Philadelphia: Lippincott-Raven.)*

the ulnar shaft. After an internal fixation and closure, the elbow is usually immobilized in a posterior splint with the elbow in 90 degrees of flexion. In approximately 7 to 10 days, active and active assisted exercises are started. Between exercise periods, the elbow is still supported by the splint. Support is usually continued until the fourth week, though maximum function may not return for 6 to 12 months. Pronation and supination are seldom permanently limited to any extent, although flexion and extension may be. The speed with which motion returns and the final range of motion depend on the extent of injury to the joint surfaces.

RADIAL HEAD FRACTURES

Fractures of the head of the radius are common in adults and usually occur as a result of a fall on an outstretched hand. There is swelling at the elbow joint, tenderness over the head of the radius, and limitation of elbow function, especially pronation-supination. Because these fractures tend to cause joint stiffness if immobilized, the key to successful treatment is to allow early motion. The treatment method and ultimate prognosis depend on the amount of damage to the joint articular cartilage, the type of fracture, and the degree of displacement. Fractures of the head and neck of the radius are classified as (1) undisplaced fractures, (2) marginal fractures, (3) comminuted fractures, and (4) fractures associated with dislocations of the elbow. Undisplaced or impacted fractures are usually treated by supporting the elbow in a comfortable degree of flexion in a collar and cuff or in a posterior splint until the pain disappears (usually several days to a week). The arm may then be placed in a sling and active movement of the elbow started. Displaced fractures involving less than a third of the articular surface are treated by reduction and early motion. Marginal fractures with displacement and comminuted fractures are treated by early excision of the radial head. The end result of excision of the radial head is generally satisfactory, but a normal elbow is not achieved. Some 50% of those patients later develop subluxation and pain at the distal radioulnar joint. With recent developments and improvements in implants, those patients might have a Silastic radial head prosthesis inserted.

RUPTURE OF THE BICEPS TENDON AT THE ELBOW

The biceps tendon may be ruptured or avulsed at or near its insertion to the bicipital tuberosity of the radius. The injury is usually associated with forcible flexion of the elbow against strong resistance, for example, when a worker who is assisting in lifting a heavy object suddenly has to bear its full weight alone. The worker will feel a painful snap or tearing sensation at the elbow, followed immediately by weakness during active flexion of the elbow and supination of the forearm. The biceps tendon is normally a flexor for supination or semisupination of the forearm but provides little or no flexor power when the forearm is pronated. The antecubital space will be tender, but swelling is usually minimal because of the strong overlying fascia. When attempting active flexion, a bulbous swelling forms on the upper arm, caused by the retracted belly of the biceps. If the tendon is partially torn, but not yet completely ruptured, it may produce symptoms of localized pain during motions requiring lifting and supination. If a surgical procedure is necessary, the recovered tendon is sutured to the insertion of the brachialis. Postoperatively, the elbow is immobilized in a posterior splint with the elbow flexed just beyond a right angle and the forearm in moderate supination. After 5 to 6 weeks, exercises are instituted.

ARTHROPLASTY

An arthroplasty of the elbow is performed to relieve patients with a severely painful elbow and humeroulnar joint destruction caused by trauma or rheumatoid arthritis (Fig. 13–34) and to restore stability and improve mobility of the elbow joint. A total arthroplasty is usually not indicated for traumatic arthritis patients because of their high activity level (Dale, Orr, & Harrell 1992); hemiarthroplasties have proven more successful with traumatic elbow problems.

In the past, constrained hinge and surface replacement devices were designed for a total elbow arthroplasty. Many of those hinged joints loosened because of the stress placed on the joint with forearm rotation. However, the hinged prosthesis is still being used in the treatment of intra-articular fractures and nonunions of the elbow in the elderly population (Fig. 13–35). To correct loosening, the total elbow arthroplasty prosthesis evolved into a nonconstrained resurfacing implant (Fig. 13–36) without a hinge. The humeral and ulnar components are not attached to each other, which allows rotation of the forearm and reduces stress on the cemented prosthesis. Today, the most effective implants resurface the capitellum and trochlea of the humerus and the trochlear notch of the ulna. The humeral and ulnar components are metal with an inserted articulating surface of polyethylene. However, a requirement for the prosthesis is that there be sufficient bone stock and soft-tissue support to provide joint stability and prevent

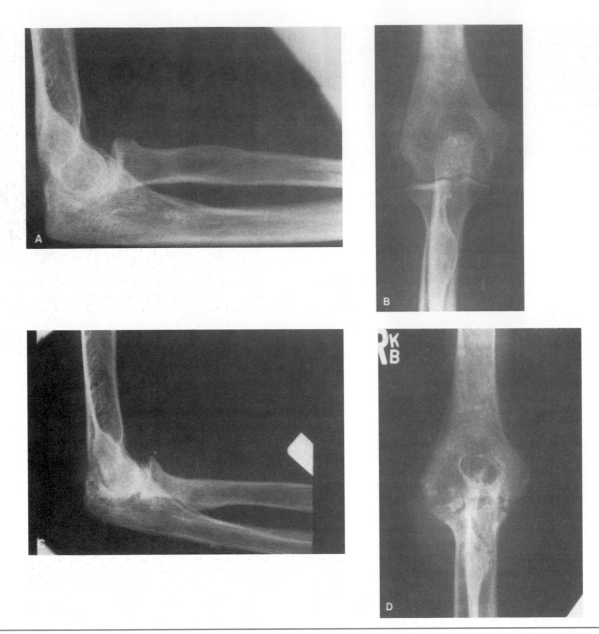

Figure 13–34   Significant rheumatoid destruction in this elbow occurred over a 3-year period. In the initial films (A and B), the joint appears normal except for slight anterior subluxation of the radius on the capitellum. In the later films (C and D), cartilage loss is noted both in the radial capitellar joint and in the ulnar trochlear portions of the joint, along with further deformity of the radial head.   *(Weinstein & Buckwalter (1994). Turek's Orthopaedic: Principles and Their Applications Philadelphia: Lippincott-Raven.)*

dislocation of the prosthesis. Semiconstrained types of elbow arthroplasties (Fig. 13–37) are also available.

NURSING PROCESS (Patient with a Total Elbow Arthroplasty)

The following nursing process is presented to demonstrate the nursing care of a patient with a total elbow arthroplasty. The nursing process begins when the patient returns to the nursing unit.

ASSESSMENT

The initial assessment of the patient involves assessing the level of consciousness and the patient's ability to follow directions. There will be a large bulky dressing on the arm that includes a long arm posterior splint with the elbow at 90 degrees of flexion. Assess the neurovascular status of the arm, especially the ulnar nerve (see Chapter 2). Check the position of the arm, and make sure it is elevated on a pillow. The wrist should not be flexed, as that would put pressure on the arm at the distal end of the splint. Check for skin irritation under or at the edges of the splint. Look for drainage from the

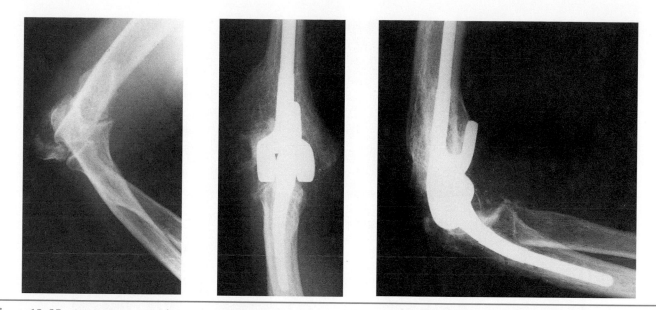

Figure 13–35 (A) An intra-articular nonunion in an 84-year-old woman (B, C) treated with a total elbow arthroplasty. *(Koval & Zuckerman (1998). Fractures in the Elderly. Philadelphia: Lippincott-Raven.)*

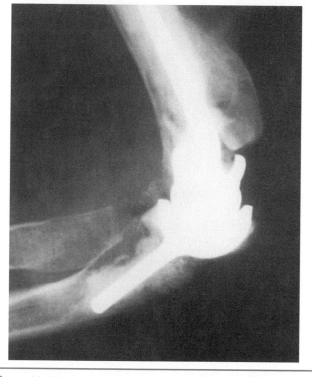

Figure 13–36 A nonconstrained total elbow replacement has been performed for rheumatoid arthritis. The patient's natural ligaments provide support for this resurfacing type of arthroplasty. *(Weinstein & Buckwalter (1994). Iurek's Orthopaedic: Principles and Their Applications. Philadelphia: Lippincott-Raven.)*

incision, and check the wound catheters for patency and the amount of drainage. Observe for signs of infection, and check the patient's vital signs. Assess the location, duration, and severity of pain.

NURSING DIAGNOSIS

Based on all of the assessment data, the major nursing diagnoses for a typical patient with an elbow arthroplasty may include the following:

- Pain and discomfort related to the surgical procedure
- Impaired physical mobility related to lack of elbow joint stability
- Increased anxiety related to knowledge deficit about the surgical procedure and the rehabilitation process

COLLABORATIVE PROBLEMS

- Infection
- Loosening of one or both components
- Ulnar nerve injury

GOAL FORMULATION AND PLANNING

The goals are to have the patient experience (1) a decrease in the amount of pain, (2) an increase in joint stability and mobility, (3) a decrease in anxiety through increased knowledge about the surgery and rehabilitation process, and (4) an absence of complications from surgery and decreased activity. Long-term goals are to have the patient pain free with return of function in the elbow.

INTERVENTIONS

ALLEVIATE PAIN

Pain control with narcotics is essential during the first 24 hours, and in most instances a PCA pump is utilized. During surgery, there is resection of bone, so that the prosthetic components can be cemented into place.

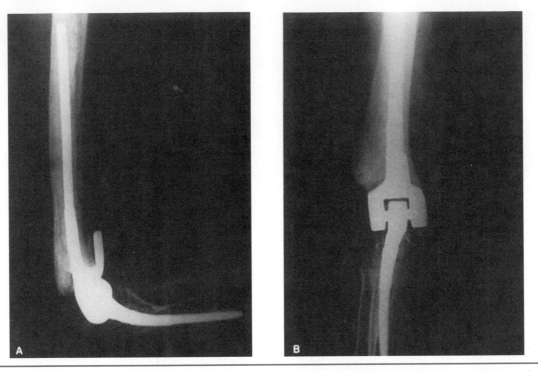

Figure 13–37   Because of markedly deficient distal humeral bone, a semiconstrained type of arthroplasty has been performed in this elbow. The metallic stems of the humeral and ulnar components are fixed to bone with methyl methacrylate cement. Together, the components function as a loose hinge.   *(Weinstein & Buckwalter (1994).* Turek's Orthopaedic: Principles and Their Applications. *Philadelphia: Lippincott-Raven.)*

Nonetheless, the joint pain following surgery may be less than that experienced before surgery. Determine measures that the patient has used in the past to relieve pain in the elbow, and use those measures as well as elevating the arm, applying ice as needed, and having the patient do finger and hand exercises when allowed. Keeping the patient's arm elevated on a pillow helps to prevent and/or reduce the swelling and thus helps to reduce pain.

Most patients with a total elbow arthroplasty have RA. Some physicians withhold the patient's nonsteroidal anti-inflammatory drugs and immunosuppressive medications for 2 to 4 weeks before and after surgery (Dale, Orr, & Harrell 1992). These patients may have stiffness and/or pain in their other joints. Without their normal medications to control inflammation and the stress of surgery, some RA patients will experience an exacerbation of their disease. Corticosteroids are given to try to help counteract the effects.

INCREASE MOBILITY
Nursing interventions to increase mobility focus on correct positioning, exercises, and ambulation.

Position.   The position that is usually most comfortable for the patient is supine with the head of the bed elevated. The patient needs to keep the arm elevated on a pillow for the first 24 hours or until the potential for swelling has decreased. The affected arm will also be supported in a sling. The patient may use the trapeze to change position and get on and off the bedpan, but they can not use their affected arm in any way. Dale, Orr, & Harrell (1992) restrict the patient from using a bedpan because they feel the patient will use their affected arm. The patient may turn to their unaffected side, but they must make sure their affected arm is positioned correctly and secured safely.

Exercises.   Only mild finger exercises are allowed until the wound catheters are removed, approximately 24 hours after surgery. Exercises of all unaffected joints are encouraged to prevent stiffness and reduced function. The posterior splint is discontinued 24 to 72 hours after surgery. Once the splint is removed, the patient will wear a sling to keep the forearm and hand elevated and elbow immobile, except during exercise periods. The occupational therapist begins with a program of passive and active range-of-motion exercises for flexion, extension, and forearm rotation. Exercises are then gradually increased, and by 2 weeks after surgery the patient is encouraged to do active exercises of the hand and shoulder. Some physicians utilize an elbow exerciser (CPM) for passive exercises.

Rehabilitation for the patient following total elbow arthroplasty varies greatly. The following discussion gives only one example of the rehabilitation and exercise regime; the patient must follow their therapist's and physician's preference. To overcome shortening of arm muscles, active exercises of the elbow, the wrist, and the forearm are usually done twice a day. To help loosen the muscles before beginning the exercises, the patient can place hot packs over their biceps and triceps and then massage the arm muscles with long rhythmic strokes toward the shoulder.

The following are some exercises for elbow extension and flexion that prevent compensatory shoulder movement and produce a reflex relaxation of antagonistic muscles that makes active motion of the elbow easier. To promote elbow flexion, place the patient in a supine position on a firm surface with the affected arm extended. Place a folded towel under the affected triceps, and stabilize the affected shoulder by placing your palm over the shoulder with your thumb on the insertion of the biceps. Tell the patient to try to flex the affected elbow while you supply slight resistance by holding the wrist with your other hand. To promote elbow extension, place the patient in the same position, but have the patient flex their arm with the wrist toward the shoulder. Then have the patient attempt to extend their forearm while you provide slight resistance to the back of the wrist and forearm.

The amount of exercise is increased gradually, but if there is even the slightest pain, the exercises should be stopped. If the elbow becomes stiff and sore, the arm should be placed back in the sling, and splinting may be necessary for a few days. In addition to those exercises, some daily activities that increase elbow flexion are eating, hair combing, writing, and turning the pages of a book. Walking with the arm at one's side increases elbow extension. Active range-of-motion exercises of the shoulder, the wrist, and the fingers, however, should be continued.

Ambulation. Ambulation is usually allowed by the afternoon of the first or the second day after surgery but may be postponed until the wound catheters are removed. At first, the patient will need assistance in getting out of bed without putting stress on the affected arm and elbow and in balancing while walking with a bulky dressing and posterior splint.

PATIENT TEACHING AND HOME CARE CONSIDERATIONS
Following an arthroplasty of the elbow, the patient must know how to recognize the signs and symptoms of infection and whom to notify if one should occur.

Activities of daily living discussions are initiated preoperatively and reinforced postsurgery by the nurse and the occupational therapist. Patients may need to learn eating, dressing, grooming, and hygiene tasks while adhering to the total elbow restrictions on avoiding lateral torque, the most stressful force on the elbow. To avoid lateral torque on the elbow during activities of daily living, patients are instructed to use the affected arm with the elbow adducted to their side and to reach forward, not out to the side.

Discuss with the patient the results to be gained from an elbow arthroplasty. The goal of a total elbow arthroplasty is to decrease the patient's pain and to increase range of motion. A review of the literature indicates that the patient can expect (1) a significant reduction in pain, as patients reported a reduction from moderate and severe pain before surgery to absent or mild pain postsurgery; (2) elbow range of motion to improve considerably, with active pronation improving from 12 to 35 degrees; (3) improvement in strength, with flexion strength improving as much as 92%, pronation strength improving 63%, supination strength improving 69%, and grip strength improving 53% (Dale, Orr, & Harrell, 1992). However, the patient must realize that time and effort are needed before he or she can regain function in the elbow. The prescribed exercises, and only those, should be done as indicated. The patient should not force the elbow to bend or straighten and should not lift objects until authorized to do so.

MONITORING AND MANAGING POTENTIAL PROBLEMS

Potential complications following an elbow arthroplasty are (1) infection, (2) loosening of one or both components, (3) ulnar nerve injury, (4) rupture of the triceps, (5) fracture of the bone surrounding the prosthesis, and (6) contractures of the elbow. Patients who have sustained a rupture of the triceps or a fracture of the surrounding bone may need added or extended immobilization. The elbow does not tolerate surgery and immobilization well. Following the prescribed exercise regime is necessary to prevent elbow contractures.

INFECTION
Observe for signs and symptoms of infection. Wound catheters are utilized to prevent the pooling of blood and the development of an abcess. During the first 24 hours, the normal amount of drainage following a total elbow replacement is approximately 250 ml. The patient may also have their immunosuppressive medications discontinued before surgery and for a period after surgery. The reason for this is to reduce the patient's risk of infection, because suppressing the immune system increases the patient's risk of infection. Most patients will be on antibiotic therapy immediately after surgery. Infection at the sites where the prosthesis is inserted can cause a loosening of the prosthesis, which can necessitate surgical removal and an elbow arthrodesis.

LOOSENING OF THE COMPONENT(S)
The patient is placed in a posterior splint with the arm flexed at approximately 90 degrees of flexion. The splint helps to protect the triceps repair and minimizes loosening of the components. An infection in the prosthesis can lead to loosening.

ULNAR NERVE INJURY
During a total elbow arthroplasty, the ulnar nerve is particularly vulnerable to injury because of its normal anatomical location along the ulnar groove of the medial humeral epicondyle. Care is taken during the surgery to dissect the ulnar nerve out of the ulnar groove to help protect it from injury, since an injury can cause intrinsic hand muscle weakness, loss of thumb and index pinch, and the inability to adduct the fourth

and fifth digits. Doing neurovascular assessment post-surgery is essential and ongoing.

EVALUATION/OUTCOMES

The patient should have minimal pain that responds to medication and exercises that reduce the swelling. A slow return to normal function in the elbow is to be expected. The patient should be encouraged to continue with the required exercises and should understand that he or she should not try to rush matters by increasing the level of exercise or by forcing the elbow to flex or extend. There should be no signs of infection.

CLINICAL PATHWAY (Patient with a Total Elbow Arthroplasty)

A generic clinical pathway for a patient with a total elbow arthroplasty is shown in Figure 13–38.

Figure 13–38
Clinical Pathway: Elbow Arthroplasty

Admission Date: _____   Discharge Plan: _____ Home _____ Skilled Nursing _____ Extended Care Facility

Pathway	Preadmission Office/OP clinic	Admission Day Op day	Discharge Postop 1	Postop 2	Postop 3	Postop 4	Outcomes Rehabilitation
Consultation	Primary Care/ Medical physician/ Rheumatologist	Case Manager Anesthesia, OT					Postoperative appt. with physician Return for OT appts.
Assessment	Nrsg database H & P exam. by MD, NP, or PA Including normal activity & elbow strength	PT, if necessary Review & add Review H & P Postop routine N/V status affected arm X-ray in OR	Cont. Cont.	Cont.			No complications
Tests	ECG/blood/UA/ Elbow x-rays	✓ preadm meds					
Medications	D/C NSAIDs/ASA 10 days b/4 OR Analgesics as needed	Routine meds PCA IV pain med Oral narcotic meds/ analgesics as needed IV Antibiotics	Cont. Cont. D/C antibiotics	D/C start oral meds Cont.			Pain relieved with oral medications
Diet	Instruct on preop meds b/4 OR Assessment wt. Balanced diet	NPO b/4 OR (Min. 8 hours)	Advance as tol.				Tolerating diet
Activity	Preop mobility	ROM exercises to unaffected joints Posterior plaster splint with elastic wrap HOB elevated	Cont. Cont.	D/C splint & A & P ROM started Sling applied Cont.			Exercises continued @ home Cont. with exercises & sling @ home Position of comfort
Treatments		Exercises— Finger Wound catheters Dressing dry	Cont. D/C Changed	Cont. Change PRN			Cont. finger exercises @ home No signs of infection

(continued)

Figure 13–38

Clinical Pathway: *(continued)*

Pathway	Preadmission Office/OP clinic	Admission Day Op day	Discharge Postop 1	Postop 2	Postop 3	Postop 4	Outcomes Rehabilitation
Education	Teach pre & postoperative teaching regarding surgical preparation	Reinforce					Reduced anxiety and able to follow exc. regime
	Rev. hosp routine						
	Finger exercises	Demonstrate exercises					
	Review hosp LOS						
D/C Plan	Include exercises & activity level, signs of infection, & when to notify their physician	Rev. restricted activities					Knows activity level
	LOS usually 3–4 days	Rev. signs of infection					Knows signs & symptoms of infect.
							Knows when to contact physician

SPECIAL CONDITIONS

TENNIS ELBOW

The syndrome of chronic disabling pain in the region of the lateral epicondyle of the humerus, which radiates down the extensor surface of the forearm, is referred to as "tennis elbow." That condition is brought on by activities that combine excessive pronation and supination of the forearm with an extended wrist. It is particularly frequent after such activities as playing tennis or racquetball or using tools such as a screwdriver, especially among persons not used to those activities. However, it is also common in individuals whose occupations require the frequent rotary motion of the forearm (e.g., tennis players, plumbers, computer operators, and carpenters). It is often associated with tendonitis of the shoulder, fibrositis of the back, and other collagenous degenerative conditions occurring in young and middle-aged adults.

The onset of the condition is usually gradual. An ache appears over the outer aspect of the elbow and is referred into the forearm. It is persistent and is intensified by grasping or twisting motions. Grasping requires tightening the extensor carpi radialis brevis and longus muscles, while rotary or twisting motions of the forearm toward supination require active contraction of the supinator longus and brevis. A well-localized point of tenderness exists at one of the following sites: the epicondylar ridge, lateral epicondyle, anterior lower edge of the capitellum, the lateral radiohumeral interval, or near a portion of the circumference of the radial head. Most commonly, it is over the anterior aspect of the radial head when the forearm is in full supination. Swelling is rarely present, and the range of motion is normal. The patient complains of weakness of grasp, particularly with the forearm pronated. A clinical test consists of reproducing the pain by completely extending the elbow, pronating the forearm, and forcibly flexing the wrist. Active attempts to dorsiflex the wrist and supinate the forearm against resistance will also intensify the discomfort.

Conservative treatment with forearm support, (Fig. 13–39) anti-inflammatory drugs, rest, and ice is effective most of the time, but recurrences are common. For a few patients, conservative treatment will be unsuccessful and an operative procedure will become necessary. One surgical procedure is to transversely divide the fascial covering of the tendons and then divide the intramuscular septum. The conjoined tendons are then severed at the epicondyle and the epicondylar ridge, and the remaining fibers are detached from the anterior joint capsule. The tendons and the extensor muscles are then allowed to displace distally. Another surgical procedure for tennis elbow is the elevation of the conjoined tendons at the epicondyle and the curettage of cortical bone to expose cancellous bone. Crisscross sutures of heavy silk are then made through the tendons, which are then sutured to the cancellous bone through holes that have been drilled into the bone. The procedure helps to avoid weakening of the extensor muscles by reducing the distance between origin and insertion. Postoperatively, the arm is immobilized for 6 weeks with the elbow flexed, the forearm supinated, and the wrist dorsiflexed.

OLECRANON BURSITIS

A bursitis is an inflammation of the sac (bursa) covering a bony prominence. Trauma to the point of the elbow

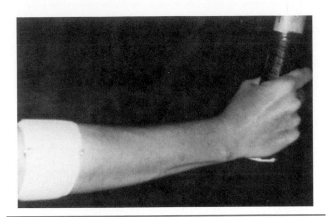

Figure 13–39   Trial of a forearm support band is a useful conservative treatment for lateral epicondylitis (tennis elbow). *(Weinstein & Buckwalter (1994). Turek's Orthopaedic: Principles and Their Applications. Philadelphia Lippincott-Raven.)*

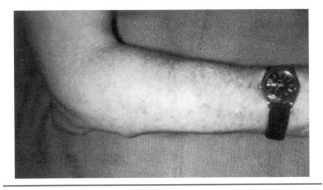

Figure 13–40   Ocleranon bursitis causes a tender enlargement over the subcutaneous portion of the proximal ulna. It must be distinguished from rheumatoid nodule formation, which generally occurs along the subcutaneous border of the ulna more distally.   *(Weinstein & Buckwalter (1994). Turek's Orthopaedic: Principles and Their Applications. Philadelphia: Lippincott-Raven.)*

often results in marked swelling of the olecranon bursa, giving rise to a large knob (or goose egg) at the elbow (Fig. 13–40). Following trauma, the fluid contained in the bursal sac is frequently bloody. Tenderness and swelling of the bursa may also be seen with gout, RA, and infections, all of which lead to a thickening of the bursal walls.

Treatment consists of aspiration of the fluid and local instillation of corticosteroids, followed by application of a pressure dressing. If this problem cannot be controlled conservatively, surgical removal of the thickened bursa may be necessary.

THE FOREARM

The forearm includes the area between the elbow and the wrist and involves the radial and ulnar bones.

FRACTURES OF THE FOREARM

Fractures of the forearm include fractures of the radius, fractures of the ulna, fractures of the shaft of the ulna

with a dislocation of the head of the radius (Monteggia's fracture-dislocation), and fractures of the radius with a dislocation of the lower end of the ulna (Galeazzi's fracture). If there is a fracture of only one bone, angulation and overriding are usually prevented by the other, but if angulation or overriding occurs, it indicates that there is a dislocation of one of the radioulnar joints. The displacement of the fragments depends upon the relationship of the fracture site to the attachments of the pronator and supinator muscles.

FRACTURES OF THE RADIUS

Fractures of the radius are the most common fractures of the forearm. In fractures of the upper third of the shaft of the radius, the proximal fragment is supinated and the distal pronated. Treatment therefore involves immobilizing the forearm, the wrist, and the hand in full supination so that the lower fragment is aligned with the upper one. Fractures of the middle and lower thirds of the radius are immobilized with the hand, the wrist, and the forearm midway between full supination and full pronation. If that procedure is not followed, there may well be permanent limitation of supination and pronation.

FRACTURES OF THE RADIUS AND ULNA

Forearm fractures of the ulna alone are rare, but fractures of both the ulna and the radius can occur at any age. In children they may be greenstick fractures, but in adults they are usually associated with considerable displacement. Pronation and supination are the essential functional motions of the forearm. To preserve those functions after a fracture, the two bones must be replaced so that they will be in correct relative alignment. The width of the interosseous space varies according to the tension or relaxation of the muscles that rotate the forearm from pronation to supination. Therefore, the governing factor determining the position in which the distal fragments of the fractures are placed in relation to the proximal fragments is the location of the muscle attachments relative to the fracture site.

In fractures above the pronator radii teres, there is outward rotation of the upper fragment of the radius by the biceps tendon. Therefore, the forearm must be placed in outward rotation (supination). In fractures below the pronator radii teres, the forearm must be placed in a position of inward rotation (pronation) to match the muscle action above. When there is a fracture of both bones, it is usually difficult to achieve and maintain a satisfactory reduction by closed manipulation and immobilization in a long arm cast. This is especially true for the ulna, which is not as well supplied with blood as the radius. A surgical procedure that involves bone grafting and the possible use of bone plating or intermedullary nailing may be necessary to repair the fractures.

OPEN FRACTURES

As a general rule, internal fixation is not used initially in the treatment of open fractures of the forearm. To reduce complications, the wound is usually first treated by irrigation and débridement. This allows the wound to either reveal itself as infected or heal. Once the wound is healed (10 to 21 days in the absence of infection), surgery may be done to insert an appropriate internal fixation device (e.g., a compression plate), or an external fixation device may be utilized (see Chapter 7).

In single bone fractures of the forearm, a cast with a window over the open wound may be used, because it can provide sufficient external fixation until the wound is healed and internal fixation can be inserted. Shortening from overriding, resulting from a delay in inserting internal fixation, is not a problem in a single bone fracture. To prevent shortening in both bone open fractures, pins are inserted through the proximal ulna and the bases of the second and third metacarpals, traction is applied to restore length, and the pins are then incorporated in a plaster cast that is windowed to allow treatment and inspection of the wounds. An external fixation apparatus such as a Wagner or Hoffmann device is also satisfactory for reduction and skeletal fixation when extensive soft-tissue wounds are involved or skin grafts may be necessary. A medullary nail through the ulna is another means of stabilizing the forearm. Skin grafting and similar procedures on soft tissues are almost impossible to carry out unless the forearm is stabilized by either external or internal methods.

MONTEGGIA'S FRACTURE-DISLOCATION

A Monteggia's fracture-dislocation is the combination of a fracture of the ulna with a dislocation of the proximal end of the radius, with or without a fracture of the radius. There are two different types. One is an anterior dislocation of the radial head with the accompanying ulnar fracture producing an anterior and lateral angulation. The other, less-common type is a posterior dislocation of the radial head with the ulnar fracture producing a posterior angulation.

Monteggia's fracture-dislocations are fairly rare but extremely difficult to treat. Manipulative reduction may be successful, but open reduction and internal fixation of the ulna are generally necessary. If there is an open reduction of the ulna, a compression plate is utilized for fixation. A closed reduction of the radius is then attempted by supining the forearm and applying pressure on the head of the radius. If that is not successful, an open reduction is done to reduce the radius. If an open radial reduction is needed, it is usually necessary to do a reconstruction of the annular ligament.

Postoperatively, the patient's arm is either placed in a posterior splint for 2 weeks (see Chapter 5) and then in a cast or is immediately placed in a long arm cast. In both procedures, the patient's arm is immobilized for 4 to 6 weeks in a position of 100 to 120 degrees of flexion at the elbow, which relaxes the biceps and helps keep the radial head reduced. The cast is then removed, and the arm is supported with a collar and cuff sling, still maintaining the elbow at 100 to 120 degrees of flexion. Gentle pronation and supination motions are permitted, but extension beyond 90 degrees is not allowed until at least 6 weeks after surgery.

GALEAZZI'S FRACTURE OF THE RADIUS

A Galeazzi's fracture is a fracture in the middle or distal thirds of the radius combined with a subluxation-dislocation of the inferior (distal) radioulnar joint. The triangular fibrocartilage of the radioulnar joint and the tip of the ulnar styloid process may be avulsed and the ligaments of the inferior radioulnar joint torn. A Galeazzi's fracture occurs in about 5% of all forearm fractures.

Treatment usually involves nonoperative manipulative reduction followed by a cast from the upper arm to the metacarpal heads. The elbow is flexed at a right angle, the forearm is held in midposition, and the hand is held in full ulnar deviation. An alternative method is to treat a Galeazzi's fracture as a displaced fracture of the radius. The arm is immobilized in supination for 6 weeks and then immobilized in a neutral position for another 6 weeks or until the fracture has united. The inferior radioulnar joint must be kept reduced during the immobilization period. If the cast becomes loose after the swelling subsides, a new cast should be applied. If closed reduction is not effective, an open reduction and an internal fixation with a plate and screws are used. The arm is then immobilized in a cast until the fracture heals.

References

Berg, E. E. (1992). Radiology review: Olecranon fracture. *Orthopaedic Nursing, 11*(5), 19–21.

Berg, E. E. (1993). Anterior shoulder dislocation. *Orthopaedic Nursing, 12*(3), 51–53.

Berg, E. E. (1995). Posterior shoulder (glenohumeral) dislocation. *Orthopaedic Nursing, 14*(1), 47–49.

Berg, E. E. (1997). Calcific tendonitis of the shoulder. *Orthopaedic Nursing, 16*(6), 68–69.

Bigliani, L. U., Flatow, E. L., & Pollock, R. G. (1996). Fractures of the proximal humerus. In C. A. Rockwood, D. P. Green, R. W. Bucholz, & J. D. Heckman (Eds.), *Rockwood and Green's fractures in adults* (4th ed., pp. 1055–1091). Philadelphia: Lippincott-Raven.

Bilyeu, P., & Hoshowsky, V. M. (1995). Shoulder. In V. M. Hoshowsky (Ed.), *NAON: Orientation to the orthopaedic operating room* (pp. 887–100). Pitman, NJ: National Association of Orthopaedic Nurses.

Campbell, R. L., & Hoshowsky, V. M. (1995). Elbow and forearm. In V. M. Hoshowsky (Ed.), *NAON: Orientation to the orthopaedic operating room* (pp. 887–100). Pitman, NJ: National Association of Orthopaedic Nurses.

Cornell, C. N., & Schneider, K. (1998). Proximal humerus. In K. J. Koval & J. D. Zuckerman (Eds.), *Fractures in the elderly* (pp. 85–92). Philadelphia: Lippincott-Raven.

Craig, E. V. (1994). The shoulder and arm. In S. L. Weinstein & J. A. Buckwalter (Eds.), *Turek's orthopaedics: Principles and their application* (5th ed., pp. 359–396). Philadelphia: J. B. Lippincott Company.

Craig, E. V. (1996) Fractures of the clavicle. In C. A. Rockwood, D. P. Green, R. W. Bucholz, & J. D. Heckman (Eds.), *Rockwood and Green's fractures in adults* (4th ed., pp. 1109–1122). Philadelphia: Lippincott-Raven.

Dale, K. G., Orr, P. M., & Harrell, P. B. (1992). Total elbow replacement. *Orthopaedic Nursing, 11*(5), 23–28.

Deuschle, J. A. & Romeo, A. A. (1998). Understanding shoulder arthroplasty. *Orthopaedic Nursing, 17*(5), 7–15.

Georgiadis, G. M., & Behrens, F. F. (1998). Humeral shaft. In K. J. Koval & J. D. Zuckerman (Eds.), *Fractures in the elderly* (pp. 93–106). Philadelphia: Lippincott-Raven.

Heveron, B., & Kaempffe, F. A. (1995). Tears of the rotator cuff. *Orthopaedic Nursing, 14*(6), 38–41.

Hotchkiss, R. N. (1996). Fractures and dislocations of the elbow. In C. A. Rockwood, D. P. Green, R. W. Bucholz, & J. D. Heckman *Rockwood and Green's fractures in adults* (4th ed., pp. 929–1014). Philadelphia: Lippincott-Raven.

Johnson, R. L. (1993). Total shoulder arthroplasty. *Orthopaedic Nursing, 12*(1), 14–22.

Lee, D. H. (1996a). Fractures and dislocations of the shoulder. In V. R. Masear (Ed.), *Primary care orthopaedics* (pp. 142–155). Philadelphia: W. B. Saunders.

Lee, D. H. (1996b). Injuries to the humerus and elbow. In V. R. Masear (Ed.), *Primary care orthopaedics* (pp. 156–164). Philadelphia: W. B. Saunders.

Leininger, S. M. (1997). *Building clinical pathways*. Pitman, NJ: National Association of Orthopaedic Nurses.

Long, J. S. (1996). Shoulder arthroscopy. *Orthopaedic Nursing, 15*(2), 21–31.

McFarland, E. G., Leigh, A. C., Urquhart, M. W., & Kellam, K. (1997a). Shoulder immobilization devices. Part 1: Shoulder immobilizers. *Orthopaedic Nursing, 16*(5), 66–71.

McFarland, E. G., Leigh, A. C., Urquhart, M. W., & Kellam, K. (1997b). Shoulder immobilization devices. Part 2: Shoulder immobilizers. *Orthopaedic Nursing, 16*(5), 66–71.

McFarland, E. G., Leigh, A. C., Urquhart, M. W., & Kellam, K. (1997c). Shoulder immobilization devices. Part 3: Abduction pillows and braces. *Orthopaedic Nursing, 16*(6), 47–54.

Meals, R. A. (1994). The elbow and forearm. In S. L. Weinstein & J. A. Buckwalter (Eds.), *Turek's orthopaedics: Principles and their application* (5th ed., pp. 401–417). Philadelphia: J. B. Lippincott Company.

Richards, R. R., & Corley, F. G. (1996a). Fractures of both bones of the forearm. In C. A. Rockwood, D. P. Green, R. W. Bucholz, & J. D. Heckman (Eds.). *Rockwood and Green's fractures in adults* (4th ed., pp. 869–910). Philadelphia: Lippincott-Raven.

Richards, R. R., & Corley, F. G. (1996b). Isolated fractures of the ulnar shaft and Monteggia fractures. In C. A. Rockwood, D. P. Green, R. W. Bucholz, & J. D. Heckman (Eds.), *Rockwood and Green's fractures in adults* (4th ed., pp. 911–923). Philadelphia: Lippincott-Raven.

Salmond, S. W., Mooney, N. E., & Verdisco, L. A. (1996). *NAON: Core curriculum for orthopaedic nursing* (3rd ed.) Pitman, NJ: National Association of Orthopaedic Nurses.

Weirich, S., & Jupiter, J. (1998). Elbow. In K. J. Koval & J. D. Zuckerman (Eds.), *Fractures in the elderly* (pp. 107–126). Philadelphia: Lippincott-Raven.

Amputation is the surgical or traumatic removal of a part of an individual's body through bone. Disarticulation is the removal of a part of the body through a joint space. Amputations range from removal of part of a digit to the removal of half of the patient's entire body. Surgical amputations are not as common as they were even 20 years ago due to better patient education, improved treatment of underlying pathologies, and alternative treatments.

Amputations are done for many reasons. Sometimes they are viewed as a result of a "failure," that is, that other methods of care have failed and an amputation was done as a last resort. Some of those procedures may have been unsuccessful attempts at revascularization, limb salvage surgery, or total joint replacements. However, amputations can be considered as a type of drastic reconstructive surgery, removing a pathologic condition or a congenital abnormality. Amputations are used to relieve symptoms, improve function, and save or improve the patient's quality of life. It is essential that members of the health team communicate a positive attitude to help the patient adjust to the amputation more readily and to encourage active participation in the rehabilitation plan.

INDICATIONS FOR AMPUTATION

Hippocrates described three indications for amputations: to remove useless limbs, to reduce invalidism, and to save the patient's life (Williamson, 1998). Today, elective amputations of the lower extremity are often performed as a result of (1) a progressive peripheral vascular disease (PVD) and arteriosclerosis (often secondary to diabetes mellitus); (2) infection (due to gangrene and osteomyelitis); (3) trauma (including crushing injuries, thermal and electrical burns, and frostbite); (4) congenital deformities; or (5) malignant tumors. However, PVD and arteriosclerosis account for the majority of lower-extremity amputations. Upper-extremity elective amputations are most often per-

formed as a result of (1) severe trauma (acute injury, thermal and electrical burns, frostbite); (2) malignant tumors; (3) infection (fulminating gas gangrene and chronic osteomyelitis); and (4) congenital deformities. Traumatic amputations of upper or lower extremities occur when a portion of the body is unexpectedly severed. Common instances in which that occurs are accidents with (1) saws, (2) knives, (3) machinery, and (4) vehicles. In some instances, the severed part may be reattached.

The surgical evaluation of a patient for an amputation involves a number of variables. The major factors are the patient's condition, the type of amputation, the level of amputation, and the patient's rehabilitation potential.

WHETHER TO AMPUTATE OR NOT

The first issue is whether to amputate or not. The patient's condition is the primary focus, and that is based on a physical assessment of the patient, results of diagnostic tests, and the patient's emotional status. Diagnostic tests may involve skin temperature studies, tests for intermittent claudication, angiography, oscillometry, and palpation of the pulses, among others.

TYPE OF AMPUTATION

The second decision is to determine the type of amputation the patient will need. There are basically two types of amputations, open or guillotine amputation and closed or flap amputation. The *open method* is used for patients who have or are likely to develop an infection. The wound remains open with drains to allow secretions to escape from the site until the infection has been eradicated. Later, during a second surgical procedure, the skin flaps are sutured over the wound and the suture line is prepared as though it were a closed amputation. In the *closed method,* skin flaps are pulled over the bone end and are sutured in place as part of the amputation procedure.

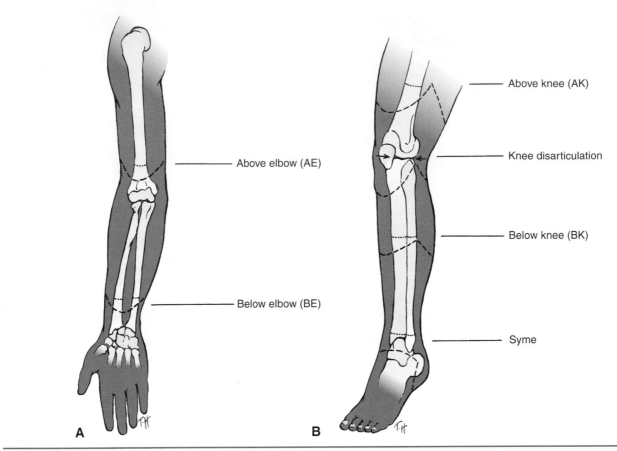

Figure 14–1   Levels of amputation are determined by circulatory adequacy, type of prosthesis, function of the part, and muscle balance. (A) Levels of amputation of upper extremity. (B) Levels of amputation of lower extremity.   *(Smeltzer & Bare (1996). Brunner & Suddarth's Textbook of Medical-Surgical Nursing. 8th ed. Philadelphia: J.B. Lippincott.)*

LEVEL OF AMPUTATION

The third consideration is the level of the amputation. Taking into consideration both the local and systemic condition of the patient, the objective is to amputate at the most distal level that will heal and be functional. In the determination, there are three criteria used by most physicians: (1) the proposed amputation level will have sufficient blood supply, (2) a prosthesis can fit on the residual limb, and (3) all necrotic and/or infected tissue is removed. The major levels of amputations (Fig. 14–1) are discussed in more depth later in this chapter, but a brief definition and a list of the most common reasons for the amputations follow:

- *Toe.* Loss of any or all of the toes is usually due to trauma or as a sequela to diabetes mellitus, trauma, or frostbite.
- *Metatarsal.* Metatarsal or midfoot amputation is performed as a result of trauma or PVD secondary to diabetes mellitus. Metatarsal amputation is performed over removal of toes to gain assurance of a good blood supply. A prosthesis, if needed, is included in the shoe.
- *Syme.* Syme or foot amputation is the removal of the foot at the ankle (sometimes also referred to as an ankle disarticulation).

- *Below the knee (BK or BKA).* Below-the-knee amputations preserve the knee joint and make prosthetic fitting and ambulation easier.
- *Knee disarticulation (KD).* Knee disarticulation removes the lower leg through the knee joint. The procedure is rarely used today because of the difficulty in fitting a prosthesis.
- *Above the knee (AK or AKA).* Above-the-knee amputations do not preserve the knee; they are usually performed for trauma or PVD.
- *Hip disarticulation (HD).* Hip disarticulation is the removal of a leg through the hip joint and occurs more commonly in younger patients due to trauma or neoplasm.
- *Hemipelvectomy (HP).* Hemipelvectomy is an amputation that removes half of the patient's pelvis and all of the patient's leg and is usually performed because of neoplasm.
- *Hemicorporectomy.* Hemicorporectomy is the removal of the lower half of the body, which includes the loss of the lower extremities, a colostomy, a urinary diversion, and the loss of sex organs. It is usually performed for advanced pelvic cancer or pelvic sepsis.
- *Finger and thumb.* Finger and thumb amputation includes all or only a portion of the digit; it is usually due to trauma or frostbite.

- *Wrist disarticulation.* Wrist disarticulation is the removal of the hand through the wrist joint.
- *Below the elbow (BE or BEA).* Below-the-elbow amputation is usually performed as the result of trauma or congenital deformities.
- *Elbow disarticulation.* Elbow disarticulation is the removal of the arm through the elbow.
- *Above the elbow (AE or AEA).* Above-the-elbow amputation is usually performed as the result of trauma or a congenital deformity.
- *Shoulder disarticulation.* Shoulder disarticulation is the removal of an arm through the shoulder joint.
- *Forequarter amputation.* Forequarter amputation removes a large portion of the patient's shoulder and an arm. It is usually performed as the result of trauma or neoplasm.

REHABILITATION POTENTIAL

The fourth factor in deciding to amputate is the patient's rehabilitation potential. Rehabilitation requires the patient's cooperation, patience, and willingness to do the exercises necessary to regain function. The patient will need good coordination, mental alertness, and the ability to follow directions. Consideration of impairments by age or disease must be evaluated. Patients who will have great difficulty in learning to walk with a prosthesis after an amputation are ones with (1) severe neurologic disease; (2) disorientation, senility, psychosis, or severe mental retardation; (3) chronic heart failure with decreased cardiac reserve; and (4) severe chronic obstructive pulmonary disease (COPD).

Taking into consideration the patient's overall physical and mental health, the question becomes, does the patient have the energy and ability to use a prosthesis? For example, with a unilateral BKA, the patient will expend 10% more energy than they normally do to walk; with bilateral BKAs, the patient will expend an additional 20%; and with a unilateral AKA, the patient will expend 60% more energy to walk. Someone once stated, walking after an AKA is like changing from walking on a flat surface to walking up stairs all of the time. If the patient is a frail elderly person with a severe heart condition or chronic obstructive pulmonary disease, they may not be able to walk with the prosthesis.

A question the patient always has is, "Will I walk again?" This question is always difficult to answer, and in most instances cannot be answered definitively. However, there are some broad guidelines that can be used. If the patient has a unilateral BKA, there is a very good chance they will be able to walk. If they have bilateral BKAs, they will be able to walk but will need to work to accomplish the goal. For patients with a unilateral AKA, it will take lots of work but they can walk, although some may walk with a cane. Individuals with bilateral AKAs normally do not walk if they are elderly, because it takes a lot of work to learn to walk and it also takes a lot of energy.

OTHER FACTORS

Although not primary factors involved in the decision to amputate, the following factors impact how well the patient adjusts to the rehabilitation process and to living with a disability. These factors are (1) personal characteristics (i.e., age, sex, marital status, occupation, educational level, personality); (2) characteristics of the disability (onset, severity, prognosis, degree of physical dependence); and (3) environmental factors (family and community support, socioeconomic status).

RESIDUAL LIMB MANAGEMENT

The major objective is to achieve healing of the amputation site, yielding a nontender stump with healthy skin for prosthetic fitting. The immediate postoperative dressing and care of the residual limb are not always the same, even for the same type of amputation. The postsurgical dressing varies, depending on the type of amputation and the patient's rehabilitation potential and goals. Dressings include soft dressings and rigid dressings. Soft bandage dressings are used if frequent dressing changes are anticipated, if further surgery is necessary (such as in an open method amputation), and if frequent assessments of the surgical site are required. Rigid dressings are used following a closed amputation to help control edema, but they need to be changed to be effective as shrinkage of the stump occurs. The rigid dressing applies uniform compression to support the soft tissue and thereby control pain and prevent contractures. Though rigid dressings may be used even if there are no plans for the patient to wear a prosthesis, the initial rigid dressing is equipped to attach a temporary prosthetic extension (pylon) and an artificial foot for early ambulation (Fig. 14–2).

Williamson (1992) states that there is another device that is effective in controlling edema, the Jobst air splint. The Jobst air splint is a plastic transparent inflatable cone-shaped device that is inflated to 20 mm Hg for 22 of 24 hours a day. At the time of Williamson's writing, the splint had some problems, one being leakage of air so that constant pressure on the residual limb was not maintained. This inconsistency in pressure hampered adequate shaping and shrinkage of the stump. Whatever the bandage, it must provide coverage of the surgical wound, stay in place despite the patient's movements, help control/reduce edema, shrink the stump, and help to mold the residual limb to facilitate a prosthesis. The choice between using a stump sock or a stump wrapping with elastic bandages is still controversial. A stump sock is easier to apply and maintain, but some physicians believe that it is not as effective in reducing edema and shaping and molding the residual limb. To be effective, the elastic bandages must be reapplied every 4 to 6 hours, because they become loose and even slip off.

Elastic bandaging has been used for many years and still remains effective, but for some patients it is difficult to apply and maintain. To be effective, the bandage is attached to the joint proximal to the stump (AKA, hip; BKA, above the knee; BEA, above the elbow; and AEA,

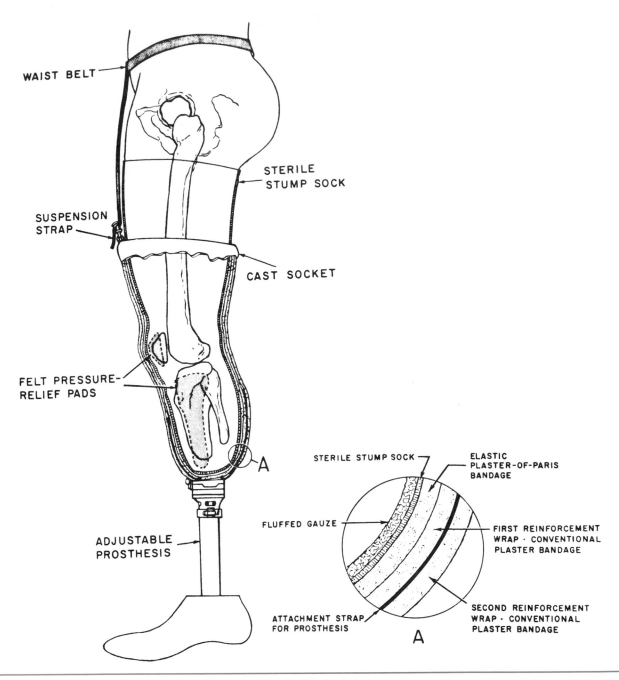

Figure 14–2   Plaster-and-pylon preparatory BK prosthesis. (*A*) Detail of circled area.   *(Scully & Barnes* Physical Therapy. *Philadelphia: Lippincott.)*

shoulder) and is applied with figure-of-eight turns, with decreasing pressure from the distal end to the proximal end of the residual limb. Effective bandaging is crucial to prevent compromised venous return, increased edema, retarded wound healing, poorly shaped residual limbs, and further shrinkage once the prosthetic socket is applied.

MAJOR PHYSICAL AND EMOTIONAL CONCERNS

The loss of an extremity requires major adjustments. The patient's perception of the amputation must be

understood. The patient must adjust to (1) a permanent change in body image, which must be incorporated in such away that self-esteem is not lost; (2) an alteration in physical mobility or ability to perform activities of daily living; and (3) modifications of activities and the environment to accommodate the use of mobility aids and assistive devices. To help the patient prevent problems and achieve the highest possible level of function and participation in life activities, the rehabilitation team must be multidisciplinary. See Chapter 1 for a discussion of a patient adjustment to a disability.

Some of the major nursing diagnoses that, to some degree, affect all patients following an amputation are (1) disturbance in self-concept, which includes body image, self-esteem, and role performance; (2) dysfunctional grieving; (3) sensory/perceptual alteration (phantom pain); (4) pain; (5) impaired skin integrity; (6) impaired physical mobility; and (7) self-care deficit. Pain and self-care deficit as they relate to patients with specific amputations are presented in the appropriate nursing processes later in this chapter.

DISTURBANCE IN SELF-CONCEPT

Self-concept reflects self-view, encompassing body image, self-esteem, role performance, and personal identity (Carpenito, 1993, p. 651). Self-concept is in constant evolution and change and is influenced by interactions with the environment and other persons and by perceptions of how others view you. Self-concept disturbance is a state in which individuals experience or are at risk of experiencing a negative change in the way they feel, think, or view themselves. This may include a change in (1) body image, (2) self-ideal, (3) self-esteem, (4) role performance, or (5) personal identity (p. 650). Following an amputation, patients may develop self-concept disturbance in one or more of those five components.

In caring for the patient, note signs that would indicate that the patient is having a disturbance in self-concept. For the patient with an amputation, note whether the patient refuses to touch or look at the amputated area or whether they are willing to let the family or significant others see the amputated area. Has the patient become overly dependent on the staff or members of the family for their care, refusing to take responsibility for care that they can do for themselves? Some patients are no longer willing to participate in family discussions or decisions. Rehabilitation activities are where a disturbance in self-concept is demonstrated most strongly. The patient may be unwilling to discuss their limitations, the amputation, care of the amputation, or their body disfigurement. The patient refuses to cooperate or participate in the rehabilitation plan. In the hospital, the patient may become abusive to others; and, when out of the hospital, they may develop abusive behaviors toward themselves (i.e., alcohol and drug abuse). There may also be periods when the patient shows anger or emotional distress (e.g., crying).

Nursing interventions for a variety of self-concept concerns are very similar. First is to try to build a trusting relationship with the patient by (1) providing a safe and private environment for them to talk; (2) encouraging them to express their feelings, especially how they view themselves; (3) encouraging them to ask questions about the treatment and rehabilitation process; (4) providing correct information and reinforcing information already provided; and (5) clarifying any misconceptions, while avoiding criticism of the patient. The second intervention is to assess for signs and symptoms of self-concept disturbance. The third is to initiate health teaching and to provide resources within the community, if needed.

DYSFUNCTIONAL GRIEVING

Grieving is defined as a state in which an individual or family experiences a natural human response involving psychosocial and physiologic reactions to an actual or perceived loss (Carpenito, 1993, p. 347). Dysfunctional grieving represents a maladaptive process occurring when grief work is suppressed or absent or when a person exhibits a prolonged, exaggerated response (p. 248). Individuals respond to a loss in different ways, but following an amputation a grief response is to be expected. Dysfunctional grieving involves excessive emotional reactions.

American society is focused on having a youthful and beautiful body, and an amputation destroys that image for the patient. An individual's grief is affected by such factors as (1) personality, (2) previous losses, (3) intimacy of personal relationships, and (4) personal resources. Other factors that contribute to dysfunctional grieving are the presence of guilt and lowered self-esteem. Guilt is an issue, especially if the patient received the amputation due to trauma caused by their carelessness or while doing recreational activities and now cannot return to their job or support their family. Observe the patient for some of the following signs of pathologic grieving when the grieving is profound, increases in intensity, and perseveres: (1) anger and denial, (2) depression and regression, (3) isolation, (4) obsession, (5) worthlessness, (6) hallucinations, (7) delusions, (8) guilt, (9) suicidal thoughts, and (10) stoicism or absence of emotion.

Nursing interventions to assist the patient are (1) to provide a safe and private environment for the patient to talk; (2) to promote a trust relationship; (3) to support the grief reaction of the patient, the patient's family, and significant others; (4) to promote family cohesiveness; (5) to promote grief work in response to denial, isolation, depression, and anger; (6) to provide correct information and reinforce information already provided; and (7) to clarify any misconceptions while avoiding criticism of the patient. Assess for signs and symptoms as an ongoing process. Initiate health teaching, and provide resources within the community, if needed.

PHANTOM PAIN

Phantom pain may begin immediately after surgery, or it may occur 2 to 3 months later. An immediate postsurgical prosthetic fitting usually helps to decrease phantom pain, but having the patient describe the pain in detail may be the most beneficial intervention. Although health personnel refer to such sensations as phantom pain, the sensation of pain is real to the patient and might better be referred to as *phantom sensations* in discussions with the patient. Some physicians do not want phantom pain discussed with the patient before it occurs, believing that if it is not discussed it is less likely to occur. In such instances, if phantom pain does occur, the patient may become frightened of what is happening and hesitant to mention it for fear that people will think their mental status is impaired. Since it does occur in 80% of the patients, most authorities believe it should be discussed with the patient before it occurs (Williamson, 1992). For further discussion on phantom pain, see Chapter 2.

IMPAIRED SKIN INTEGRITY

To prevent problems of impaired skin integrity, it is imperative that good stump care be instituted from the very beginning. Stump hygiene involves meticulous skin care as well as the maintenance of stump socks, elastic wraps, and prosthetic sockets and is crucial in avoiding skin breakdown. There are a number of skin lesions that can occur due to wearing a prosthesis. Measures that help to prevent skin breakdown on and around the stump are to establish a routine of (1) daily cleansing (preferably at night) with soap and water and drying thoroughly; (2) daily inspection of the stump for redness, abrasions, and irritations; and (3) daily changing and washing of the stump socks and elastic wraps with mild soap and water (preferably at night so they are completely dry by morning). Instruct the patient to never apply the shrinkage device unless both the stump and the sock/wrap are thoroughly dry. Massaging the stump is essential to help desensitize the residual limb and prevent scar tissue formation. Friction massage can break up scar tissue should it occur. The skin must be mobile and not adhere to the underlying tissue, or it can tear when stressed by wearing a prosthesis.

Even though all of these measures are followed, the patient may still develop skin lesions (Fig. 14–3). One that is quite common is an epidermoid cyst that occurs at the prosthetic socket brim and is usually the result of pressure. Socket modification is necessary to resolve the problem. Verrucous hyperplasia is a painful condition involving wart-like overgrowths of skin that may progress to fissuring, oozing, and infection. The cause of verrucous hyperplasia has been identified as a lack of contact between the end of the stump and the prosthetic socket. Abrasions, blisters, and infected hair follicles also occur as a result of pressure from a malfitting prosthesis.

IMPAIRED PHYSICAL MOBILITY

Following an amputation, efforts need to focus on preventing the development of contractures. Hip and knee contractures are potential problems following most lower-extremity amputations. Abduction-adduction, external-internal rotation, and flexion-extension exercises are important to maintain or restore as much function in the extremity as possible. The patient should not be allowed to leave their extremity in a position of abduction, external rotation, or flexion once the exercises are completed. Range of motion to all unaffected joints is started on the operative day and encouraged throughout the rehabilitation process. The patient needs to do upper-extremity exercises to increase strength in their arms for crutch walking following a lower-extremity amputation (see Chapter 4). Further discussion regarding impaired mobility as it relates to specific amputations is presented in the appropriate nursing process later in this chapter.

LOWER–EXTREMITY AMPUTATION

Amputations and disarticulations affecting the lower extremity are briefly discussed, and a nursing process is presented to assist the nurse in caring for patients with a hip disarticulation, above-the-knee amputation, and below-the-knee amputation.

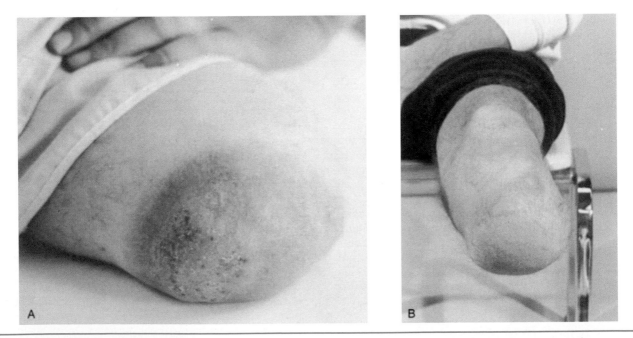

Figure 14–3   (A) Stump edema syndrome and (B) epidermoid cysts result from a poorly fitting, non-total-contact socket.   *(Scully & Barnes Physical Therapy. Philadelphia: Lippincott.)*

HEMIPELVECTOMY

If an amputation is done for a malignant tumor in or about the hip, it is usually a hemipelvectomy. It is a radical and infrequently done procedure known by many names, including interinnominoabdominal, interabdominal, interpelviabdominal, iliabdominal, transiliac, transpelvic, and hindquarter amputation. Because of the proximity of the hip joint to the upper part of the femur, a hip disarticulation is usually not appropriate for hip tumors. A hemipelvectomy is not usually done for tumors of lower grade malignancies such as chondrosarcomas occurring in areas where complete removal of the intact tumor is possible. Although a benign tumor, which is destroying function, can be removed from the head and neck of the femur and replaced by a prosthesis, or the acetabulum can be removed and replaced, these instances are rare.

HIP DISARTICULATION

Amputations through the proximal thigh and disarticulation at the hip joint are generally the result of trauma or neoplastic disease. A hip disarticulation may be indicated for malignant tumors, especially lesions of the femoral shaft below the trochanter. The distal femur is a common site for osteogenic sarcoma. Occasionally, a disarticulation may be necessitated by infection or by the restructuring of a severe congenital anomaly to fit a prosthesis. Surgical removal proximal to the bone in which the tumor occurs has resulted in statistically superior outcomes when compared to amputation through the same bone at a higher level. Thus a hip joint disarticulation is the level of choice for most malignant bone tumors of the thigh.

The objective of postoperative medical management is to provide firm support to the operative site. In the past, this was commonly accomplished by soft compression dressings. If soft-tissue compression dressings alone are used, they should be adequately reinforced by pressure bandaging and kept under sufficient tension to control and hasten stump maturation. Today, it is common practice to utilize a rigid dressing and a postsurgical prosthetic fitting so that walking with progressive weight bearing can be started within a few days. The only absolute contradictions to immediate postsurgical prosthetic fitting are an actual or potential infection at the site of the amputation or an open amputation.

The prosthetic fitting, usually applied by a prosthetist, consists of a rigid plaster of Paris dressing, a pylon going from the stump to the ankle with no hip or knee joints, and a foot-ankle assembly. The rigid dressing is applied to the hip in such a way that compression is firmly and evenly distributed over the end of the stump, both iliac crests, and the ischial tuberosity on the affected side. The initial rolls of plaster are of elastic plaster of Paris, because it conforms to the contour of the stump better and permits easier control of tension. The outer rolls are of regular plaster of Paris, because the elastic plaster is not as strong as the conventional type. The prosthetic pylon and the foot-ankle assembly are aligned to allow a smooth gait that will not be fatiguing and will avoid excessive pressure on the stump.

To make a swing-through gait easier, the length of the prosthetic fitting is 0.9 to 1.3 cm shorter than the length of the opposite leg. However, some physicians do not use immediate postsurgical prosthetic fitting following hip disarticulations or hemipelvectomy amputations because the available components (1) do not allow the patient to sit comfortably and (2) require ambulation on a pylon without a movable hip or knee joint. Furthermore, the hip disarticulation stump matures rapidly when treated by conventional methods, allowing early fitting with a properly articulated definitive prosthesis. After a minimum of 6 to 12 weeks following a hip disarticulation or hemipelvectomy, a Canadian hip disarticulation prosthesis, or a modification of it, can be fitted.

NURSING PROCESS (Patient with a Hip Disarticulation)

The following nursing process demonstrates the care of a patient following a hip disarticulation. The nursing process begins after the patient returns to the nursing unit.

ASSESSMENT

Before surgery, the patient's general condition should be thoroughly evaluated. In all elective amputations, the prosthetist as well as the surgeon should evaluate the patient before surgery so that necessary measurements can be made and a shoe for the prosthetic foot can be obtained if an immediate postsurgical prosthetic fitting is to be utilized. Preoperative psychological assessment of the patient will greatly enhance postoperative nursing assessment and intervention. Even though the amputation may be elective, the operation may be a lifesaving measure or a first step toward regaining function and decreasing pain. It is important that the patient understand the operation before it occurs to foster a positive attitude toward rehabilitation. Let the patient ask questions, and make the patient comfortable enough to express fears, anxieties, and negative feelings. Opportunities should also be given to the family and significant others to express their fears and anxieties. Observe interactions between the patient, the family, and significant others, specifically with regard to the topic of amputation. A visit by a person who has had an amputation or a family member of an individual who has had amputation may also be helpful.

Postoperatively, assess the patient's level of consciousness. Auscultate the patient's chest for clearness of the lungs and any heart abnormalities. Check vital signs, and note any signs of pain or discomfort. Special assessment concerns focus on fluid and electrolyte balance, bleeding, and shock. Look for signs of bleeding along the incision line and posterior to it. Note the amount of drainage from the wound drains, assess for urinary output, and check the drying of the plaster cast if an immediate postsurgical prosthetic fitting was utilized. Note the location and intensity of pain. Observe the emotional responses to the surgery and attitudes toward the hip; most patients or family members will not look at the area.

Ongoing assessment needs to include observation for signs of symptoms of infection, impaired skin integrity, and emotional responses by the patient to the loss of a limb.

NURSING DIAGNOSIS

Based on all of the assessment data, the major nursing diagnoses for a typical patient following a hip disarticulation include the following:

- Pain and discomfort related to soft-tissue trauma from surgery
- Impaired physical mobility related to the loss of a leg
- Impaired skin integrity related to the surgical procedure and the prosthetic fitting
- Disturbance in self-concept related to a change in body image
- Grieving related to the loss of a leg
- Increased anxiety related to knowledge deficit about the rehabiliation process

COLLABORATIVE PROBLEMS

- Postoperative hemorrhage
- Infection

GOAL FORMULATION AND PLANNING

The immediate goals are to have the patient experience (1) a decrease in the level of pain through repositioning and prescribed medications; (2) an increased potential for ambulation through bed exercises, transfers, and sitting; (3) no impaired skin integrity; (4) a positive self-concept related to body image and role performance through open discussions; (5) normal grieving for the loss of a leg; (6) a decreased anxiety through increased knowlege about the rehabilitation process and mobility capabilities; and (7) an absence of complications related to surgery. Long-term goals are (1) to have the patient free of physical and emotional complications, (2) to maintain full functional capabilities of the rest of the body, and (3) to restore as much function as possible by the use of a prosthesis.

INTERVENTIONS

ALLEVIATE PAIN

Routine nursing measures and prescribed medications may be utilized for pain relief. The surgical pain that occurs following a disarticulation usually requires strong opiates for only a few days. If the patient had a lot of pain before surgery, some patients will see the postoperative pain as being less severe and will require less medication. Other patients may experience pain in combination with their expression of grief and concern about the alteration of their body image, and thus the pain is not relieved by medications. Patients who are managed with an immediate postoperative rigid cast usually have less pain. Phantom pain (i.e., pain in the amputated limb) is usually not relieved by medications. (For a discussion of phantom pain, see the discussion earlier in this chapter and in Chapter 1.)

INCREASE MOBILITY

To increase mobility, nursing interventions focus on exercises, ambulation, and sitting to help the patient develop a sense of balance before starting to walk.

Exercises. To increase the potential for ambulation and decrease complications, bed exercises such as coughing, deep breathing, and the use of the trapeze should be started as soon as the patient is awake after surgery. It will be easier for most patients to turn to the nonoperative side, but as the pylon is removed when they are in bed, they may turn to the operative side if the remaining leg is supported by pillows. Exercises to increase arm strength are also encouraged (see Chapter 4).

Ambulation. Early ambulation with limited weight bearing on the prosthetic fitting is very beneficial psychologically and lessens the emotional trauma from the loss of a limb. Most patients are up by at least 12 to 24 hours (or even sooner) after surgery, even though the pylon fitting is often not applied until the drains are out, some 24 to 36 hours after surgery. Most younger patients will be able to stand in parallel bars or with crutches on the second or third postoperative day. Many are able to leave the hospital within 5 to 9 days (or earlier) but will probably not be able to resume their occupation with the temporary prosthesis because of difficulties in sitting. (See Chapter 4 for crutch walking.) It is important to recognize that some patients may have a weakened general physical condition and weak upper-extremity muscles. Such patients may not be able to utilize crutches immediately and may need to use a wheelchair.

Sitting. Sitting with an immediate postsurgical prosthetic fitting following a hip disarticulation or a hemipelvectomy is difficult, because the rigid dressing covers both iliac crests, the ischial tuberosity on the amputated side, and the stump area. Because there is no hip or knee joint, the patient is unable to bend from the iliac crest down on the affected side. Positions in which the patient could sit are those in which the patient is able to flex the uninvolved hip. In the hospital, a total hip chair may be available, and it will usually be easy for the patient to use. Continue to work with the patient on methods of using other chairs and what might be done at home. If a conventional soft dressing is used or if the prosthetic fitting is removed, the patient will have difficulty in learning to sit without support, because there is no femur on the involved side to help with balance. Special exercises and techniques need to be learned and practiced for patients to balance themselves and sit correctly. The nurse needs to work closely with the patient and the physical therapist regarding those exercises.

SKIN INTEGRITY

Following a disarticulation, the goal is to have the residual limb develop healthy skin and be well prepared for prosthetic application. During prosthetic use, the skin must remain intact and be free of irritation or abrasion. (See impaired skin integrity and residual limb management earlier in this chapter.)

SELF-CONCEPT

Self-concept reflects a self-view encompassing body image, self-esteem, role performance, and personal identity. In preparation for and/or following a disarticulation, the patient may experience a negative view of how they feel, think, or even view themselves as a person. (See disturbance of self-concept earlier in this chapter.)

GRIEVING

The loss of an extremity may come as a shock to the individual even though they have been prepared preoperatively. This is especially true if the patient has lost the complete leg and is even having trouble being able to balance themselves to sit. The patient may show a wide variety of behaviors (from crying, withdrawal, and apathy to anger) and express many different feelings (of depression, fear, and helplessness) as they are coping with the loss and working through their grieving. The major role for the nurse is to acknowledge the loss and to listen and support the patient, the family, and significant others. (See dysfunctional grieving earlier in this chapter.)

PATIENT TEACHING AND HOME CARE CONSIDERATIONS

Initially, it may be difficult for the patient to look at the stump, let alone handle the dressing or the prosthesis. It will take time, but the patient's acknowledgment is an important step in the rehabilitation process. The term *stump* may cause anxiety or feelings of degradation to the patient, so it is advisable to try to avoid the word, even though it seems to be the most descriptive term available. Allow time for frank and open discussions about what the remaining portion of the hip looks like. Discuss the immediate prosthetic fitting, and note that although the pylon does not look like a leg, it does allow for ambulation and, with pajamas on, it can be less noticeable in the hospital. Discussions with nurses, a rehabilitated amputee, and the prosthetist about what the final prosthesis will look like (color, joints, and so on), how it will function, and what the patient will be able to do can be helpful.

Decrease fear about future role performance by health education and candid discussions of what to expect from the permanent prosthesis. Discuss the requirements of the patient's present job and the patient's potential to return to it or to another related job. The social worker should work with the nurse, the physical therapist, the prosthetist, and the physician to help the patient deal with job-related problems.

To increase the patient's self-esteem, provide opportunities for patients to be alone with their families. Encourage the patient to express concerns about any impairment in family roles. Treat the family as the unit of care, and enlist the family's support of the patient by supporting them in adjusting to the patient's surgery. Help them communicate with the physician, and keep them informed of the patient's daily progress. Utilize the patient's concern for the family to motivate the patient to actively participate in the rehabilitation process.

MONITORING AND MANAGING POTENTIAL PROBLEMS

Observe for signs and symptoms of hemorrhage and shock, which are special concern with a hip disarticulation, and implement nursing measures to prevent infection and problems with elimination.

SHOCK

Following a hip disarticulation, there is less chance for hemorrhage than with a hemipelvectomy, but there is still a concern. Observe the patient's vital signs, and note the amount of drainage on the dressing or from the wound catheter. Keep accurate intake and output records, and note abnormalities in the balance totals. (See Chapter 4 for further discussion.)

INFECTION

The skin is prepared preoperatively from the costal margins proximally to both knees distally. In surgery, the scrotum may be either stitched or strapped to the uninvolved thigh. Implement nursing measures to prevent skin infection. The incisional sutures are usually removed on the fourteenth day. If the patient has a postsurgical prosthetic fitting, the cast will be changed at that time. Casts may also be changed if they are too loose. (For further information on casts and cast care, see Chapter 5.) If the patient has a soft dressing, make sure the patient is cleansed well after bowel or bladder elimination and change soiled dressings.

ELIMINATION

Preoperatively, the patient was given enemas to cleanse the bowel. (The patient with a hemipelvectomy may have the anus temporarily sutured closed or sealed off with oiled silk during surgery.) Defecation is encouraged after the second day, aided by the use of neostigmine and a gentle enema on the fourth or fifth day if needed. A Foley catheter is usually inserted preoperatively and removed about the fourth or fifth day postoperatively.

EVALUATION/OUTCOMES

In the evaluation of the patient with a hip disarticulation, the patient is relieved of surgical pain through medications and nursing interventions. Determine whether the patient is having phantom pain and their understanding of their pain. The patient is able to do exercises without supervision, walk with crutches, transfer to a chair, and balance to sit with correct posture. The patient should be free of any break in skin integrity or infection. Finally, the patient, the patient's family, and significant others are in the early stages of adjusting to the loss, change in body image, and working effectively toward acceptance at the time they leave the hospital.

ABOVE-THE-KNEE AMPUTATION

Above-the-knee (AK) amputations of the lower extremity may be the result of a number of disorders, including infections, neoplasms, and traumatic injuries. Most, however, are the result of peripheral arterial disease. By far the most frequently encountered form of peripheral arterial disease is arteriosclerosis obliterans or peripheral arterial insufficiency, an organic disease of the arteries of the legs. The disease causes the arteries to become narrowed and obstructed so that the legs and feet do not receive enough blood. The obstructions usually are permanent, and the disease is therefore chronic. Arteriosclerosis obliterans is a disease restricted almost exclusively to adults and is usually manifested at ages over 50. Diabetes mellitus appears to increase the prevalence and severity of the disease, as does cigarette smoking. Circulation to the legs can be improved by growing (or grafting) new blood vessels and by increasing the volume of blood carried by unblocked arteries. Femoral-popliteal bypass surgery is also used to relieve this condition. If these methods fail, however, an amputation may be necessary.

The nursing assessment of the patient before surgery emphasizes a circulatory assessment of the lower extremities. Probably the most important assessment is for arterial pulsation. The assessment proceeds from the dorsalis pedis to the posterior tibial, the popliteal, and finally the femoral artery. Note how you were able to detect a pulse distally, bearing in mind that in the normal healthy population, 7% lack a dorsalis pedis pulse and 3% lack a posterior tibial pulse (Maher, 1998). Use a Doppler to help in the assessment of the pulse. Note any intermittent claudication, that is, a pain, ache, cramp, or feeling of severe fatigue that affects the muscles distal to the occluded artery after exercise and that is usually relieved by rest. Assess skin temperature, looking for alterations in the skin temperature of the patient's lower extremities by using the dorsum of your hand or the back of a finger. Compare one extremity to the other, unless both are involved. Note the skin color changes that occur in various positions. Abnormal postural color changes are pallor, which indicates a cessation of capillary flow; cyanosis, which indicates an obstruction to the outflow of blood; and rubor, which indicates an excessive flow of blood because of arterial and capillary dilation. Note any ulceration or gangrenous appearance, especially in the terminal segment of the toes or the heel.

After the patient's general physical condition is determined, assess the psychological status of the patient. A psychological assessment of the patient preoperatively will greatly enhance postoperative nursing assessments and interventions. Even though the amputation is elective, it is the first step in regaining function and decreasing pain. It is important that the patient understand the operation before it occurs to foster a positive attitude toward rehabilitation. Let the patient ask questions, and make the patient comfortable enough to express fears, anxieties, and negative feelings. Opportunities should also be given to the family and significant others to express their fears and anxieties. Observe interactions between the patient, the family, and significant others, specifically with regard to the topic of amputation. A visit by an amputee or an amputee's family may also be helpful. A number of physicians/institutions also arrange to have the prosthetist meet and evaluate the patient before surgery to begin the working relationship. The patient can provide the prosthetist with a necessary shoe, and the prosthetist can make the necessary measurements.

SURGICAL PROCEDURE

Amputation through the thigh (AK amputation) is the second most frequent kind of amputation, exceeded only by BK procedures. Because in the AK amputation the patient's knee joint is lost, it is extremely important that the stump provide a good fit for the prosthesis. The conventional constant friction knee joint in most AK prostheses extends 9 to 10 cm distal to the end of the prosthetic socket, so the femur must be amputated sufficiently proximal to the knee to allow room for the joint in the prosthesis. Thus, most AK amputations are performed anywhere from 10 cm above the knee joint to 10 cm below the hip joint.

In a closed AK amputation, the skin flaps are usually equal; hence, the suture line divides the anterior and posterior portions of the stump. The femur is severed about 5 cm proximal to the muscles and skin, the blood vessels are ligated and cut, and the sciatic nerve is ligated and cut approximately 5 to 7.5 cm proximal to the end of the bone. The muscles are either sutured over the distal end of the femur or holes are made in the distal end and the muscles are sutured to the bone (myoplasty). Penrose drains or plastic tubes for suction drainage are placed deep into the wound, and the skin flaps are closed. An immediate postsurgical fitting (see Fig. 14–2) is then applied to the femur, with one strap going around the waist and a second going over the shoulder. (See residual limb management earlier in this chapter for further details on immediate postsurgical prosthetic fittings and dressings.) For patients without an immediate postsurgical fitting, a pressure dressing is applied and a procedure for stump wrapping is instituted (Fig. 14–4).

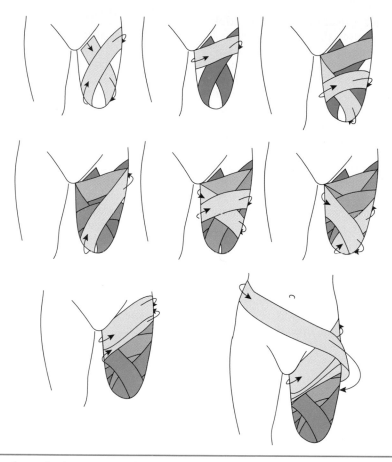

Figure 14–4 Bandaging an above-the-knee amputation.

Begin by explaining to the patient that the purpose of the procedure is to help reduce swelling and shape the stump for a prosthesis. Explain the procedure to the patient as you are doing the bandaging, as the patient must learn to do it by him/herself.

Sew three 4-inch elastic bandages together end-to-end, and roll them into one long bandage, or use a special elastic bandage designed for stump wrapping. Make figure-of-eight turns with the bandage, wrapping around the top of the patient's leg, downward under the stump, and back to the groin area. Keep the bandage roll away from the stump and avoid going straight around the stump, as that is apt to interfere with circulation.

To begin, have the patient in a semi-Fowler's position or sitting on the side of the bed. Hold the end of the elastic bandage at the top medial anterior surface of the patient's leg or, even better if the patient is able, ask the patient to hold the bandage. Bring the bandage diagonally downward toward the distal end of the patient's stump and loop the bandage around the end of the stump (A).

While applying even pressure, bring the bandage diagonally upward over the anterior of the stump up to the groin (B), and bring the bandage around the back of the stump and across the front to (C) anchor the proximal ends of turns (A) and (B). That completes the first figure-of-eight, and it will no longer be necessary to hold the end of the bandage.

Continue around the back of the patient's stump once again and bring the bandage from high on the medial side down to the lateral aspect of the distal end of the stump (D). Bring the bandage about halfway up the back toward the medial side of the stump, and continue across the front going slightly upward (E).

Then bring the bandage down the back to the end of the stump on the medial side and up the front diagonally toward the hip on the lateral side (F). (Turns D, E, and F make the second figure-of-eight.)

Continue around the back of the leg and up on the medial side, and then bring the bandage across the front, going slightly downward (G). Next, bring the bandage around the back going slightly upward, and continue that upward motion across the front of the stump (H).

Bring the bandage downward across the back to the end of the stump on the medial side, and then bring it halfway up the front toward the lateral side (I). Continue the upward motion around the back of the stump to the upper medial side, and then angle the bandage downward across the front to the end of the stump on the lateral side (J). Repeat the figure-of-eight turns at least once more to the groin to cover all of the fatty tissue high on the inside of the thigh.

To prevent the bandage from slipping, bring it diagonally over the patient's buttocks to the opposite iliac crest and then diagonally across the lower abdomen toward the lateral side of the stump, resuming figure-of-eight until the stump is completely covered and the elastic bandage is exhausted.

Finally, secure the bandage with clips, safety pins, or adhesive tape. If clips or safety pins are used, make sure they are on the anterior surface of the stump to prevent pressure areas from developing. Chart the procedure, the patient teaching, and the patient's response.

When there is a previous infection or a potential infection due to an open fracture, an alternative procedure known as a guillotine or open amputation is usually done. In a guillotine amputation, the bone, skin, and muscle tissues are all resected at the same level. The blood vessels are ligated, but the skin is not sutured closed to allow for open drainage of any purulent exudate. The stump is then covered with a bulky compression dressing. To prevent the skin and muscles from receding from the end of the bone, the extremity is put in skin traction with approximately 5 pounds of weight. There are a number of methods for applying the traction. One is to apply three or four strips of adhesive tape over the dressing and attach them to a piece of wood distal to the end of the stump, which is then connected by a rope and pulley to weights at the foot of the bed. Another is to put a stockinette over the dressing and tie a knot in the end of the stockinette, which is connected to the rope leading to the traction apparatus. (For further discussion on the principals of traction and the care of a patient in traction, see Chapter 6.) After a period of antibiotic therapy and skin traction, the patient returns to surgery for a closed amputation.

NURSING PROCESS (Patient with an Above-the-Knee Amputation)

The following nursing process demonstrates the nursing care of a patient following an above-the-knee amputation. The nursing process begins after the patient returns to the nursing unit.

ASSESSMENT

The postoperative assessment focuses on fluid and electrolyte balance, bleeding, and shock. Look for signs of bleeding along the incision line and posterior to it. Note the amount of drainage from the wound drains, assess for urinary output, and check the drying of the plaster cast if an immediate postsurgical prosthetic fitting was utilized. Check the patient's vital signs, and auscultate the chest for any lung or heart abnormalities. Note the location and intensity of pain. Observe the emotional responses to the surgery and attitudes toward the amputated extremity; most patients or family members will not look at the stump.

If the patient has had an open amputation, check the position of the patient and the traction apparatus to make sure the pull is correct. Note the color and the amount of drainage. Assess the emotional status of the patient. If the patient has had a closed amputation because of peripheral vascular disease, the patient will have had preoperative teaching. For patients with traumatic injuries, however, there is frequently little time to prepare them and their family.

NURSING DIAGNOSIS

Based on all of the assessment data, the major nursing diagnoses for a typical patient following an above-the-knee amputation include the following:

- Pain and discomfort related to bone and soft-tissue trauma from surgery
- Impaired physical mobility related to the loss of a leg
- Disturbance in self-concept related to self-esteem, body image, and role performance
- Impaired skin integrity related to the surgical procedure and the prosthetic fitting
- Grieving related to the loss of a leg
- Increased anxiety related to knowledge deficit about the rehabilitation process and future walking

COLLABORATIVE PROBLEMS

- Hemorrhage
- Infection

GOAL FORMULATION AND PLANNING

The goals are to have the patient experience (1) a decrease in the level of pain through repositioning and prescribed medications; (2) an increase in mobility through exercises (plus traction, if an open amputation), ambulation with a prosthetic fitting (if appropriate), and crutches; (3) a positive self-concept through communication and education; (4) no break in skin integrity related to bed rest or the prosthetic fitting; (5) going through the normal stages of the grieving process; (6) a decrease in anxiety related to patient teaching about the surgical procedure and the rehabilitation process; and (7) an absence of complications related to surgery. Long-term goals are (1) to have the patient free of physical and emotional complications, (2) to maintain full functional capabilities in the rest of the body, and (3) to restore as much function as possible with the use of a prosthesis.

INTERVENTIONS

ALLEVIATE PAIN

Nursing measures and prescribed medications are utilized for pain relief. With the use of a rigid dressing, there is usually a decrease in the severity of pain after surgery. Strong opiates are often unnecessary or are only used for a few days. If the extremity is elevated to prevent edema and reduce pain, this should only occur for the first 24 hours as it can lead to the development of flexion contractures. The traction used in an open amputation, by applying a continuous pull, helps to prevent or reduce pain from muscle spasms.

Phantom pain (i.e., pain in the amputated limb) is usually not relieved by medications. An immediate postsurgical prosthetic fitting usually helps to decrease phantom pain, but having the patient describe the pain in detail may be the most beneficial treatment. Although health personnel refer to such sensations as phantom pain, the sensation of pain is real to the patient and might better be referred to as *phantom sensations* in discussions with the patient. Some physicians do not want phantom pain discussed with the patient before it occurs, believing that if it is not discussed it is less likely to occur. In such instances, however, if phantom pain does occur, the patient may become frightened about what is happening and hesitant to mention it for fear that people will think their mental status is impaired. (For further discussion on phantom pain, see the phantom pain section earlier in this chapter and in Chapter 2.)

INCREASE MOBILITY

To increase the patient's physical mobility, nursing interventions focus on exercises and ambulation.

Exercises.   To increase the potential for mobility and to decrease complications, the patient needs to start exercising all uninvolved joints and utilizing the trapeze to change positions as soon as they have recovered from anesthesia. Upper-extremity exercises are needed to assist the patient with ambulation. The patient with an immediate postsurgical fitting can turn to either side. Put a pillow between the legs and keep the stump in correct alignment when turning or resting on a side. Most patients will not want to turn and will need encouragement. Some may prefer lying on the uncasted extremity.

Even after ambulation has begun, patients still need to remember proper positioning in bed and must continue to exercise. One recommended exercise is to squeeze a pillow between the legs. (Once the exercise is done, remove the pillow to prevent abduction, and place a trochanter roll or sandbag along the side of the affected leg to prevent abduction or external rotation.) Encourage the patient to have the bed flat several times a day while they are supine. They should also lie prone for at least 30 minutes twice a day. These two procedures help to prevent hip flexion contractures. The patient is encouraged to work on upper-extremity exercises to assist with ambulation. Once patients have developed good balance when standing, they should stand with proper supports and swing the affected extremity back and forth. This procedure helps with hip flexion and extension. Other exercises may be required by the patient's physician and the physical therapist.

Ambulation.   For patients with an immediate postsurgical prosthetic fitting, early ambulation with limited weight bearing on the prosthetic fitting (utilizing a three-point crutch gait) is very beneficial psychologically and also lessens the emotional trauma from the loss of a limb. Most patients are up as soon as the drains are removed, 24 to 48 hours after surgery. Patients generally start ambulating early, although their pylon fitting does not have a knee joint and requires them to walk stiff-legged. Later, the patient progresses to a pylon fitting with a knee component (Fig. 14–5) before a permanent prosthesis.

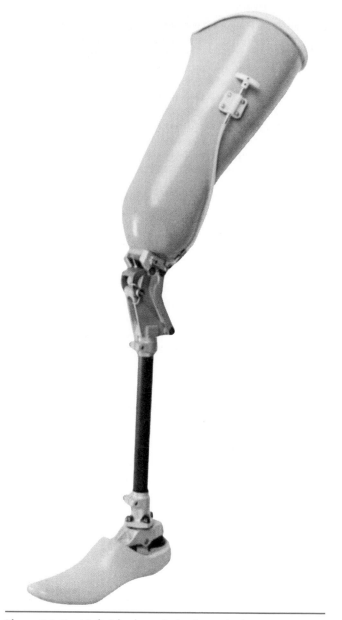

Figure 14–5   Unfinished exoskeletal prosthetic components. Note their overly large shape and rough appearance, which permits contour and color customization for each amputee. *(Scully & Barnes* Physical Therapy. *Philadelphia: Lippincott.)*

Traction.   For patients with an open amputation and skin traction, maintain the traction as though it were skeletal traction. Do not release the traction without a physician's order. (For more details on traction, see Chapter 6.)

PATIENT TEACHING AND HOME CARE CONSIDERATIONS

The areas covered in the care of a patient with a hip disarticulation also apply here. Discuss with the patient how to dress with the rigid dressing in place and the types of chairs that would be the easiest to get out of without knee flexion. Teach or have physical therapy teach how to go up and down stairs and how to get in and out of a chair, and make sure the patient demonstrates safe crutch walking behaviors.

Until the rigid dressing is removed, the patient will not be allowed to shower or to get the rigid dressing wet. Once the rigid dressing is removed, most physicians will allow the patient to shower and use a mild soap to wash the residual limb. However, the most important aspect about showering is safety. Since the patient has had an AK amputation, they will need to use a stool in the shower at least until they have developed strength in their back, abdomen, and other leg.

An open amputation may be particularly traumatic, and it is important to spend time with the patient discussing the traction, how long it will be on, and the treatments that will follow. Remember, these patients will have to return to surgery for a closed amputation.

MONITORING AND MANAGING POTENTIAL PROBLEMS

Potential for shock/hemorrhage and infection are the two major concerns postsurgery. Infection or potential infections are of special concern for a patient with an open amputation. If the amputation resulted from osteomyelitis, the patient may be placed in isolation.

SHOCK

Patients who have had an AK amputation have had the major arteries of their leg cut and sutured and thus are at risk for hemorrhage and shock if a suture should release. (See Chapter 4 for further discussion regarding shock.)

INFECTION

Infection is a frequent complication following amputation. Many of the patients having an AK amputation have poor circulation and other health conditions that place them at risk for a systemic infection. Most patients will be on antibiotic therapy for the first few days. Observe for signs and symptoms of infection, and teach the patient so they can be alert for any signs of infection. The patient needs to check pressure areas (Fig. 14–6) to prevent the development of a decubitus or an infection.

EVALUATION/OUTCOMES

The patient will have the surgical pain controlled with medication and understand the cause of the phantom pain. The patient will be able to do exercises and will be able to ambulate safely using crutches. The patient demonstrates a positive attitude toward the rehabilitation process and willingly participates. During discussions with the patient, the patient's family, and significant others, there will be verbalization of working through to the stage of acceptance of the amputation. If the patient has an open amputation, the residual limb shows signs of being free of infection.

KNEE DISARTICULATION

A disarticulation of the knee or a knee-bearing (KB) amputation is relatively rare. Physicians are reluctant to

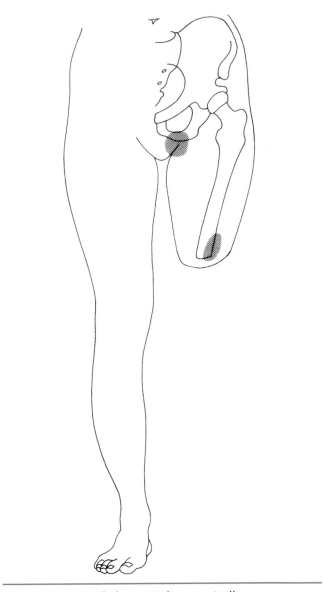

Figure 14–6 Stippled areas indicate typically pressure-sensitive AK residuum tissue. *(Scully & Barnes* Physical Therapy. *Philadelphia: Lippincott.)*

amputate the leg at that level because of difficulties in fitting a functional prosthesis to half a joint. With advances in prosthetic devices, those difficulties are being reduced and knee disarticulations may in the future replace some AK amputations. Nursing care is similar to the care of a patient with an AK amputation.

BELOW-THE-KNEE AMPUTATION

The most common type of amputation today is the below-the-knee (BK) amputation, where the remaining tibia is 12.5 to 17.5 cm long, depending on the patient's height. Usually 2.5 cm of bone length remains for each 30 cm of body height. Most physicians agree that the ideal level for a prosthetic fitting is about 15 cm below the knee. Below-the-knee amputations are the result of a number of disorders, including infections, neoplasms (see Chapter 3), and traumatic injuries. Most, however, are the result of peripheral arterial disease.

The surgical procedure is similar to the open or closed method of AK amputation, except that there are two bones involved. The myoplasty attaches the muscles to the tibia because it is the weight-bearing bone. The fibula is usually severed proximal to where the tibia is severed so that the prosthesis will fit better. Following a closed method of amputation, the physician may use a compression dressing with ace bandages (Fig. 14–7), but more likely there will be an immediate postoperative prosthetic fitting (see Fig. 14–2). Although the patient may not wear a prosthesis, most physicians will have an immediate postsurgical fitting applied that will extend from the stump to midthigh. The straps will go along the sides of the cast portion of the fitting and attach to the strap that goes around the patient's waist. No shoulder strap is necessary.

NURSING PROCESS (Patient with a Below–the–Knee Amputation)

The following nursing process demonstrates the nursing care of a patient following a below-the-knee amputation. The nursing process begins after the patient returns to the nursing unit.

ASSESSMENT

Before surgery, the patient's general condition should be thoroughly evaluated. In all elective amputations, the prosthetist as well as the surgeon should evaluate the patient before surgery so that necessary measurements can be made and a shoe for the prosthetic foot can be obtained if an immediate postsurgical prosthetic fitting is to be utilized. Preoperative psychological assessment of the patient will greatly enhance postoperative nursing assessments and interventions. Even though the amputation may be elective, the operation may be a lifesaving measure or a first step toward regaining function and decreasing pain. It is important that the patient understand the operation before it occurs to foster a positive attitude toward rehabilitation. Let the patient ask questions, and make the patient comfortable enough to express fears, anxieties, and negative feelings. Opportunities should also be given to the family and significant others to express their fears and anxieties. Observe interactions between the patient, the family, and significant others, specifically with regard to the topic of amputation. A visit by a person who has had an amputation or a family member of an individual who has had an amputation may also be helpful.

Postoperatively, assess the patient's level of consciousness. Auscultate the patient's chest for clearness of the lungs and any heart abnormalities. Check vital signs, and note any signs of pain or discomfort. Special assessment concerns focus on fluid and electrolyte balance, bleeding, and shock. Look for signs of bleeding along the incision line and posterior to it. Note the amount of drainage from the wound drains, assess for urinary output, and check the drying of the plaster cast if an immediate postsurgical prosthetic fitting was utilized. Note the location and intensity of pain. If the amputation was a traumatic amputation or the result of a trauma, observe for any other possible injuries. Observe the emotional responses to the surgery and attitudes toward the residual limb; most patients or family members will not look at the area.

Ongoing assessments need to include observation for signs and symptoms of infection, impaired skin integrity, and emotional responses by the patient to having an amputation.

NURSING DIAGNOSIS

Based on all of the assessment data, the typical nursing diagnoses for a patient with a BK amputation includes the following:

- Pain and discomfort related to bone and soft-tissue trauma from the surgery
- Impaired physical mobility related to the loss of the lower leg
- Impaired skin integrity related to the surgical incision and the prosthesis
- Disturbance in self-concept related to self-esteem, body image, and role performance
- Increased anxiety related to knowledge deficit about the rehabilitation process and future mobility

COLLABORATIVE PROBLEMS

- Hemorrhage
- Infection

GOAL FORMULATION AND PLANNING

The goals are to have the patient experience (1) a decrease in the level of pain through repositioning, therapeutic communication, and prescribed medications; (2) an increase in mobility through bed exercises and early ambulation; (3) no abrasions or breaks in skin integrity; (4) a positive self-concept through communication; (5) a decrease in anxiety through increased knowledge and open discussions; and (6) an absence of complications. Long-term goals are (1) to have the patient free of physical and emotional complications, (2) to maintain the full functional capabilities of the rest of the body, and (3) to restore as much leg function as possible by the use of a prosthesis.

INTERVENTIONS

ALLEVIATE PAIN

Nursing interventions for pain relief used in the care of patients following a BK amputation are medications and nursing measures. With the use of a rigid dressing, strong opiates are often unnecessary. The patient may

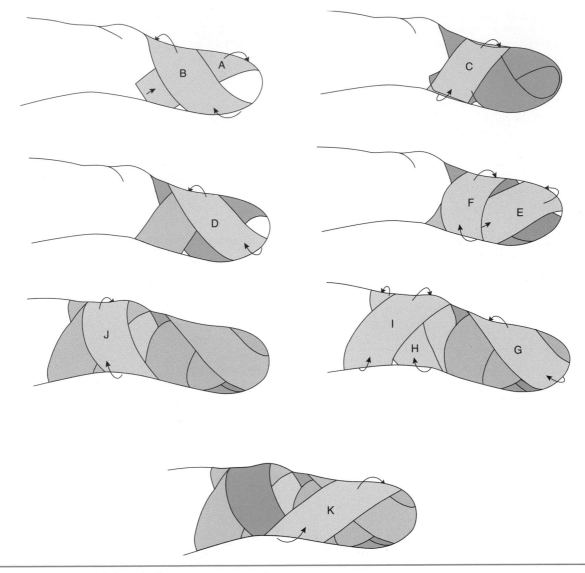

Figure 14–7   Bandaging a below-the-knee amputation.

Begin by explaining to the patient that the purpose of the procedure is to help reduce swelling and to shape the stump for a prosthesis. Explain the procedure to the patient as you are doing the bandaging, as the patient must learn to do it by him/herself.

Sew two 4-inch elastic bandages together end-to-end, and roll them into one long bandage, or use a special elastic bandage designed for stump wrapping. Make figure-of-eight turns with the bandage, wrapping around the upper portion of the patient's leg downward under the stump, and back to the upper portion. Keep the bandage roll away from the stump, and avoid going straight around the stump, as that is apt to interfere with circulation. There should be more pressure at the end of the stump than at the top to ensure proper venous blood return, but firm pressure should be used throughout.

To begin, place the patient in a semi-Fowler's position or have the patient sit on the side of the bed. With one hand, hold the end of the bandage on the medial side of the leg, just below the knee. With the other hand, bring the bandage across the front and downward to the distal end of the stump (A). Bring the bandage across the back to the medial side, and then bring it up and across the front of the patient's leg (B).

Bring the bandage across the back to the medial side and then bring it down and across the front of the stump (C) to anchor turns (A) and (B). That completes the first figure-of-eight, and it will no longer be necessary to hold the end of the bandage.

Continue around the stump, down the back to the medial end, and then up the front to the lateral side (D).

Continue diagonally up the back toward the medial side of the knee and then diagonally downward across the front of the leg to the lateral end of the stump (E). Bring the bandage up the back and across the front just below the knee (F).

Continue around the leg and down the back to the medial end of the stump, and then go up the front to the lateral side of the knee (G). Continue across the back of the leg and upward to above the knee cap (H). Bring the bandage across the back again, and then cross the front of the leg in a downward fashion (I).

Bring the bandage across the back and then upward across the front to the lateral side just above the knee (J).

Bring the bandage down the back of the knee and then down the front of the stump (K). Continue with figure-of-eight turns (D, E, F, and G) as long as the bandage permits.

Anchor with clips, safety pins, or adhesive tape. Chart the procedure, the patient teaching, and the patient's response.

complain of phantom pain, which medications do not relieve. (See the care of the patient with an AK amputation as well as the discussion on phantom pain earlier in this chapter and in Chapter 2.)

INCREASE MOBILITY
Measures that help the patient to regain their physical mobility include correct positioning, exercises, and ambulation with crutches.

Position. Immediately after surgery, the patient's affected leg may be elevated to reduce swelling and pain, but only for the first 24 hours. The patient should be encouraged to use the trapeze—initially with assistance—to change position in bed. The patient can turn to either side, but the patient will probably prefer turning to the unaffected side with pillows between the legs for comfort. The pillows help to protect the unaffected leg from the immediate postoperative fitting, and the pillows also help reduce any feelings of stress the patient may have from where the cast is applied to their leg.

Exercises. The patient must do exercises to strengthen the triceps of their arms for crutch walking. The patient must start doing quadriceps- and gluteal-setting exercises and straight leg raises with the affected extremity as soon as possible.

Ambulation. Early ambulation with limited weight bearing on the prosthetic fitting is beneficial psychologically, as it helps to lessen emotional trauma from the loss of the limb. Most patients are up with assistance within 24 hours after surgery. A patient with a BK amputation and an immediate postsurgical dressing will walk like a patient with an AK amputation, because the cast covers the knee, limiting flexibility in mobility. Once the cast is removed and the prosthesis is applied, the patient regains the use of their knee; the prosthesis will supply a hinge joint for the ankle (Fig. 14–8).

PATIENT TEACHING AND HOME CARE CONSIDERATIONS
Before a patient can accept a change in body image, he or she must first understand what has happened and what the prognosis is. The patient, the family, and significant others need time to adjust to the amputation. The adjustment to a disability, discussed in Chapter 1, comes more easily to some patients than to others. The age of the patient and the reasons for the amputation influence the adjustment process. For most patients following a BK amputation, the chances of returning to near normal activities are very good. Many are able to ambulate to a gait that is about indistinguishable from normal.

See patient teaching and home care considerations for a patient following an AK amputation earlier in this chapter. The teaching for cast care is the same as that for a patient with a long leg cast (see Chapter 5). Crutch walking will initially use a four-point gait, and the patient should know how to go up and down stairs before leaving the hospital (see Chapter 4).

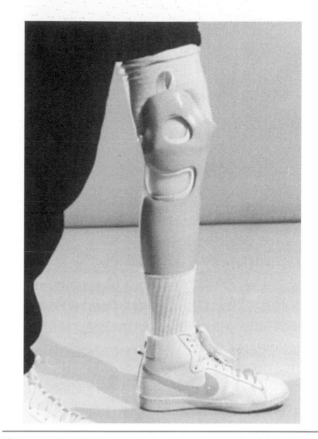

Figure 14–8 The BK socket is a transparent, flexible socket supported by a rigid frame, which may attach to any exoskeletal or endoskeletal shank. *(Scully & Barnes* Physical Therapy. *Philadelphia: Lippincott.)*

MONITORING AND MANAGING POTENTIAL PROBLEMS

Complications from surgery and bed rest should be minimized by early ambulation for the patient with a BK amputation, but the customary preventive measures need to be employed. Other potential complications are hemorrhage and infection. Observe for signs and symptoms of bleeding that could lead to shock since the major vessels in the lower extremity have been severed and sutured.

INFECTION
Infection or potential infections are of special concern for a patient with a BK amputation, especially if the reason for the amputation was trauma or osteomyelitis. The patient with osteomyelitis may even be put in isolation. The amputation was performed high enough to gain a good blood supply and to remove any necrotic tissue. However, there is always the chance the procedure was not sufficient to eradicate the osteomyelitis or prevent infection from contamination. The patient is placed on IV antibiotic therapy. Observation for the signs and symptoms of infection needs to be enforced and the patient instructed on these signs and symptoms. The patient must also check the residual limb for pressure areas (Fig. 14–9).

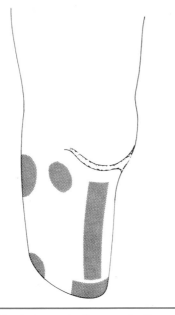

Figure 14–9 Stippled areas indicate typically pressure-sensitive BK residuum tissue. *(Scully & Barnes* Physical Therapy. *Philadelphia: Lippincott.)*

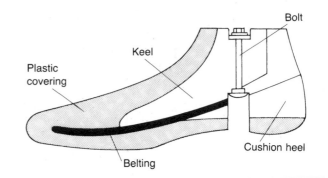

Figure 14–10 SACH foot cross section. Foam rubber composes the cushion heel, and wood or hard plastic composes the solid ankle and keel. *(Scully & Barnes* Physical Therapy. *Philadelphia: Lippincott.)*

EVALUATION/OUTCOMES

A typical patient following a BK amputation should be free of surgical pain and have an understanding of phantom pain. Note how well the patient is able to ambulate and sit with the immediate postsurgical fitting. The patient is able to go up and down stairs with the use of crutches and continues to do arm and leg exercises to regain strength for walking. Determine how well the patient, the family, and significant others are adjusting to the change in body image and progressing toward the stage of acceptance.

ANKLE AMPUTATION (SYME)

Amputations near the ankle are relatively infrequent, but may be done for severe trauma or infection. The most common such amputation, the Syme amputation, is done at the level of the distal tibia and fibula, 0.6 cm proximal to the ankle joint. The durable skin of the heel flap is used to provide the weight-bearing skin.

The amputation must leave a weight-bearing stump and enough space between the end of the stump and the ground so that a prosthesis with a functioning ankle joint can be worn The prosthesis, which must accommodate the distal tibial metaphysis, is rather large and bulky. For that reason, a BK amputation is often recommended for women. The prosthesis is a molded plastic socket, with a removable medial window to allow passage of the bulbous end of the stump through its narrow shank, and a solid-ankle-cushion-heel (SACH) foot (Fig. 14–10).

Most patients following a Syme amputation have a cast. Sutures are usually removed after 2 weeks. Weight

bearing is not allowed for up to 8 weeks. A walking cast is then applied and left on until healing is complete. The focus of nursing care is in helping the patient and significant others to adjust to the change in body image and in teaching the patient to walk with or without a prosthesis. The two most common causes of an unsatisfactory Syme amputation are the posterior migration of the heel pad and skin slough.

AMPUTATION THROUGH THE FOOT

Amputation of a single toe, with few exceptions, usually causes little disturbance in stance or gait. Amputation of the great toe does not materially affect standing or walking at a normal pace. If the patient walks rapidly or runs, however, a limp appears because of the loss of pushoff normally provided by the great toe. Amputation of the second toe is always followed by severe hallux valgus because the great toe tends to drift toward the third to fill the gap left by the amputation.

Amputation of any of the other toes causes little disturbance. Of these, the fifth toe is most commonly amputated, usually because it overlaps the fourth toe. Amputation of all the toes causes little disturbance in ordinary slow walking and usually requires no prosthesis other than a shoe filler. It is somewhat disabling for a more rapid gait, when spring and resilience in the foot are required, and when squatting or "tiptoeing."

An amputation through the metatarsals is disabling in proportion to the level of amputation. The more proximal the level, the greater the disability. The loss of pushoff due to the absence of a positive fulcrum in the ball of the foot is chiefly responsible for gait impairment. Again, no prosthesis is usually required other than a shoe filler.

Amputations more proximal than the transmetatarsal level (e.g., tarsometatarsal) result in considerable awkwardness in walking because of the loss of support and pushoff. Consequently, amputations of the forefoot have been largely replaced by amputation at the ankle or below the knee.

UPPER–EXTREMITY AMPUTATION

AMPUTATION ABOUT THE SHOULDER

Shoulder amputations are usually necessitated by malignancy or severe trauma. The types of amputations are (1) through the anatomical neck of the humerus, (2) disarticulation at the shoulder, and (3) forequarter amputation. Any amputation performed at the level of the axillary fold or more proximally requires the same prosthetic fitting as a shoulder disarticulation. Although prosthetic devices are available for these amputees, they are only able to perform limited functions.

An amputation at the neck of the humerus is usually done for severe trauma. The humerus is resected at the level of the anatomical neck, and the end of the humerus is smoothed with a rasp. The long head of the triceps, both heads of the biceps, and the coracobrachialis are then sutured over the end of the humerus. Other muscles are then sutured, and a skin closure that allows accurate opposition of the skin edges is done. Disarticulation is a very similar procedure, except that the head of the humerus is also removed, and in some instances a partial excision of an unduly prominent acromion process may be done to give the shoulder a more smooth and rounded contour.

A forequarter (shoulder girdle or interscapulothoracic) amputation consists of the removal of the entire upper extremity and shoulder girdle in the interval between the scapula and the thoracic wall. It is performed only for the removal of malignant tumors when the tumor extends to or through the region of the shoulder joint or extensively infiltrates the deltoid, pectoral, or subscapular muscles. Because of the nature of the operation and the disease for which it is performed, an atypical skin flap is often done. Closure is somewhat difficult and often requires auxiliary skin grafts.

The primary focus of nursing care in all three of these amputations is to help the patient adjust to a change in body image, assist in rehabilitation with or without a prosthesis, and, depending on the prognosis, help the patient adjust to impending death.

ABOVE-THE-ELBOW AMPUTATION

Amputations through the arm, or above-the-elbow (AE) amputations, are defined as those between the axillary fold and the distal supracondylar region of the humerus. These amputations are usually done because of trauma or malignancy. Arm prostheses contain an elbow lock mechanism to allow movement and stabilize the joint in flexion and extension and a turntable mechanism to substitute for humeral rotation. The elbow lock mechanism usually extends 3.8 cm distally from the end of the prosthetic socket and should be at the level of the elbow on the opposite arm. Therefore, the AE amputation should be at least 3.8 cm proximal to the elbow joint. Nursing care focuses on helping the patient and significant others adjust to the change in body image and on

assisting with rehabilitation. See Figure 14–11 for bandaging an AE amputation.

CINEPLASTIC PROCEDURE

A cineplastic amputation is one in which the stump is formed so that the patient may activate the prosthesis by muscular action. The cineplastic procedure consists of surgically constructing a canal transversely through a muscle, usually the biceps brachii. A rod is inserted into the canal and attached to an external cable, which connects with the mechanism of the artificial hand. Contraction of the muscle is effective in producing flexion in the artificial hand. With advances in prosthetic techniques, however, this procedure is rarely used.

ELBOW DISARTICULATION

A disarticulation of the elbow is the removal of the arm at the level of the distal condyles of the humerus. The elbow joint is believed to be an excellent level for a disarticulation because the broad flair of the humeral condyles can be firmly grasped by the prosthetic socket, and humeral rotation can be transmitted to the prosthesis. In more proximal amputations, humeral rotation cannot be transmitted, and a prosthetic elbow turntable is necessary. Most authorities believe disarticulation of the elbow is preferable to a more proximal amputation. The focus of nursing care is to help the patient adjust to a change in body image and to assist in rehabilitation with or without a prosthesis.

AMPUTATION THROUGH THE FOREARM (BELOW THE ELBOW)

Amputations through the forearm, known as below-the-elbow (BE) amputations, are the result of neoplasms or trauma. Such amputations usually preserve as much length as possible, because today almost any well-constructed, well-healed, and satisfactorily padded stump can be fitted with a functional prosthesis. The more distal underlying soft tissue consists primarily of relatively avascular structures such as fascia and tendons. Thus, with few exceptions, an amputation at the junction of the middle and distal thirds of the forearm is preferable to more proximal amputations. Even a very short (3.8 cm) BE stump is preferable to an amputation through or above the elbow. From a functional standpoint, preserving the patient's elbow joint is extremely important. Improved prosthetic fitting techniques, such as the Munster or a split socket with step-up hinges, can provide even a very short BE stump with an excellent prosthetic device. The focus of nursing care is to help the patient adjust to a change in body image and to assist in rehabilitation with or without a prosthesis.

AMPUTATION ABOUT THE WRIST

Whenever feasible, a transcarpal amputation or a disarticulation of the wrist is preferable to an amputation through the forearm, because pronation and supination

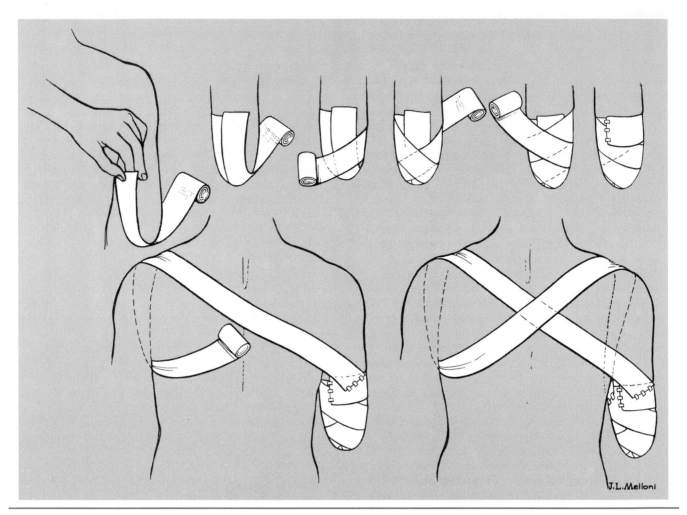

Figure 14–11 Wrapping above-the-elbow residual limb. An elastic bandage wrapping for an above-the-elbow residual limb minimizes edema and shapes it for a prosthesis. The bandage may need to be secured by wrapping across the back and shoulders. *(Suddarth (1991). The Lippincott Manual of Nursing Practice. 5th ed. Philadelphia: J.B. Lippincott.)*

are preserved as long as the distal radioulnar joint remains normal. Although only 50% of any pronation and supination is transmitted to a prosthesis, those motions are extremely valuable to the amputee. Furthermore, when compared to more proximal amputations, the longer lever arm left by amputation at the wrist increases the ease and power with which the prosthesis can be used. In transcarpal amputations, flexion and extension of the radiocarpal joint are preserved, and these motions can be utilized prosthetically. Prosthetic fitting for transcarpal amputation stumps is difficult but possible. Wrist disarticulation prostheses are not available, and thin prosthetic wrist units are now being used that allow the arms to be of equal length. Postoperative care focuses on helping the patient adjust to a change in body image and facilitating the rehabilitation of the patient, regardless of whether a prosthesis is involved.

METACARPAL AMPUTATION

Surgical amputation through the fingers or metacarpals is a salvage procedure, usually following trauma. The objective of the amputation is to preserve as much function as possible in the hand while shortening the time required for healing, decreasing the permanent disability, and preventing the continuation of pain. Every effort is usually made to maintain the length of the bony structures, the mobility of the joints, and the sensibility of the skin. In amputations of several digits, pinch and grasp are the chief functions to be preserved.

The only absolute indication for a metacarpal amputation is an irreversible loss of blood supply. Other factors to be considered, however, are (1) the prognosis for function; (2) the soundness of other digits; (3) the extent of the involvement of the five tissue areas (i.e., skin, tendon, nerve, bone, and joint); (4) the time since injury; and (5) the ability to salvage the thumb.

AMPUTATION OF THE FINGERTIP

Amputations of the fingertips vary markedly in level depending on the amount of skin lost, the depth of the soft-tissue defect, and whether the phalanx has been partially amputated. When skin alone has been lost, a free skin graft may suffice. When there is deep soft-tissue defect, however, several methods are available. One is amputation of the finger proximal to the defect. This provides ample skin and other soft tissues for closure but does shorten the finger. Another is a free skin graft, but this normally does not restore sensibility. Many different flap skin grafts and surgical techniques, including cross finger grafts, have also been used. Occasionally, a severed fingertip is recovered and replaced as a free graft. Although the graft usually survives in children, the results in adults have been poor.

INDEX FINGER AMPUTATION
An amputation of the index finger at its proximal interphalangeal joint, or at a more proximal level, leaves an unsightly, useless stump that may hinder the pinch between the thumb and middle finger. Therefore, an amputation should be through the shaft of the second metacarpal.

After surgery, the hand is elevated for 48 hours. Because an amputation through the second metacarpal involves hand tissues, it may cause stiffness in the other fingers. Because a branch of the median nerve is in the first web space, the nerve may become damaged. One potential residual effect may be a sunken scar on the dorsum of the hand.

MIDDLE OR RING FINGER AMPUTATION
The amputation of either the middle or ring finger leaves a gap in the hand through which small objects can drop when the hand is used in a scooping maneuver. The space also lets the remaining fingers deviate toward the midline. In multiple amputations, the third and fourth metacarpal heads are important because they help stabilize the metacarpal arch; but in single finger amputations, that is of less importance.

In some middle finger amputations, the third metacarpal head is excised and the index ray (the index finger and second metacarpal) is transposed ulnarward. That procedure has been done with good results, because it leaves a natural symmetry and makes the presence of only three fingers less obvious. However, removing the third metacarpal head weakens the pinch. When the ring finger is amputated, transposing the little finger ray is rarely done. In most instances, the fourth metacarpal is resected at its base, which permits a "folding in" of the fifth digit to close the gap.

Postoperatively, drains and a soft pressure dressing are usually applied. On the second day, the drains are removed; and 8 to 10 days postoperatively, the dressing is usually changed and the sutures removed. A light volar plaster splint (see Chapter 5) is then applied to keep the wrist in a neutral position and support the hand. The splint is worn for about 4 weeks but must be removed daily to cleanse the hand and exercise the small joints.

LITTLE FINGER AMPUTATION
An amputation of the little finger should save as much tissue as possible. Often the little finger survives when all of the other fingers have been destroyed, and it then becomes important in forming the pinch with the thumb. When the little finger alone is amputated, the fifth metacarpal shaft may be divided and the abductor digiti quanti transferred to the proximal phalanx of the ring finger. That procedure smooths the ulnar border of the hand.

AMPUTATION OF THE THUMB
The lack of a thumb causes a severe deficiency in hand function and is usually considered to constitute a 40% disability of the hand as a whole. If there is a traumatic amputation of the thumb, reamputation to obtain closure is not considered because the thumb should never be shortened. The wound is initially closed using a free skin graft, pedicle graft, or a local or distant flap graft. When the thumb has been severed at the MCP joint or a more proximal level, reconstruction of the thumb is usually indicated.

Reconstruction surgery of the thumb should meet five requirements. They are (1) the presence of sensation in the thumb, (2) sufficient stability so that pinch pressure does not cause the thumb joints to deviate or collapse, (3) sufficient mobility to enable the hand to flatten and the thumb to oppose for pinch, (4) sufficient length to enable the opposing digital tip to touch the thumb, and (5) a satisfactory appearance.

Acceptable reconstructive procedures include (1) lengthening the thumb using a short bone graft and transferring local skin for sensibility; (2) the pollicization of a digit (i.e., transpositioning a finger to replace an absent thumb); and (3) the direct free transfer of a toe to the hand with anastomosis of both the vessels and nerves by microsurgical techniques.

REPLANTATION/ REVASCULARIZATION

The following is a brief description of replantation and revascularization of an amputated part. Revascularization is the reattachment of a part that has been incompletely amputated, even if the remaining structures have no blood supply. Replantation is the reattachment of a body part that has been completely severed from the body. There are two types of replantation, major and minor. A major replantation is the reattachment of a part proximal to the wrist or ankle, and a minor replantation is the reattachment of a part distal to the wrist or ankle. The success of revascularization or replantation is measured by the degree of return of useful function, which may not be evident for many months because of the slow regeneration of the peripheral nerves.

Patients usually view replantation as preferable to amputation or prosthesis, even with the risk, time, and expense involved. Replantation is generally more successful for children, for multiple digit amputations, for thumb amputations proximal to the interphalangeal joint, for clean guillotine amputations, for amputations with minimal contamination, and for digits that are available for replantation 6 hours or less after amputation. Replantation is less effective in patients over 50 years of age, in single digit amputations, in severe crush or avulsion injuries, and in the presence of associated injuries.

The time interval from the accident to arrival at the replantation facility is critical and should be reduced to a minimum because of ischemia. The amputated part should be wrapped in gauze and placed in a plastic bag inside an iced container. Muscle tissue begins to deteriorate after only 4 to 6 hours at room temperature. That time may be increased to 12 hours (30 hours for digits) or more by cooling the part as described, with care taken to avoid freezing the amputated part. (Freezing will eliminate any possibility of later replantation.) There should be no attempt to wash, irrigate, or perfuse the amputated part prior to transportation. Care for the patient after the amputation involves controlling the bleeding by direct pressure and elevation and NOT using a clamp. The clamp may crush and damage exposed blood vessels and nerves, and the need to excise the crushed ends further shortens the vessels. When the bleeding vessels are so large that direct pressure and elevation of the part with the patient lying supine are inadequate, a pneumatic tourniquet should be used. The wound can be irrigated with isotonic saline and wrapped in a dry, bulky dressing for patient transport or stabilization.

Authorities do not agree on many preoperative, intraoperative, and postoperative aspects of replantation surgery but do agree on certain basic principles. First, the history and general physical assessment of the patient should indicate that the patient can tolerate surgery that may last 10 or more hours. Second, the patient and the family need to understand the possibility of complications, including the loss of the amputated part and the probable need for multiple surgeries.

When a patient returns from surgery after a replantation, there will be a bulky dressing and dorsal and volar plaster splints on the affected hand. Most physicians apply a layer of petroleum gauze directly over the skin wound, followed by layers of gauze dressing over the dorsal and volar surfaces. Cotton soaked in a physiologic solution is then applied to keep the dressing moist. The dorsal and volar plaster splints are applied over the cotton dressing to hold the wrist and fingers in functional position and are held in place by a circular bandage. During the first week, the splints are removed and the dressing is soaked with a physiologic solution every 8 hours to prevent drying of blood or crust formation that may constrict the vascular flow.

The replanted part is held at heart level for approximately a week after surgery, while the patient is kept on bed rest. Frequent evaluations of the circulation of the replanted part are carried out on the fingertips and small areas of the skin that were left exposed. Should a vascular occlusion occur, the patient may have to return to surgery. Some physicians may utilize leeching. The purpose of the leech is to help drain replanted or transplanted tissue engorged with venous blood and allow the body time to restore normal venous circulation, especially in replanted digits. Leeches will not usually attach to ischemic (arterially impaired) tissue. The leech's salivary glands secrete a local anesthetic that helps to mask the sensation of the leech's bite when they are attached to the patient's skin. The leech's saliva also contains an anticoagulant and a vasodilator, both properties that make the leech a suitable and important aspect of microsurgery and revascularization/replantation. Forceps, not fingers, are used to attach the leech to the wound where it will remain in place for 10 to 15 minutes. After a leech is attached, it will withdraw an average of 5 to 10 ml of blood. Because of the hirudin in the leech's saliva, a wound has been known to ooze up to an additional 50 ml of blood over the 24 to 48 hours after the leech has been removed, which helps to relieve congestion in the revascularized area. Care must be taken in removing the leech to prevent regurgitation of gut contents back into the wound. Each leech is used for only one patient and used only once.

The environment of the patient should be kept reasonably warm to avoid vasoconstriction of the replanted part, and smoking must be prohibited to prevent vasoconstriction from nicotine. Sedation of the patient relieves anxiety and assists peripheral vasodilation. Systemic heparin, low molecular-weight dextran, aspirin, and stellate ganglion blocks have been advocated postoperatively; but some authorities routinely use only aspirin and low-molecular-weight dextran. Dressings are changed infrequently to avoid manipulation of the replanted part. The first dressing change is best delayed for 7 to 10 days, and active motion should not be started for at least 3 weeks after surgery.

References

Carpenito, L. J. (1993). *Nursing diagnosis: Application to clinical practice* (5th ed.). Philadelphia: J. B. Lippincott Company.

Casady, L., & Scaduto, J. (1991). Thumb replantation: A case study. *Orthopaedic Nursing, 10*(3), 24–25.

Ellwood, L. (1998). Disorders of the hand and replantation. In A. B. Maher, S. W. Salmong, & T. A. Pellino (Eds.), *Orthopaedic nursing* (2nd ed., pp. 859–898). Philadelphia: W. B. Saunders.

Higgins, R. M. (1991). Replantation of digits. *Orthopaedic Nursing, 10*(3), 11–18.

Krebs, D. E. (1989). Prosthetics and orthotics. In R. M. Scully and M. R. Barnes (Eds.), *Physical therapy* (pp. 998–1051). Philadelphia: J. B. Lippincott Company.

Maher, A. B. (1998). Assessment of the musculoskeletal system. In A. B. Maher, S. W. Salmond, & T. A. Pellino (Eds.), *Orthopaedic nursing* (2nd. ed., pp. 168–189). Philadelphia: W. B. Saunders.

Roundsville, C. (1992). Phantom limb pain: The ghost that haunts the amputee. *Orthopaedic Nursing, 11*(2), 67–70.

Salmond, S. W., Mooney, N. E., & Verdisco, L. A. (1996). *NAON: Core curriculum for orthopaedic nursing* (3rd ed.). Pitman, NJ: National Association of Orthopaedic Nurses.

Smeltzer, S. C., & Bare, B. G. (1996). *Brunner and Suddarth's textbook of medical-surgical nursing* (8th ed.). Philadelphia: Lippincott-Raven.

Williamson, V. C. (1992). Amputation of the lower extremity: An overview. *Orthopaedic Nursing, 11*(2), 55–65.

Williamson, V. C. (1998). Amputation. In A. B. Maher, S. W. Salmond, & T. A. Pellino (Eds.), *Orthopaedic nursing* (2nd ed., pp. 718–745). Philadellphia: W. B. Saunders.

Yetzer, E. A. (1996). Helping the patient through the experience of an amputation. *Orthopaedic Nursing, 15*(6), 45–49.

Yetzer, E., Kauffman, G., & Sopp, F. (1994). Development of a patient education program for new amputees. *Rehabilitation Nursing, 19*(6), 355–358.

Yetzer, E., Winfree, M., & Scaglione, C. (1989). An amputee support group. *Rehabilitation Nursing, 14*(3), 141–142.

Index